*304 illustrations, 7 in color*

*Second Edition*

# A Manual of Tropical Medicine

THOMAS T. MACKIE, M.D., Colonel, M.C., A.U.S. (Retired)

*Chairman, The American Foundation for Tropical Medicine*
*Consultant in Tropical Medicine, The Roosevelt Hospital, New York City,*
*The Veterans Administration Hospital, West Haven, Connecticut, and*
*The Norwalk Hospital, Norwalk, Connecticut*

*Formerly Professor of Preventive Medicine, Wake Forest College, The*
*Bowman Gray School of Medicine*

GEORGE W. HUNTER, III, Ph.D., Colonel, M.S.C., U.S.A.

*Chief, Section of Parasitology-Entomology, Fourth Army Area Medical*
*Laboratory, Brooke Army Medical Center, Fort Sam Houston, Texas*

*Professor of Parasitology, Affiliated Units of the Graduate School, Baylor*
*University*

*Formerly Chief, Department of Medical Zoology, 406th Medical General*
*Laboratory, Tokyo, Japan*

C. BROOKE WORTH, M.D.

*Field Staff Member, Division of Medicine and Public Health, The Rocke-*
*feller Foundation*

*W. B. Saunders Company, Philadelphia & London, 1954*

# List of Collaborators

R. TUCKER ABBOTT, M.S.

Lt. U.S.N. (Reserve).
Associate Curator, Division of Mollusks, U.S. National Museum, Smithsonian Institution.

*Contributing to:* MOLLUSCS.

EDWARD W. BAKER, PH.D.

Acarologist, Division of Insect Detection and Identification, Bureau of Entomology and Plant Quarantine, U. S. Department of Agriculture, U.S. National Museum, Washington, D.C.

*Contributing to:* THE ACARINA (MITES).

E. J. BELL, Sc.D

Senior Scientist, Rocky Mountain Laboratory, National Institutes of Health, National Microbiological Institute, Hamilton, Montana.

*Contributing to:* RICKETTSIAL DISEASES.

GEORGE R. CALLENDER, M.D.

Brig. General, M.C., U.S.A. (Retired).
Director, Pathology and Applied Sciences Service, Veterans Administration; Member, Scientific Advisory Board of the Armed Forces Institute of Pathology; Consultant, Gorgas Memorial Institute; Consultant, Walter Reed Memorial; Consultant, American Board of Preventive Medicine.

*Contributing to:* DIARRHEAL DISEASES.

NORMAN F. CONANT, PH.D.

Professor of Mycology and Associate Professor of Bacteriology, School of Medicine, Duke University; Member, Advisory Panel for Microbiology, Office of Naval Research; *Ad Hoc* Committee on Sectional Research in Microbiology, National Institutes of Health; Member, Subcommittee on Cutaneous System, National Research Council, Division of Medical Sciences.

*Contributing to:* MYCOTIC DISEASES.

GORDON E. DAVIS, Sc.D.

Principal Medical Bacteriologist, Rocky Mountain Laboratory, National Institutes of Health, National Microbiological Institute, Hamilton, Montana; Consultant, Naval Medical Research Unit, No. 3, Cairo, Egypt.

*Contributing to:* RELAPSING FEVERS; THE ACARINA (TICKS).

## WILLIAM S. GOCHENOUR, JR., V.M.D.

Lt. Colonel, V.C., U.S.A.

Chief, Liaison, Standards and Animal Branch, Office of The Surgeon General, Department of the Army; Member, *Leptospira* Subcommittee, International Committee on Nomenclature, International Congress for Microbiology.

*Contributing to:* LEPTOSPIRAL DISEASES; RAT-BITE FEVER.


## ROBERT L. HULLINGHORST, M.D.

Colonel, M.C., U.S.A.
Assistant Chief of Infectious Disease Section, Armed Forces Institute of Pathology; Associate Member, Commission on Hemorrhagic Fever; Chairman, Committee for Follow-Up of Epidemic Hemorrhagic Fever.

*Contributing to:* RABIES; EPIDEMIC HEMORRHAGIC FEVER.


## GLEN M. KOHLS, M.S.

Senior Sanitarian (Reg.), U.S. Public Health Service, Rocky Mountain Laboratory, National Institutes of Health, National Microbiological Institute, Hamilton, Montana.

*Contributing to:* THE ACARINA (TICKS).


## WILLIAM H. W. KOMP, M.S.

Medical Entomologist, Laboratory of Tropical Diseases, National Institutes of Health; Consultant in Malaria, Division of Health and Sanitation, Institute of Inter-American Affairs.

*Contributing to:* MOSQUITO VECTORS OF DISEASE.


## ARTHUR P. LONG, M.D., D.P.H.

Colonel, M. C., U.S.A.
Assistant Chief, Preventive Medicine Division, Office of The Surgeon General, Department of the Army.

*Contributing to:* SMALLPOX.


## JEAN MAYER, PH.D., SC.D.

Associate Professor of Nutrition, Harvard University; Consultant in Nutrition for United Nations; Member, Editorial Staff of *Nutrition Reviews*.

*Contributing to:* NUTRITIONAL DISEASES.


## ARTHUR P. MOON, M.S.

1st Lt., M.S.C., A.U.S. (Reserve).
Section of Parasitology-Entomology, Fourth Army Area Medical Laboratory, Brooke Army Medical Center, Fort Sam Houston, Texas.

*Contributing to:* LABORATORY DIAGNOSTIC METHODS.

## JOHN P. O'BRIEN, M.D.

Major (Reserve), Australian Military Forces.
Post-Graduate Lecturer in Pathology, The University of Sydney, Australia; Pathologist, Lewisham Hospital, Sydney.

*Contributing to:* TROPICAL ULCER; DESERT SORE; CUTANEOUS DIPTHERIA; EFFECTS OF HEAT.

## CORNELIUS B. PHILIP, PH.D., SC.D. (HONORARY)

Principal Medical Entomologist and Assistant Director, Rocky Mountain Laboratory, National Institutes of Health, National Microbiological Institute, Hamilton, Montana; Member, Editorial Committee, *Experimental Parasitology* and *Journal of Parasitology.*

*Contributing to:* RICKETTSIALPOX.

## ALBERT M. RICHMOND, M.D.

Colonel, M.C., U.S.A.
Commanding, Fourth Medical Field Laboratory, A.P.O. 180, N.Y., N.Y.; Consultant, Pathology and Laboratory Service, U.S. Army, Europe.

*Contributing to:* BRUCELLOSIS; PLAGUE; TULAREMIA.

## ALBERT B. SABIN, M.D.

Professor of Research Pediatrics, University of Cincinnati College of Medicine; Member, Commission on Virus and Rickettsial Diseases of the Armed Forces Epidemiological Board; Consultant, Epidemiology, U.S. Public Health Service.

*Contributing to:* VIRUS DISEASES; TOXOPLASMOSIS.

## ARVEY C. SANDERS, B.S.

Lt. Colonel, M.S.C., U.S.A.
Department of Bacteriology, Army Medical Service Graduate School.

*Contributing to:* DIAGNOSIS OF DIARRHEAL DISEASES.

## FREDERICK J. STARE, PH.D., M.D.

Professor and Chairman, Department of Nutrition, Harvard University; Senior Associate in Medicine, Peter Bent Brigham Hospital; Consultant in Nutrition to The Surgeon Generals of the Army and U.S. Public Health Service; Editor, *Nutrition Reviews.*

*Contributing to:* NUTRITIONAL DISEASES.

## ALAN STONE, PH.D.

Entomologist, Division of Insect Detection and Identification, Bureau of Entomology and Plant Quarantine, U.S. Department of Agriculture, U.S. National Museum, Washington, D.C.

*Contributing to:* MOSQUITO VECTORS OF DISEASE; PHLEBOTOMUS VECTORS OF DISEASE.

## Phillips Thygeson, M.D., Oph.D.

Clinical Professor of Ophthalmology, University of California Medical School; Editorial Staff, *American Journal of Ophthalmology;* Consultant, Ocular Research Unit, U.S. Army; Medical Consultant, Expert Committee on Trachoma, World Health Organization.

*Contributing to:* TRACHOMA.

## H. W. Wade, M.D.

Associate Medical Director and Pathologist, Leonard Wood Memorial, Culion Leper Colony, Palawan, Philippine Islands; Editor, International Journal of Leprosy; President, International Leprosy Association.

*Contributing to:* LEPROSY.

## Luther S. West, Ph.D.

Lt. Colonel, M.S.C., A.U.S. (Reserve).
Head, Department of Biology, Northern Michigan College of Education, Marquette, Michigan; Lecturer, Rackham School of Graduate Studies, University of Michigan; Consultant, World Health Organization.

*Contributing to:* DIPTERA; MYIASIS.

## Robert H. Yager, V.M.D.

Lt. Colonel, V.C., U.S.A.
Director, Veterinary Division, Army Medical Service Graduate School.

*Contributing to:* LEPTOSPIRAL DISEASES; RAT-BITE FEVER.

# Preface to the Second Edition

The first edition of the Manual of Tropical Medicine was published during World War II as one of a group of volumes prepared under the auspices of the National Research Council to meet the needs of the Armed Forces in the tropics. The requirements of military medicine were necessarily controlling factors in the planning, and the contents were based largely upon the curriculum of the Course in Tropical and Military Medicine as presented at the Army Medical School, Army Medical Center, Washington, D.C. The primary objective was concise presentation of the essential practical aspects of the epidemiology, diagnosis, treatment, control and prophylaxis of the more important tropical diseases.

Throughout the past decade a variety of factors have been continuously operative focusing world attention on many areas in which these conditions are endemic. Political unrest, the growth of nationalism, the threat of Communism, the dependence of modern industrial economies upon raw materials and other products of the warm countries are augmenting the importance of these regions to the world as a whole. Similarly, they have increased the responsibilities of physicians and public health workers to control preventable endemic and communicable diseases.

These various factors have proved to be effective stimuli to constructive research in the fields of medicine and public health in the tropics. Much new and important information has been obtained and great progress has been made especially in the fields of epidemiology, treatment and disease control. This accumulation of new knowledge has rendered obsolete much of the first edition.

In the preparation of the second edition, the authors have adhered to the fundamental objectives of the original volume. Military medicine continues to be of importance and again effort has been directed to condense information essential for the Armed Forces, the clinician, the field worker and the student of tropical medicine. Substantial changes have been made throughout to include important advances in knowledge and to provide the most recent information relating to the practice of tropical medicine and tropical public health. New and pertinent observations in many fields have necessitated both deletion and substitution in the original text. Several of the sections have been largely or entirely rewritten by collaborators distinguished in their respective fields so that the current presentations represent the views of recognized authorities. The shifting emphasis on some diseases and the field experience of the authors has led to the inclusion or substitution of new chapters on the virus encephalitides, trachoma, rickettsialpox, trench fever, leptospiral diseases, leprosy, toxoplasmosis, gnathostomiasis, trichostrongyliasis, the nutritional diseases, effects of heat, epidemic hemorrhagic fever and medically important molluscs. Other chapters have been extensively revised, particularly those dealing with the rickettsial diseases, relapsing fever, the dysenteries, malaria, schistosomiasis, filariasis and laboratory techniques.

It is obvious that the diseases dealt with in this volume are not restricted to the tropics and the subtropics or other geographically limited regions. Although the climatic conditions characteristic of the equatorial zone are essential factors determining the prevalence of certain of them, others are encountered in the temperate zone and still others occur both in the hot and humid countries and in the colder regions of the world. The limiting and determining factors of prevalence include not only climatology, but sanitation and hygiene. Historically, however, these so-called exotic diseases have been grouped together under the generic title of Tropical Medicine. This second edition of the Manual of Tropical Medicine is presented with the hope that those who are interested in the regions where these diseases are prevalent and in the welfare of their people will find it of assistance in their work.

THOMAS T. MACKIE
GEORGE W. HUNTER, III
C. BROOKE WORTH

# Acknowledgments for the Second Edition

It is regretted that the necessity for limiting the size of the volume has had to take precedence over the inclusion of bibliographies. The listing of the many contributors to tropical medicine in the past decade would have forced abandonment of the original concept of a compact single volume of practical and useful information. Material has been drawn from many sources including recent specialized texts, numerous medical and technical journals, and abstracting journals such as the Tropical Diseases Bulletin, without which this revision would have proved an impossible undertaking.

We wish to express once more our deep appreciation to those individuals cited in the acknowledgments to the first edition of the Manual of Tropical Medicine. Our particular thanks are due to Major General George E. Armstrong, Surgeon General of the United States Army, for his interest and vision which were important factors in making this revision possible.

We are deeply indebted to our collaborators who furnished the basic manuscripts for the presentation of subjects in their special fields. In many instances they provided original material. Dr. Marion P. Sulzberger of New York University Medical School and Dr. Donald M. Pillsbury of the University of Pennsylvania Medical School rendered valuable assistance by their critical reading of the section on Effects of Heat; also Major Donald H. Hunter in connection with the section on Bacterial Diseases. Expression of our appreciation is likewise due to Colonel Tom F. Whayne, M.C., Colonel Calvin H. Goddard, M.C., and Lieutenant Colonel Ralph W. Bunn, M.S.C.; to Colonel Emory C. Cushing (M.S.C. retired); Lieutenant Colonel Samuel O. Hill, M.S.C.; Lieutenant Colonel Joseph E. Webb, Jr., M.S.C.; Captain Robert M. Altman, M.S.C.; Captain A. A. Therrien, M.S.C.; and Lieutenant Myron G. Radke, M.S.C., for aid in the revision of certain textual material. Valuable assistance has been rendered by Miss Aimee Wilcox and Miss Katherine A. Patterson by their critical evaluation of certain portions of the text dealing with the diagnosis of malaria, and by Dr. W. H. Wright and Dr. Myrna F. Jones by their assistance with the chapter on Helminthic Diseases. Dr. Marshall Hertig, Dr. W. M. Mann, Director of The National Zoological Park, Washington, D.C., Dr. Redginal Hewitt of Lederle Laboratories, Dr. Orrin P. Wilkins, Dr. Harvey Blank of E. R. Squibb and Sons, Dr. Harry A. Feldman of University Hospital, Syracuse University, Pfc. David H. Shamer, Mr. Flournoy M. Philips and Mrs. Dorothy F. Shelton most generously gave their assistance and advice in the presentation of material in their particular fields. For the preparation of the section on Laboratory Diagnostic Methods, we are indebted to Dr. Paul C. Beaver, Tulane University School of Medicine; to Dr. M. M. Brooke, Communicable Disease Center, the United States Public Health Service; to Lieutenant Colonel Kenneth F. Burns, V.C.; and to Captain James J. Sapero, M.C., U.S.N., who provided respectively the material for the Stoll and Beaver egg counting methods, the PVA technique, the complement fixation and hemagglutination inhibition reactions, and the MIF technique.

Greatful appreciation is extended to the Armed Forces Institute of Pathology for most of the illustrations of pathology. All cuts not bearing a special acknowledgment were furnished through the courtesy of this institution. We also wish to express our thanks to Dr. M. S. Ferguson of the Communicable Disease Center; Dr. E. C. Faust of Tulane University; Dr. T. B. Magath of the Mayo Clinic; Dr. Cornelius B. Philip, the Rocky Mountain Laboratory; Lieutenant Colonel Walter J. LaCasse, M.S.C., U.S.A.F.; Lieutenant L. W. Shatterly, M.S.C., U.S.A.F.; and Mr. Ralph E. Duxbury, Army Medical Service Graduate School, for certain illustrations. Others are acknowledged in the text.

Although it has not proved practicable to include a general bibliography, the following publications must be mentioned as major sources from which much of the material for this volume has been gathered.

Strong: *Stitt's Diagnosis, Prevention and Treatment of Tropical Diseases,* 2 vols., 7th ed. Philadelphia, The Blakiston Company, 1944.

Manson-Bahr: *Manson's Tropical Diseases*, 13th ed. Baltimore, The Williams and Wilkins Company, 1950.

Napier: *The Principles and Practice of Tropical Medicine,* 2 vols. New York, The Macmillan Company, 1946.

Ash and Spitz: *Pathology of Tropical Diseases.* Philadelphia, W. B. Saunders Company, 1945.

Conant, Smith, et al.: *Manual of Clinical Mycology,* 2d ed. Philadelphia, W. B. Saunders Company, 1954.

Pillsbury, Sulzberger, and Livingood: *Manual of Dermatology.* Philadelphia, W. B. Saunders Company, 1942.

Craig and Faust: *Clinical Parasitology,* 5th ed. Philadelphia, Lea & Febiger, 1951.

Chandler: *Introduction to Parasitology,* 8th ed. New York, John Wiley and Sons, 1949.

Faust: *Human Helminthology,* 3d ed. Philadelphia, Lea & Febiger, 1949.

Belding: *Textbook of Clinical Parasitology,* 2nd ed. New York, Appleton-Century-Crofts Company, Inc., 1952.

Herms: *Medical Entomology,* 4th ed. New York, The Macmillan Company, 1950.

Riley and Johannsen: *Medical Entomology,* 2d ed. New York, McGraw-Hill Book Company, Inc., 1938.

Simmons and Gentzkow: *Laboratory Methods of the United States Army*, 5th ed. Philadelphia, Lea & Febiger, 1944.

Moulton et al.: *A Symposium on Human Malaria.* Washington, American Association for the Advancement of Science, 1941.

Moulton et al.: *A Symposium on Relapsing Fever in the Americas.* Washington, American Association for the Advancement of Science, 1942.

Hackett: *Malaria in Europe.* London, Oxford University Press, 1937.

Wenyon: *Protozoology*, 2 vols. New York, William Wood and Company, 1926.

Brumpt: *Précis de Parasitologie.* Paris, Masson et C$^{ie}$.

James A. Oliver's and Dudley Jackson's treatises on snakebite in Bercovitz: *Clinical Tropical Medicine.* New York, Paul B. Hoeber, Inc., 1944.

Boyd: *Malariology*, 2 vols. Philadelphia, W. B. Saunders Co., 1949.

Dawson, et al.: *Report of Proceedings, Third International Congress for Microbiology.* New York, International Association of Microbiologists, 1940.

Shattuck: *Diseases of the Tropics.* New York, Appleton-Century-Crofts, Inc., 1949.

Simmons, et al.: *Global Epidemiology.* Philadelphia, J. B. Lippincott Co., Vol. I, 1945; Vol. II, 1951.

Sawyer, W. A., et al.: *Transactions, Fourth Internation Congress on Tropical Medicine and Malaria.* 2 vols. Washington, U.S. Government Printing Office, 1948.

Numerous publications and periodicals of the Army, Navy and United States Public Health Service, and innumerable other books, journals, monographs and papers in the field of tropical medicine and parasitology which for reasons of space it is impossible to cite in detail were also consulted.

Special gratitude and appreciation are due Adelaide W. Hunter for critical reading of the entire galley and page proof. Likewise our sincere thanks are extended to Miss Shirley Damon, Mrs. Ann Forbush and Mrs. Norma J. Swaney for their aid in preparation of the typescript.

Finally, the authors wish to express their deep appreciation to the publishers, W. B. Saunders Company, for their interest and invaluable assistance which made this Second Edition possible.

THE AUTHORS

# Contents

## Section II    Rickettsial Diseases

*Section VII*    **Helminthic Diseases**

*Section VIII*    **Nutritional Diseases**

## Section IX    Miscellaneous Conditions

## *Section XII*    Some Laboratory Diagnostic Methods

# 1 Introduction

The majority of virus diseases which affect human beings everywhere in the world are acquired from other human beings. An appreciable number, however, are acquired either from animals or from insects. The virus diseases which have their reservoir in man are world-wide in distribution but the actual incidence of clinically recognized infections may differ considerably in different parts of the world, depending on such factors as hygiene, isolation of the population, and certain other characteristics of the way of life of a particular population group. This entire group of diseases is as readily encountered in the tropics as in temperate zones, although because of the factors just mentioned, the ecological pattern of the disease may be quite different in the tropics. The virus diseases which are acquired from animals or insects, with certain exceptions such as rabies, generally have a more limited distribution. Thus, certain of the insect-borne virus diseases which affect human beings are more specifically diseases of the tropical or subtropical regions because the insects which transmit them or the conditions necessary for the maintenance of the virus are found only in these regions.

Some virus diseases of man present a clinical pattern which is

1

characteristic enough to permit at least presumptive diagnosis, while others can be diagnosed specifically only with the aid of certain laboratory tests. The following outline may help the clinician to systematize his thinking and handling of the virus diseases which he may encounter in different parts of the world.

## Virus Diseases of Man Endemic in U.S.A.

### Group A: Simple, Specific Laboratory Diagnostic Tests Available

*(1) Human Reservoir.* Influenza, mumps, smallpox, vaccinia, herpes simplex, trachoma, inclusion blennorrhea, lymphogranuloma venereum, molluscum contagiosum.

*(2) Animal or Insect Reservoir.* Psittacosis-ornithosis, rabies, St. Louis encephalitis, western equine encephalitis, eastern equine encephalitis, California encephalitis, lymphocytic choriomeningitis, Colorado tick fever.

### Group B: Specific Laboratory Tests Not Available or Not Yet Developed for Routine Use

Common cold, primary atypical pneumonia, undifferentiated respiratory disease, measles, German measles, chickenpox, herpes zoster, exanthem subitum, infectious hepatitis, poliomyelitis, epidemic pleurodynia, herpangina, epidemic keratoconjunctivitis, and warts. All viruses in this group have their reservoir in man.

## Virus Diseases of Man Found Outside U.S.A.

### Group A: Viruses May Be Imported or Patients with Infection May Enter

Yellow fever, dengue, Japanese B encephalitis, Venezuelan encephalitis, Russian tick-borne encephalitis, louping ill encephalitis, West Nile fever, Bwamba fever, Rift Valley fever, sandfly (pappataci, phlebotomus) fever, and various African and South American mosquito-borne viruses whose role in human disease is still obscure. With the exception of the Bwamba and West Nile fever viruses, whose mode of dissemination in nature is unknown, all the other viruses mentioned are known to be insect borne and may have an extra-human reservoir.

### Group B: Exotic Viruses Only Occasionally Responsible for Human Infection as a Result of Exposure in Laboratory or Field

Newcastle disease of fowl, foot-and-mouth disease of cattle, vesicular stomatitis of cattle and horses, "B" virus of monkeys, ovine pustular dermatitis, infectious anemia of horses, and cowpox.

## Classification of Viruses by System Affected

At least 50 distinct viruses have been mentioned in the tabulations just given as being capable of causing human disease. The physician faced with the problem of diagnosis may find it helpful to associate certain viruses with clinical manifestations which affect predominantly one system. These may be classified as follows:

### Acute Infections of Respiratory Tract

*(1) Infections Associated with Pneumonia.*   Primary atypical pneumonia, psittacosis-ornithosis.

*(2) Infections without Pneumonia.*   Influenza, common cold, undifferentiated respiratory disease.

### Virus Disease with Special Effect on Skin

*(1) Generalized Maculopapular, Scarlatiniform or Petechial Rash.* Measles, rubella, exanthem subitum, early smallpox, systemic lymphogranuloma venereum, dengue.

*(2) Generalized or Localized Vesicular or Vesiculopustular Eruptions.*   Herpes simplex (also eczema herpeticum), herpes zoster, varicella, vaccinia (also eczema vaccinatum), smallpox.

*(3) Tumors.*   Molluscum contagiosum, warts.

### Virus Diseases with Special Effect on Mucous Membranes

*(1) Mucous Membranes of Mouth and Throat Present Lesions in the Following.*   Measles, varicella and herpes zoster, herpangina (due to Coxsackie group A viruses), herpes simplex, variola-vaccinia, and, more rarely, lymphogranuloma venereum, foot-and-mouth disease, and molluscum contagiosum.

*(2) Viruses with Special Effect on Genitalia.*   Lymphogranuloma venereum, herpes simplex, inclusion blennorrhea, mumps, molluscum contagiosum, warts.

*(3) Viruses with Special Effect on Eyes.*   Trachoma, inclusion blennorrhea, herpes simplex, herpes zoster, epidemic keratoconjunctivitis, molluscum contagiosum.

### Systemic Virus Infections

*(1) Within U.S.A.*   Mumps, infectious hepatitis, epidemic pleurodynia, Colorado tick fever, and lymphocytic choriomeningitis.

*(2) Outside U.S.A.*   Yellow fever, dengue, sandfly (pappataci, phlebotomus) fever, Venezuelan encephalitis virus, Rift Valley fever, West Nile fever, Bwamba fever, and perhaps certain others, as yet undefined or ill defined syndromes, which may be caused in Africa or South America by mosquito-borne viruses which have been re-

covered in the laboratory but whose role in human disease is as yet not established.

### Virus Diseases with Special Effect on the Nervous System

The various viruses which may play a role in infections of the human nervous system will be discussed separately.

## Laboratory Confirmation of Diagnosis

The specific laboratory confirmation of the diagnosis of human virus infections is achieved by different methods for different viruses. Demonstration of an antibody response bearing a definite time relationship to the clinical syndrome under consideration is the simplest and most convenient method from the point of view of a virus diagnostic laboratory. Complement fixation, hemagglutination inhibition, or neutralization tests may be used for demonstrating the antibody. For this purpose it is necessary to obtain an acute-phase serum specimen as soon after onset of illness as a virus disease may be suspected and another serum specimen sometime during convalescence, usually between two and four weeks after onset.

The following virus diseases are best diagnosed by serologic procedures: influenza, psittacosis-ornithosis, lymphogranuloma venereum, yellow fever, dengue, Rift Valley fever, Colorado tick fever, lymphocytic choriomeningitis, mumps, primary infection with herpes simplex virus, and all the arthropod-borne encephalitides. Simple serologic procedures for the diagnosis of infection with poliomyelitis virus have been developed recently and should soon lend themselves to routine application. It is not possible to diagnose infection by serologic procedures unless one can demonstrate that antibody for a given virus first appeared or significantly increased in titer during the course of the illness or convalescence. The mere presence of antibody for a certain virus does not mean that the current infection was caused by it because the patient might have had an inapparent infection with this virus sometime in the past.

In a few virus diseases more direct and rapid diagnosis is possible by simple laboratory procedures. For example, infection with the vaccinia-variola group of viruses may be demonstrated within a few hours, or at most within 24 hours, by testing the contents of vesicles or crusts for the presence of the specific complement-fixing antigen. Microscopic examination of conjunctival scrapings obtained in patients with suspected trachoma or inclusion blennorrhea and the microscopic examination of the contents of nodules in suspected molluscum contagiosum can provide immediate confirmation of the diagnosis. In fatal infections caused by the rabies virus, a diagnosis is also possible by the demonstration of Negri bodies.

Virus recovery is, in most instances, too laborious and time consuming a procedure for routine diagnostic purposes. However, on occasion it may be the most rapid or only way in which the diagnosis can be established. For the differential diagnosis between variola and vaccinia the virus must be recovered and identified. In persons with a history of recurrent herpes simplex, it may not be possible to establish by serologic methods whether a given eruption is caused by the virus of herpes simplex or herpes zoster, and only recovery of herpes simplex virus from some of the vesicles can establish the diagnosis. If epidemiologic circumstances should lead one to suspect that an outbreak of ill defined illness might be caused by either the Venezuelan equine encephalitis virus or Rift Valley fever virus, the fastest way to identify the agent would be by inoculating mice with blood obtained shortly after onset of illness. Such mice usually succumb in two days and a complement-fixing antigen prepared from their tissues can be used for the immediate identification of the virus.

The first cases in a developing epidemic of arthropod-borne encephalitis may be fatal and the most rapid way to identify the virus responsible for the epidemic can be by inoculation of brain tissue obtained at necropsy into mice. The most important precautions in obtaining the material for virus recovery are that the specimens be obtained as aseptically as possible and that they be kept absolutely cold during the period of storage and shipment. Tissues which cannot be inoculated immediately should either be frozen or put into 50 per cent buffered glycerol-saline and stored in an ordinary refrigerator. Body fluids should not be mixed with anything but should preferably be frozen, and, if freezing is impossible, should be kept cold by means of ordinary ice (pp. 839–840).

# 2 Systemic Virus Diseases of Special Importance or Interest in Certain Tropical or Sub-tropical Areas

## Smallpox

**Synonyms**  Variola (major and minor), alastrim, amaas, Kaffir milk pox, West Indian modified smallpox, parasmallpox.

**Definition**  Smallpox is an acute infectious, communicable virus disease, usually characterized by severe toxemia and a single crop of skin lesions which typically progress through macular, papular, vesicular and pustular stages. In the purpura variolosa variety of variola major, this skin eruption does not develop.

**Distribution**  The disease is endemic throughout the world; Asia, Africa and the Middle East are particularly important foci. It is most prevalent in those areas in which successful vaccination is not practiced.

**Etiology and Epidemiology**    Elementary or Paschen bodies, demonstrable in the fluid of the skin lesions, probably represent virus particles. When appropriately stained they are visible with the ordinary microscope and measure about 200 millimicrons in diameter. Epithelial cytoplasmic inclusions, Guarnieri bodies, found in variola infections are believed to represent intracellular aggregates of virus.

This filtrable virus is quite stable and is resistant to drying. It is present in the upper respiratory tract of the patient or in the skin lesions, which retain the virus until they are healed. Scales and desquamated epithelium harbor viable virus for long periods of time.

Transmission is from man to man, usually directly by contact or by respiratory droplets or droplet nuclei. However, indirect spread may occur through contact with contaminated clothing, bedding or other articles which have been in contact with the patient.

Smallpox is highly contagious, ranking with measles and chickenpox in this respect. All persons in the immediate environment (hotel, hospital, barracks, ship, etc.) must be considered contacts exposed to infection. Susceptibility is universal and is altered only by a prior attack of the disease or by successful vaccination.

**Pathology**    The virus enters the body through the upper respiratory tract and, in the susceptible individual, multiplies locally. Viremia follows with dissemination of the virus to the viscera, and particularly to the skin and certain other epithelial surfaces where multiplication continues.

The typical focal lesions develop in the skin. Degeneration and separation of cells of the epidermis and exudation result in vesicle formation. The vesicle is multilocular and umbilicated. The lesions are deeply situated within the skin. In the course of several days the vesicle fluid becomes cloudy and subsequently purulent, forming the pustule. This progression may be modified, however, by the use of antibiotics and the lesions may develop from the vesicular to the desiccated stage without becoming pustular.

Other organs than the skin are also affected showing inflammatory reactions, cloudy swelling, and at times focal hemorrhages.

In the severe fulminating hemorrhagic form of the disease, purpura variolosa, there is massive intracutaneous hemorrhage as well as mucosal hemorrhages in the kidney, gums and oral mucous membranes. In this form, the blood findings include thrombopenia, a high leukocytosis with many young granulocytes including blast cells, and anemia.

**Clinical Characteristics**    The incubation period is usually about twelve days with extremes of six to twenty-two days. Ordinarily the onset is abrupt with sharply rising temperature following chills or chilly sensations and accompanied by symptoms of severe toxemia, headache, nausea and vomiting, and severe general aching most pronounced in the back muscles. Marked prostration is common.

This stage of invasion usually continues for two or three days during which a prodromal flushing or rash may appear. During this period also the generalized violaceous erythematous blush of purpura variolosa appears and is an exceedingly bad prognostic omen. It is usually followed immediately by hemorrhagic phenomena and death ensues before the appearance of the typical eruption.

The characteristic skin lesions commonly appear about the fourth day accompanied by subjective and objective improvement in the patient's condition. The lesions at first are macular, soon becoming papular and, within a few days, vesicular. In the absence of anti-

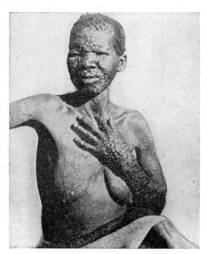

Fig. 1. Smallpox (variola major): characteristic distribution of lesions. (Courtesy of Capt. L. D. Greentree, M.C., A.U.S.)

biotic therapy the pustular stage is reached in about one week. By the tenth day, or soon after, the contents of the lesions are absorbed and desiccation with crusting and scaling follows.

The character and distribution of the skin lesions have diagnostic and prognostic significance. In contradistinction to those of chickenpox, they are deep within the skin and even in the early stages have a hard "shotty" feel; the vesicles are multilocular, tough and difficult to break; all lesions tend to be at the same stage of development; and the distribution of the smallpox lesions is peripheral. The greatest concentrations are seen on the face, forearms, wrists, palms, lower legs and feet including the soles (Fig. 1). The extensor surfaces of the extremities are frequently more heavily involved than the flexor areas. They are usually relatively sparse on the chest, abdomen and upper thighs.

When the skin lesions remain well separated, particularly on the face, the disease is referred to as "discrete" smallpox and the fatality rate averages 10 to 15 per cent. When the lesions merge or appear to coalesce the disease is spoken of as "confluent" and the mortality rates approach 50 per cent. In hemorrhagic smallpox in which there is appreciable hemorrhage into the lesions the fatality rate approximates 80 per cent. Purpura variola, in which the typical eruption fails to develop, is almost invariably fatal (Fig. 2).

**Diagnosis**   The differential diagnosis is concerned particularly with chickenpox and to a much lesser extent with generalized vaccinia. Despite the characteristic differences between the eruptions of

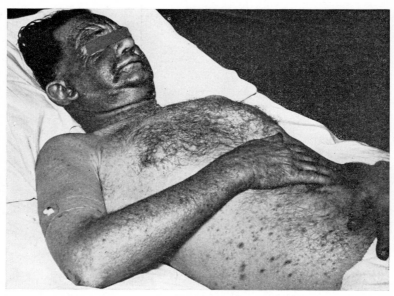

Fig. 2. Smallpox (purpura variolosa): showing skin hemorrhages but no other lesions. (Courtesy of Col. A. P. Long, M.C. and 406th Medical General Laboratory.)

smallpox and chickenpox either of the alternative diagnoses is hazardous to make in adults, particularly in areas where smallpox is known to be endemic. Under such circumstances a presumptive diagnosis of smallpox is safer.

Specific diagnosis may be made by demonstration of the elementary and inclusion bodies in material from the lesions, and by isolation of the virus on the chorio-allantoic membrane of embryonated eggs.

**Treatment**   There is no specific treatment. The antibiotics, particularly those offering broad spectrum coverage, may have some beneficial effect. However, they have not materially altered the prognosis of severe cases. General supportive treatment including good nursing care continues to be of primary importance.

**Prophylaxis**   Successful vaccination is the only method for the prevention of smallpox. In areas of high endemicity and where a virulent form of the disease is found, such as Eastern and Southeastern Asia, such vaccination should be repeated frequently, probably at least every year or two. Vaccines produced in the United States and other western countries will protect against the virulent strains of smallpox virus found in other regions. In the presence of an outbreak of the disease all known and possible contacts must be vaccinated to prevent spread.

Successful vaccination is not simple; it requires meticulous care. The essential points for successful immunization are:

    *a.* The use of a potent vaccine;

    *b.* Vaccination by the proper technique;

    *c.* Proper interpretation of the vaccination result;

    *d.* Repetition of all unsuccessful vaccinations until a successful one is obtained.

## Trachoma

**Synonym**    Granular conjunctivitis.

**Definition**    Trachoma is a specific infectious disease of the conjunctiva and cornea caused by a virus of large particle size and characterized by the presence of Halberstaedter-Prowazek cytoplasmic inclusion bodies in the conjunctival and corneal epithelial cells. It rarely heals spontaneously, is chronic in nature, and often displays acute or subacute exacerbations, due sometimes to viral activity and sometimes to superimposed bacterial infection. Visual damage results from corneal opacification due to the formation of scar tissues.

**Distribution**    Trachoma has a world-wide distribution. The prevalence is greatest in Egypt and the Middle East, where 90 to 100 per cent of the population in some villages may be affected. It is widespread throughout the Mediterranean littoral, the Balkans, Africa and Asia. Important foci exist in certain of the Pacific islands, Korea, Argentina, Brazil and Venezuela. Minor foci are present in the United States, Canada and Japan.

**Etiology**    The disease is caused by an atypical virus of large particle size belonging to the psittacosis–lymphogranuloma venereum group. It is strictly epitheliotropic and involves only the corneal and conjunctival epithelial cells, in which it appears as intracellular cytoplasmic agglomerations or inclusion bodies. In acute cases the virus can be seen free in the exudate in the form of elementary bodies.

**Epidemiology**    The infectivity of trachoma is low in the chronic stage but may be high during an acute onset, an acute exacerbation, or in the presence of secondary infection with bacteria. This is particularly true in the case of the gonococcus or the Koch-Weeks bacillus, which are so commonly associated with trachoma in Egypt and the Middle East. For the most part transmission requires close personal contact; transfer from mother to child is characteristic. Accidental infection of physicians and nurses during surgical procedures has occurred.

**Pathology** The earliest recognizable lesion is the characteristic cytoplasmic inclusion bodies which develop in the conjunctival and corneal epithelial cells. This is followed by subepithelial infiltration with inflammatory cells, particularly plasma cells, and by the development of lymphoid follicles. Follicular hypertrophy is characteristic of the chronic disease. The upper tarsal conjunctiva, the fornix and the upper limbus region are principally involved. The activity of the virus causes slow but steady necrotic changes in the subepithelial tissues.

**Clinical Characteristics** Trachoma may start acutely, especially in adults, with dense conjunctival infiltration, papillary hypertrophy, and considerable exudate. More often, especially in children, the onset is insidious and there are few external signs other than slight

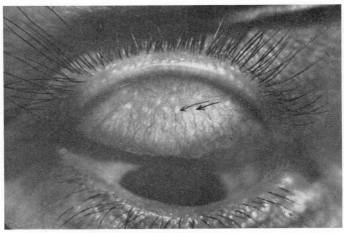

Fig. 3. Trachoma: characteristic follicles, early infection. (Courtesy of Dr. Phillips Thygeson.)

ptosis; only when the upper lids are everted are the characteristic follicles of stage I (MacCallan's classification) observed (Fig. 3). The cornea is always involved simultaneously with the conjunctiva but the first epithelial changes, consisting of minute fluorescein-staining erosions and infiltrates, are recognized only with the biomicroscope. The later changes of pannus, corneal ulceration, and scarring are grossly visible. Unlike pannus from other causes, that of trachoma begins, and is always more extensive, in the upper quadrants.

Regardless of the mode of onset, the disease progresses over a period of months or years through stage II, in which the hypertrophy is predominantly follicular (Fig. 4), to the characteristic cicatricial features of late, stage III, trachoma (Fig. 5), which include lid deformity, corneal opacity, and, in extreme cases, loss of tear function with resultant cornification of the conjunctival and corneal epithelium. Healed trachoma (stage IV) is characterized by a smooth, cicatrized conjunctiva, and a scarred but noninfiltrated cornea; mild cases may be symptom free but the complications of trichiosis and secondary infection usually produce persistent irritation.

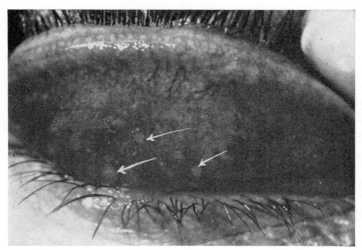

Fig. 4. Trachoma: follicular hypertrophy. (Courtesy of Dr. Phillips Thygeson.)

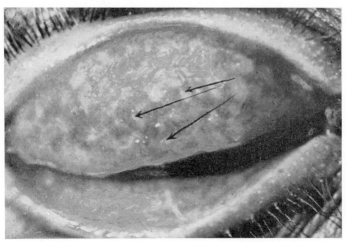

Fig. 5. Trachoma: late scarring and deformity of lid. (Courtesy of Dr. Phillips Thygeson.)

**Diagnosis** The diagnosis of trachoma is ordinarily based on clinical data alone but the finding of cytoplasmic inclusion bodies in scrapings, or of the characteristic cellular changes in expressed follicular material, may be useful in early and atypical cases. A clinical diagnosis of trachoma may be made when follicular hypertrophy or scars, involving predominantly the conjunctiva of the upper tarsus and fornix, occur in association with the characteristically patterned pannus. With the aid of the biomicroscope these diagnostic changes can be recognized early in the disease.

Acute trachoma at onset must be differentiated from the various types of acute follicular conjunctivitis, especially inclusion conjunctivitis (swimming-pool conjunctivitis) and epidemic keratoconjunctivitis. For this purpose examination of the cornea is essential since inclusion conjunctivitis does not affect the cornea and the keratitis in epidemic keratoconjunctivitis is characterized by coin-shaped opacities without pannus formation. Chronic follicular conjunctivitis is readily differentiable from chronic trachoma on the basis of its lack of pannus formation. Severe cicatricial trachoma is occasionally confused with ocular pemphigus or one of the other cicatrizing types of conjunctivitis.

**Treatment**   Prior to the introduction of the sulfonamides and the wide spectrum antibiotics, treatment consisted of cauterization of the conjunctiva with chemical agents such as copper sulfate ("blue stone"), combined with mechanical expression of the follicles. Sulfonamide treatment over periods of from two to four weeks during which low blood concentrations have been maintained has been shown to be more effective than shorter periods of high concentration. The broad spectrum antibiotics likewise have proved of value when used topically in ointment form for relatively long periods. Supplementary follicular expression may shorten the required treatment course.

Recommended therapy consists of combined antibiotic and sulfonamide treatment. A 1 per cent aureomycin or oxytetracycline (Terramycin) ophthalmic ointment should be applied topically every two or three hours during the day. Concurrently one of the less toxic sulfonamides should be administered by mouth in divided dosage sufficient to maintain a moderate blood concentration of the drug. The duration of treatment depends upon the response of the individual case.

In heavily endemic areas where mass treatment is to be undertaken the antibiotic ointment should be used four times daily for a period of two months. Cases found to be resistant on re-examination should then receive combined treatment.

**Prophylaxis**   There is no specific prophylaxis. The problem in endemic areas is essentially the control of the acute ophthalmias. This can be accomplished by mass treatments using topical antibiotic preparations. However, their effective use depends upon a network of fixed and mobile ophthalmologic diagnostic and treatment units coordinated with existing public health facilities.

## Lymphogranuloma Venereum

**Synonyms**   Climatic bubo, tropical bubo, Nicholas-Favre disease, poradenitis, lymphogranuloma inguinale.

**Definition** A specific infectious venereal disease due to a filtrable virus and characterized by transient, often unnoticed, primary lesions followed by superficial and deep lymphadenitis with eventual suppuration and fistula formation. The pelvic colon and rectovaginal septum are frequently involved in the female, producing proctitis, stricture of the rectum and rectovaginal fistula.

**Distribution** Lymphogranuloma venereum is widespread throughout the world, in both tropical and temperate regions. The infection is particularly prevalent among prostitutes and other sexually promiscuous individuals. It has become an important public health problem.

**Etiology** The etiologic agent is a filtrable virus which may be recovered from the primary genital lesions, the affected lymph nodes, inflamed tissue of the rectum, inflammatory lesions of the colon and the cerebrospinal fluid of patients with meningoencephalitis. Elementary bodies measuring 125 to 175 millimicrons may be demonstrated within the leukocytes in Giemsa-, Machiavello- or Castaneda-stained smears of pus from inguinal buboes. There is a striking morphologic resemblance between the elementary bodies of lymphogranuloma venereum and psittacosis. These viruses also possess a common antigen.

The virus may be propagated by intracerebral inoculation in mice and upon the chorio-allantoic membrane or in the yolk sac of the developing chick embryo, from which rich suspensions may be obtained. These are suitable for preparation of antigen for the Frei skin test and for the complement fixation reaction.

**Epidemiology** Although the disease is transmitted principally by sexual contact, accidental laboratory infections indicate that it may be acquired by other routes and without apparent localization or tissue reaction at the portal of entry. Cases have been reported in which invasion occurred apparently through the mucous membrane of the upper respiratory tract and through the skin of the hands. It is evident from surveys that mild, unrecognized infections are not infrequent. The disease is especially prevalent in the colored race.

**Pathology** The pathology of lymphogranuloma venereum varies with the duration and the severity of the infection. The primary lesion, which is seldom seen, is a transitory small papule, vesicle, or ulcer. From this site invasion of the lymphatics occurs. Different routes are followed in the two sexes with resultant differences in the pathology and the clinical phenomena. In the male the inguinal nodes are involved with further extension to the deep iliac nodes. In the female invasion of the inguinal nodes is uncommon, the usual pathology consisting of a pelvic lymphadenitis affecting the rectovaginal septum and producing inflammatory lesions of the rectum and rectosigmoid.

Accompanying the acute adenitis in either sex there is inflammation of surrounding tissue with matting of the lymph nodes, necrosis and stellate abscesses (which cannot be histologically differentiated from tularemia), and the development of chronic fistulas which may drain for considerable periods of time. Healing is accompanied by extensive scar tissue formation which may lead to elephantiasis of the genitalia and rectal stricture. The microscopic picture of the involved lymph nodes and adjacent tissues is that of a subacute or chronic infectious granuloma. In the rare instances in which the upper respiratory tract has apparently been the portal of entry there has been involvement of the cervical lymph nodes.

**Clinical Characteristics**    The incubation period is frequently only a few days. The primary lesion may or may not be noticed and usually consists of a small painless papule, vesicle or ulcer, often disappearing within a week or ten days, situated on the penis in the male and commonly on the vaginal wall or cervix in the female.

The secondary stage of the disease is characterized by the appearance of lymphadenitis. It begins insidiously and runs a chronic indolent course in the male, enlargement of the inguinal nodes of one or both sides is often the presenting symptom. At first they are discrete, later becoming considerably enlarged, matted, adherent to the skin and finally fluctuant. The overlying skin becomes discolored and ultimately sinus formation occurs with the discharge of a seropurulent exudate which may continue for weeks or months. In the female there are often no localizing symptoms prior to invasion of the rectum and the appearance of blood and pus in the stools. This stage may be accompanied by constitutional symptoms such as malaise, anorexia, headache and fever. In the rare instances in which infection occurs through the respiratory tract, there may be acute disease with chills, sweating, septic fever and articular rheumatism. Severe meningoencephalitis has been reported in a few patients. It can occur in individuals who exhibit minimal or negligible evidence of this infection on the genitalia or lymph nodes. Untreated it may last for many weeks.

The third stage of the disease is most striking in the female. It is characterized by chronic proctitis, and occasionally by the development of rectovaginal fistula, fistulous tracts about the rectum, and perirectal abscess. The extensive fibrosis often leads to marked rectal stricture. In both sexes the disorganization of the lymphatic structures may lead to elephantiasis of the genitalia.

**Diagnosis**    In the *differential diagnosis* the inguinal bubo of lymphogranuloma venereum must be distinguished particularly from that of mild ambulant plague (pestis minor), from syphilis, from pyogenic lesions of the lower extremities, and from chancroidal infection. In plague the affected lymph nodes are much more painful and tender and stained smears of material aspirated from them will reveal *Pasteurella pestis*. In the adenitis of syphilis the lymph nodes are discrete, not matted or adherent, and the primary lesion or the scar of such lesions is usually demonstrable. The bubo occurring in the course of a chancroidal infection should seldom cause confusion because of the extensive ulceration usually accompanying it. The rectal and colonic lesions may be confused with fistula due to other causes, perirectal abscess, and chronic infections of the rectum and colon of other types.

Meningoencephalitis due to the virus of lymphogranuloma venereum must be differentiated especially from tuberculous or influenzal meningitis. It is the only viral infection of the nervous system which in the early stages is associated with a lowered sugar content in the cerebrospinal fluid. Unusually high values for protein (250 mg. to 3570 mg. per 100 ml.) are characteristic. Pleocytosis may be as high as 4000 leukocytes per cubic millimeter, with as many as 75 per cent polymorphonuclear cells, during the early stages, and it may persist at lower levels, with a predominance of mononuclear leukocytes, for many months after clinical improvement.

The complement fixation test is most useful for diagnosis especially when a fourfold or greater rise in titer can be demonstrated by two successive tests early in the disease. A rise may not be demonstrable when the first test is performed more than a month after onset. A titer of 1:32 or more in patients exhibiting clinical manifestations compatible with lymphogranuloma venereum may be accepted as confirmatory of the diagnosis except in the presence of early syphilis.

The Frei test, using yolk sac antigen, is more specific than formerly and may be positive seven to ten days after onset of adenitis. However, a positive Frei test may not be noted for five or six weeks. The complement fixation test may become positive before the Frei test.

**Treatment** Unlike other virus infections this disease responds to sulfonamide therapy. Both rapidity of cure and ultimate prognosis are determined by the stage of the disease in which treatment is initiated. Good results may be anticipated in early cases. Later, in the presence of extensive damage with fistula formation and fibrosis, repeated courses of treatment may be required. Enlarged fluctuant lymph nodes should be aspirated but not incised. Rectal stenosis and rectovaginal fistula may require surgical intervention.

Sulfamerazine and sulfadiazine are the drugs of choice although sulfathiazole and sulfanilamide give good results. *Dosage:* 1.0 gm. by mouth every six hours for seven to ten days. Sufficient fluids must be given to maintain an urinary output of 1500 ml. per day to avoid precipitation of the drug within the renal tubules. Inadequate treatment may give rise to sulfonamide-resistant strains of the virus.

Aureomycin and chloramphenicol (Chloromycetin) have been reported to give good results in early cases.

The antimonials are not recommended. It is probable that the value ascribed to these preparations has been due to confusion of diagnosis with granuloma inguinale or chancroid, or to an effect on secondary bacterial infection.

## Infectious Hepatitis

**Definition**   Infectious hepatitis (infective hepatitis, epidemic jaundice) is an acute, diffuse hepatic infection characterized by fever, anorexia, vomiting, abdominal distress and jaundice.

**Distribution**   Probably world-wide. Although the disease is rarely recognized among the native populations of many tropical and subtropical regions, there is evidence to believe that the virus is widely disseminated among them.

**Etiology and Epidemiology**   Epidemic hepatitis is caused by a virus which is most readily demonstrated in the blood and feces of patients. No extra-human source of the virus is known; thus far, the infection has been transmitted only to human beings. Based on tests in human volunteers, the virus is known to be able to pass through bacteria-tight filters; to be resistant to heating at 56° C. for at least 30 minutes, and to one part of residual chlorine per million for the same length of time. The virus is readily transmitted to human volunteers, both by feeding and by parenteral inoculations.

Experimental evidence indicates that human feces constitute a source of virus for natural infection, and limited explosive waterborne, milk-borne and food-borne epidemics have been described. The virus is either absent or difficult to demonstrate in the nasopharyngeal washings and urine of patients. It is important to note, however, that the seasonal incidence of large scale epidemics of infectious hepatitis, although beginning in midsummer and early autumn, frequently do not reach their peak until early or middle winter, and occasionally extend well into spring. Epidemics are particularly prone to occur under conditions of poor sanitation and hygiene which favor the dissemination of human fecal material. Since the blood is infectious during the incubation period, as well as during the early stages of the disease, it is probable that transfusions, blood counts and other procedures using inadequately sterilized instruments may serve as additional means of transmitting the virus.

**Pathology**   Pathologic changes consist predominantly of an extensive necrosis of the parenchyma associated with an inflammatory response at the periphery of the lobule. Liver biopsies performed during the recovery phase of the disease reveal considerable regeneration of hepatic parenchyma and ultimately complete restoration after a period of about two to three months.

**Clinical Characteristics**   The incubation period is said to range from ten to forty days, averaging about twenty-five days. The clinical manifestations vary greatly in different individuals and tend to be less severe in children than in adults. Mild infections without manifest jaundice are common and it is probable that clinically inapparent infections occur as well.

The pre-icteric phase may vary from one to twenty-one days in duration; the average is about five days. Fever, chills, nausea and vomiting, anorexia and epigastric tenderness are the predominating signs and symptoms. They may be the only clinical features in non-icteric cases.

The icteric phase may persist from one to ten weeks. The average duration is about six weeks. The liver becomes enlarged and is usually tender and easily palpable. The stools are frequently clay colored. Restlessness, mental confusion, loss of emotional control, coma and hemorrhagic phenomena are grave prognostic signs. Recovery is gradual, convalescence is slow and relapses are not infrequent.

Death may occur within three to ten days after onset of the illness or as late as the third to the eighth week. However, the mortality rate is very low. Among military patients during World War II the case fatality rate was 1.8 per thousand.

**Diagnosis**   Definitive diagnosis is difficult in the pre-icteric or non-icteric cases since there are no specific laboratory tests for the identification of the virus. Bromsulfalein retention is the first liver function test to become positive during the pre-icteric phase, while the cephalin-cholesterol and thymol turbidity tests become positive somewhat later. The appearance of bilirubin in increasing amounts in the urine is another diagnostic aid. All of these tests may become positive in patients who never develop clinically recognized jaundice.

**Treatment**   No specific therapy is available. A highly nutritious, well balanced and palatable diet, and bed rest are recommended until clinical jaundice has disappeared and the bromsulfalein test has returned to normal.

**Prophylaxis**   The prophylaxis against infectious hepatitis entails effective protection against the transmission of human feces or of any material potentially contaminated by it from one individual to another by food, water, flies or other indirect means of transfer. Because of the presence of virus in the blood, needles and syringes which have been used for patients with the disease should be sterilized by boiling or autoclaving for at least fifteen minutes.

Normal human gamma globulin in doses of 0.06 to 0.12 ml. per pound of body weight has been shown to be effective when administered to people exposed to infection in institutional outbreaks. It is possible that even smaller amounts of gamma globulin may be effective and that the period of passive protection is at least six to eight weeks.

## Yellow Fever

**Synonyms**   Virus amaril; fièvre jaune, gelb fieber.

**Definition**   An acute infectious, endemic or epidemic disease caused by a filtrable virus transmitted by species of mosquitoes belonging chiefly to the genera *Aedes* and *Haemagogus*, characterized by hepatic necrosis which tends to be midzonal in distribution and by a solid immunity after recovery. Protective antibodies persist in the serum for many years if not for life.

**Distribution**   The disease is endemic throughout much of South

America, especially in the rain forests of the Orinoco, Magdalena, Altrato and Amazon watersheds. It is also present along the southern coast of Bahia in Brazil, northern Argentina and Ecuador. Since 1948 yellow fever has advanced westward across Panama and northward through Costa Rica into southeastern Nicaragua where it has occurred in epidemic form. In Africa it extends from the west coast south of the Sahara through the Belgian Congo into Northern Rhodesia, Nyasaland, Uganda, Kenya, and Eritrea.

**Etiology**    Strains of yellow fever virus obtained from different areas appear to be immunologically identical. Recently isolated virulent strains injected into nonimmune rhesus monkeys produce a rapidly fatal disease with the characteristic lesions of yellow fever. Intracerebral inoculation into mice produces a fatal encephalitis. Serial intracerebral passage in mice transforms the natural viscerotropic virus into a fixed neurotropic strain, which, however retains the capacity to confer immunity against infection by the natural virus. Unlike the natural virus, it is not readily transmitted by *Aedes aegypti*.

The virus multiplies in various species of the genera *Aedes, Haemagogus, Eretmapodites, Culex* and a few species of *Mansonia* (*Taeniorhynchus*). Mosquitoes of the last three genera do not transmit the virus by bite. Following the infecting blood meal there is an extrinsic incubation period of one to three weeks, depending upon conditions of temperature and humidity, in the course of which multiplication of the virus occurs. The mosquitoes which can transmit the disease then become infective to a new host and the infection persists throughout the life of the mosquito. Virus is recoverable from the blood of a patient with yellow fever during only the first three to five days of the disease.

**Epidemiology**    Yellow fever may be described as occurring in three forms. The first of these occurs in classic epidemic outbreaks which are strictly urban and *A. aegypti*–transmitted. The second, jungle yellow fever, occurs in the absence of *A. aegypti*. It is endemic in certain jungle areas in South and Central America and Africa. It becomes highly endemic or even epidemic in certain jungle regions when the human population is abundant and nonimmune. The third form is the *Aedes*-borne rural yellow fever which has occurred in certain sparsely populated areas in Brazil.

Classic epidemic yellow fever is an urban disease transmitted by *A. aegypti*; it is characterized by an interval of two to three weeks between the arrival of an infected person and the first appearance of secondary cases. This interval corresponds to the period of extrinsic incubation of the virus in the vector, *A. aegypti*. This mosquito is domestic and is always found in close proximity to man, breeding in and about houses.

Jungle yellow fever in South and Central America appears to be a disease primarily of jungle animals, especially primates and marsupials, and is transmitted by forest mosquitoes. The animals have free virus in their blood for only a few days and rapidly become immune; therefore it is improbable that there is a true animal reservoir. The principal vectors are *Haemagogus spegazzinii* and its subspecies *falco*, *H. capricornii*, and *Aedes leucocelaenus*. It is believed that the virus survives the dry season in the adult mosquito. Human disease is a casual episode occurring for the most part in persons clearing the jungle and is, in consequence, a disease primarily of young adult males, rarely affecting women and children. When the human population is abundant in an area where jungle yellow fever is endemic *Haemagogus* may act as a vector from man to man, producing epidemic outbreaks.

Jungle yellow fever in Africa is essentially a disease of monkeys. *Aedes africanus* and *A. leuteocephalus* appear to be the active vectors in the monkey population, while *A. simpsoni*, a semidomestic mosquito, transmits the virus from monkey to man.

In all areas where the disease is endemic mild unrecognized forms occur.

Since recovery from the disease is accompanied by the development of a permanent solid immunity, in both man and animals, maintenance of the virus in an area depends upon a delicate balance of many factors. The more important of these are the nature of the reservoir, the species of vectors, climatic and other factors affecting multiplication of the vectors, and the number and distribution of nonimmune hosts. Disturbance of this balance accounts for the disappearance of the disease from many areas where it has been prevalent in the past.

The recent spread of the disease into Central America, the increasing number of mosquito species which have been shown capable of harboring and transmitting the virus, and the prevalence of proven vectors in the Far East are ample indications of the ominous threat that yellow fever constitutes for India and the Orient.

However, two procedures permit accurate identification of the disease in time and place and the institution of appropriate quarantine measures and mass immunization of exposed population groups. The mouse protection test identifies immune individuals in the surviving population and analysis of the age groups from whom serum was taken indicates the time at which the infection was prevalent. Similarly, histologic examination of specimens of liver tissue obtained by the viscerotome provides conclusive proof of current disease without problems associated with routine postmortem examinations.

**Pathology**  The essential lesion is hepatic necrosis which, in the early stages, is characteristically midzonal in situation. The parenchymal cells (Fig. 6) exhibit acidophilic hyaline degeneration of the cytoplasm forming Councilman bodies. The skin and viscera are often bile-stained and degenerative changes are demonstrable in the spleen and myocardium. Hemorrhages may be present in the skin, gastro-intestinal tract, lungs and other organs.

The pathologic physiology is characteristic and important:

1. There is a rapid decrease in urinary output which may progress to severe oliguria. This is accompanied by a rapidly diminishing excretion of chlorides.

2. Increasing amounts of albumin and numbers of casts are present in the urine in the early stages.

3. In severe cases peptonuria appears about the fourth day and increases in magnitude in fatal cases.

4. Hypoglycemia may be severe and persistent.

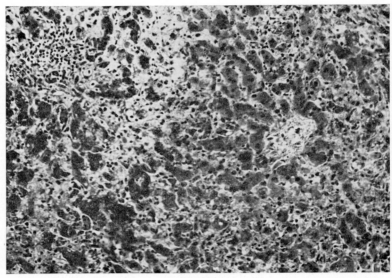

Fig. 6. Section of liver in yellow fever. Necrosis of parenchyma most intense in intermediate zones, leukocytic infiltration.

5. In severe cases there is an increase in the guanidine-like substances in the blood.

These changes revert to normal during convalescence.

**Clinical Characteristics** There is great variation in severity ranging from instances of mild transitory fever to the exceedingly acute and rapidly fatal types. The incubation period is usually three to six days. After mild prodromal symptoms a moderate rise in temperature occurs with elevation of pulse rate and blood pressure, chilliness, headache and bone aches. The fever reaches a maximum of 104° F. usually by the second day and remains elevated for another day or two. Faget's sign—a falling pulse rate in the presence of a constant or rising temperature—appears in this primary febrile period. After three to four days of fever, in some instances the temperature falls to normal to be followed shortly by a secondary rise producing the characteristic saddleback fever curve. Jaundice and hemorrhage may appear by the fourth or fifth day. Ordinarily icterus is not intense even in severe cases. Nausea and vomiting are common. Gastro-intestinal hemorrhage producing coffee ground vomitus, the classic "black vomit," occurs in severe infections and is of ominous import. The patient is usually clear mentally and often anxious and alert.

The secondary rise of fever may terminate by crisis or lysis in the second week. Most of the deaths occur from the fourth to the ninth day. Relapses are rare and convalescence is usually rapid and without sequelae. A permanent immunity is produced.

**Mortality**    The mortality rates in epidemics of yellow fever have reached as high as 50 per cent. In endemic areas the death rate among the native population is usually 7 to 10 per cent.

**Diagnosis**    The diagnosis of yellow fever on clinical grounds is easy in the presence of an epidemic. Sporadic cases, however, may present difficult diagnostic problems. The following points may be of value:

1. In the initial stage there is a polymorphonuclear leukocytosis followed at the end of the first week by leukopenia with a rise of mononuclear cells.
2. Increasing albuminuria and casts.
3. Rapidly diminishing urinary chloride excretion.
4. Hypoglycemia.
5. Peptonuria appearing about the fourth day of illness.
6. Increase of the guanidine-like substances in the blood.

In the *differential diagnosis* one should consider malaria, leptospiral jaundice, infectious hepatitis, relapsing fever and in mild cases, dengue.

**Treatment**    There is no specific treatment. Ample fluids should be administered together with glucose to combat the hypoglycemia. Calcium relieves the symptoms of guanidine intoxication and should be given in the form of the gluconate, 10 to 20 ml. of a 7.5 per cent solution in glucose solution, intravenously each day.

**Prophylaxis**    The prevention of urban yellow fever entails four essential procedures:

1. Elimination of the vector, *A. aegypti.*
2. Prevention of importation of this vector by airplane or ship.
3. Control of individuals entering from an endemic area.
4. Vaccination of nonimmune persons.

*Aedes aegypti* is a domestic insect frequenting the interior and immediate vicinity of houses, where it also lays its eggs (for the details of control measures see p. 746). Airplanes returning from endemic areas must be thoroughly sprayed with an efficient insecticide before they are opened and passengers or cargo released. Similarly, ships should be inspected and appropriate measures taken to eliminate *A. aegypti* if present. Unvaccinated individuals entering from regions where the disease is endemic should be held under control for a period equal to the incubation period of the disease: three to six days.

Efficient individual protection is conferred by administration of yellow fever vaccine. Two vaccines have been developed, each of which confers efficient and long-lasting protection. The American 17D vaccine is a living attenuated neurotropic virus grown in chick embryos. It contains no human serum. The desiccated vaccine is distributed in ampules which must be stored at a temperature below freezing until immediately before use. It is then re-hydrated with physiologic salt solution to the original volume, diluted to 1/10 with additional salt solution, agitated to ensure even suspension and must then be used within one hour.

One subcutaneous injection of 0.5 ml. is given irrespective of age. The vaccine produces an inapparent infection in most individuals. About 5 per cent, however, have a slight febrile reaction on the fifth to the seventh day. Protective antibodies are usually demonstrable in the blood about the tenth day. The vaccine virus is not infective for mosquitoes. The United States Public Health Service requires revaccination every four years.

The Dakar mouse brain neurotropic virus vaccine has advantages and disadvantages. It does not require storage under refrigeration and should be administered by scarification of the skin. Systemic reactions occur in approximately 20 per cent of individuals immunized by this preparation by the scarification method. The percentage is considerably higher when it is injected subcutaneously. Some cases of encephalitis have followed its use.

## Dengue

**Synonyms**  Dandy fever, breakbone fever, bouquet.

**Definition**  A self-limited acute febrile illness, characterized by pain in various parts of the body, prostration, rash, lymphadenopathy and leukopenia. It is transmitted by certain species of mosquitoes belonging to the genus *Aedes*.

**Distribution**  In considering the distribution of dengue virus in the world, one must differentiate between the endemic areas in which the virus is presumably constantly present, areas in which strangers and newcomers are at risk of acquiring the infection, and areas in which some of the largest epidemics have occurred by virtue of importation of the virus but in which, experience has shown, the disease is not endemic and does not constitute a danger to newcomers. Recent experience suggests that certain regions of the Southwest Pacific, Northern Australia, New Guinea, Indonesia, India, and countries bordering on the South China Sea may be considered to be endemic areas. It is also probable that some of the countries and islands in the Western hemisphere in the region of 10° North or South latitude may also constitute endemic areas. The information about Africa is sketchy and inadequate. It is known that during the period of World War II no confirmed cases of dengue were encountered among American and British troops stationed in various countries bordering on the Mediterranean.

Epidemics, due to the importation of the virus, involving hundreds of thousands of people have occurred in areas where the mosquitoes capable of transmitting dengue fever were present, notably Japan during World War II, Greece in 1927–1928, and the Gulf Coast and adjacent Southern states of the U.S.A. in 1922 (Fig. 7).

**Etiology**  The etiologic agent is a virus of the same order of magnitude as that of yellow fever, being approximately 17 to 25 millimicrons. The virus is present in the patient's blood shortly before onset and in many instances throughout the entire febrile period. The greatest concentration, however, has been found within the first twenty-four hours.

There are at least two distinct immunologic types of the virus, the Hawaiian type, and the New Guinea "C" type. All available strains which were recovered during World War II in Hawaii, New Guinea, India, and Japan were found to belong to one or the other of these two immunologic types. There is a possibility, however, that still other immunologic types may be encountered as further studies are made of viruses from other outbreaks.

**Epidemiology**  Human beings, possibly also certain species of monkeys in some regions, and certain mosquitoes of the genus *Aedes* are involved in the cycle of infection by which dengue virus is known to be perpetuated in nature. *Aedes aegypti, Aedes albopictus* and *Aedes scutellaris* (also known as *Aedes hebrideus*) are the only proved vectors of the virus. *Aedes vexans, Aedes solicitans, Aedes taeniorhynchus, Aedes cantator, Anopheles punctipennis, Anopheles quadrimaculatus* and *Culex pipiens* did not transmit the infection under experimental conditions which permitted *A. aegypti* to act as an effective vector. *Aedes aegypti* mosquitoes require a minimum extrinsic incubation period of eight days, and more usually eleven to fourteen days, before they are capable of transmitting the infection acquired in an infective blood meal. Under suitable conditions of temperature they can act as effective vectors for the rest of their lives, which may be as long as one to three months. A single infected mosquito can transmit the infection. Since the virus is present in the blood of man or monkeys for only a few days, it is clear that the disease is most likely to persist in those areas where the conditions are favorable for the survival of mosquitoes throughout the year. It is for this reason that countries near the equator are probably the true permanent reservoirs of dengue and true endemic areas of the disease. Although the new-born human population (after the first three to six months of life) in these equatorial, endemic regions may be enough to keep the cycle of infection going from year to year, it is possible that a jungle type of dengue fever, depending on mosquito transmission among susceptible monkeys, may also exist.

Recent experimental work has shown that infection with dengue

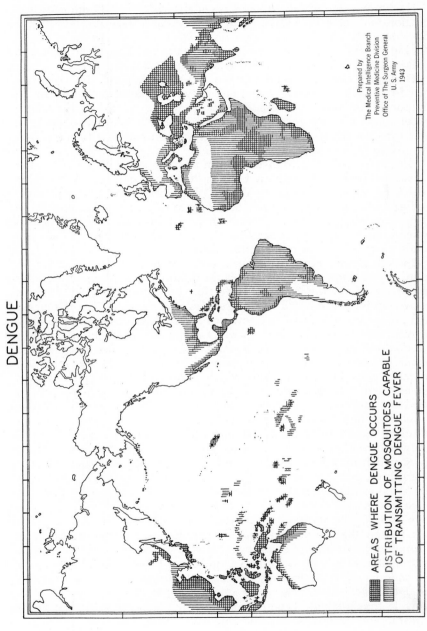

Fig. 7. Geographical distribution of dengue.

virus leaves a long-lasting immunity. Previous assumption that immunity to dengue may be variable or of short duration is probably best explained on the basis of the existence of more than one immunologic type of dengue, as well as by the fact that the clinical diagnosis of dengue may not have been reliable when multiple attacks of the disease were assumed to have occurred in human beings under natural conditions. Experimental studies on human volunteers have revealed that for a period of many months after recovery from infection with one type of dengue virus, the individual may respond in a modified way to infection with another immunologic type of dengue virus. Since at least two different types of the virus have been found to occur in a single epidemic area, many febrile illnesses, which, clinically, could not be diagnosed as dengue, have been proved to be caused by dengue virus.

**Clinical Characteristics**   The usual incubation period is from five to eight days with a range of from two and one-half to fifteen days, depending upon the amount of virus introduced. Headache, backache, fatigue, stiffness, anorexia, chilliness, malaise and occasionally rash may appear six to twelve hours before the first rise in temperature. In about half the number of patients the onset is sudden, with a sharp rise in temperature, severe headache, pain behind the eyes, backache, pain in the muscles and joints, and chilliness but only rarely a shaking chill. Fever persists for five to six days in typical cases and usually terminates by crisis. A saddleback or diphasic type of temperature curve, which is seen in some patients with dengue, is not observed in the majority and cannot be regarded as a pathognomonic sign of the disease. Anorexia and constipation are common, and epigastric discomfort with colicky pain and abnormal tenderness of the abdomen may be seen. Altered taste sensation also constitutes a common symptom early in the disease. Marked weakness and dizziness, photophobia, drenching sweats, sore throat, cough, epistaxis, dysuria, hyperesthesia of the skin, pain in the groin and testicles, and delirium are among the manifestations that are occasionally encountered. The lymph nodes are frequently enlarged, but rarely the spleen. Nuchal rigidity is absent even when the patient complains of a stiff neck.

A rash usually appears on the third to the fifth day and rarely lasts for more than three or four days. It is usually maculopapular, fading on pressure, but occasionally it may be scarlatiniform. Although it is usually first seen on the chest, trunk and abdomen, it eventually spreads to the extremities and frequently to the face. On the last day of fever or shortly after defervescence another type of eruption occurs in many patients. This consists of small petechiae over the dorsum of the feet and legs and occasionally also in the axillae, over the dorsum of the wrists, hands and fingers, and on the buccal mucosa and hard and soft palates.

A typical example of the characteristic changes in the leukocytes is shown in Figure 8. The most marked leukopenia occurs several days after onset of fever and is due to a diminution in the neutrophiles. The blood picture, as a rule, returns to normal within a week after defervescence.

This clinical picture is characteristic of a primary infection with dengue virus. It has been established, by isolation of virus in human volunteers, that mild febrile illnesses of from one to three days'

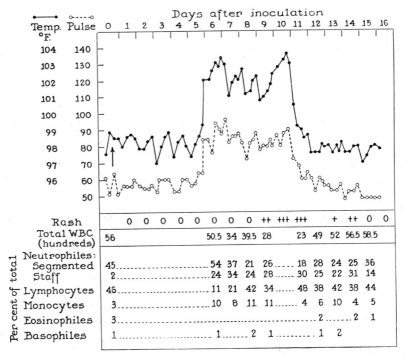

Fig. 8. Graphic representation of temperature and pulse rate of a human volunteer inoculated experimentally with the Hawaiian strain of dengue virus by means of the bites of eight infected *Aedes aegypti* mosquitoes; arrow indicates day on which the patient was bitten. Time of appearance of rash is also indicated, as well as total and differential blood counts. (Sabin in Viral and Rickettsial Infections of Man, edit. by T. M. Rivers. J. B. Lippincott Co. 2nd ed. 1952: by permission of the National Foundation for Infantile Paralysis.)

duration without rash may also be dengue. Experimental work in human volunteers suggests that the most probable explanation for this is that such individuals possess a partial immunity resulting from previous infection with another immunologic type of the virus.

**Diagnosis**   Dengue should be suspected among newcomers in endemic areas; among recent arrivals from an area where the disease is endemic; and during epidemics in nonendemic regions due to importation of the virus and the presence of the vector mosquitoes.

The virus in human blood is best preserved in the frozen or

lyophilized state, but it can also remain active for several weeks when it is stored at the temperature of ordinary melting ice. Both immunologic types of dengue virus have now been thoroughly adapted in mice and suitable antigens for neutralization, complement fixation and hemagglutination tests are available. The dengue viruses have also been shown to have a group relationship not only with the virus of yellow fever but also with the viruses of West Nile, Japanese B encephalitis and St. Louis encephalitis. These relationships are more readily demonstrable by the hemagglutination inhibition and complement fixation tests than by the neutralization test. However, the neutralization test with specific antisera permits the specific identification not only of the two individual types of dengue but also of the other viruses in this group. The complement fixation and hemagglutination inhibition tests are probably more suitable for use in the field because the group specificity of their antigens is not likely to miss an infection with a hitherto unrecognized immunologic type of dengue virus.

In the *differential diagnosis* one must consider influenza, typhus, measles, rheumatic fever, malaria and sandfly fever. In endemic areas dengue may be difficult to distinguish from the early stages of yellow fever.

**Treatment**  Treatment is symptomatic.

**Prophylaxis**  Passage of the dengue virus in mice has produced a variant which still produces rash and immunity but has lost its capacity to cause any significant disease in human beings. Although dengue vaccine prepared with such modified virus has proved effective in experimental studies, it has not yet been tested in the field. The type of anti-mosquito measures to be used are determined in large measure by whether or not *A. aegypti* or *A. albopictus*, or both, are the predominant mosquitoes in the area.

## Sandfly Fever

**Synonyms**  Phlebotomus fever, pappataci fever, three-day fever, summer influenza of Italy.

**Definition**  A self-limited, *Phlebotomus*-transmitted illness characterized by fever of short duration, severe headache, pain in the eyes, conjunctival injection, malaise and leukopenia.

**Distribution**  Since the clinical diagnosis of sandfly fever is not always reliable, one cannot be certain that the disease has occurred outside areas in which its definitely established vector, *Phlebotomus papatasi* is known to occur. The distribution of *P. papatasi* is restricted to certain parts of Europe, Africa and Asia that lie between 20° and 45° north latitude. The disease is definitely known to occur in Italy, along the Adriatic Coast of Yugoslavia, Greece, Malta, Crete, Cyprus, Egypt, Palestine (Israel), Syria, Iraq, Iran, the coast of Crimea, the Azov and Black Sea littoral, certain provinces of central Asia in the U.S.S.R., and the northwest and central provinces of India. Although other species of man-biting *Phlebotomus* flies are known to occur in South America and some also in North America, there is no evidence that sandfly fever occurs in the Western Hemisphere.

**Etiology and Epidemiology** The disease is caused by a virus which is present in the blood of patients during a period of approximately twenty-four hours before onset of fever. The virus is not greater than 40 to 60 millimicrons in size and may be smaller. It has been preserved for many years in the frozen or lyophilized state.

The only valid information about this virus thus far has been derived from experimental work on human volunteers. Reports that the virus has been cultivated in the chick embryo have not been confirmed. All previous attempts to transmit it to laboratory animals, including monkeys, have been unsuccessful. Recently a virus was

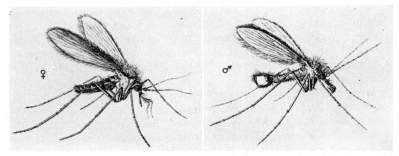

Fig. 9. Male and female of *Phlebotomus papatasi*, the vector of sandfly fever. (Sabin, Philip and Paul. J.A.M.A., *125:* 1944.)

recovered from the serum of experimentally infected human beings by blind passage in newborn mice. This virus has unique properties and has been shown to be neutralized by convalescent serum from human beings experimentally infected with the human virus. Residents in *Phlebotomus*-free areas develop a solid immunity to reinfection with the same strain of sandfly fever virus. However, there is evidence that there may exist more than one immunologic type of sandfly fever virus since an agent recovered during an epidemic in Naples, possessing the properties of sandfly fever virus, did not cross immunize with two other strains which were recovered from Sicily and the Middle East. The two latter strains did cross immunize, one against the other. There is no immunologic relationship between the viruses of sandfly fever and dengue.

*Phlebotomus papatasi* is the only proved vector of the virus. Secondary cases do not arise by contact in the absence of the vector. *Phlebotomus papatasi* is a sand-colored, hairy midge, about 2 to 3 mm. long and 1 mm. thick (Fig. 9). It can be recognized by the position of its wings, which are usually elevated and spread to form a V. Only the female of the species bites; the usual biting hours are during the night and early morning. Their flight, which consists more of a series of hops, is said to be not more than fifty to one hundred yards from their breeding ground. They alight on stones and other obstacles in their approach to a house, and after entry continue to hop about with long pauses before biting. These peculiarities of the flight and movement of sandflies make them particularly vulnerable to residual DDT spray. Although breeding spots are difficult to demonstrate, typical sites are said to be rubble, loose soil, cracks in embankments and other dark, protected spots containing sufficient moist organic matter to provide a suitable place for the development of their larvae. Sandflies thrive during the hot, dry seasons, the precise period varying in different parts of the world. Thus, the season of the disease in different regions may vary from April or early May through early October. Some evidence has been presented for the transovarial transmission of the virus among sandflies. However, this is not easy to demonstrate or repeat. Consequently, the ultimate reservoir of the virus is still in doubt.

The disease is probably widespread early in childhood in the indigenous populations of endemic areas and is largely unrecognized. Sandfly fever has been a problem particularly among recently arrived immigrants and troops. Under suitable conditions the vast majority of newcomers to endemic areas develop the disease during the course of the season.

**Clinical Characteristics**  The average incubation period is from three to four days, the range being from two and one-half to nine days. The onset, as a rule, is sudden. The following signs and symptoms may be encountered: headache, burning sensation or pain in the eyes, photophobia, stiffness in neck and back, backache, pains in the joints and extremities, anorexia, nausea, vomiting, abdominal distress, alteration or loss of taste, sore throat, epistaxis, profuse sweating, and chills or chilliness. Constipation may occur during the first few days and diarrhea during convalescence. In approximately 85 per cent of the patients the fever is of two, three or four days' duration. Fevers that are of less than one day's duration and occasionally as long as five to nine days may occur. The pulse rate is at first elevated but then drops more rapidly than the temperature. During convalescence an actual bradycardia may be present.

There are probably no characteristic physical signs, but conjunctival injection, which is occasionally limited to the exposed portion of the ocular conjunctiva (Pick's sign), may be observed. The exposed parts of the neck and chest appear erythematous, often as though the patient had just been severely sunburned. Although reactions to the bites of sandflies, and occasionally urticaria or erythema multiforme, may be encountered, there is no true rash.

Changes in the leukocyte count are similar to those encountered in dengue and other viral infections accompanied by leukopenia (Fig. 10). The picture is somewhat different at different stages of the illness. During the first day of the fever, the total count may be,

within normal limits, associated with a relative and sometimes absolute increase in the neutrophiles which is due to an increase in immature cells. During the first day, however, a relative and absolute
decrease in the lymphocytes occurs. During the next two or three
days the number of neutrophiles begins to drop and the immature

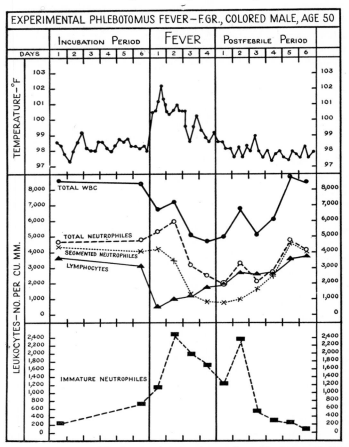

Fig. 10. Differential white blood count in experimental sandfly fever. (Sabin, Philip
and Paul: J.A.M.A. *125:* 1944.)

cells increase to a point where they may outnumber the segmented
cells (Fig. 10). The greatest decrease in the total number of leukocytes may not be observed until the end of the febrile period or after
defervescence. While the neutrophiles are decreasing, the lymphocytes are rising to a point where they may constitute as much as 40 to
65 per cent of the total number of leukocytes. The changes in the
proportions of the different cells at different stages of the disease are
more important for diagnostic purposes than is a single total leukocyte count.

No evidence of hepatic damage has been found by liver function tests. Although there have been reports of pleocytosis during certain outbreaks of the disease, there is no evidence that the virus of sandfly fever is responsible for it. The duration of convalescence varies with the individual and the climate. Marked uncontrollable, transitory mental depression is occasionally encountered. One or two cycles of recurrent fever during convalescence have been reported and similar febrile cycles have been encountered in approximately 5 per cent of the human volunteers. The cause of these recurrent cycles of fever is unknown, since no virus has been found in the blood. There have been no fatalities among thousands of uncomplicated cases of the disease.

**Diagnosis**    There are no specific laboratory procedures for the confirmation of the diagnosis of sandfly fever. Repeated differential leukocyte counts revealing the characteristic changes in the relative proportions of the different cells at different stages of the disease constitute the most valid diagnostic evidence.

During the hot dry seasons of the year a febrile illness among newcomers in an endemic area should arouse suspicion of sandfly fever. Differential diagnosis may be difficult. The aseptic meningitis syndrome caused by poliomyelitis virus, the pre-icteric or non-icteric forms of infectious hepatitis, and influenza without associated respiratory signs may readily be confused with sandfly fever.

**Treatment**    Treatment is symptomatic.

**Prophylaxis**    Adult sandflies are very susceptible to DDT residual sprays, and large areas in Palestine and Italy were freed of the disease when DDT was used primarily to control adult *Anopheles*. Spraying of the breeding places with DDT may also kill the immature stages. Spraying indoors with aerosol bombs containing pyrethrum will kill the adults. Rubble, stone walls, etc., within 100 to 200 yards of human habitations should be removed to eliminate breeding places or be sprayed with DDT. Suitable insect repellents applied to exposed skin areas will provide temporary individual protection.

## Rift Valley Fever

**Definition**    A self-limited febrile illness of several days' duration characterized by severe headache, malaise, leukopenia and rapid recovery. It is primarily a disease of sheep, cattle and other lower animals.

**Distribution**    Rift Valley fever is restricted to certain parts of Africa. Recently a sizable epidemic has occurred among both cattle and human beings in South Africa.

**Etiology and Epidemiology**    The virus is present in the blood of patients and is highly infectious for mice by inoculation by any route. The mice usually succumb within about two days after inoculation. The most marked pathologic changes are in the liver.

Except under special circumstances, it is inadvisable to work with this virus in the laboratory or to attempt virus isolation from the blood of patients because of the extremely high incidence of laboratory infection among individuals working with it.

The virus has been recovered from mosquitoes in nature belonging to several species of the genera *Eretmapodites* and *Aedes; E. chrysogaster* has been shown to be capable of transmitting the infection under experimental conditions.

**Diagnosis** Rift Valley fever should be suspected in the presence of a self-limited febrile illness in endemic or potentially endemic areas. The diagnosis can best be established by demonstrating the appearance of complement-fixing or neutralizing antibodies in patients suspected of this infection. Antibodies have been demonstrated as early as four days after defervescence and are known to persist for many years.

**Treatment** Treatment is symptomatic.

**Prophylaxis** Mosquito control where practical.

## Colorado Tick Fever

Colorado tick fever is caused by a virus which is transmitted by the wood tick *Dermacentor andersoni*. The disease has been recognized not only in Colorado but also in Oregon, Utah, Idaho and Wyoming and, more recently, in the Bitter Root Valley of Western Montana, where a virus has been recovered from *D. andersoni* and the disease has been specifically diagnosed in a human being. The virus has recently also been recovered from dog ticks, *Dermacentor variabilis*, collected on Long Island, New York, but, thus far, no human cases have been recognized in this area.

The disease should be suspected during the tick season in patients with a self-limited, febrile, nonexanthematous illness, characterized by two bouts of fever and associated with leukopenia and malaise. As a rule, an initial bout of fever of two or three days' duration is followed by an afebrile interval of approximately the same length. A second febrile period then ensues, also lasting two to three days.

The diagnosis can be confirmed by the demonstration that complement-fixing antibodies for the virus, which were absent during the acute phase, have appeared during convalescence. The second serum specimen should be collected approximately two weeks after onset of the illness. Control measures are limited to protection against attachment by ticks.

## Bwamba Fever

Bwamba fever is a febrile illness of four to five days' duration associated with headache, generalized malaise and conjunctivitis which has been observed among native Africans of the Bwamba region in Uganda. A virus having a diameter of 100 to 150 millimicrons has been recovered from the blood of clinical cases. It is pathogenic for mice by intracerebral inoculation, while rabbits and guinea pigs have not been found to be susceptible. Neutralizing antibodies for the virus have been shown to develop during convalescence. Antibodies for this virus have been found to be widespread among native Africans in East and West Africa. This virus must, therefore, be considered as one of the potential etiologic agents of febrile illnesses of relatively short duration and of unknown etiology.

## Undefined or Ill Defined Syndromes Caused by African and South American Mosquito-borne Viruses

A number of new viruses have been discovered in Africa and in South America in the course of a search for the virus of yellow fever. Semliki Forest virus was recovered from *Aedes abnormalis* in Uganda. A certain proportion of Africans, resident in Uganda and without any special history of suggestive disease, have been found to have neutralizing antibodies for this virus. Among other viruses recovered in Africa, mostly in Uganda and adjacent regions, are the Bunyamwera, Ntaya, Zika, Uganda S, and Kumba viruses.

Whether or not any of these agents is capable of producing a clinically recognizable illness in man is at present unknown. They will have to be considered, however, whenever certain undefined or ill defined clinical syndromes of potential viral etiology are encountered in Africa for which no etiologic agent can be found among the better known viruses.

The West Nile virus was originally recovered in Uganda from the blood of a woman with mild fever. It has since been found in the blood of several children residing in the vicinity of Cairo, Egypt, during the course of routine serologic surveys. During the course of experimental studies with this virus as a potential therapeutic agent in cancer patients, it has been found that certain strains are capable of producing a severe encephalomyelitis. This virus is antigenically related not only to the viruses of Japanese B and St. Louis encephalitis, but also to those of dengue and yellow fever. It is obvious that only awareness of the existence of this virus will permit the establishment of its role in human disease.

Four viruses known as *Anopheles A, Anopheles B, Wyeomyia* and *Ilheus* have been recovered from mosquitoes in South America. The latter virus is a distinct entity related to the West Nile, St. Louis and Japanese B group. Neutralizing antibodies for it have been found in human beings residing in the Ilheus region of Brazil. The role of these viruses in human disease also remains to be established.

# 3 Virus Diseases with Special Effect on Nervous System

The viruses which have a special effect on the human nervous system, with the possible exception of rabies, are generally capable likewise of producing pathologic effects in the human body outside of the central nervous system. Again with the possible exception of rabies, it is a characteristic of this entire group of viruses that the vast majority of individuals infected by them either exhibit no clinical manifestations of the infection or very mild signs of disease. These inapparent or clinically unrecognized infections, or very mild infections, are partly due to the fact that the nervous system is not invaded by these viruses in all instances and partly that in many individuals the multiplication of the viruses within the nervous system may be of a sufficiently low order of magnitude not to give rise to clinical manifestations.

The viruses which affect the human nervous system are either arthropod-borne (mosquitoes or ticks) or originate from lower animals, whose infected secretions or excreta are transmitted to man by bite or some other manner, or from other human beings. The geographic distribution of the arthropod-borne encephalitis viruses is limited by the distribution of the vector and natural reservoir of the virus. These will be considered in greater detail with the individual viruses. Viruses originating from animals may occur anywhere in the world where these infected animals are present. It is also obvious that certain parts of the world have succeeded in ridding themselves of these infections either by natural isolation or by artificial quarantine. As an example, one may mention the absence of rabies from Britain.

The viruses which have their origin in other human beings are limited in their geographic distribution only by the size of the population group that is needed for their maintenance and by the isolation of a given population group from the outside world.

Viral infection of the nervous system must be considered whenever nuchal or spinal rigidity or more severe signs indicating involvement of the central nervous system appear in the course of an acute febrile illness unaccompanied by the cerebrospinal fluid changes which are ordinarily associated with bacterial or mycotic infection. The findings in the cerebrospinal fluid and the severity of the clinical manifestations may be used as helpful guides in arriving at a clinical suspicion of the virus that may be involved. Thus, when the cerebrospinal fluid is normal on at least two examinations several days apart and there are clinical manifestations pointing to involvement of the spinal cord or medulla or both, rabies and poliomyelitis which has passed the acute phase must be suspected. When pleocytosis is present and the sugar is low, only lymphogranuloma venereum need be considered. When pleocytosis is associated with normal sugar and the clinical manifestations are so mild that only the aseptic meningitis syndrome is suspected, the following viruses must be considered: (*a*) poliomyelitis, which, in general, is probably the most common cause of the aseptic meningitis syndrome and is most common during the summer and autumn in temperate zones; (*b*) mumps, which is probably the next most common cause of the aseptic meningitis syndrome and in temperate zones is most often encountered during the winter and spring months; (*c*) the virus of lymphocytic choriomeningitis, only rarely the cause of this syndrome and, in temperate zones, almost never encountered during the summer and autumn months; (*d*) the viruses of herpes simplex and herpes zoster, which may on rare occasions be the etiologic agents.

The extent to which the arthropod-borne encephalitis viruses may be a cause of the aseptic meningitis syndrome remains to be elucidated. During some outbreaks of Japanese B encephalitis among American troops, none of the patients exhibiting only signs of the aseptic meningitis syndrome yielded evidence of infection with this virus, while in other outbreaks a certain proportion showed serologic evidence of recent infection with Japanese B virus. However, it should be noted that an almost similar proportion of other Americans who were in the same area and remained well also developed antibodies for the Japanese B virus. Accordingly, it is quite possible for a certain proportion of people who develop the aseptic meningitis syndrome owing to infection with poliomyelitis virus to develop antibodies for any of the arthropod-borne encephalitis viruses that might be undergoing simultaneous dissemination among the population. Since epidemics caused by the arthropod-borne encephalitis viruses usually coincide with the higher seasonal incidence of poliomyelitis, it is evident that before an individual case of the aseptic meningitis syndrome can be considered as being caused by one of the encephalitis viruses, it must be demonstrated by appropriate serologic tests that concurrent infection with poliomyelitis virus had not occurred. There is no adequate evidence at the present time that the arthropod-borne encephalitis viruses are among the causes of the aseptic meningitis syndrome.

When pleocytosis is present in association with more severe signs of involvement of the central nervous system, the following viruses come up for consideration: poliomyelitis, the arthropod-borne encephalitis viruses in endemic areas, rabies, and occasionally also the virus of herpes simplex. The disease known as von Economo's encephalitis or encephalitis lethargica, which gained prominence during the period of 1916 to 1926 and then apparently disappeared, is mentioned here chiefly to indicate that it is still an etiologic and epidemiologic enigma. At this time one would probably suspect it only when an encephalitis of chronic course is followed by parkinsonism.

In general, the virus diseases which attack the human nervous system are characterized by a relatively brief course. As a rule there is either a fatal outcome within a period of about two weeks or defervescence and improvement within seven to fourteen days after onset. Clinically, the differential diagnosis between poliomyelitis and the encephalitis caused by the arthropod-borne viruses is aided by the fact that the most severe involvement of the nervous system in poliomyelitis is invariably ushered in by paralysis of some part of the body supplied by either spinal or cranial nerves, while the more severe involvement of the nervous system resulting from an attack by the arthropod-borne viruses is generally ushered in by psychotic manifestations, convulsions, muscle twitching, disorientation and sometimes coma.

All of the viruses which give rise to clinically recognizable disease of the human nervous system, with the exception of mumps and lymphocytic choriomeningitis, attack the neurons directly. The clinical effects are the expression of the attack upon neurons situated in different anatomic areas. The basic character of the lesions produced by the viruses of poliomyelitis and the arthropod-borne encephalitis viruses is essentially the same. Pathologic differentiation between these must be based on the distribution of the lesions in the nervous system. Thus, both the poliomyelitis viruses and the arthropod-borne encephalitis viruses can attack neurons in the spinal cord, with the production of neuronophagia and inflammatory lesions which cannot be distinguished one from the other. While it is true that the spinal cord is more commonly and extensively attacked in poliomyelitis than in the diseases produced by the arthropod-borne encephalitis viruses, it is also true that by the examination of the spinal cord alone it is not possible either to confirm or reject the diagnosis of one or the other group of viral agents. Only an examination which includes multiple areas of the cerebral cortex and cerebellum permits such a differentiation. The anterior frontal, temporal and occipital portions of the cortex, and the molecular and Purkinje cell layers of the cerebellum, show no significant lesions in poliomyelitis. In the arthropod-borne viral encephalitides, however, lesions are almost invariably present in these areas. While it is true that in infections caused by the viruses of louping ill, Russian spring-summer encephalitis, and Japanese B encephalitis, the molecular and Purkinje cell layers of the cerebellum may be more frequently and extensively involved, it is not possible to make a diagnosis of infection by these viruses based on the pathologic findings alone.

The diagnosis of rabies is aided by the finding of Negri bodies, particularly in the various cells of Ammon's horn and other portions of the temporal cortex, while the actual destruction of neurons and inflammatory reactions may be minimal or absent. In the encephalitis caused by the virus of herpes simplex, the attack is not only on the neurons but also on the glial and other cells of the supporting structures of the nervous tissue. Here the presence of acidophilic, intranuclear inclusions associated with diffuse areas of softening and inflammation are helpful guides to the diagnosis, which, however, must be confirmed by animal inoculation. The viruses of mumps and of lymphocytic choriomeningitis attack the meninges or the choroid plexus or both.

## Arthropod-borne Encephalitis Viruses

Some of the arthropod-borne encephalitis viruses are transmitted to human beings by the bites of mosquitoes and others by ticks. Mosquito-transmitted viruses include the St. Louis, western equine, eastern equine, California, Venezuelan, and Japanese B viruses. The Russian spring-summer encephalitis and the louping ill viruses are tick transmitted.

**Distribution**    The St. Louis, western equine, eastern equine, California and Venezuelan viruses are known to occur only in the Western Hemisphere. The Japanese B virus is restricted to the far Pacific, certain Pacific islands and the Orient. It is probable that it is present in Australia as well. The extent to which the West Nile virus and some of the mosquito-borne viruses that have recently been discovered in Africa are responsible for disease of the human nervous system in Africa is as yet unknown.

**Etiology**    All of the arthropod-borne viruses are relatively small, ranging from about 15 to 30 millimicrons in size. They may be separated into two groups on the basis of their pathogenicity for small laboratory animals. The St. Louis, California, Japanese B, Russian spring-summer and louping ill viruses produce fatal, clinically recognizable infection in mice but not in guinea pigs or rabbits.

The viruses of the other group, which includes western equine, eastern equine and Venezuelan encephalitis, are highly pathogenic for guinea pigs and rabbits as well as for mice.

A multiplication inhibiting genetic factor in certain mice affects the St. Louis, Japanese B, Russian spring-summer and louping ill viruses. It is without effect on the viruses of western equine, eastern equine and Venezuelan encephalitis.

**Epidemiology**    Human beings are only incidental hosts of the arthropod-borne encephalitis viruses and probably play a negligible role in the natural history of the infection cycle which maintains the viruses in nature.

Identification of the ultimate reservoir of the viruses transmitted by mosquitoes to man and to other hosts still presents an unsolved problem. There is no adequate evidence that the mosquitoes themselves are capable of maintaining the virus in nature from winter to summer and from year to year. In fact, the available evidence suggests that the mosquitoes are infected during a particular time of the year by feeding on some other host which has a viremia for a limited period of time.

The demonstration of the viruses of St. Louis encephalitis and western equine encephalitis in certain species of chicken mites or bird mites gave rise to the hypothesis that such mites, in fact, might be the ultimate reservoir of all the mosquito-transmitted viruses, because it has been shown that viruses infecting mites may be transmitted from generation to generation by way of the ova. Thus far it has not been possible to confirm that mites which harbor the virus can produce a viremia in chickens or birds and thus provide a source of virus for mosquitoes. It is not as yet clear whether the mites are merely an incidental host for the virus because they happen to have fed on birds or chickens that had virus in their blood, or whether they actually serve as the important reservoirs for maintaining these viruses in nature.

It is quite clear that the ticks themselves constitute the ultimate reservoir of the viruses of the tick-borne Russian spring-summer encephalitis and of louping ill. The ticks are also the only known vectors of these viruses and the seasonal incidence of these infections corresponds quite closely to the attachment periods of the ticks.

**Prophylaxis**   The control and prevention of disease caused by the arthropod-borne encephalitis viruses presents many difficult problems. In general, protection against ticks should provide a suitable barrier against infection by the viruses which cause Russian spring-summer encephalitis and louping ill. In the mosquito-borne viruses only the St. Louis, western equine and Japanese B viruses have produced epidemics affecting thousands of human beings at a time. Attempts to control established epidemics caused by the mosquito-transmitted encephalitis viruses have met with little success because by the time the epidemic is recognized the vast majority of individuals have already been infected and, with certain exceptions, such epidemics are usually of limited duration. Eradication of the mosquitoes which are the potential vectors, in an attempt to prevent the unpredictable epidemics, is both very difficult to achieve and economically not quite feasible.

While Formalinized vaccines are available for a number of these viruses their use during an epidemic is impractical because it takes too long for immunity to develop. Since even the better vaccines produce immunity for only a limited period of time not exceeding one or two years, and since only a very small portion of the population is affected even during the most severe epidemics, which occur at unpredictable times, it is not as yet practical to use vaccines in an attempt to immunize, and maintain in an immune state, the entire population at risk. While there is experimental evidence that the administration of small amounts of potent antibody for these viruses can impart a passive immunity which might be useful during an epidemic, there are at present no available sources of such antibody which might be used in human beings during epidemic periods.

### St. Louis Encephalitis

This virus occurs in midwestern and southwestern United States. It has been demonstrated in *Culex tarsalis* mosquitoes in nature. This mosquito is believed to be its most common vector although it is possible that in certain areas *Culex pipiens* and certain other culicine mosquitoes may also serve as vectors. Although this virus is endemic in certain parts of California, its occurrence in other areas is quite unpredictable. Thus, there was the large epidemic in the St. Louis area in 1933 followed by a smaller one in 1937. There has not been another outbreak of this disease in that area between 1937 and 1952.

**Diagnosis** The diagnosis of the disease is made by serologic methods or by the recovery of virus from the central nervous system of a fatal case. Neutralizing, complement-fixing and hemagglutination inhibition antibodies develop early in convalescence. Hemagglutination inhibition antibodies are as a rule the first ones to appear and a presumptive diagnosis may be made by finding them in high titer during the latter part of the active infection period. Definitive diagnosis, however, is best made by demonstrating a significant rise in titer in paired sera of complement-fixing or hemagglutination inhibition antibodies.

## Western Equine Encephalitis

While the principal endemic area for this virus is in the United States west of the Mississippi River, it has also been reported recently from Michigan, Alabama and Florida and is also known to occur in adjacent areas of Canada, as well as in Argentina. It is prevalent in certain parts of California where outbreaks of considerable magnitude have occurred. However, the largest single epidemic caused by this virus developed in 1941 in Minnesota, North Dakota and the adjacent provinces of Canada in which several thousand people were attacked during a relatively short period of time.

*Culex tarsalis* mosquitoes have been shown to harbor this virus in nature and they are also believed to be the vectors under natural conditions.

**Diagnosis** The specific diagnosis of infection by this virus is accomplished by the same procedures used for the identification of the St. Louis encephalitis virus.

## Eastern Equine Encephalitis

This virus occurs in the eastern United States, Canada, Mexico, Cuba, Panama, the Dominican Republic and Brazil. It has also been recognized in recent years in Alabama, Michigan, Arkansas and Texas. Although epizootics of the disease in horses and pheasants occur with considerable frequency in the eastern United States only two small outbreaks have been recorded in human beings. One occurred in Massachusetts in 1938 and involved 34 persons; another one in 1947 in Louisiana involved about 15 persons.

The virus has been shown to be capable of multiplying in *Aedes sollicitans* and has been isolated from wild *Mansonia perturbans*, but the actual vectors of this virus in nature are as yet unknown.

**Diagnosis** The specific diagnosis of the infection is made by demonstrating a significant rise in titer of complement-fixing antibodies in paired sera.

## California Encephalitis

The California virus has been recovered from *Aedes dorsalis* and *Culex tarsalis* mosquitoes caught in the San Joaquin Valley of California, but not yet from man, other mammals or birds. Serologic survey data suggest that clinically inapparent infection has occurred in human beings, horses and certain other mammals in California. On the basis of such data it is believed that at least one severe case of encephalitis in an infant, and possibly two others, in Kern County, California, were caused by this virus.

## Venezuelan Equine Encephalitis

This virus is known to occur in Venezuela, Ecuador, Trinidad, Panama, and possibly also Colombia. It is highly infectious for human beings. With few exceptions, individuals who have worked with this virus in the laboratory have developed clinically recognized illnesses. In none of the many laboratory infections reported thus far has there been definite involvement of the central nervous system. Only two fatal infections, both with central nervous system involvement, have been reported and both of them occurred in Trinidad among Americans. The extent to which this virus is responsible for disease among human beings residing in the endemic areas of Central and South America is not yet known.

Although *Aedes taeniorhynchus* and *Mansonia titillans* have been considered as potential vectors of this virus, there is as yet inadequate information on the mode of transmission in nature.

**Diagnosis** Diagnosis of this infection may be made most rapidly by the inoculation of mice with blood obtained during the early febrile stage of the illness. The mice succumb within two to three days and the virus can be quickly identified by preparing a complement-fixing antigen from the brain or liver for test with known antiserum. For practical purposes, however, it is advisable to establish a diagnosis by the demonstration that antibodies, either complement-fixing or neutralizing, which were absent during the acute phase, appeared or increased in titer during convalescence. Neutralizing antibody can appear within five days after onset.

## Japanese B Encephalitis

This virus has been recovered from human beings in Japan, particularly south of Hokkaido, and in Okinawa, Guam, Korea, China, Manchuria and the neighboring maritime provinces of the Soviet Union. The virus of Australian X disease corresponds in most of its characteristics to that of Japanese B encephalitis, and the Murray

Valley encephalitis virus recently recovered in Australia is either identical or very closely related to it.

**Epidemiology** Epidemics affecting thousands of people have occurred at varying and unpredictable intervals in Japan, and lesser outbreaks have also been described from Okinawa, Korea and Manchuria. Although a high incidence of inapparent infection has been shown to occur among the native Chinese population, the incidence of clinically recognized cases of encephalitis is very low and no epidemics have been described. Antibody studies on the native populations suggest that infection with Japanese B encephalitis has probably also occurred on Formosa and in Indo-China, Java, the Philippines, the Malay Peninsula and Sumatra. However, since the virus has not yet been recovered from those areas, one cannot be certain that those antibodies may not be due to infection with a related virus.

Extensive studies performed in Japan indicate that *Culex tritaeniorhynchus* is the only mosquito from which the virus has been definitely and unequivocally recovered in nature. There is no evidence that *Culex pipiens pallens* or other mosquitoes are infected under natural conditions. The seasonal incidence of epidemics of Japanese B encephalitis bears a precise relationship to the rise and fall of the numbers of *C. tritaeniorhynchus* mosquitoes. As one might expect, the peak of the epidemic period is separated from the peak of the mosquito population by a period of one to two weeks, which corresponds in part to the extrinsic incubation period of the virus in the mosquitoes and in part to the intrinsic incubation period of the infection in man. By the time an epidemic is thoroughly established the number of *C. tritaeniorhynchus* mosquitoes may already be quite small and at the termination of the epidemic it may be difficult to find these mosquitoes in appreciable numbers.

**Diagnosis** It has not proved possible to confirm reports that the virus can be recovered from the blood, cerebrospinal fluid, urine, feces or saliva of patients with the disease. Complement fixation and hemagglutination inhibition tests are the serologic procedures of choice for establishing the diagnosis. A significant rise in titer of these antibodies may be demonstrated as early as seven to ten days after onset of the first symptoms. The diagnosis of the infection in a fatal case may be established most rapidly by transmitting the infection to mice by intracerebral inoculation of human brain tissue and then preparing a complement-fixing antigen from the brains of mice which succumb.

## Russian Spring-Summer Encephalitis

The virus is definitely known to occur only in the far eastern provinces of the U. S. R. It is not quite clear whether the agent which has been recovered in certain European parts of Russia is the same as that found in far eastern regions or is in effect the virus of louping ill.

The virus has been demonstrated in the wood tick *Ixodes persulcatus*. The prevalence of the disease corresponds to the distribution and seasonal activity of this vector. Thus the disease is most common in May and June, particularly among workers in lumber camps and other forest workers living in adjacent villages. It is rare in urban areas. The diagnosis is established by serologic methods, although differentiation between infection by this virus and the virus of louping ill may be difficult or impossible.

### Louping Ill

Sporadic cases of encephalitis have been observed in human beings where the virus is known to be enzootic among sheep of North England and Scotland. Similar sporadic cases have recently been reported from Czechoslovakia and White Russia.

The tick *Ixodes ricinus* is the vector of the disease among sheep in England and Scotland and the same species has also been reported as harboring the virus in White Russia. The louping ill and Russian spring-summer encephalitis viruses are so similar that they are either different strains of the same virus, or perhaps immunologically related types of the same virus.

## Viruses Transmitted by Animal Secretions or Excretions

### Rabies

**Synonyms**  Hydrophobia, rage, lyssa, rabbia, raiva, tallwut.

**Definition**  Rabies is an acute infectious disease caused by a filtrable virus, primarily involving the central nervous system and characterized by hyperexcitability, pharyngeal spasm, convulsions, and death.

**Distribution**  The disease is widely disseminated throughout all areas of the world, with the exception of Australia and Hawaii where enforcement of quarantine measures before large urban centers developed prevented its entry. Scandinavia and the British Isles have eradicated the disease and the Netherlands, Switzerland, and Canada are also relatively free of it.

**Etiology and Epidemiology**  Rabies exists in an enzootic form in wild animals and in the dog. The virus present in the saliva is transmitted by the bite of an infected animal. An increased prevalence of human cases of the disease often is a reflection of epizootic conditions in the dog population or the sylvan reservoir. Vampire bats are a source of human infection in Trinidad.

**Pathology**  Lesions characteristic of neurotropic viral infections are present in the central nervous system, chiefly in the medulla, the basal ganglia motor cortex, and the posterior horns of the spinal cord. When present, the characteristic inclusions, Negri bodies, are pathognomonic. They are frequently absent in infections with certain strains of virus.

The Negri body is a globular or ovate, acidophilic, intracytoplasmic structure with maximum size approximating that of a red blood cell. The larger bodies often contain basophilic material.

**Clinical Characteristics**    The incubation period is highly variable, ranging from ten days to more than seven months. It is believed that the virus reaches the brain along neural pathways and that the location of the bite is a factor determining both incubation period and severity. Slight to moderate fever, occipital headache, malaise, anorexia, vomiting and abnormal sensations in the region of the infecting bite mark the onset of disease. Hyperesthesia and mental and neuromuscular hyperexcitability develop rapidly, together with stiffness of the neck and violent spasms of the pharynx and the accessory muscles of respiration. The mere sight, smell or sound of liquid stimulates this reflex. The acute excitability progresses to gen-

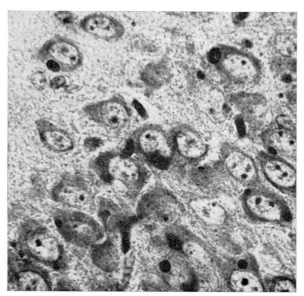

Fig. 11. Intracytoplasmic inclusion bodies: Negri bodies of rabies.

eralized convulsions, and death usually occurs during a seizure. A clinical variant, often associated with bites on the toes, particularly those inflicted by vampire bats, presents the picture of an ascending paralysis with little or no hyperexcitability or difficulty in swallowing. In both forms the disease is invariably fatal.

**Diagnosis**    The characteristic clinical picture and history of exposure should suggest rabies. Definitive intra-vitam diagnosis may be made by isolation of the virus from saliva or by demonstration of neutralizing antibodies when vaccine has not been administered. Demonstration of Negri bodies in autopsy material and recovery of the virus establish the diagnosis (Fig. 11).

The intermittent nature of the muscle spasm aids in the differentiation from tetanus.

**Treatment**    Treatment is supportive and symptomatic. Barbiturates are recommended in preference to morphine for sedation. An attempt should be made to maintain fluid balance.

*Prophylaxis*   1. *Local treatment of wounds* inflicted by rabid animals is probably highly effective. Some authorities consider thorough washing with 20 per cent medicinal soft soap sufficient for open wounds; however, cauterization with concentrated nitric acid is recommended for deep puncture wounds or for those more than two hours old.

2. *Disposition of Suspect Animal.* It is imperative that an effort be made to catch but not destroy the dog or other animal that has inflicted the bite. It should be observed, preferably by a veterinarian, and if typical signs are not apparent or death does not occur within ten days, rabies is not present. When clinical disease is fully developed, the animal should be sacrificed and the intact head frozen and delivered to a laboratory providing rabies diagnostic facilities for the area. Definitive diagnosis may be established rapidly by recognition of Negri bodies in impression smears of the animal brain, usually from the region of Ammon's horn, or by their presence in the brains of mice inoculated with a suspension of the suspect brain.

3. *Active immunization* is recommended and in an endemic area should be started immediately, when

(*a*) the animal is apprehended and presents clinical signs of rabies;

(*b*) the animal is killed and the brain found positive for rabies by microscopic examination;

(*c*) the animal is killed and despite negative findings on microscopic examination, the animal is suspected of being rabid;

(*d*) the animal escaped, or was an unidentifiable stray.

Such treatment consists of fourteen daily subcutaneous injections of a commercially available rabbit brain suspension. Since rare but serious reactions do occur from sensitization to rabbit brain tissues, vaccine should not be administered without evidence of exposure as outlined in the criteria listed. Improvement in the recently developed chick embryo–adapted vaccine may remove this objection.

4. *Passive immunization* by administration of hyperimmune serum offers promise, but currently this is being used in conjunction with vaccine prophylaxis.

*Control*   Effective measures for control include licensing of dogs, destruction of strays, quarantine of imported dogs, confinement and observation of a dog guilty of unprovoked biting and of all canine contacts of a rabid animal, quarantine or muzzling of all dogs for six months after the last reported case, reduction of the wild animal reservoir, and compulsory vaccination of dogs where quarantine cannot be effectively enforced or where exposure to an endemic wild animal reservoir exists.

## Lymphocytic Choriomeningitis

The virus of lymphocytic choriomeningitis has its reservoir in wild mice and possibly also in dogs. It is excreted in the urine and feces.

Human beings may therefore acquire the virus by direct or indirect contact and possibly also by breathing in the dried virus contained in dust. It has been demonstrated that *Trichinella spiralis* may pick up the virus, when it is present in infected animals, and then transmit it to other animals through its larvae.

This virus is responsible for only a small proportion of cases exhibiting the aseptic meningitis syndrome and it is doubtful whether it has ever been the cause of more severe central nervous system involvement. Experimental studies on human volunteers suggest that infection with this virus may take the form of two or three waves of fever during a two- or three-week period unaccompanied by localizing symptoms. Fatal cases of the acute systemic type of the disease have been reported and in them the lungs and liver exhibited inflammatory changes.

**Diagnosis** The diagnosis can best be established by the complement fixation test using serum specimens obtained during the acute phase of the illness and about three weeks after onset. Neutralizing antibodies appear later than the complement-fixing antibodies and may be used to establish the diagnosis by tests of serum specimens obtained at the beginning of convalescence and late in convalescence. Virus isolation is not recommended as a routine procedure, although the virus can be recovered from the blood and cerebrospinal fluid.

### B Virus of Monkeys

The B virus, endemic among certain types of monkeys, is a relative of the herpes simplex virus of man. At least two fatal cases of the disease, characterized chiefly by an encephalomyelitis, have been observed in human beings after bites by rhesus monkeys. The appearance of vesicular lesions at the site of a monkey bite, followed by central nervous system involvement, should lead to suspicion of the infection.

**Diagnosis** The virus can be isolated from fatal cases by inoculation of brain tissue and viscera into rabbits.

## Viruses Originating in Human Beings

### Poliomyelitis

**Synonyms** Acute anterior poliomyelitis, infantile paralysis.

**Distribution** Poliomyelitis occurs throughout the world wherever human beings live in large enough numbers, or in sufficient contact with other regions to maintain the chain of transmission.

**Etiology** At least three distinct immunologic types of poliomyelitis virus are known. There is evidence to suggest, however, that not all strains belonging to the same immunologic type are of the same virulence or have the same capacity for producing the severe paralytic sequelae of infection.

*Epidemiology*  Poliomyelitis in human beings appears to be primarily an infection of the alimentary tract and only occasionally a clinically recognized disease of the nervous system. Human stools are the richest source of the virus in nature. Although the virus can be demonstrated in material obtained by swab or washings from the posterior pharyngeal wall, there is reason to doubt that under ordinary conditions it reaches the external environment by means of droplets from the mouth. The many direct and indirect routes by which human feces may be transmitted from one individual to another constitute the potential modes of transmission of the infection among human beings.

Experimental evidence has demonstrated that dosage is an important factor determining the outcome of infection. The incidence of paralysis following ingestion of large doses of virus is very much higher than after ingestion of small doses. Conversely, the incidence of inapparent or clinically mild or unrecognized types of infection is very much greater after the repeated ingestion of minute amounts of virus.

There are data to suggest that the genetic constitution of the host, and severe physical exertion or fatigue during the early stages after invasion of the nervous system, may determine whether the outcome of a given infection will be paralytic or nonparalytic. However, there is reason to believe that factors relating to the virulence of the various strains of virus and the amount ingested play a more important role in determining the incidence of paralysis and the occurrence of epidemics.

The incidence of paralytic poliomyelitis in certain population groups over a period of many years appears to be inversely proportional to the amount of virus that is being disseminated among them. This is one of the seeming paradoxes in the epidemiology of the disease. Thus, antibody studies have shown that the incidence of paralytic poliomyelitis among populations exhibiting the highest incidence of inapparent or clinically unrecognized infections in the very early age groups is relatively much lower than in countries with advanced sanitation and hygiene. In the former areas epidemics or large outbreaks of the disease are rare or practically unknown. It has been suggested, therefore, that poor sanitation and hygiene which afford ample opportunity for transmission of the virus likewise provide a greater opportunity to acquire the inapparent or very mild type of infection by exposure to strains of low virulence and repeated exposure to small doses of virus. This would create a population predominantly immune at a time when more virulent strains of virus were introduced. It would explain the relative absence of outbreaks or epidemics in such communities at a time when newcomers resident in the same areas experience a high attack rate of paralytic poliomyelitis.

According to this view epidemics occur when strains of virus of higher virulence invade population groups that have been insufficiently immunized by strains of lower virulence belonging to the same immunologic type.

**Diagnosis** The diagnosis of poliomyelitis can be made with assurance on clinical grounds alone only when characteristic paralysis of muscles supplied by spinal or cranial nerves develops during the course of an acute febrile illness associated with pleocytosis. During epidemic periods, the vast majority of cases of the aseptic meningitis syndrome are caused by poliomyelitis virus. There is likewise abundant evidence to indicate that the minor febrile illnesses without signs of nervous system involvement which occur among contacts of poliomyelitis cases are due to infection by poliomyelitis virus.

The recent development of tissue culture methods for the detection of poliomyelitis virus in the stools, as well as for the measurement of antibody against the several immunologic types of poliomyelitis virus, has introduced procedures by which it is now possible to confirm in the laboratory the clinical diagnosis of suspected infection with poliomyelitis virus. It may be some time, however, before these have been sufficiently developed to permit their use for routine diagnostic purposes.

**Treatment** While the treatment of poliomyelitis in the acute stage is still chiefly symptomatic, there are certain important guiding principles which may be helpful. When the disease is suspected, bedrest during the entire febrile phase and for at least several days thereafter is of great importance in the attempt to prevent or diminish the paralytic consequences of the infection. This also applies to patients with the aseptic meningitis syndrome who require no other care beyond the relief of pain when it is present. In paralytic patients who have an involvement of the spinal cord which may lead to paralysis of the muscles of respiration, the availability of proper respirator care may prove to be lifesaving. In patients with manifestations which make it difficult to keep the airway patent, performance of a tracheotomy may be indicated.

**Prophylaxis** Prevention of infection with poliomyelitis virus by attempts to interrupt the chain of transmission is difficult to achieve because of the many ways in which the infectious agent in human stools may be contracted by human beings. When it becomes necessary to protect individuals passing through, or temporarily residing in, areas of poor sanitation and hygiene the same precautions which are observed in guarding against other infectious agents transmitted by human feces may also be employed with reference to poliomyelitis. Recent experiments suggest that human gamma globulin containing a high concentration of antibodies for the different types of poliomyelitis virus may prove to be useful in providing temporary protection against the paralytic infection. While the dosage that might prove to be effective obviously depends on the concentration of antibody in the preparation used, the dosage employed in the one field trial which yielded suggestively positive results was 0.28 ml. per kilogram of body weight.

### Mumps

This virus should be suspected as a cause of the aseptic meningitis syndrome in individuals with or without evidence of involvement of the salivary glands when they give a history of recent exposure to a case of mumps or during a period when mumps is epidemic in the community.

*Diagnosis*   The diagnosis can best be established by complement-fixation or hemagglutination inhibition tests on serum specimens obtained during the acute phase of the illness and early during convalescence. Although the virus can be recovered from the cerebrospinal fluid in mumps meningitis, it is not recommended as a diagnostic procedure for routine purposes.

### Herpes Simplex

There are no specific clues for suspecting this virus as a cause of either the aseptic meningitis syndrome or severe encephalitis, because patients with these diseases have exhibited neither the skin nor mucous membrane manifestations of infection by herpes simplex virus. It should be kept in mind, however, as a possible cause of severe and often fatal meningo-encephalitis, not only in children but also in adults.

*Diagnosis*   In surviving patients the diagnosis can be established by serologic procedures and in fatal cases by the demonstration of acidophilic intranuclear inclusions in various types of cells in the nervous system and by isolation of the virus in mice or eggs.

# 4   Diseases Caused by Coxsackie Viruses

*Definition*   The name Coxsackie was originally applied to viruses which were highly pathogenic for newborn mice and hamsters after inoculation by peripheral routes and nonpathogenic for older animals of the same species. The characteristic lesion in the newborn animals is extensive necrosis of the muscles which produces paralysis of the extremities.

*Distribution*   The Coxsackie viruses are as common as or more common than the viruses of influenza and poliomyelitis. They are found throughout the world.

*Etiology*   These viruses are among the smallest known. They are highly resistant to treatment with ether, various antibiotics and a variety of other chemical agents. There are now at least fifteen immunologically distinct Coxsackie viruses (Fig. 12). They do not exhibit identical properties nor do all of them produce extensive destruction of muscle and the characteristic paralysis of the extremities. These fifteen serologically distinct strains are further classified into groups A and B, principally on the basis of the clinical and pathologic manifestations of infection in mice. The group A and group B viruses likewise are associated with different clinical manifestations in man.

There is no evidence of etiologic relationship between these viruses and such diseases as poliomyelitis, the aseptic meningitis syndrome or certain other ill defined syndromes in human beings.

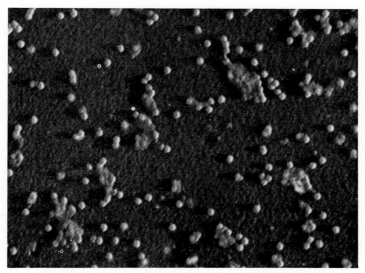

Fig. 12. Electron photomicrograph of Coxsackie virus, Dalldorf type 2. Prepared from amniotic fluid. (Magnification 48,000 ×.) (Briefs, Breese, Warren and Huebner. J. Bact., *64*(2):242, 1952.)

The group A viruses produce extensive paralysis and necrosis of skeletal muscle and almost no other significant pathologic change in sucking mice and hamsters. Mice and hamsters which are older than two to three weeks can no longer be infected by group A viruses. The group B viruses, on the other hand, not only produce slight or moderate focal lesions in the muscles, but also cause characteristic lesions in the brain, subcutaneous fat, pancreas and occasionally in the liver and heart muscle. Most of the group B viruses can be propagated in adult mice and large doses can produce fatal infections, with pancreatitis as a striking manifestation.

**Epidemiology**   Man is the only known reservoir. These viruses have been found among human beings in almost every part of the world where search has been made. They are present in greatest concentration in the stools and a simple rectal swab may provide sufficient material for isolation of the virus. Although they have also been recovered from material obtained from the posterior pharyngeal wall, there is at present no certainty that these viruses occur in man elsewhere than in the alimentary tract. They have been demonstrated with great ease in filth, in flies and in sewage.

There is good evidence that two clinically distinct diseases of man are caused by infection by the Coxsackie viruses. The clinical syndrome, herpangina, has been proved to be etiologically associated with several immunologic types of the group A viruses. There is equally good evidence that epidemic pleurodynia is associated with several immunologic types of the group B viruses.

However, studies of family and neighborhood contacts and of members of the general population have shown that many, if not most, of the individuals infected with these viruses do not suffer clinical disease.

### Herpangina

**Definition**   Herpangina is a self-limited, febrile illness of several days' duration associated with vesicular or ulcerative lesions in the posterior region of the mouth and in the throat.

**Clinical Characteristics**   The disease occurs predominantly among children, generally during the summer and early autumn months in the temperate zone. The characteristic lesions appear as minute vesicles or small punched-out ulcers surrounded by red areolas. From two to twenty may be present on the anterior pillars of the fauces, the pharynx and the palate. Dysphagia may be marked. Systemic manifestations may include anorexia, vomiting and occasionally prostration. The prognosis is good and no fatalities have been reported.

**Diagnosis**   The clinical manifestations are so pathognomonic that presumptive diagnosis may be made immediately. Laboratory confirmation of infection by the Coxsackie viruses is still a problem for research laboratories because of the large number of immunologic types.

**Treatment**   Treatment is symptomatic and should include proper oral hygiene.

### Epidemic Pleurodynia

This is a self-limited, acute febrile illness characterized by severe pain in the chest or abdomen, or both, and associated respiratory distress. The disease has a sudden onset, and other systemic manifestations may include headache and anorexia. Fatalities are unknown. A sporadic case may be difficult to diagnose, but the diagnosis is not difficult during epidemics.

# 5   Introduction

## Description of Rickettsiae

The pathogenic rickettsiae are minute, pleomorphic, mostly obligate intracellular parasites living and multiplying in arthropod tissues. Their characteristics as a group place them between bacteria and viruses. They resemble viruses particularly in their requirement of living host cells for growth, and resemble bacteria by virtue of their morphology and microscopic visibility. They occur as minute coccoid or rod-shaped organisms, frequently occurring in pairs, and sometimes in filamentous forms. The electron microscope has shown what appears to be a limiting membrane surrounding a protoplasmic substance containing one or more dense granules.

Rickettsiae stain poorly with the ordinary aniline dyes but well by Giemsa's method and most of them especially well with the Macchiavello stain. The organism of scrub typhus does not take the Macchiavello stain but stains best by the Giemsa technique. When stained by Giemsa's method rickettsiae appear reddish purple, while with the Macchiavello technique they stain red and the cell which contains them stains blue (Figs. 13, 14, 15).

The pathogenic rickettsiae have been cultivated only in the pres-

**51**

ence of living tissue cells. The yolk sac of developing chick embryos has proved the most successful medium. Agar tissue cultures have provided rich growths of the rickettsiae of the spotted fever group. Such cultures are convenient for the study of intranuclear parasitism, so characteristic of this group of organisms. Certain experi-

Fig. 13.

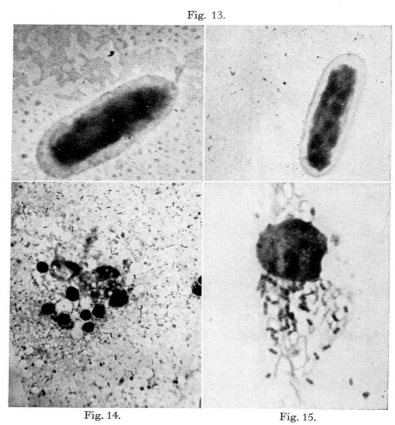

Fig. 14.                                        Fig. 15.

Fig. 13. *Rickettsia prowazekii*, electronic photomicrographs. (Courtesy U.S.A. Typhus Commission.)

Fig. 14. *R. prowazekii*, yolk sac culture. (Courtesy U.S.A. Typhus Commission.)

Fig. 15. *R. tsutsugamushi*, agar tissue culture. (Courtesy U.S.A. Typhus Commission.)

mental evidence suggests that in tissue cultures, the growth of rickettsiae is best when tissue metabolism is at a low level, while growth of most viruses is best in actively growing cells.

The known common reservoir hosts include ticks, mites, small domestic and wild rodents, other small mammals, and some of the larger domestic mammals, *viz.*, cattle, sheep, goats, and dogs. Man is almost certainly a reservoir of *Rickettsia prowazekii* as indicated by the recent all but conclusive evidence that Brill's disease is a recrudescence of epidemic typhus fever (Table 1).

While the rickettsiae of epidemic typhus prove fatal to their arthropod vector, the louse, those of murine typhus are not harmful to the flea which maintains the infection throughout its lifetime. The rickettsiae of the spotted fever group may live for years in the tissues

### Table 1  Rickettsial Diseases of Man

| DISEASE | ETIOLOGIC AGENT | USUAL VECTOR TO MAN | RESERVOIR |
|---|---|---|---|
| *Typhus group:* | | | |
| A. Epidemic (Brill's disease) | *Rickettsia prowazekii* | *Pediculus humanus* | Man |
| B. Murine | *R. typhi* | *Xenopsylla cheopis* | Rat |
| *Spotted fever group:* | | | |
| A. American spotted fevers (including spotted fevers of U.S.A., Canada, Mexico, Panama, Colombia and Brazil) | *R. rickettsii* | *Dermacentor andersoni, D. variabilis* and *Amblyomma americanum* (U.S.A.). *Rhipicephalus sanguineus* (Mexico). *A. cajennense* (South America and ? Mexico) | Ticks, rodents (?), rabbits(?) |
| B. Fièvre boutonneuse (including Kenya typhus, South African tick-bite fever, and Indian tick typhus) | *R. conorii* | *Rhipicephalus sanguineus* in Mediterranean Basin, Kenya and possibly India. *R. evertsi, A. hebraeum, Haemaphysallis leachi* in South Africa | Ticks, dogs(?), rodents(?) |
| C. North Queensland tick typhus | *R. australis* | *Ixodes holocyclus*(?) | Unknown (complement fixation antibodies in rats, bandicoots, and other small mammals |
| D. Rickettsialpox | *R. akari* | Mites: *Allodermanyssus sanguineus* | House mice (*Mus musculus*) |
| *Scrub typhus* (*Tsutsugamushi disease*) | *R. tsutsugamushi* | Trombiculid mites: *Trombicula akamushi, T. deliensis* | Mites, field rats and mice, and small mammals |
| *Q fever* | *Coxiella burnetii* | Infection of man probably by inhalation of contaminated air-borne droplets or dust | Ticks, cattle, sheep, goats, and certain wild animals |
| *Trench fever* | *R. quintana* | *P. humanus* | Man |
| *Unclassified:* | | | |
| Siberian tick typhus | *R. sp.* | *D. silvarum, D. nuttalli, H. concinna* | Ticks, rodents(?) |

of their tick vectors and are passed through the eggs from generation to generation.

In susceptible experimental animals the rickettsiae accumulate in cells of mesothelial origin, especially the lining cells of serous cavities and those of the intima and media of blood vessels. The organisms of epidemic, murine and scrub typhus and of Q fever are intracytoplasmic in position, while those of the spotted fever group may appear both in the cytoplasm and in the nucleus.

## Diagnostic Features of the Rickettsial Diseases

The rickettsial diseases of man have been separated into five distinct groups by virtue of their epidemiologic and immunologic characteristics.

The definitive diagnosis of the rickettsial diseases is made by laboratory procedures: (1) the serologic reaction of the patient's blood (Table 2) and (2) the isolation of the specific agent in experimental animals (see Table 3).

The Weil-Felix reaction is based upon the production by certain of the pathogenic rickettsiae of nonspecific agglutinins against the "O" nonmotile variant of certain strains of *Proteus X*. The three type strains in general use for this test are the OX19, OX2 and OXK. Living or phenol-, Formalin- or alcohol-killed cultures may be used. Twenty-four hour culture suspensions of these organisms, adjusted to a density of a MacFarland nephelometer reading No. 3, are used for the usual macroscopic agglutination test with serial dilutions of the patient's serum. The tubes are incubated at 37.5° C. for two hours, are held in the ice box overnight and then read (pp. 840–842).

With the exception of Q fever, rickettsialpox, and trench fever, a rise in Weil-Felix titer is characteristic of the rickettsial infections. It is important that this rise in antibody titer be demonstrated, and no single titer should be regarded as significant, since Weil-Felix titers may sometimes be encountered in sera from persons with illnesses unrelated to the rickettsial diseases. Louse-borne relapsing fever produces relatively high titers to the OXK strain of *Proteus* organisms in a large proportion of cases. It is impossible to differentiate epidemic typhus, murine typhus and Rocky Mountain spotted fever by means of the Weil-Felix reaction since high OX19 titers may occur in all these diseases. When a high OX2 agglutination is obtained it is suggestive of an infection with a member of the spotted fever group but an absolute diagnosis cannot be made. The Weil-Felix reaction usually shows a rise in titer in the late febrile period and in early convalescence but decreases in titer in late convalescence. Sera from guinea pigs that have been infected with these diseases do not give a Weil-Felix reaction but complement fixation and agglutination are obtained with rickettsial suspensions.

OXK is the only strain that is agglutinated in scrub typhus, and a rising titer for this strain is considered as diagnostic, provided an infection with louse-borne relapsing fever is ruled out.

The complement fixation test provides a means for specific diagnosis of epidemic typhus, murine typhus, Rocky Mountain spotted

*Table 2   Rickettsial Diseases—Diagnostic Features in Man*

| DISEASE | WEIL-FELIX | SPECIFIC COMPLEMENT FIXATION* | EARLY DISTRIBUTION RASH | PRIMARY ULCER— LOCAL ADENOPATHY |
|---|---|---|---|---|
| *Typhus group:* | | | | |
| A. Epidemic (Brill's disease) | OX19 | *Rickettsia prowazekii* | Trunk | 0 |
| B. Murine | OX19 | *R. typhi* | Trunk | 0 |
| *Spotted fever group:* | | | | |
| A. American spotted fevers (including spotted fevers of U.S.A., Canada, Mexico, Panama, Colombia and Brazil) | OX19 OX2 | *R. rickettsii* | Extremities | 0 |
| B. Fièvre boutonneuse (including Kenya typhus, South African tick-bite fever and Indian tick typhus) | OX19 | *R. conorii* | Extremities | + |
| C. North Queensland tick typhus | OX19 OX2 | *R. australis* | General | + |
| D. Rickettsialpox | Occas. OX19 | *R. akari* | Trunk, varicelliform rash | + |
| *Scrub typhus* (*Tsutsugamushi disease*) | OXK | *R. tsutsugamushi* | Trunk | + |
| *Q fever* | None | *C. burnetii* | No rash | 0 |
| *Trench fever* | None | ? | Trunk | 0 |
| *Unclassified:* Siberian tick typhus | OX19 | ? | Extremities | + |

* It is only by the use of washed rickettsial suspensions and by comparison of serum titers that specific complement fixation may be observed in the typhus group and in the spotted fever group.

fever, and Q fever. For within-group differentiation (*e.g.*, epidemic and murine typhus) it is necessary to use type specific antigens prepared by removing soluble antigens from the rickettsial organisms by repeated washing. With the rickettsial suspensions, differences between epidemic and murine typhus are often greater in rickettsial agglutination than by complement fixation. The soluble antigens are

*Table 3  Rickettsial Diseases—Usual Reaction in Laboratory Animals*

| DISEASE | GUINEA PIG | | | | |
| --- | --- | --- | --- | --- | --- |
| | INCU-BA-TION | FEVER | SCROTAL SWELLING | Mooser CELLS | INTRA-NUCLEAR RICKETTSIAE |
| *Typhus group:* | (days) | (days) | | | |
| A. Epidemic (Brill's disease) | 5–8 | 6 | Rare | None | None |
| B. Murine | 3–5 | 5 | Swelling | Usual | None |
| *Spotted fever group:* A. American spotted fever including spotted fe-vers of U.S.A., [virulent strain] | 3–4 | 5–9 | Scrotal necrosis | Endothelial cells with few rickett-siae | Present |
| Canada, Mexico, Panama, Colombia, and Brazil) [mild strain] | 4–6 | 4–5 | Rare | | Present |
| B. Fièvre boutonneuse (including Kenya ty-phus, South African tick-bite fever, and In-dian tick typhus) | 3–6 | 2–4 | Swelling | Endothelial cells with few rickett-siae | Present |
| C. North Queensland tick typhus | 4 | 2–4 | Swelling | Endothelial cells with few rickett-siae | Present in tissue culture |
| D. Rickettsialpox | 4–6 | 3–5 | Swelling and redness | Endothelial cells with few rickett-siae | Present in tissue culture |
| *Scrub typhus* (*Tsutsugamushi disease*) | 6–12 | 5–7 | None | None. Peri-toneal exu-date with rickettsiae | None |
| *Q fever* | 5–7 | 5–12 | None | None | None |
| *Trench fever* Usual laboratory animals not susceptible | | | | | |

S.E. = slightly enlarged   V.L. = very large   E. = enlarged

It should be pointed out that this chart represents *usual* reactions with *adapted* strains following *intraperitoneal* inoculation in laboratory animals. The period of in-cubation in original isolations is always longer than is recorded here for adapted

| GUINEA PIG | | | | WHITE RAT | WHITE MOUSE |
|---|---|---|---|---|---|
| SPLEEN | OUTCOME | IMMUNITY | ORGAN USED FOR PASSAGE | | |
| S.E. | Survives | To each other in this group, but not to members of other groups | Brain | In apparent infection, cannot be maintained in rats | Same as rat |
| S.E. | Survives | | Tunica exudate | Fever, scrotal swelling; Mooser cells; persists in brain | Infection; usually survives |
| E | 50–80% mortality | That of A and B of this group is complete to each other, incomplete or questionable to other members of this group, and negative to members of other groups | Blood | No disease | No disease |
| E | Survives | | Blood | | |
| S.E. | Survives | | Tunica exudate | No disease | Inapparent infection |
| S.E. | Survives | ? | Tunica exudate | ? | Inapparent infection |
| S.E. | Survives | ? | Tunica exudate | ? | Infection; usually survives |
| S.E. | 10–20% mortality | To scrub typhus but not to members of other groups | Brain, spleen, peritoneal exudate | Same type reaction as guinea pigs; persists in brain | 85% mortality in 7–21 days, peritoneal exudate with rickettsiae |
| V.L. | 10–20% mortality | To Q fever but not to members of the other groups | Blood or spleen | Mild reaction | Infected; usually survives. Very large spleen with rickettsiae |

strains. Likewise the period of incubation as well as the febrile reaction with adapted strains will vary with the amount of infectious material used for inoculation. There is a great variation in strain virulence with different strains and the reactions they induce in the experimental animal will vary.

group specific and have been demonstrated for the agents of epidemic and murine typhus, scrub typhus, and several of the spotted fever group. A soluble antigen has recently been demonstrated for the agent of Q fever, but is not of diagnostic significance.

The rickettsial agglutination test likewise has diagnostic value but for the present large amounts of pure suspension are difficult to obtain.

Strains of most of these organisms can be maintained in large male guinea pigs. The rickettsiae of scrub typhus are more easily isolated and maintained in mice. Certain host reactions in the infected male guinea pig, after intraperitoneal inoculation, may be useful in differentiating rickettsial diseases. These reactions are not in-

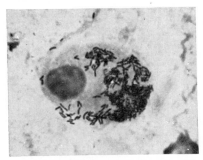

Fig. 16. Murine typhus, Mooser cell. Intracytoplasmic rickettsiae in large serosal cell of tunica vaginalis. (Courtesy U.S.A. Typhus Commission.)

variably obtained and the virulence of the strain for the guinea pig does not necessarily parallel that for man.

Characteristically the reactions described in Table 3 may be observed after inoculation with strains virulent for guinea pigs:

1. In Rocky Mountain spotted fever and most other strains of American spotted fever a scrotal swelling and skin necrosis are produced in animals that survive for a sufficient time. Later sloughing of the scrotum and necrosis of the skin of the feet and ears may occur. The primary pathologic lesion is an endothelial proliferation followed by thrombosis and necrosis. In smears of the tunica vaginalis rickettsiae may be seen in both the cytoplasm and the nucleus of large mononuclear cells.

2. Murine typhus characteristically produces a nonreducible scrotal swelling with erythema of the scrotum appearing on the first or second day of fever—the Neill-Mooser reaction. This is essentially an inflammatory reaction of the tunica vaginalis. The inflammatory exudate consists of large mononuclear (serosal) cells filled with rickettsiae which are intracytoplasmic in position. These heavily infected cells are referred to as "Mooser cells" (Fig. 16). In contrast to the characteristic findings in American spotted fever infections, rickettsiae are not found within the nucleus.

3. Epidemic typhus and Q fever usually produce no scrotal reaction.

Certain clinical features of the rickettsial diseases have diagnostic value. In scrub typhus, fièvre boutonneuse, North Queensland tick typhus, and rickettsialpox, there is a characteristic local reaction at the site of inoculation, an ulcer often covered by a black adherent crust (eschar, tâche noir). This is followed by local or regional lymphadenitis.

The characteristic initial distribution of the rash is likewise helpful in differential diagnosis. In epidemic typhus, murine typhus, scrub typhus and trench fever the rash appears first on the trunk and later spreads to the extremities. In diseases of the spotted fever group the rash appears first on the extremities, ankles and wrists, and may then spread to the entire body. The rash in rickettsialpox is characteristic, and resembles that seen in chickenpox. The individual lesions of this rash begin as small erythematous papules which, as they increase in size, acquire a centrally located vesicle.

# 6 Epidemic Typhus

**Synonyms**   Jail fever, ship fever, typhus exanthematicus, louse typhus. Fleckfieber (German); typhus exanthematique (French); tabardillo (Spanish).

**Definition**   An acute infectious disease caused by *Rickettsia prowazekii* transmitted by the human louse, *Pediculus humanus*. It is characterized by fairly abrupt onset, continuous fever of about two weeks' duration accompanied by severe headache and marked prostration, a characteristic rash appearing about the fifth day, first in the axillae, on the loins, abdomen and back which frequently becomes petechial, and terminating by crisis or rapid lysis. In epidemic outbreaks the mortality has reached 70 per cent.

**Distribution**   Typhus fever, in the epidemic form, has appeared in all continents with the exception of Australia. It is prevalent chiefly in cooler areas including the higher altitudes of the tropic zone, especially where heavier clothing is worn and change of clothing is infrequent. It was a disease of ancient times, when it was frequently confounded with typhoid and plague. The great epidemic center has been Europe. During and following World War I extensive epidemics appeared in Poland, Russia, Serbia and Rumania. In parts of Europe, especially in Poland and Rumania, and during the Italian campaign in Abyssinia, typhus was accompanied by relapsing fever. Recent epidemics have occurred in Morocco, Algiers, Tunis, Italy and Egypt. It has also been prevalent at times in several areas in southern Africa. (Fig. 17.)

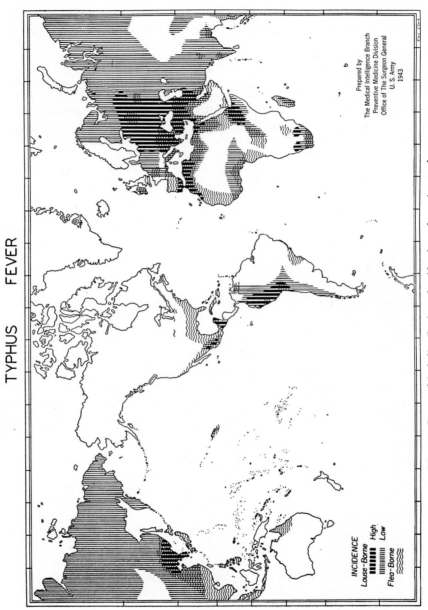

Fig. 17. Geographical distribution of epidemic and murine typhus.

In Asia the northern part of the continent and the mountainous area toward the south are chiefly affected. In Latin America the disease prevails in parts of Mexico, Central America and in the western countries of South America. No epidemic has occurred in Canada or the United States in recent years.

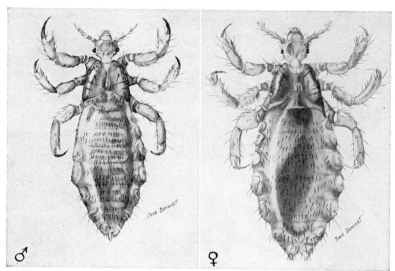

Fig. 18. *Pediculus humanus* var. *corporis:* male and female. (Courtesy National Institute of Health, U.S. Public Health Service.)

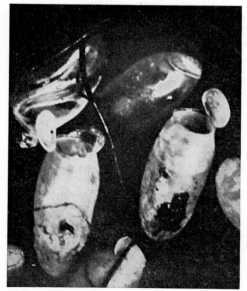

Fig. 19. Nits of *Pediculus humanus* var. *corporis*.

**Etiology**  *Rickettsia prowazekii* invades the cytoplasm of cells. It does not invade the cell nucleus.

**Epidemiology**  Epidemic typhus is a disease of louse-infested populations under conditions of famine, crowding, and generally un-

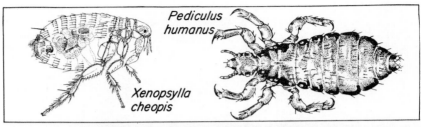

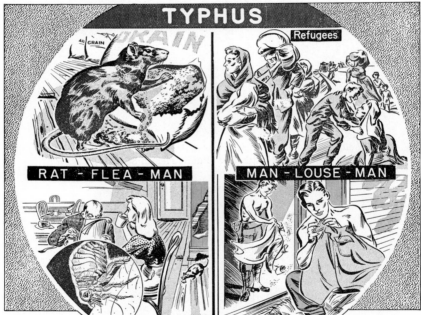

|  MURINE | EPIDEMIOLOGY | EPIDEMIC |
|---|---|---|
| 1. Reservoirs: Rats, mice | | 1. Reservoir: Man |
| 2. Vectors: Fleas, rat louse, rat mite | | 2. Vector: *Pediculus humanus* |
| Rat to rat — *Nosopsylla, Xenopsylla, Polyplax, Liponyssus* | | 3. Louse-infested population |
| | | 4. Famine |
| Rat to man — *Xenopsylla* | | 5. Crushed lice — abraded skin |
| 3. Rat transportation, migration | | 6. Louse feces — abraded skin; mucous membranes |
| 4. Infected rat urine, feces, in food, drink | | 7. Dust from infested clothing, bedding |
| 5. Flea feces — abraded skin, inhalation | | |

Fig. 20. Epidemiology of epidemic and murine typhus.

hygienic surroundings. The body louse, *P. humanus* var. *corporis* (Figs. 18, 19), is the common vector; man is the probable reservoir. The saliva, urine and feces of the patient are not infectious. It is now known that transmission is not effected by the bite of the louse but rather by contamination of the abraded skin with the body fluid of the crushed louse or by louse feces through the abraded skin, or through mucous membranes. Dried louse feces from clothing or bedding may be a source of infection by inhalation or by contamination of the conjunctivae. It has been reported that the rickettsiae retain their virulence in dried louse feces for many months (Fig. 20).

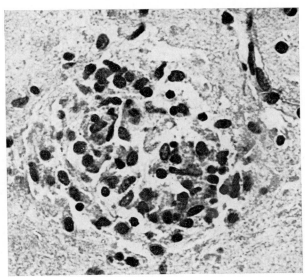

Fig. 21. Typhus nodule in brain showing necrosis and accumulation of mononuclear phagocytes. (Courtesy of U.S.A. Typhus Commission.)

Epidemic typhus appears most frequently during the winter and spring months, since the heavier clothing worn during these seasons and infrequent bathing afford opportunity for the rapid multiplication of lice.

**Pathology** The specific pathologic lesions of typhus consist of proliferation of the endothelium of arterioles and capillaries, leading to thrombosis, hemorrhagic manifestations, secondary necrosis and gangrene. There is an accompanying perivascular round-cell infiltration. These changes are found particularly affecting the vessels of the skin, the central nervous system, and the myocardium. In some areas they resemble early miliary tubercles, the Fraenkel typhus nodules of the skin, while in the brain the perivascular cell accumulations are suggestive of the pathology of encephalitis. Thrombosis of larger blood vessels is rare. (Fig. 21).

Cloudy swelling of the myocardium is frequently observed. The spleen may be slightly enlarged, is often extremely friable, and commonly shows diminution of lymphoid elements. The liver and kidneys likewise show cloudy swelling. Numerous miliary lesions are frequently observed in the basal ganglia, the medulla and the cerebral cortex. These present varying stages of the basic pathology consisting of proliferation of vascular endothelium, thrombosis, perivascular infiltration, necrosis, and neurogliar proliferation.

Bronchitis, bronchopneumonia and nephritis are frequent and often fatal complications. Secondary parotitis is common, especially in the absence of proper care of the mouth.

The rash is often evident after death and hemorrhagic areas in the skin and subcutaneous tissues are common, especially in areas which have been subjected to pressure and trauma. Areas of skin necrosis or gangrene are frequently present.

**Clinical Characteristics**    After an incubation period averaging five to fifteen days the disease sets in abruptly, or more commonly with a prodromal period of one to two days in which headache, vertigo, backache, anorexia and general malaise are prominent. Usually the temperature rises rapidly by the end of the second day, reaching 103° to 104° F. by the third or fourth day, then remaining continuously elevated. With the rise of fever the face becomes flushed, the conjunctivae injected, the expression apathetic, and the headache usually severe. Conjunctivitis is frequent in the early stages. Consciousness is commonly dulled and prostration is marked. Early and persistent circulatory weakness is usual.

The characteristic eruption appears on the third to the seventh day, first in the axilla and on the flanks, then extending to the abdomen, chest and back, and later to the extremities. It is most marked on the back. The palms and soles are rarely affected and the face remains clear. Initially it consists of slightly raised rose spots which blanch on pressure, but these soon become permanent and later purpuric. During convalescence the rash fades to a brownish pigmentation which gradually disappears (Fig. 22).

With the appearance of the rash, prostration and cardiac depression become more evident. Headache is severe and the patient becomes stuporous, sometimes as markedly so as in plague. The mouth is foul and cough frequently develops. Constipation is usual. The temperature remains elevated except for slight morning remissions. The pulse is weak and irregular and the blood pressure is low. The white blood count is not characteristic, rarely exceeding 12,000 with a differential count of about 80 to 85 per cent polymorphonuclear cells.

In nonfatal cases about the end of the second week a critical change occurs in the apparently grave condition of the patient. The temperature falls accompanied by marked diaphoresis, stupor disappears, consciousness clears and the urinary output improves. Circulatory weakness may continue, however, for sometime during convalescence. In other instances following the fall in temperature severe and increasing signs of involvement of the central nervous system continue, progressing to death.

Bronchitis, bronchopneumonia and nephritis are common complications, and parotitis and otitis media are not infrequent. Gangrene of the toes, less often of the fingers, and of the skin over the sacrum is not uncommon.

In uncomplicated cases convalescence is usually rapid and complete. Recovery is followed by longstanding immunity.

Previous immunization with an effective vaccine may greatly modify the clinical picture of classic typhus fever. The rash may be

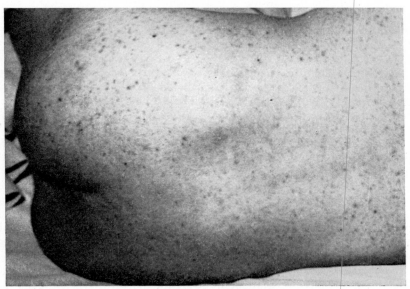

Fig. 22. Erythematous and petechial rash, epidemic typhus. (Courtesy of U.S.A. Typhus Commission.)

absent or of very short duration, the symptoms are less severe and fever may be present no more than three to five days.

**Diagnosis** The clinical diagnosis of typhus is often difficult in children and in the early stages of an epidemic. During the prodromal period as well as in the pre-eruptive days following the onset a variety of acute infectious diseases may be considered; among these are typhoid fever, relapsing fever, malaria, influenza and, in appropriate regions, Rocky Mountain spotted fever or scrub typhus. The exanthem and subsequent course, however, make clinical differentiation from nonrickettsial diseases possible. Murine typhus, although generally a milder disease, can be ruled out definitely only by isolation and identification of the rickettsiae or by the complement fixation test. Lice, if detected on the patient or in his clothes, should cause early suspicion of relapsing fever or epidemic typhus.

In all isolated cases, or in the absence of a recognized epidemic, the clinical diagnosis should be confirmed by serologic tests (see Table 2, p. 55). The Weil-Felix reaction becomes positive in 50 per cent of cases by the eighth day of the disease and by the thirteenth day it is positive in all instances. This test provides the earliest presumptive evidence although it does not exclude murine typhus or Rocky Mountain spotted fever. To have diagnostic significance it is necessary to demonstrate a rise in the antibody titer of the patient's serum. A single positive test is only suggestive. The reaction becomes negative in late convalescence and, therefore, cannot be used to determine past infection.

The complement fixation test is highly specific. It becomes positive about the end of the first week and the highest titer is reached during the first two or three weeks of convalescence. It remains positive indefinitely and, therefore, may be used to identify past infection.

Rickettsial agglutination is likewise a specific diagnostic procedure. Agglutinins appear in the patient's blood about the end of the first week or early in the second week. They disappear in late convalescence after the Weil-Felix reaction has become negative. A suspension of killed rickettsiae is used as antigen for the test.

Blood specimens for serologic tests, especially the Weil-Felix reaction, should be obtained as early as possible after the onset and at intervals during the course of the disease and into convalescence.

The rickettsiae may be isolated from the patient's blood during the acute stage of typhus fever by intraperitoneal inoculation of guinea pigs with ground-up clot. In contrast with murine typhus, epidemic typhus typically produces no tunica reaction in these animals, or, if a mild swelling occurs in the first passage, there are no tunica reactions in passages from the first guinea pig to subsequent animals.

**Treatment**    In no other disease is good nursing care more important. Symptomatic management should be directed primarily to the control of toxemia by ample fluid administration, the maintenance of bowel function by enemata, strict oral hygiene, great care to protect the skin against bed sores, and protection of the circulatory system.

Delirium may be controlled by sponge baths and the application of ice bags to the head, although severe cases may require hyoscine with or without morphine. Lumbar drainage may be useful in some instances.

The circulatory system must be watched carefully and cardiac stimulants are often indicated.

Preliminary experience indicates that certain of the antibiotics may prove to be valuable specific therapeutic agents. They are rickettsiostatic and not rickettsiocidal. Chloramphenicol (Chloromycetin) is the preparation of choice although both aureomycin and oxytetracycline (Terramycin) appear to be of some value. The recommended dosage of chloramphenicol is an initial dose of 2 to 4 gm. and thereafter 3 gm. daily in divided doses at intervals of four hours.

Treatment should be continued until the patient has been afebrile for at least forty-eight hours.

In the majority of cases antibiotic therapy is associated with cessation of fever within three to five days and marked reduction in the incidence of complications.

**Prophylaxis** All persons entering a typhus area should be immunized with an effective vaccine made from killed *R. prowazekii*. The Cox type yolk sac vaccine was extensively used during World War II. Although it did not completely eliminate infection among exposed personnel, the course of the disease among vaccinated individuals was much shorter and milder, the incidence of serious complications greatly reduced, and the mortality practically nil. It is recommended that two doses each of 1 ml. be given subcutaneously at intervals of ten to fourteen days. Thereafter a booster dose of 1 ml. should be given at the beginning and in the middle of the typhus season.

Since this vaccine contains egg, protein sensitivity must be watched for and the vaccine must be administered with caution to egg-sensitive individuals.

It must be remembered that whereas a clinical attack of epidemic typhus confers protection against murine typhus, immunization with the killed rickettsiae of epidemic typhus does not produce such cross immunity.

The mass protection of population groups in the presence of epidemic typhus involves the extensive application of delousing measures with adequate police support to ensure treatment of all members of the community and to prevent ingress of louse-infested individuals into cleaned areas. Immediate delousing of all contacts of acute cases is of the utmost urgency in the control of an epidemic. This in turn entails an effective case finding and reporting mechanism.

Mass disinfestation is easily and rapidly accomplished by the use of louse powders blown into each individual's clothing by hand or power dusters. DDT 10 per cent in an inert base such as talc or pyrophyllite has proved most effective and the lethal effect on lice persists for more than two weeks. When a DDT-resistant strain of lice is encountered, as was the case in Korea, lindane 1 per cent in inert dust should be substituted. Three applications are desirable at seven day intervals, each not to exceed 60 gm. lindane per person (Table 69, p. 749).

Medical and control personnel working in an epidemic area must exercise great care to avoid infection. Lousy clothing should be removed and sterilized and the patient himself should be thoroughly deloused. Attendants should wear clothing impregnated with a lousicide and, in view of the infectiousness of dried louse feces, they should wear protective masks, goggles and gloves while they are in a potentially infected environment.

Important subsidiary measures include improvement of living

conditions, provision of adequate bathing and laundering facilities, and the dispensing of additional supplies of clothing and food.

## Brill's Disease

Brill's disease, formerly considered to be a form of murine typhus, has been shown by serologic studies and by recovery of *R. prowazekii* from patients to be an avirulent form of epidemic typhus fever. It is clinically milder than epidemic typhus and is attended by no mortality.

Cases are invariably single, sporadic, not associated with louse infestation, not related to outbreaks of murine typhus, and occur in individuals, principally of Russian birth, many of whom have had epidemic typhus fever prior to emigrating from Europe.

# 7 Murine Typhus

**Synonyms** Endemic typhus, flea typhus, Brill's disease (incorrect usage, Southern U. S. A.).

**Definition** A mild febrile disease of about fourteen days' duration, caused by *Rickettsia typhi* and transmitted by flea bites, by contact with flea feces, or by the ingestion of food contaminated by rat urine.

**Distribution** Murine typhus is world-wide in distribution.

**Etiology** The morphology and staining reactions of *R. typhi* are similar to other species of the genus. These rickettsiae are found in large numbers in the cytoplasm of the serosal cells of the tunica vaginalis of the infected male guinea pig (Neill-Mooser reaction).

**Epidemiology** Murine typhus is associated with the brown rat, *Rattus norvegicus*, and possibly other small rodents which act as reservoirs. Rat fleas, lice and mites transmit it from rat to rat. (Fig. 20.) The tropical rat flea, *Xenopsylla cheopis*, and other species of the genus are considered the most important vectors. The temperate zone rat flea, *Nosopsyllus fasciatus*, the rat louse, *Polyplax spinulosus*, and the tropical rat mite, *Liponyssus bacoti*, play similar roles. Infection in man probably takes place chiefly by rubbing flea feces into the skin while scratching. The inhalation of dry flea feces or ingestion of food contaminated by rat urine may also result in infection. *Nosopsyllus fasciatus* seldom, if ever, feeds on man. Murine typhus is not fatal to the rat, and consequently, the rapid transfer of fleas from the dead rat host to man, as in plague, does not occur. Although the rat louse does not bite man, the rat mite attacks man readily and may be considered a potential vector.

Transmission of murine typhus from man to man by the body louse, *P. humanus* var. *corporis*, has been demonstrated.

The majority of cases occur in the summer and fall; epidemic typhus, however, appears chiefly in the winter and spring months.

In the southern United States the incidence of murine typhus is twice as high in males as in females.

**Pathology**  The pathology of murine typhus in general is similar to that of epidemic typhus. However, it is not known in detail since fatalities are uncommon (less than 5 per cent in the U. S. A.). It is probable that histopathologic changes in the small vessels, similar to the alterations seen in epidemic typhus, occur. Cutaneous petechiae are infrequent and large areas of skin necrosis have not been reported.

**Clinical Characteristics**  Except in persons over fifty, murine typhus is in general a milder disease than the epidemic variety. The onset follows an incubation period of six to fourteen days and may be either abrupt or gradual. In the latter case the temperature rises to 102° to 105° F. during the first week and remains elevated until about two weeks after onset. The rash, usually limited to the chest, abdomen and inner surfaces of the arms, resembles that of epidemic typhus with the exception that petechiae are rare. The macules, appearing about the fifth day, at first fade on pressure but soon lose this character. After two to ten days they disappear. The temperature usually falls by rapid lysis, recovery being complete, although convalescence may be delayed. Mental symptoms are not marked and complications are rare.

**Diagnosis**  The diagnosis and differential diagnosis of murine typhus present problems similar to those of epidemic typhus. Serologic reactions and animal inoculation must be depended upon to distinguish this disease from other rickettsial infections.

The Weil-Felix test does not differentiate murine typhus from epidemic typhus or from Rocky Mountain spotted fever. Complement fixation, however, is highly specific for each of the three diseases.

The reaction of inoculated male guinea pigs, when typical, is of value in the diagnosis. The scrotal swelling without necrosis and with numerous rickettsiae in the serosal cells of the tunica vaginalis —the Neill-Mooser reaction—is characteristic.

**Treatment and Prophylaxis**  The treatment of murine typhus is the same as that for epidemic typhus.

Since rats constitute the primary reservoir in nature, rat control through poisoning, trapping, and rat-proofing are logical procedures for control. Rat-proofing is the only measure of permanent value. Particular attention should be paid to granaries and storehouses, thereby depriving rats of their major food supply.

# 8 American Spotted Fevers

**Synonyms**   Rocky Mountain spotted fever, exanthematic typhus of São Paulo, Tobia fever, Choix fever, pinta fever.

**Definition**   An acute febrile disease caused by *Rickettsia rickettsii* and transmitted by the bite of certain ticks. It is characterized by a rash first appearing on the wrists and ankles and later, in some cases, over the entire body including the face, the palms of the hands and soles of the feet.

**Distribution**   Formerly thought to be restricted to certain areas of the Rocky Mountain states, it has since been reported from British Columbia, Alberta, and Saskatchewan (Canada), from forty-four states (U. S. A.), and from Brazil, Colombia, Mexico, and Panama. In Brazil the disease was originally reported as exanthematic typhus of São Paulo and in Colombia as Tobia fever. Choix fever or pinta fever in northern Mexico has recently been identified with spotted fever.

**Etiology**   *Ricksettia (Dermacentroxenus) rickettsii* has the general characteristics of the subgenus and is capable of invading the cell nucleus.

The spotted fever diseases of the United States, Canada, and the various Latin American countries represent a single disease entity as indicated by specific serologic tests or other laboratory studies.

**Epidemiology**   Spotted fever is essentially a rural disease occurring in areas where ticks and their rodent hosts are prevalent. However, in the eastern United States the tick vector is frequently brought into yards by dogs and foci of infection have thus been established in some suburban areas. Since the tick is not an habitual parasite of man the disease does not, as a rule, appear in epidemics; but in some heavily tick-infested areas in Colombia it has reached almost epidemic proportions and in other areas multiple infections in the same family are not as infrequent as they were once thought to be.

The severity of the disease may vary greatly in areas separated by only short distances. The degree of virulence within each of these areas appears to be relatively constant, although unexplained.

*Tick vectors* may be considered in two groups: (1) ticks which feed both on wild rodents and on man, and (2) ticks which serve as vectors among wild rodents but do not feed on man or seldom come in contact with him.

(1) The common vectors of the human disease are: in western Canada and the western United States, the wood tick, *Dermacentor andersoni* Stiles (Fig. 23); in the eastern United States, the dog tick, *D. variabilis* (Say); and in Texas and Oklahoma, the Lone Star tick, *Amblyomma americanum* (Linn). As a rule only the adults of the two species of *Dermacentor* feed on man; nymphs, however, may in rare instances feed on children. On the other hand, larvae, nymphs

and adults of *A. americanum* are reported to use man as a host. In Mexico, *Rhipicephalus sanguineus* (Latr.) is the only proved vector to man, but *A. cajennense* has also been found naturally infected there. In Colombia and Brazil, *A. cajennense* (Fabr.) is the accepted vector.

Several other species of ixodid ticks and at least three species of argasid ticks are efficient *experimental* vectors (see p. 644).

(2) The rabbit tick, *Haemaphysalis leporis-palustris* (Packard), an important vector of *Pasteurella tularensis* among rabbits, is also

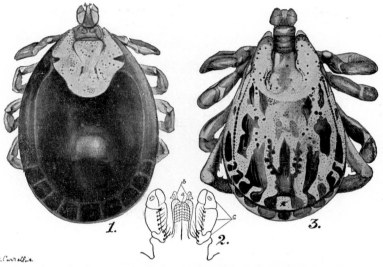

Fig. 23. *1.* Female *Dermacentor andersoni*. *2.* Mouthparts showing (*a*) hypostome, (*b*) chelicerae, (*c*) palps. *3.* Male. (Strong: Stitt's Diagnosis, Prevention and Treatment of Tropical Diseases. The Blakiston Co.)

considered an important vector of spotted fever among these animals. This tick does not feed on man. Rabbits however are hosts also to *D. andersoni*, a common vector to man. The argasid tick, *Ornithodoros parkeri* Cooley, may play an equally important role in nature. This tick has a wide distribution in nine western states, has several hosts in common with *D. andersoni*, and transmission through the egg to the fourth generation with no reduction in the virulence of the rickettsiae over a period of five years has been demonstrated. This tick feeds readily on man but seldom comes in contact with him.

The infection is commonly transmitted to man by the bite of the infected tick. Occasional instances of infection have occurred, however, following contamination of the hands by crushing ticks while removing them from domestic animals.

**Pathology** The pathology of Rocky Mountain spotted fever resembles that of typhus in that the chief lesions are found in small blood vessels. There are distinct differences, however, in the histopathology and in the structures affected. There is greater destruction of the deeper layers of the vessel walls and less perivascular infiltration. The rickettsiae invade both the vascular endothelium and smooth muscle fibers of the vessel wall, causing endothelial proliferation, necrosis of the wall, thrombosis and infarction with hemorrhage into the surrounding tissues. These lesions occur predominantly in the skin and subcutaneous tissues, the voluntary muscles, and the testes, with resulting areas of necrosis. There are no distinctive changes in the viscera; the spleen is commonly much enlarged,

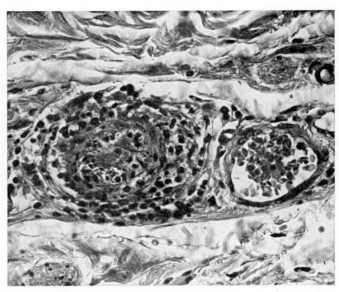

Fig. 24. Rocky Mountain Spotted fever: lesion of skin showing thrombosis, necrosis of vessel wall and perivascular infiltration.

firm and dark red in color. Lesions of the central nervous system are uncommon (Fig. 24).

In fatal cases the rash is hemorrhagic and necrosis of the scrotum or vulva is frequent. There may likewise be necrosis of the prepuce or of the fingers or toes, lobes of the ears, or of the soft palate. Hemorrhages into the muscles and subcutaneous tissues are widespread.

**Clinical Characteristics**   Both mild and virulent strains of Rocky Mountain spotted fever are well known, and contrary to former belief, are both found in all regions where the disease occurs. Depending on the virulence of the strain, the incubation period varies from three to fourteen days. In the severe type the onset is sudden with headache, chills, marked pains in the joints and generalized body pains. The fever rises gradually or fairly rapidly to about 104° F. and remains elevated without morning remissions. On the third or fourth day the rash makes its appearance. At first it closely resembles that of measles, but unlike the latter exanthem, it remains discrete in its subsequent course. The eruption begins as macules on the forearms and ankles, later spreading inward along the extremities to the trunk and forehead (Fig. 25). There is a still later spread to the palms, soles and scalp, when mucous membranes may also be involved. The mature lesions frequently become petechial. There is a moderate leukocytosis and the differential count is not characteristic.

The height of the illness is reached in the second week. At this time the pulse becomes rapid and weak and nervous symptoms, espe-

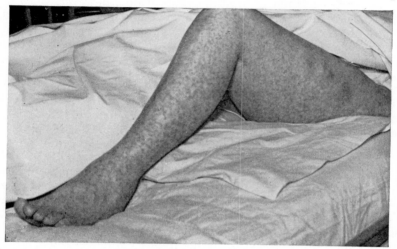

Fig. 25. Generalized rash of Rocky Mountain spotted fever. (Courtesy U.S.P.H.S., Rocky Mountain Laboratory.)

cially delirium, may appear. It is during this period that necroses and deaths occur. If the patient survives the fourteenth day, his chances for recovery are excellent.

The temperature shows a gradual fall during the third week. Areas in which the rash was most petechial often show scaly exfoliation or occasionally cast-like desquamation. There may be residual cicatrices in such areas of the skin. Complications such as deafness and visual disturbances may follow severe attacks but are not permanent. Convalescence is rapid in uncomplicated cases.

The *mortality* depends on the virulence of the rickettsial strain and on the age of the patient. Fatality rates as high as 80 per cent are known for some strains; others do not exceed 5 per cent. Persons over fifty years of age are particularly prone to die of Rocky Mountain spotted fever, while children are but slightly affected as a rule. The over-all case fatality rate from this disease in the United States was previously about 19 per cent, but has recently become practically nil with the introduction of the newer antibiotics into the treatment of the disease.

**Diagnosis**   A history of recent contact with ticks, especially in regions where the prevalence of this disease is recognized, should direct suspicion toward a diagnosis of Rocky Mountain spotted fever. In the absence of such evidence the physician must rely principally upon laboratory tests. The initial distribution of the rash on wrists and ankles is suggestive, but the clinical distinction between Rocky Mountain spotted fever and epidemic or murine typhus is frequently very difficult and often impossible.

The Weil-Felix test usually becomes positive at the end of the second week. It is not of final diagnostic value, however, since it is positive also in epidemic and murine typhus. The fact that Rocky Mountain spotted fever sometimes gives a positive reaction to *Proteus* OX2 is likewise only partially helpful, since some cases of typhus give a similar reaction. Complement fixation becomes positive during the second week. This test is highly specific in differentiating Rocky Mountain spotted fever from both epidemic and murine typhus. In both the above serologic tests, it is the *rise* in titer of the second and subsequent blood samples that is of significance. There is accumulating evidence that specific therapy with antibiotics often inhibits the formation of complement-fixing antibodies while not appreciably affecting the results of the Weil-Felix test (p. 840).

Since the rickettsiae are present in the blood of man throughout the febrile course of the disease, intraperitoneal inoculation of male guinea pigs with ground-up clot of the patient's blood may have diagnostic value. Strains of rickettsiae virulent for guinea pigs typically produce a characteristic scrotal necrosis; mild strains, however, do not. The rickettsiae in cells of the tunica vaginalis exudate are intranuclear as well as intracytoplasmic in position, an important diagnostic point.

The severity of the infection for man bears no relation to the intensity of the reaction in the inoculated guinea pig. A strain of rickettsiae that is virulent for man may be virulent or mild for the laboratory animal, and conversely a strain that produces mild disease in man may be extremely virulent for the guinea pig.

**Treatment**   Aureomycin, oxytetracycline (Terramycin), and chloramphenicol (Chloromycetin) have all proved highly effective in the treatment of Rocky Mountain spotted fever. With each of these drugs clinical manifestations of the illness have been arrested in about two to three days.

Therapeutic regimens are similar for each of the drugs, the general schedule used satisfactorily at present being as follows: An initial dose for adults of about 3 to 4 gm. is given orally, and this is followed by a similar amount daily in divided doses until the temperature returns to normal levels. With aureomycin and Chloromycetin the daily schedules have generally consisted of 0.25 gm.

doses every two or three hours, while with Terramycin 1.0 gm. every eight hours has proved satisfactory.

Sole reliance upon the antibiotic in seriously ill patients late in the course of their disease is inadequate. Treatment utilizing transfusions of saline, glucose, plasma and whole blood is vital for support of the embarrassed circulatory system.

**Prophylaxis**   In areas where Rocky Mountain spotted fever commonly occurs it has been found practicable to immunize large groups of the population by the inoculation of a skilled suspension of the specific rickettsiae. Such vaccination reduces the incidence and also lessens the severity of those attacks which may subsequently occur. The injections should be repeated yearly in those likely to be exposed.

Temporary area control may be secured by applying DDT, 50 per cent wettable powder at 8 pounds per 100 gallons of water, applied at the rate of 4 pounds actual DDT per acre.

Other preventive measures are related to contact with ticks. Tick-infested areas should be avoided if possible; if not, protective clothing should be worn. Careful inspection of the entire body surface should be made every few hours in order to remove such ticks as may have entered the clothing. Infected wood ticks may inoculate the individual within six hours after attachment; hence regular de-ticking is an important measure in avoiding infection.

Clothing treated with a newly developed, all-purpose repellent protects individuals from ticks, chiggers, and fleas (see p. 751). Insecticides such at DDT, chlordane, dieldrin and toxaphene are effective in controlling ticks in localized areas, and on vegetation along roadsides, pathways, and other places where ticks concentrate.

Ticks should be removed from dogs with forceps or a piece of paper rather than by grasping them between the unprotected fingers. The hands should be carefully washed with soap and water after contact with them.

# 9   Related Spotted Fevers

## Boutonneuse Fever

**Synonyms**   Fièvre boutonneuse; fièvre exanthematique de Marseille; escarro-nodulaire (French).

**Definition**   A disease of the spotted fever group caused by *Rickettsia conorii* which is transmitted in the Mediterranean area chiefly by the tick *Rhipicephalus sanguineus* (Latr.). A "tâche noir" is present. The rash appears on the trunk and may subsequently involve the entire body.

**Distribution**    First reported from Tunis in 1910, boutonneuse fever is now known to be endemic in most countries of the Mediterranean Basin and in the Crimea. It is probable that similar infections reported in Kenya, Ethiopia, Belgian Congo, and certain other places in Africa are the same disease. Present evidence from specific serologic and other laboratory investigations suggests that South African tick-bite fever, and a similar rickettsiosis occurring in the Northwestern Frontier Province and Kumaon Hills of India, may be identical with boutonneuse fever.

**Etiology**    *Rickettsia* (*Dermacentroxenus*) *conorii* (Syn. *Dermacentroxenus rickettsia* var. *pijperi*) is the etiologic agent. Intranuclear rickettsiae have been reported but the organisms are much less regularly seen in this position than are the rickettsiae of the American spotted fevers.

**Epidemiology**    The usual host of *R. sanguineus* is the domestic dog, which is probably the chief animal reservoir of the disease. The epidemiology of the disease, especially in areas where this tick species is involved, is therefore comparable to that of spotted fever in the eastern United States, where dogs are prominent hosts of the adult tick vector. In Kenya, *Rhipicephalus simus* Koch and *Haemaphysalis leachi* (Audouin) are also reported as vectors in addition to *R. sanguineus*.

South African tick-bite fever has nearly as varied an epidemiology as American spotted fever. In South Africa infections are contracted more often in the fields or veld than in urban areas. The larvae of *Rhipicephalus evertsi* Neumann and *Amblyomma hebraeum* Koch are the common vectors in certain rural areas, while the dog tick *H. leachi* seems to play an important role in the dissemination of the infection into the suburbs. This latter tick, in which hereditary transmission of the agent has been demonstrated, constitutes a natural reservoir of this rickettsia.

From *R. sanguineus* ticks caught on the premises of a former tick-typhus patient in Kashmir, northern India, a strain of rickettsia has been isolated which appears to be immunologically closely related to, or identical with, the agent of boutonneuse fever.

**Pathology**    The detailed pathology in boutonneuse fever, Kenya typhus, and South African tick-bite fever has not been reported.

Boutonneuse fever, South African tick-bite fever and Kenya typhus differ from the spotted fever of the Americas in the frequent occurrence of a primary lesion (tâche noir) supposedly at the site of the infective bite. This is a granulomatous process which frequently ulcerates and which is accompanied by regional lymphadenitis.

Histologic examination of the maculopapular rash of boutonneuse fever is said to reveal swelling of the vascular endothelium with perivascular infiltration; purpuric lesions show congestion and hemorrhages.

**Clinical Characteristics**    These typhus-like diseases are very much alike from the clinical point of view, although variations in their severity have been noted. After an incubation period of about a week there is usually an abrupt onset with chills and a rapid rise of temperature to about 104° F. At this time the tâche noir is already present. Except for persistent insomnia, headache and muscular pains, the febrile course is accompanied by less extreme symptoms than in the other rickettsial diseases. Prostration and delirium are not marked. The fever usually lasts one to two weeks and the temperature then drops rapidly to normal. The mortality is low.

On the second to fourth day the rash appears on the trunk and extremities. It is macular or maculopapular and may become hemorrhagic but not coalescent. The palms, soles and face are involved later; the abdomen, however, may show few lesions.

**Diagnosis** Clinical diagnosis of these three diseases is simplified by a history of tick bite. The discovery of a tâche noir and its associated regional lymphadenopathy is of great diagnostic significance. The rash and the typhus-like clinical course of the diseases are likewise significant.

The Weil-Felix test usually becomes positive late in the second week. In all three there is agglutination of *Proteus* OX19. A specific complement fixation test for boutonneuse fever has recently been devised.

Guinea pig inoculations result in nonfatal, typhus-like reactions which vary in intensity and regularity according to the particular strain of the rickettsia injected. In this animal, boutonneuse fever can not be distinguished from other spotted fever strains of low virulence, except possibly by cross vaccination or complement fixation tests. It cross immunizes with Rocky Mountain spotted fever strains of both high and low virulence, and with tick bite fever of South Africa. However, Rocky Mountain spotted fever vaccine, which affords complete protection against the homologous disease in guinea pigs, gives no protection against boutonneuse fever.

**Treatment** Treatment with the antibiotics aureomycin, oxytetracycline (Terramycin) or chloramphenicol (Chloromycetin), as described in the chapter on American Spotted Fevers, has yielded favorable results. As in other typhuslike illnesses, good nursing care is important. Palliative measures and sedation are indicated in the more severe cases.

**Prophylaxis** Ticks and tick-infested areas should be avoided when possible. Since dogs are the usual hosts of several of the vector ticks of boutonneuse fever and related diseases, especial care should be exercised in preventing tick infestation of such pets and human habitations. Effective tick repellents and insecticides for such purposes are available (see p. 751). The short-haired type of dog might be considered a more desirable domestic animal in endemic areas. Strays or wild dogs should be exterminated. The preventive measures advocated for Rocky Mountain spotted fever apply also in the prevention of this disease. Immunizing vaccines have been reported only for the American spotted fevers, but vaccines against these rickettsial agents do not confer protection against boutonneuse fever.

## North Queensland Tick Typhus

A mild rickettsial disease has been reported from both northern and southern areas of Queensland, Australia. This disease, designated as North Queensland tick typhus, produces in man a syndrome resembling boutonneuse fever. The etiologic agent is capable of intranuclear growth, a characteristic of the agents of the spotted fever group. Although North Queensland tick typhus is antigenically related to this group, it is differentiated by specific complement fixation. The etiologic agent is *Rickettsia australis* Philip.

Tick transmission of this disease has been assumed on circumstantial evidence. The first described infections occurred in troops undergoing training in restricted, tick-infested areas in North Queensland. A history of tick bite was obtained from a majority of the patients, some of whom developed eschars at the site of tick bite. *Ixodes holocyclus* Neumann is suspected of being the most probable vector of the disease. Specific complement-fixing antibodies have been found in four species of small marsupials (two bandicoots, kangaroo rat and brush-tail opossum), and in one rat, all taken in endemic environs where human cases had been contracted.

The diagnosis of this disease is aided by the presence of an eschar associated with regional lymphadenopathy, rash, and a typhuslike clinical course. The Weil-Felix reaction is positive for *Proteus* OX19 and OX2. The complement fixation test has not been thoroughly studied in human cases of North Queensland tick typhus. However, in the guinea pig the disease can be differentiated from other rickettsial diseases by specific complement fixation.

## Siberian Tick Typhus

A tick-borne rickettsial disease, designated by this name, has been reported from eastern and central Siberia. The illness is mild and characterized by the occurrence of a lesion at the site of the tick bite, regional lymphadenitis, headache and rash. *Dermacentor nuttalli* Olenev, *D. silvarum* Olenev, and *Haemaphysalis concinna* Koch are the reported vectors. Natural infection with the causative rickettsia and its transovarial transmission have been demonstrated in these three tick species. It is important to note that the etiologic relationship of Siberian tick typhus to other rickettsioses has not been established. Newer serologic methods have so far not been applied to agents definitely known to bear an etiologic relation to the disease designated as Siberian tick typhus.

# 10   Scrub Typhus

**Synonyms**   Tsutsugamushi, Japanese river fever, Japanese flood fever, kedani fever, mite typhus, rural typhus, tropical typhus.

**Definition**   An acute, febrile, rickettsial disease transmitted by larval mites (chiggers). The site of infection is usually marked by an eschar.

**Distribution**   Scrub typhus has a wide distribution in eastern and southern Asia and the islands of the southwest Pacific. It extends

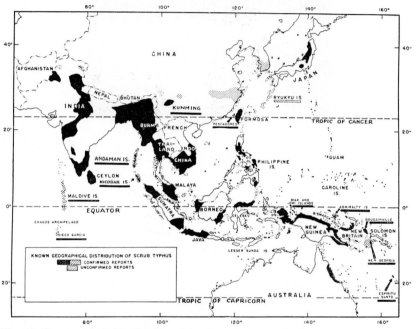

Fig. 26. Geographical distribution of scrub typhus. (Modified from Philip in Pullen's Communicable Diseases, p. 755. Lea and Febiger, 1950.)

from Japan, where a new endemic area was found near Mt. Fuji, south through Formosa, the Philippines, Borneo, Celebes, Indonesia, New Guinea, the northeast coast of Australia and the adjacent island groups as far east as Espiritu Santo. It is likewise endemic in Indo-China, Malaya, Thailand, Burma, India, China, Ceylon, and islands in the Indian Ocean and the Bay of Bengal. Cases have recently been reported from Korea but it is possible that these were ferried from Japan. Unconfirmed cases have been found in the lower Yangtse Valley and the Ryukyus (Fig. 26).

**Etiology**   *Rickettsia tsutsugamushi* (= *R. orientalis*) (Fig. 27).

**Epidemiology**   Although the disease is most prevalent in midsum-

**79**

mer in Japan, there is no seasonal prevalence in the subtropics and tropics. Scrub typhus is a "place" disease, its local distribution depending upon the distribution of the vector mites, and infected areas are frequently extraordinarily discrete and circumscribed. Commonly these are grassy or covered with scrub underbrush often associated with flooded river banks, although infected mites have been collected in primary jungle.

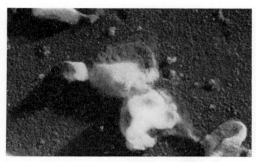

Fig. 27. Electron photomicrograph of *Rickettsia tsutsugamushi* prepared from yolk sac suspension. 23,000 ×. (Courtesy Department of Virus and Rickettsial diseases, Army Medical Service Graduate School.)

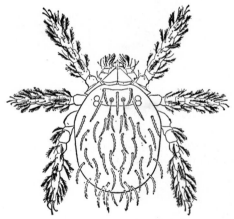

Fig. 28. *Trombicula akamushi* larva (greatly enlarged). (Nagayo et al.: Am. J. Hyg.)

Only two species of mites belonging to the subfamily TROM-BICULINAE have been incriminated as vectors, *Trombicula akamushi* (= *T. fletcheri*) and *Trombicula deliensis* (= *T. walchi*) (Fig. 28).

The infecting agent is acquired and transmitted by the mite in only the larval stage. The rickettsiae then survive in the mite through its nonparasitic nymphal and adult stages and are passed through the eggs to the next generation of larvae, which are infective and transmit the organisms to new hosts.

Field mice, rats, voles, shrews and other small animals which are hosts to the larval mite may act as reservoirs of the disease.

**Pathology** The most characteristic feature of the pathology of scrub typhus is the primary ulcer or eschar resulting from the attachment of the infecting mite. The regional lymph nodes are markedly enlarged, some of them at times showing central necrosis, and generalized lymphadenopathy is common. The body cavities contain moderate amounts of serofibrinous fluid. The lungs usually show hemorrhagic pneumonia with secondary lobular pneumonia.

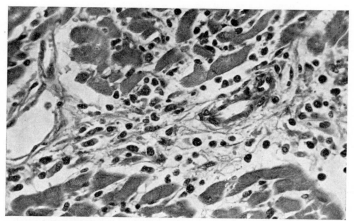
Fig. 29. Scrub typhus, monocytic infiltration of heart muscle.

The liver and spleen are enlarged and there is congestion of the parenchymatous organs.

Histologic examination reveals that the vascular system is primarily affected as in other rickettsial diseases. There is widespread focal vasculitis and perivasculitis with accumulations of monocytes, plasma cells and lymphocytes. The most striking damage is found in the heart, lung, brain and kidney (Figs. 29, 30). Focal and diffuse myocarditis is characteristic; interstitial and lobular pneumonia is usual in fatal cases. Meningitis and encephalitis may occur with degeneration, and there may be monocytic infiltration and nodule formation in the brain. The kidneys show congestion and focal interstitial lesions.

**Clinical Characteristics** The primary lesion or eschar may be found in over 60 per cent of cases. It may be located on any part of the body, particularly on the clothed surfaces, but careful and complete examination of all skin areas may be necessary to find it. It begins as a painless papule which slowly enlarges. On the moist surfaces of the body such as the axilla, scrotum and perineum it develops into a punched-out shallow ulcer with flat, greyish yellow base surrounded by an elevated pink areola. On the drier areas of the skin the ulcer is covered with an adherent blackish scab. Occasionally there may be more than one eschar. They range in size from 0.3 to 2.0 cm. in diameter (Fig. 31).

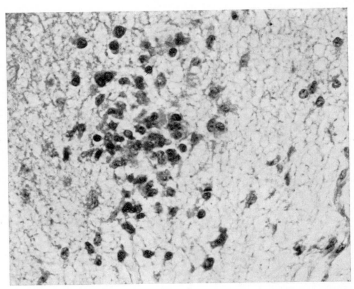

Fig. 30. Scrub typhus, nodule in brain showing edema, degeneration and monocytic infiltration.

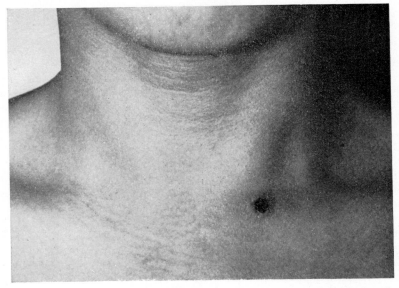

Fig. 31. Eschar or primary lesion of scrub typhus. (Courtesy U.S.A. Typhus Commission)

Since attachment of the larval mite does not produce irritation or itching and since no local symptoms accompany the developing primary lesion, the individual frequently is unaware both of exposure to infection and of the existence of the eschar.

After an incubation period of from seven to eighteen days, the disease begins acutely with severe headache, fever, chilliness and malaise. During the first week the fever rises progressively, reaching 104° to 105° F. while the pulse remains relatively slow, seldom exceeding 100. The regional lymph nodes draining the area of the pri-

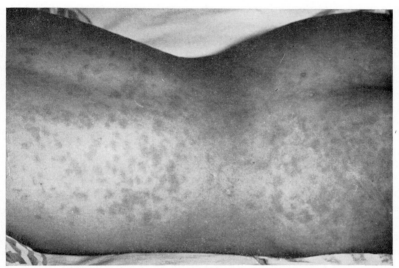

Fig. 32. Rash of scrub typhus. (Courtesy U.S.A. Typhus Commission.)

mary lesion are enlarged and tender, there is frequently less marked generalized lymphadenopathy and the spleen may be palpable. Between the fifth and the tenth day the characteristic red macular rash appears on the trunk and may extend to the arms and legs. It usually persists for several days (Fig. 32).

Signs of respiratory involvement appear early with cough, and in more than half the cases accompanied by physical signs indicative of pneumonitis.

During the second week the temperature remains elevated, the pulse rate ranges at a higher level, and headache, apathy, conjunctival congestion and varying degrees of deafness are common. In severe cases there may be evidence of involvement of the central nervous system with the development of delirium, stupor and muscle twitching. The systolic blood pressure is commonly below 100 mm. Hg.

In nonfatal cases the temperature falls by lysis at the end of the second or the beginning of the third week. The pulse and blood pressure return to normal and the abnormal physical findings disappear. Convalescence is generally prolonged. Sequelae in the form of psychiatric difficulties or persisting deafness are not unusual.

The mortality has ranged as high as 60 per cent in certain outbreaks. However, among United States forces during World War II it varied from 0 to 25 per cent.

Experimental infections in human volunteers indicate that recovery is followed by lasting immunity against a homologous strain of *R. tsutsugamushi* but that there is little or no immunity to heterologous strains after one or two years.

**Diagnosis** Differential diagnosis may be difficult in some of the regions where scrub typhus is endemic. The clinical picture may suggest other rickettsial infections, dengue, infectious hepatitis, typhoid and malaria; often malaria is a concomitant infection, or a latent malaria may be activated during the acute clinical phase of scrub typhus. However, the association of a primary lesion or eschar with regional lymphadenitis, headache, prostration, disproportionately low pulse rate, fever and leukopenia is highly suggestive. Definitive diagnosis must be based on laboratory tests.

Until recently the Weil-Felix reaction has been considered specific, giving a positive reaction to *Proteus* OXK but negative ones to OX19 and OX2. However, the reaction may be negative in well established cases, or, on the other hand, relapsing fever may evoke a false positive reaction. Nevertheless the Weil-Felix reaction is of great value in the diagnosis of scrub typhus. OXK agglutinins are generally present in the patient's serum by the end of the second week but none develop against the OX19 strain. Maximum titer is reached by the end of the third week, after which they decline rapidly, often disappearing by the fifth or the sixth week. To have diagnostic significance, the Weil-Felix reaction must show a rising titer in serially taken serum specimens.

Satisfactory antigen for complement fixation is not generally available. Unequivocal diagnosis of scrub typhus, therefore, is based upon recovery of the rickettsiae from the patient's blood or tissues or from laboratory animals (see Table 3, pp. 56, 57).

Many strains of scrub typhus rickettsiae will not survive in guinea pigs, but it appears that all are pathogenic for laboratory mice. The tsutsugamushi strain after several passages kills about 85 per cent of white mice within fourteen days. The peritoneal exudate in these animals contains *R. tsutsugamushi*.

**Treatment** Chloramphenicol (Chloromycetin), aureomycin and oxytetracycline (Terramycin) are rapidly acting and highly effective therapeutic agents. The average time interval between initiation of therapy and completion of defervescence is respectively thirty-one, twenty-five and thirty-seven hours. However, rickettsemia is demonstrable for thirty to forty-eight hours after the start of treatment. Furthermore, when treatment of infected human volunteers is initiated within the first three days of the disease, relapses or recrudescences occur in about 50 per cent. These respond promptly to further treatment and they may be prevented by a supplementary dose given on the eighth or ninth day after onset. The rickettsiostatic effect of the antibiotics apparently persists for a week after the last dose.

Administration of Chloromycetin is not associated with toxic or disagreeable side effects and is the drug of choice. Both aureomycin and Terramycin may cause gastric irritation, nausea and vomiting.

DOSAGE, CHLOROMYCETIN AND AUREOMYCIN. An initial dose of 3.0 gm. should be given by mouth followed by an additional 3.0 gm. in divided doses during the subsequent twelve to twenty-four hours.

DOSAGE, TERRAMYCIN. 1.5 gm. by mouth every six hours until a total of 6.0 gm. has been given.

During World War II para-aminobenzoic acid (PABA) proved of value, and it should be used in the event that the antibiotics are not available. However its effect upon the fever is much slower. It must be used with caution because of toxic hematologic and renal reactions, and administration must be prolonged.

DOSAGE, PABA. After an initial oral loading dose of 4.0 to 8.0 gm., 2.0 gm. should be given every two hours day and night until the blood level reaches 20 to 40 mg. per 100 ml. Thereafter from 1.0 to 3.0 gm. must be given every two hours to maintain the blood level until at least the fourteenth day.

The drug is rapidly excreted, consequently repeated blood level determinations are necessary. These should invariably be performed immediately prior to the time an additional dose is due.

The general treatment of scrub typhus is directed to maintenance of fluid balance and protection of the myocardium.

**Prophylaxis** No effective vaccine is available. However, when it is necessary for an individual to enter mite-infested areas in a region where scrub typhus is endemic, a high degree of protection may be obtained by rigorous application of three procedures. Camp sites should be burned, the surface vegetation removed by bulldozer or the area sprayed with dilutions of lindane or dieldrin emulsions. All clothing should be impregnated with a 5 per cent dimethyl phthallate emulsion, which gives excellent protection against the larval mites until the clothes are washed, or with the new U. S. Army preparation, M-1960 (see Table 69, p. 751). Exposed skin areas should be treated every two to three hours with an insect repellent such as dimethyl phthallate, dibutyl phthallate, M-2020 or M-2043 (see Table 69, p. 751).

Although effective chemoprophylaxis has been obtained using Chloromycetin in doses of 3.0 to 4.0 gm. every four to seven days and continued over a period of four to six weeks after the last potential exposure, it is not free from risk and should be used with caution if at all. Such long-continued administration may contribute to severe secondary infection by monilia and to the development of serious blood dyscrasia, particularly agranulocytosis.

# 11 Q Fever

**Synonyms**  Nine-mile fever (United States), Balkan grippe (Greece).

**Definition**  An acute febrile illness caused by *Coxiella burnetii*. Rickettsemia occurs during the febrile phase and interstitial pneumonitis usually develops. There is no rash, and the Weil-Felix reaction is negative.

**Distribution**  Practically world wide—Australia, North America to Panama, central and western Europe, Africa, and southern Asia.

**Etiology**  *Coxiella burnetii* (= *R. burnetii*, *R. diaporica*) possesses the general characteristics of the rickettsiae as regards association with arthropods, cultural characteristics, morphology and staining reactions, but possesses some distinguishing features. This agent passes Berkefeld N filters or collodion membranes with an average pore diameter of 400 millimicrons, is more resistant to certain physical and chemical agents, persists for months to years in tick feces, has distinct immunologic properties, and does not produce agglutinins for *Proteus X* strains. Such characteristics of the etiologic agent together with the lack of the usual typhuslike rash and Weil-Felix serology, plus failure of arthropods to play an important role in human infection, have resulted in the differentiation of *C. burnetii* on a generic level. Various strains of *C. burnetii* have exhibited only minor differences. The agent does not invade the nuclei of host cells.

**Epidemiology**  There is considerable evidence indicating that Q fever in man is a respiratory disease caused by the inhalation of dust particles contaminated with material from infected animals. The great majority of cases have occurred among persons exposed to domestic livestock, cattle, sheep, or goats, or their products; *e.g.*, slaughterhouse employees, dairy workers, and those living in the neighborhood of dairies or in households using raw milk. Except for a few reported instances, secondary infections have not occurred from contact with patients ill with Q fever under conditions where other sources of infection could be ruled out.

*Coxiella burnetii* has been isolated repeatedly from raw milk of infected dairy cows, sheep and goats, and, on autopsy, from the mammary gland and adjacent lymph nodes of dairy cows. Infected cows may shed the organisms in the milk for long periods of time. Placental membranes from some infected, parturient cows and sheep have been demonstrated to be highly infectious. The agent has also been isolated from air samples from areas occupied by infected cattle or sheep.

Ticks are the only known arthropod host of *C. burnetii*, and natural infection with this agent has been found in at least seventeen species from various parts of the world. However, arthropods apparently are of little, if any, importance in direct transmission of the disease to man, nor do they appear necessary for maintenance of the disease in domestic animals.

**Pathology**    Histopathologic reports are available on three of the nine fatal cases of Q fever which have been recorded in the literature. In these former cases, a state of red and grey consolidation was noted in the lung. The exudate of the consolidated areas was predominantly of the mononuclear cell type, most of the cells being swollen and degenerate macrophages in which coccoid or bacillary forms of *C. burnetii* may be demonstrated. These organisms may be either intra- or extracellular. The rickettsiae have also been found in macrophages of the spleen and testes, in neuroglial cells in the brain, and in kidney cells.

**Clinical Characteristics**    Following an incubation period which varies from twelve to thirty days, with an average of about eighteen days, Q fever presents a fairly consistent syndrome characterized by acute onset with fever, headache, weakness, malaise, chilly sensations, sweats, and considerable variation in severity and duration. The acute stage lasts from a few days to several weeks. A pneumonitis is revealed in the majority of cases examined by x-ray, and is attended by mild cough, scanty expectoration, chest pain and minimal physical findings. Complications and sequelae are occasionally reported, and mortality is less than one per cent. With few exceptions, patients do not develop a cutaneous rash.

Roentgenographic findings resemble those seen in cases of primary atypical pneumonia. They are first revealed on the third or fourth day, and usually persist beyond termination of the febrile period. Evidence of pulmonary involvement may occur with mild or inapparent illnesses.

**Diagnosis**    The diagnosis of Q fever can be established with certainty only by demonstrating a substantial rise in titer in the specific complement fixation or rickettsial agglutination tests, or by recovery of the agent from the patient. The cold hemagglutinin and other agglutination tests, including the Weil-Felix reaction, are negative.

With suitable antigens, significant complement fixation titers usually appear during the second week of the illness, and may persist for several years. About 90 per cent of patients develop specific agglutinins by the end of the fourth week. Strains of *C. burnetii* vary in their sensitivity as antigens in the complement fixation and agglutination tests, and only those of high sensitivity produce satisfactory antigens. Some strains appear to maintain a low degree of such sensitivity even after adaptation to egg culture. On the other hand, other strains of this agent become sensitive antigens upon adaptation to chick embryos, which in some cases require several passages beyond those in which large numbers of organisms are first visible in stained smears of infected yolk sac tissue.

Isolation of the agent by inoculation of guinea pigs or mice with blood of the patient is usually successful. Guinea pigs respond with high fever and splenomegaly, and rickettsiae may be found in the spleen and in the inflammatory exudate covering this organ. Identification of Q fever in this animal is made by serologic tests, or by immunity tests with a known strain of *C. burnetii*. A characteristic, nonfluctuant, indurated skin lesion in which rickettsiae can be demonstrated develops in subcutaneously inoculated animals.

**Treatment**    Aureomycin, oxytetracycline (Terramycin), and chloramphenicol (Chloromycetin) have been reported to be of value in treatment of Q fever. Aureomycin is not invariably effective.

Treatment of a few cases of Q fever with Terramycin has been reported. The drug was administered orally. Good results were obtained when treatment consisted of an initial dose of 3 gm., which was followed twenty-four hours later by a daily dose of 1.5 gm. given in divided doses every six hours for three days. In such cases clinical response with relief of symptoms began after twenty-four hours and was complete in forty-eight to seventy-two hours. The average febrile period after Terramycin was given was two days, while the average length of fever before treatment was three days. Favorable results have also been reported in some cases in which treatment was begun as late as the seventh day after onset of the acute illness.

**Prophylaxis**    Wholly effective means for control of endemic Q fever are not at hand. Efforts for their development must be directed against the major animal sources of human infection, *i.e.*, dairy cows, sheep, and goats, but such efforts must await additional information on the modes of transmission of infection and the effect of vaccination in these animals. Vaccination of special personnel intensely exposed to infection (*e.g.*, laboratory personnel), is of proved protective value and is recommended. Milk should be pasteurized. Careful sterilization of the sputum and excreta of patients is desirable. Possible infection from domestic animal pelts which may contain infective tick feces should be considered, and mechanical transportation of infective material by flies has been demonstrated in the laboratory.

# 12    Trench Fever

**Synonyms**    Wolhynia fever, Meuse fever, quintan or five-day fever.

**Definition**    Trench fever is a specific relapsing, infectious disease transmitted from man to man by the body louse, *Pediculus humanus*, and caused probably by *Rickettsia quintana*. Blood and urine of convalescents are infectious over a long period.

**Distribution**    The disease occurred in epidemic form in many parts of Europe and in Mesopotamia and Egypt during World War I, and in troops on the German-Russian frontier in World War II.

**Etiology**   *Rickettsia quintana* (= *R. pediculi, R. weiglii, R. wolhynica*) is probably the causative agent, as suggested from evidence obtained by infection of human volunteers and transmission by clean laboratory-bred lice. However, inability to grow this agent in laboratory animals or in tissue culture has caused some persons to consider the evidence for the rickettsial etiology of trench fever as incomplete.

*Rickettsia quintana* grows extracellularly in the lumen of the gut of lice fed on a patient, or injected intrarectally with the patient's blood. The agent is nonpathogenic for the louse, which, once infected, remains so for life, but does not pass the agent transovarially. *Rickettsia quintana* is fairly resistant to the usual environmental factors and louse feces may remain infectious for several weeks, or longer.

**Epidemiology**   Epidemics of trench fever have occurred in troops during World Wars I and II, and in laboratory personnel on whom lice were being fed in the process of making typhus vaccine by the Weigl method. No other outbreaks among the civilian population have been described, although recent work indicates that endemic foci of this disease exist in certain regions such as Volhynia, the Ukraine, and Bessarabia.

Transmission of trench fever from man to man takes place through the agency of the infected body louse, either through its bite alone, or by contamination of the abraded skin with the infective louse feces. Man is probably the reservoir of this disease, since *R. quintana* may be recovered from the blood of convalescents for long periods, although the length of such periods varies considerably. Although in nearly all convalescents the organism is present in the blood during the illness and for a few weeks afterwards, its subsequent presence in this tissue may be transitory, or may last for several months or even years, or may be periodic in which case the agent appears for a few weeks at a time at various intervals one or more times a year. *Rickettsia quintana* has been demonstrated in the blood of otherwise normal convalescents one, three, four, five, and even eight years after cessation of acute symptoms. It also appears that this rickettsia may remain latent in some convalescents for long periods during which the agent cannot be recovered from the blood. Latent infections, manifested by either frank illness or merely an active blood carrier state, have been reported to occur following some unrelated stimuli such as other infections, or injections of typhus or anti-typhoid vaccines.

**Pathology**   Biopsy of the exanthematic lesion of trench fever reveals a perivascular infiltration, principally of lymphocytes, but the vascular intima is normal and there is no thrombotic process. The causative organism apparently does not invade cells, having been demonstrated only in the circulating blood.

There are no autopsy reports on trench fever.

**Clinical Characteristics**   The symptomatology of trench fever is extremely variable, making a clinical diagnosis of many cases difficult or impossible. Headache, malaise and body pains may appear as prodromes toward the close of the ten- to thirty-day incubation period. The actual onset is nevertheless sudden. Headache, vertigo, pain in the back and legs, especially in the shins, postorbital pain on movement of the eyes, often nystagmus on lateral gaze, and injection of the eyes accompany a rapid rise of temperature to 103° or 104° F. The primary fever continues for several days to a week, less often for several weeks. The leukocyte count is variable, some cases presenting a leukocytosis; in others the count is normal or a leukopenia may be present. Albuminuria is usual and polyuria common.

The initial febrile episode is followed in about 50 per cent of cases by a regularly or irregularly relapsing type of fever curve. Three to five such relapses are usual although as many as seven may occur.

A distinctive rash is a quite constant feature of the disease but is irregular in the time of its appearance. It is usually associated with an acute febrile phase, however, manifesting itself early in the initial attack or in a relapse. The rash consists of small erythematous macules—occasionally papules—that blanch on pressure. They are relatively few in number and often disappear within twenty-four hours. Their distribution is characteristic, including particularly the chest, back and abdomen.

*Convalescence* is frequently prolonged and complicated by a variety of symptoms among which those of functional derangements of the circulatory system and neurasthenia are the most common. The mortality is negligible.

*Immunity* appears to be variable in duration, but its actual development is a controversial question, in view of the relapsing character of the disease, the periodic nature of the blood carrier state in some individuals, and the evidence for the existence of latent infections with *R. quintana.*

**Diagnosis**   The differential diagnosis of trench fever may include influenza, dengue, the dengue-like fevers, malaria and brucellosis. Laboratory tests present the best diagnostic aid and consist of isolation of the agent in lice, and of specific serologic tests.

Isolation of *R. quintana* from the patient in clean, laboratory-bred lice has provided the most practical means of diagnosis. This may be accomplished either by feeding the lice on the patient, or by injecting lice with the patient's blood intrarectally according to Weigl's method. Within four to twelve days after the blood meal, or two to four days after injection, organisms appear in the louse excreta. Histologic examination of the intestinal lining of the louse is necessary to ascertain that the organisms develop extracellularly. Repeated feedings are usually required to infect more than a small percentage of lice. Demonstration of *R. quintana* in the blood of a suspected patient does not always constitute a definite diagnosis of trench fever, since this organism is known to persist for long periods in the blood of convalescents. A negative history of past illness with this disease or of residence in louse-infested environment where people are lousy aids in the diagnosis.

Complement fixation and agglutination employing washed suspensions of *R. quintana* prepared from dried infected louse excreta are of reported value as specific diagnostic aids. The Weil-Felix reaction is negative.

Attempts to isolate the agent in the usual laboratory animals, or to cultivate it in fertile hen's eggs, have so far been unsuccessful.

**Prophylaxis** The prophylaxis of trench fever depends upon effective measures for louse control. The infectious agent is present in the patient's urine during the acute stages of the disease; suitable precautions in the disposal of excreta must therefore be emphasized. The agent also may persist in the blood for almost a year; individuals recovered from this disease should consequently not be used as blood donors.

# 13 Rickettsialpox

**Synonym** Kew Gardens spotted fever.

**Definition** Rickettsialpox is a relatively mild to moderately severe, nonfatal, typhuslike disease accompanied by a varicelliform rash, lymphadenopathy and leukopenia. It is preceded by an initial lesion or eschar at the portal of entry at the site of attachment of a mite.

**Distribution** Proved cases have been restricted to certain urban communities on the North Atlantic seaboard of the United States. Under the name "rickettsiose vesiculeuse" the disease has been reported, but not confirmed, in French Equatorial Africa.

**Etiology** The intracytoplasmic agent *Rickettsia* (*Dermacentroxenus*) *akari* is capable of invading the nucleus of infected host cells (Fig. 33). Cross reactions in the complement fixation tests indicate a relationship to the spotted fever group of tick-borne rickettsiae.

In addition to man, wild and laboratory mice, guinea pigs, and chick embryos, but not monkeys, have been shown to be susceptible.

**Epidemiology** Proved cases have been resident in house-mouse–infested dwellings in urban areas, including modern apartment developments. In some instances outbreaks have approached epidemic proportions.

The natural vector is a widespread, though not common, mite parasite of mice, *Allodermanyssus sanguineus* (Fig. 34). However, the more ubiquitous tropical rat mite, *Liponyssus bacoti*, can transmit the disease experimentally. Natural infection has been demonstrated in mice and in *A. sanguineus*.

Patients are not aware of attachment by the rapidly feeding mites and are probably attacked while asleep. Prevalence of the disease according to age, sex and occupation is proportionate to these char-

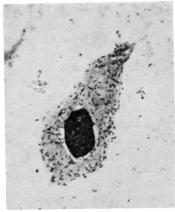

Fig. 33. *Rickettsia akari*, the agent of rickettsialpox, in a cell from the peritoneum of an infected white mouse. (Courtesy Rocky Mountain Laboratory, photo by N. J. Kramis.)

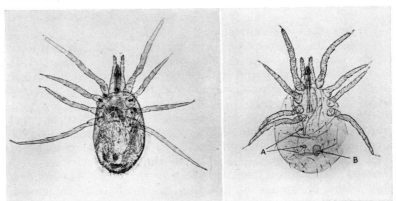

Fig. 34. Photomicrographs of *Allodermanyssus sanguineus*, the mite vector of rickettsialpox; adult ♀ (left, 108 ×), and nymph (150 ×, with 2 dorsal shields (*A*) and anal plate (*B*), retouched for emphasis). (Courtesy Rocky Mountain Laboratory, photo by N. J. Kramis.)

acteristics in the residents of the endemic loci. Ages of patients have ranged from less than one year to over fifty years.

**Pathology**   Reports of the human pathology are confined to biopsy studies of the histopathology of primary and secondary cutaneous lesions. During the fastigium of the disease the initial lesion at the site of attachment of the infected mite consists of a shallow ulcer approximately 0.5 cm. to 1.5 cm. in diameter. It is covered with a brown to black crust and is surrounded by an erythematous area about 2.5 cm. in diameter. The lesion may occur on any part of the body.

**Clinical Characteristics** The incubation period has not been accurately determined. The initial lesion appears as a round firm papule. Five to ten days later the clinical syndrome appears suddenly. It is characterized by fever, chills, sweating, headache, backache and lassitude. Typically, these symptoms persist for a week or ten days. Regional or generalized lymphadenopathy and a maculopapular and papulovesicular rash, usually appearing early in the course of the disease but occasionally not until the fifth or sixth day, are nearly constant features. The cutaneous lesions may be scanty or profuse. They never become confluent. They do not involve the plantar surfaces of the feet nor the palmar surfaces of the hands, and seldom the mucous membranes. Temperatures are especially elevated in the afternoons and frequently fluctuate between 98° and 104° F. in the course of a day. Photophobia is not infrequent.

The symptoms subside by lysis, generally from one to two weeks after onset. Convalescence may be protracted in severe cases. It is possible that a lasting immunity is produced, since no second attacks have been reported, and recovered laboratory animals resist attempted re-infection.

**Diagnosis** The clinical syndrome accompanied by eschar, rash and lymphadenopathy, together with residence under potentially endemic conditions, should direct attention to this disease. Up to the present time the geographic distribution eliminates the clinically similar fièvre boutonneuse and scrub typhus. The constant occurrence of the primary lesion, a vesicular rash, and vector considerations will aid in differentiation from the other rickettsioses. The rash of chicken-pox is more superficial and the vesicles are thin and easily broken. The lesions of smallpox, though initially quite similar to those of rickettsialpox in their deeper, firmer character, have a different maturation, usually becoming pustular with eventual scar formation.

Leukopenia is the only significant blood change.

Recovery of the infectious agent by inoculation of blood from the patient into white mice is desirable for conclusive laboratory diagnosis of sporadic cases. A specific antigen prepared from yolk sacs of infected chicken eggs fixes complement in higher dilutions of convalescent serum than in sera from the related spotted fever group, although some cross reaction occurs. There is no cross fixation with the other typhuslike diseases. A rising complement fixation titer against the spotted fever group of antigens will differentiate rickettsialpox from other conditions with which it might be confused. Increased *Proteus* OX19 agglutinins have seldom been observed.

**Treatment**    Oxytetracycline (Terramycin), aureomycin, and chloramphenicol (Chloromycetin) are reported to have beneficial effects against *R. akari* in experimental infections. Preliminary observations have shown that as little as 2.5 gm. of Terramycin, administered early in the disease with an initial dose of 0.5 gm. and 0.25 gm. thereafter every six hours, induce defervescence in about twenty-four hours without relapse.

**Prophylaxis**    Prevention of infection is dependent upon elimination of mice from residential buildings.

# 14  The Relapsing Fevers

**Synonyms**  Tifo recurrente, fiebre recurrente, febris recurrens, fièvre recurrente, rückfall fieber, rückfall typhus, garapata disease, kimputu, spirillum fever, famine fever, tick fever.

**Definition**  The relapsing fevers are acute infectious diseases characterized by alternating febrile and afebrile periods, caused by spirochetes transmitted through the agency of the louse, *Pediculus humanus* var. *corporis* and by ticks of the genus *Ornithodoros*.

**Distribution**  Louse-borne relapsing fever has been reported from all continents. It has disappeared from the United States but frequently occurs in parts of South America, Europe, Africa and Asia. Isolated cases in Cuba, Brazil and Australia occurring in recently arrived immigrants are said to be louse-borne.

The tick-borne relapsing fevers are widely distributed throughout the Eastern and Western Hemispheres. In the *Americas* endemic centers are known in southern British Columbia, Canada; in thirteen of the western states of the U. S. A.; in Aguascalientes in the plateau regions of Mexico; in Guatemala and Panama in Central America; and in South America chiefly in Colombia, Ecuador and Venezuela. An endemic focus has also been reported from northern Argentina (Fig. 35).

**95**

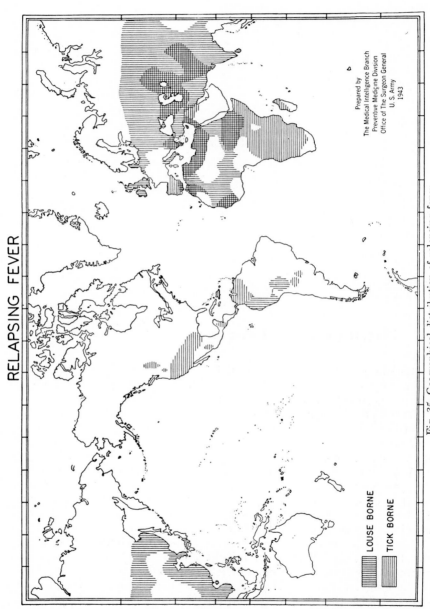

Fig. 35. Geographical distribution of relapsing fever.

In *Africa*, with the exception of the Sahara and the rain forest belt, the tick-borne disease is present from the Mediterranean to Cape Colony and from the Atlantic Ocean to the Red Sea.

In *Europe* it is reported from Spain, Portugal and the Caucasus. In Asia it occurs in Cyprus, Israel, Syria, Iraq, Iran, in the southern U.S.S.R. as far east as the western border of China, in Afghanistan, and in Kashmir and Jammu, India.

**Etiology** Relapsing fever spirochetes are loosely wound, flexible coils with tapering ends. The number of turns in the coil may vary widely in different strains or in the same strain under varied conditions. Multiplication is by transverse fission. These spirochetes stain

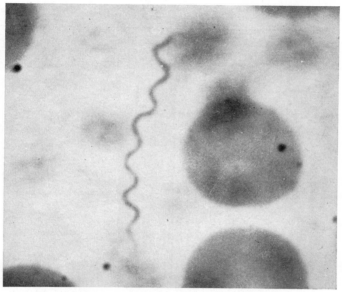

Fig. 36. Spirochete of relapsing fever in blood film.

readily with ordinary bacterial stains and especially with the Romanowsky blood stains. Attempts to maintain cultures by bacteriologic methods have not met with success. Strains are conserved only by frequent animal passage; in the developing chick embryo; or in the specific tick host, where they survive for years even in unfed ticks (Fig. 36).

Although it is generally agreed that the relapsing fever spirochetes constitute a single *genus* there is little agreement as to the acceptance of any one of the generic names variously designated as *Protomycetum, Spirochaeta, Spirillum, Spironema, Treponema* and *Borrelia.* The term *Borrelia* is gaining acceptance.

Similarly, there are no generally accepted criteria for *species* determination. Morphology, the standard basis for classification of higher forms, and the reactions in various media used for the differentiation of bacteria of similar morphology afford no basis for classification. Staining reactions, cross immunity tests, serologic reactions, and pathogenicity for different animals have likewise proved unsatisfactory. Recently, the specific relationship which has been

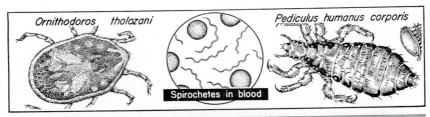

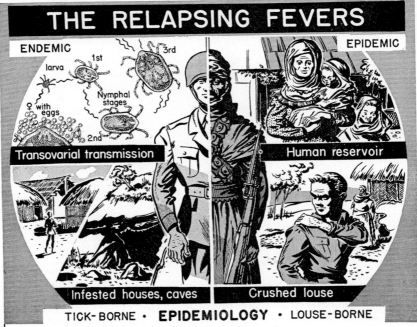

Fig. 37. Epidemiology of the relapsing fevers.

shown to exist between the several species of *Ornithodoros* and their respective spirochetes has been proposed as a more accurate method of approach.

*Borrelia recurrentis* (= *obermeieri*) is quite generally accepted as the louse-borne type although other specific names have from time to time been used, as *B. carteri* in India, and *B. berbera* and *B. aegyptica* in Africa.

**Epidemiology**    To a considerable extent the vector determines the *epidemicity* or *endemicity* of the disease. Louse-borne relapsing fever is typically epidemic; the tick-borne disease is endemic. Infection of man by the louse is generally considered to occur through crushing of the insect and the resulting contamination of the abraded skin rather than by direct inoculation by the bite. The life span of the louse is short, transovarial transmission has not been demonstrated, and man is its only host (Fig. 37).

Ticks, on the other hand, utilize man and a variety of animals as hosts. They are not permanent ectoparasites but leave their hosts after each blood meal. The *Ornithodoros* ticks are biologic vectors of the spirochetes of relapsing fever and experimental evidence indicates that some of them may constitute the most important reservoir of infection. The spirochetes are passed to successive generations through the eggs. Thus 100 per cent of the progeny from the first oviposition of the fifth generation of *O. turicata* have been shown to be infective. Local rodent populations which serve as hosts for the tick have been incriminated in certain instances as reservoirs of the infection (Fig. 37).

The method of infection of man by *Ornithodoros* varies with different species. *Ornithodoros moubata* infects through the secretions of the salivary and coxal glands. In dissected specimens, spirochetes are more numerous in the salivary glands in the nymphal stages and in the coxal glands in the adult stage. *Ornithodoros turicata*, *O. parkeri*, *O. hermsi*, *O. tholozani*, and probably others, infect definitely by *bite*. In experimental studies with *O. turicata* mice have become infected in less than one minute of tick feeding, long before coxal fluid appears. Furthermore, the "coxal fluid" in *O. hermsi* is not fluid but appears as a dry white deposit; in ticks of this genus defecation does not take place during feeding.

There is little agreement of opinion concerning the transmissibility of tick-borne spirochetes by lice, or of louse-borne spirochetes by ticks. The potential role of ticks as initiators of epidemics of relapsing fever in poorly nourished, crowded, and louse-infested populations may be important in the epidemiology of the disease. In fact, recent studies have demonstrated a relatively long survival of some tick-borne spirochetes within the body louse.

LOUSE-BORNE RELAPSING FEVER. The louse-borne form occurs under the same conditions as epidemic typhus and the two diseases not infrequently appear together. It has often been a scourge of armies in the field. Its prevalence depends upon the relative resistance of the human host and upon ecologic and sociologic conditions that favor rapid multiplication and frequent transfer of the louse vector. Undernourishment, over-crowding, lack of personal hygiene—especially in bathing and changing of clothes—are contributing factors. The relative humidity and temperature markedly influence the degree of louse infestation. High temperatures retard reproduction of the insect vectors. The disease is, therefore, often seasonal. Furthermore, the heavy clothing usually worn throughout the coldest months favors lousiness. Among the scantier clothed populations of equatorial Africa the louse-borne disease is seldom seen.

The great epidemics in Poland, Central Russia, Serbia, Rumania, India and across central Africa were louse-borne. In the Rumanian epidemic of World War I there were an estimated 1,000,000 cases of typhus in a population of 5,000,000 and an even higher incidence of relapsing fever. Lesser epidemics have occurred in Edinburgh, Dublin, in the coastal cities of the eastern United States and at Oroville, California. The extensive apparently louse-borne epidemic which appeared in French Guinea in 1921, spreading eastward to the western border of the Anglo-Egyptian Sudan and southward into Nigeria and the Gold Coast, resulted in some areas in a case mortality of nearly 75 per cent. Over a two year period 80,000 to 100,000 deaths are estimated to have occurred.

TICK-BORNE RELAPSING FEVER. A number of species of *Ornithodoros* in various parts of the world has been shown to transmit relapsing fever. Other species have not been investigated or their relationship to the incidence of the disease is not known with certainty.

In British Columbia, *O. hermsi* must be considered the vector as it is the only known species of the genus present and is the proved vector in the contiguous areas of northern Idaho and eastern Washington.

In the United States there are three species known to be vectors in definite areas: viz., *O. hermsi* in California, Colorado, Idaho, Nevada, Oregon and Washington; *O. turicata* in New Mexico, Kansas, Oklahoma and Texas; and *O. parkeri* in Stanislaus county in California. However the distribution of *O. turicata* and *O. parkeri* is much wider than is indicated by these known endemic areas. *Ornithodoros turicata* is present in nine states and extends as far east as Florida. *Ornithodoros parkeri* has a quite general distribution in nine western states, and spirochetes which produce typical reactions in laboratory animals have been recovered from ticks of this species collected in California, Idaho, Montana, Nevada, Oregon, Wyoming and Utah. Although *O. talaje* has been reported from various areas and spirochetes producing characteristic disease in experimental animals have been recovered from ticks of this species collected in Arizona, Kansas and Texas, it has not been shown to be a vector of relapsing fever north of Guatemala.

In Mexico, *O. turicata* has a wide distribution and is the only known vector. Spirochetes have been recovered from *O. dugesi*, a

## Table 4 The Relapsing Fever Spirochetes and Their Tick Vectors

| DISTRIBUTION | NAMED SPIROCHETES | VECTORS |
|---|---|---|
| Western Canada<br>British Columbia | Borrelia hermsii | Ornithodoros hermsi |
| Western United States | B.turicatae<br>B. hermsii<br>B. parkeri<br>? | O. turicata<br>O. hermsi<br>O. parkeri<br>O. talaje |
| Mexico | B. turicatae<br>B. dugesii | O. turicata<br>O. dugesi |
| Central America | B. venezuelensis<br>? | O. rudis<br>O. talaje |
| South America<br>Colombia, Ecuador and Venezuela | B. venezuelensis | O. rudis |
| Africa | B. duttonii<br>B. persica<br>B. hispanica<br>B. normandi<br>B. crocidurae  (Senegal)<br>B. merionesi  (Morocco)<br>B. dipodilli  (Kenya) | O. moubata<br>O. tholozani<br>O. erraticus<br>O. normandi<br>O. erraticus*<br>O. erraticus*<br>O. erraticus* |
| Asia | B. persica<br>B. latychevi<br>?<br>?<br>B. microti  (Iran) | O. tholozani<br>O. tartakovskvi<br>O. crossi<br>O. neerensis<br>O. erraticus* |
| Europe | B. hispanica<br>B. caucasica | O. erraticus<br>O. verrucosus |

* Represents the small form; see explanatory note below for detailed explanation.

EXPLANATORY NOTE: *Borrelia novyi*, which has been used widely in experimental studies, is not included as its origin is unknown in relation to vectors. There is no valid reason for its designation as "the American strain." It is believed that *O. talaje* spirochetes have never been given an authentic name. Although *B. venezuelensis* is, at times, used indiscriminately for the spirochetes transmitted by *O. rudis* and by *O. talaje*, *O. talaje* spirochetes are not transmitted by *O. rudis* in the laboratory. *Ornithodoros crossi* spirochetes have characteristics of *B. persica* and *O. crossi* is considered a synonym of *O. tholozani* by some workers while others give it a subspecific status. The term. *O. crossi* is used here as it thus appeared in the literature on relapsing fever in Kashmir and Jammu. There are two so-called "forms" of *O. erraticus*, the large and the small. It is possible that when further biologic studies have been made it will be necessary to revert to *O. erraticus* for the small form from which it was originally described and *O. marocanus* for the large form. For sometime *O. marocanus* has been considered a synonym of *O. erraticus* on the basis of priority. In the table, the vectors marked "*" are the small form. *Borrelia merionesi* and *B. microti* may be synonyms of *B. crocidurae* on the basis of priority. *Borrelia dipodilli* seems to stand apart from the others. Little is known concerning the relation of some of the spirochetes to the disease in man. This holds true of *O. talaje* spirochetes as there has been much confusion between *O. talaje* and *O. rudis*, although they are quite distinct biologically.

At present, the borrelias of prime importance are: *B. turicatae*, *B. hermsii*, *B. venezuelensis*, *B. persica*, *B. hispanica* and *B. duttonii*.

*O. tholozani* = *O. papillipes*<br>
*O. rudis*     = *O. venezuelensis*<br>
*B. persica*   = *B. sogdiana* and *B. usbekistanica*

species very closely related morphologically and biologically to *O. talaje*.

In Guatemala, where the disease has been reported sporadically, *O. talaje* is the only known species of the genus present.

In Panama, both *O. rudis* and *O. talaje* are reported as transmitters although it seems that the former is the more important.

In South America, there are numerous endemic areas in Colombia, Venezuela and Ecuador, where *O. rudis* is the principal vector. *Ornithodoros furcosus* is abundant in houses in the interior valleys of Ecuador and *O. amblus* in coastal areas of Peru, but neither species has been incriminated although both bite man readily. The reported distribution of relapsing fever in Bolivia suggests the tick-borne disease but a tick vector has not been found. Sporadic cases in Peru are reported to be louse-borne. A single case report has come from Argentina and *O. talaje* is said to be present in this republic.

In Africa, *O. moubata* is recognized as the most important vector. This species has been reported from as far west as Sierra Leone, across the continent from west to east, southward to Cape Colony and in Madagascar. This tick is a parasite essentially of man although its recorded hosts are being extended. *Ornithodoros savignyi* has an even wider distribution and is reported as being parasitic chiefly on man although it has been taken in large numbers in a camel yard in the environs of Cairo. However, there are no available authentic records of spirochetes ever having been recovered from ticks of this species as collected in nature.

*Ornithodoros erraticus*, both large and small forms, has a general distribution in northern Africa and spirochetes have been repeatedly recovered from ticks collected over a wide area. The tick vectors in Tunisia and northern Libya have not been definitely determined. However, *O. normandi*, which feeds on man and from which spirochetes have been recovered, is reported to be numerous in rodent burrows near Kef in Tunisia where *O. erraticus* is at times found in the same burrows. *Ornithodoros tholozani* has been reported from the western Egyptian Desert, which extends this species as a potential vector over a considerable area.

In the areas east of the Mediterranean, *O. tholozani* is the recognized vector in Israel, Syria, Iraq and Iran. It has also been reported responsible for an outbreak of relapsing fever in the Island of Cyprus. *Ornithodoros tartakovskyi* has recently been found in Iran and spirochetes have been recovered from it.

In the U.S.S.R., *O. tholozani* and *O. tartakovskyi* are the reported vectors although little is known concerning the latter species in relation to the disease in man. *Ornithodoros tholozani* extends to the western border of China and into Afghanistan.

In northern India, especially in Kashmir and Jammu, the tick-borne disease is endemic. Here, *O. crossi* (*O. tholozani?*) is the proved vector.

In Europe, *O. erraticus* is the only known vector in Spain and

Portugal and *O. verrucosus* in the North Caucasus. The tick-borne disease has been reported from Jugoslavia and Greece but these reports cannot be confirmed.

The importance of the several species of *Ornithodoros* as vectors varies directly with their frequency of contact with man. *Ornithodoros hermsi* is found in wooded areas at relatively high elevations in the western United States and is brought into houses by tree squirrels (*Tamiasciurus*) and chipmunks (*Eutamias*) from their nests in decaying logs and trees where these ticks have been found in large numbers. Once established in dwellings the tick constitutes a perma-

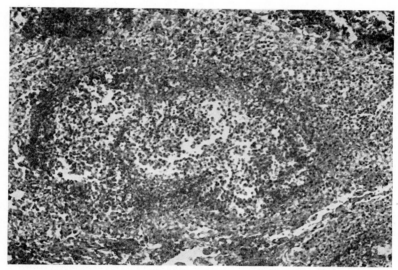

Fig. 38. Miliary lesion in spleen with central necrosis and mononuclear exudate. Spirochetes in surrounding zone of infiltration.

nent reservoir of infection. Other house-dwelling ticks, notably *O. moubata* in tropical Africa and *O. rudis* in northern South America, are in close contact with their human hosts and under such conditions the tick-borne disease may approach epidemic proportions in a changing population. *Ornithodoros parkeri*, found chiefly in the burrows of ground squirrels and prairie dogs (*Cynomys* species) comes in contact with its human host less often and although spirochetes causing typical reactions in laboratory animals have been recovered from ticks of this species collected over a wide area in the western United States human cases attributable to *O. parkeri* are rare. *Ornithodoros turicata* and *O. tholozani*, when infesting caves or burrows or recesses under overhanging ledges, may cause numerous infections among groups of people visiting such areas or using them as a refuge in inclement weather or under the exigencies of war.

**Pathology** The most striking and constant pathologic changes are encountered in the spleen and liver; less often lesions are present in the kidney, myocardium and central nervous system. Jaundice is common in fatal cases and there may be numerous small hemorrhages in the skin, stomach, intestine and kidneys. The spleen is usually enlarged and soft and often presents multiple areas of infarction. Characteristic miliary lesions are commonly visible in the gross specimen (Figs. 38, 39). These consist of a zone of congestion and cellular infiltration in which spirochetes are particularly numerous surrounding the malpighian bodies. The liver may be enlarged and may present parenchymatous degeneration. Spirochetes are commonly demonstrable within the reticulo-endothelial cells. Areas of degeneration may likewise be found in the kidney and the myocardium. Rarely, a hemorrhagic meningitis is present and spirochetes may be demonstrable in the parenchyma of the brain.

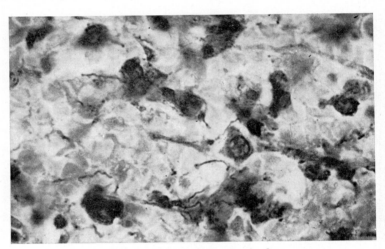

Fig. 39. Spirochetes in lesion of spleen.

The majority of deaths are due to complications, particularly pneumonia.

**Clinical Characteristics**   Relapsing fever is characterized clinically by recurring periods of fever and toxemia, each of a few days' duration separated by afebrile intervals of about a week or ten days. Two to ten or more relapses may occur in untreated or improperly treated cases.

There is no clinical distinction between the louse-borne and tick-borne forms of the disease although in general the louse-borne variety is said to have a lesser tendency to multiple relapses. The mortality, usually from 2 to 5 per cent, has reached nearly 75 per cent in a serious West African epidemic outbreak.

There seem to be rather characteristic variations in the severity of the disease in different areas; these variations have led to the consideration of the relapsing fevers in terms of specific geographic regions. However there are great variations in severity and in the clinical phenomena in different cases even within a given area.

Thus certain special types have been described, such as African tick fever, and North African, Persian, Indian, European, and American relapsing fever. In North Africa the disease is said to be of relatively short duration but frequently complicated by involvement of the central nervous system. Facial and ocular palsies are said to be of common occurrence in this form. Jaundice and a somewhat high mortality rate are rather frequent in the Indian form. The Persian type of the disease is characteristically mild and the relapses not numerous. Relapsing fever in Europe and the Americas is commonly a moderately severe disease; however the relapses seldom exceed two or three in number.

The incubation period varies from three to ten days. The onset is usually sudden, associated with vertigo, headache, myalgia and fever which rises rapidly to 104° to 105° F. or even higher. The temperature remains elevated with slight daily remissions throughout the primary febrile period. Vomiting is common. A slight icteric tint of the sclerae is usual. In severe cases there may be marked jaundice by the time of the crisis. A diffuse bronchitis is frequently present especially in the first febrile episode. Transitory erythematous or petechial eruptions are quite common during the initial fever. Characteristically they are most marked about the neck and shoulder girdle, extending later to the chest and abdomen. Herpes and epistaxis are also not unusual. The spleen is often somewhat enlarged and tender. A polymorphonuclear leukocytosis is present from the onset and, in cases experiencing high fever and bronchitis, may be marked. The urine commonly contains albumin and casts, and in severe cases hematuria may occur. Spirochetes are usually demonstrable in the blood during the febrile periods, but not in the apyrexial intervals.

After four or five days of severe illness the temperature falls by crisis accompanied by profuse sweating and not infrequently by prostration and signs of cardiac weakness. The afebrile period lasts three to ten days during which time there is usually marked clinical improvement.

The relapse sets in acutely and the subjective and objective phenomena are quite similar to those of the initial attack. In the relapses conjunctivitis and iritis are often seen and there may be transitory or permanent cranial nerve palsies. Deafness likewise is not uncommon and may persist. Uterine hemorrhage is not unusual and the pregnant woman frequently aborts. Again after a few days of illness the attack terminates by crisis.

There are usually four to five such recurrences although occasionally there may be as many as ten or more. Late in the course of the disease peripheral neuritis may be persistent and troublesome.

**Diagnosis**   In the differential diagnosis, relapsing fever may have to be distinguished particularly from malaria, dengue and typhus. When jaundice is present it may be confused with yellow fever and leptospirosis.

The clinical picture and leukocytosis may be suggestive. Definitive diagnosis, however, depends upon detection of the spirochetes. These are demonstable in the blood stream only during the pyrexial period. In some instances they may be seen easily in Giemsa-stained blood films. In others, when the organisms are scanty, intraperitoneal inoculation of blood into white mice or young white rats is useful since the spirochetes are easily found in their blood within twenty-four to forty-eight hours. With some strains there may be a continuous spirochetemia for many days and spirochetes may be recovered from the brain of some experimental animals several months after the initial infection.

The disease produced in monkeys and guinea pigs resembles the human infection. Although guinea pigs are resistant to infection with some strains, other strains produce typical febrile relapses with a disappearance of spirochetes from the peripheral blood during the afebrile periods and reappearance at the time of the rise in temperature. Hemoperitoneum has been reported as a constant reaction with some tick strains from north Africa. Hamsters have been used extensively in the experimental studies.

In instances of the louse-borne disease spirochetes may be demonstrated by removing lice from the patient, grinding them up and inoculating the suspension into mice. The demonstration of spirochetes in ticks from the patient, however, affords only presumptive evidence, since some ticks carry spirochetes which they cannot transmit.

The Wassermann reaction is positive at times in the acute stage of the disease.

**Treatment**   The susceptibility of the spirochetes of relapsing fever to certain drugs and antibiotics varies widely. The former concept that arsenicals, particularly neoarsphenamine, are specific therapeutic agents in a high proportion of cases has been seriously questioned, especially during World War II.

Two arsenical drugs may prove useful. They should be administered intravenously during a rise in temperature as follows:

Neoarsphenamine 0.3 to 0.9 gm. for adults, and 0.005 to 0.01 gm. per kilogram of body weight for children, for two successive days. It is frequently followed by vomiting, elevation of temperature, and aggravation of other symptoms.

Mepharsen 0.04 to 0.06 gm. should be given intravenously on three successive days.

Therapy should be instituted as early as possible but should be limited to the early hours of one of the paroxysms. Late in the pyrexial period there may be serious reactions to the drug and in the apyrexial intervals it is ineffective.

In the louse-borne type of relapsing fever, penicillin has proved very effective when administered in a dosage of 25,000 units every three hours until 1,000,000 units have been given.

In experimental studies in white mice infected with *B. novyi*, aureomycin was found to be more effective than penicillin and streptomycin less so. However, these antibiotics have not been used on a sufficient scale in the human disease to warrant definite conclusions.

Recovery is followed by immunity which appears to last about one year.

**Prophylaxis** Approved methods of protection against ixodid ticks are not applicable to ticks of the genus *Ornithodoros*. Biotopes and feeding habits of the two groups differ widely. For the most part, argasid ticks remain within, or in close proximity to, their host habitats, such as burrows, caves, hollow logs or stumps, or in dwellings. Wattle huts, cracks and crevices in adobe huts, floor matting, beds fashioned of bamboo or the rustic bark shingles of more pretentious summer homes afford excellent harborage for these ticks.

Some species feed readily in all stages on man. Feeding is rapid and infection may take place in less than one minute following attachment. The larvae are extremely small and go unnoticed until the engorged tick appears red with blood. Some species are definitely night feeders and may not be discovered until intensive search has been made. A house once infested may be considered always infested. It may be necessary to destroy the more primitive huts by burning. Modern homes should be proofed to prevent ingress of rodent hosts. Some of the newer insect repellents may afford protection under bivouac or semi-bivouac conditions.

Avoidance of lice constitutes full prophylaxis against louse-borne relapsing fever. Since the spirochetes are not found in louse feces, it is necessary to make contact with body fluids of crushed lice to acquire the disease. Louse control should be rigidly practiced.

# 15  Yaws and Bejel

## Yaws

**Synonyms** Framboesia, pian.

**Definition** Yaws is an infectious, contagious, nonvenereal, spirochetal disease caused by *Treponema pertenue*. It is characterized by three stages: an initial cutaneous lesion, the "mother yaw"; nondestructive secondary lesions of the skin, bones and periosteum; and finally destructive deforming lesions of the skin, bones and periosteum. Onset is rare before the age of eighteen months. The disease may extend over forty years or more, causing ill health and disability. Infection produces a slowly developing relative immunity.

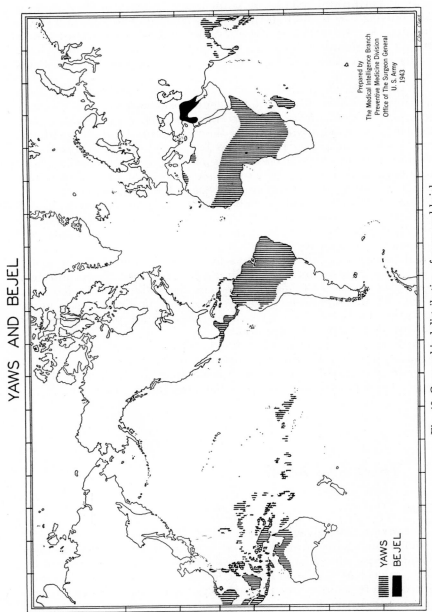

Fig. 40. Geographical distribution of yaws and bejel.

**Distribution**  Yaws is restricted to the tropical zones where it is widespread in many areas of the world, being especially prevalent in hot, moist, lowland countries. It is common in the West Indies, tropical America, throughout equatorial Africa, Ceylon, Malaya, Burma. Thailand, French Indo-China, Indonesia, the Philippines, Samoa, and other Pacific Islands. It is also present in northern Australia but is relatively uncommon in India and China (Fig. 40).

**Etiology**  The etiologic agent, *T. pertenue*, is a rigid, spiral organism with attenuated extremities which is morphologically indistinguishable from *T. pallidum*. Infection is accompanied by positive serologic reactions as in syphilis. The organism has not been grown in artificial culture media. It is present in great numbers in the discharges from open primary and secondary lesions.

**Epidemiology**  For many years there has been a sharp difference of opinion as to the identity of yaws and syphilis, and the exact relationship between these two diseases is still controversial. The conservative view, however, holds that yaws is due to infection by a different but closely related strain of organism. It has frequently been observed that syphilis is rare or unknown among populations in which yaws is prevalent.

There are important clinical and epidemiologic differences between the two diseases. Yaws is not a venereal disease, it is not hereditary, and it is predominantly a disease of childhood. The primary lesion of yaws is almost invariably extragenital and is similar to the lesions of the secondary stage. In moist skin areas, however, the "mother yaw" may closely resemble a chancroid.

Yaws is a disease strictly of the tropical zones. In the colder climates within the tropics it occurs in modified form and it does not spread when introduced into the temperate zones. The incidence is highest among native populations whose level of personal hygiene is low, and Europeans are rarely infected. It is more common in males than in females.

The spirochetes are unable to penetrate the unbroken skin and infection occurs directly through contact of cuts, abrasions or other cutaneous lesions with an open yaws lesion on another individual, or indirectly through soiling of the broken skin with contaminated material. It is commonly communicated by person to person contact, and primary yaws in an adult is usually confined to nursing mothers who are infected by their infants.

Flies, especially species of *Hippelates*, may be mechanical vectors in some areas. In general, however, insects are of no importance in transmission.

Yaws tends to be a seasonal disease. Cases presenting the lesions of the primary and the secondary stages are much more numerous during the rainy season than at any other time of year.

**Pathology**  The most characteristic feature of the pathology of yaws is the predominant involvement of the skin. The organisms are most abundant in the epidermis.

The cutaneous lesions consist of granulomatous papules and macules. In the papules, or framboesiform lesions, the epidermis is greatly thickened by epithelial hyperplasia, by cellular infiltration, and by exudation of serum. The papillae are elongated and infiltrated and there are often hyperplasia and thickening of the interpapillary pegs. The infiltration consists of plasma cells, lymphocytes, polymorphonuclear leukocytes, eosinophils and some increase of large mono-

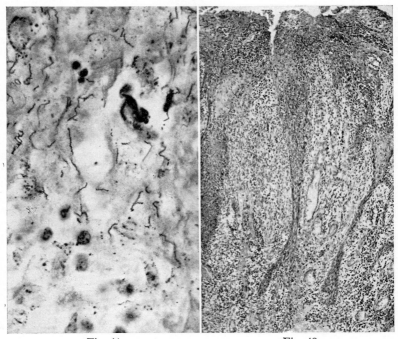

Fig. 41.                                          Fig. 42.

Fig. 41. *Treponema pertenue* in epidermis.
Fig. 42. Papular lesion of yaws showing thickening of epidermis, elongation and infiltration of papillae and hyperplasia of interpapillary pegs.

nuclears and fibroblasts. Perivascular cell accumulations in the corium are not as characteristic as in syphilis (Figs. 41, 42).

This process, leading to the formation of a smooth papule, may be followed by hyperkeratosis of the overlying epithelium and by superficial erosion. The eroded yaw exudes a yellowish secretion which dries to form a crust. The underlying ulcer is shallow, sharply defined, and the floor of granulation tissue bleeds easily. Progressive overgrowth of granulation tissue then produces the characteristic fungating more or less ulcerated framboesiform lesion which is covered with a dirty yellow crust of dried exudate. The epidermis at the margin of the granuloma is thickened and contains many spirochetes.

The later lesions of the disease include ulcerating granulomatous nodules of the skin and subcutaneous tissues and indolent ulcers (Fig. 43). Invasion of skeletal tissues produces osteitis and periostitis leading to bony deformities. Less often there may be extensive destructive lesions of the nose and hard palate producing the condition known as gangosa (Fig. 44).

**Clinical Characteristics** After an incubation period of three weeks to a month, the initial lesion appears at the site of some pre-existing break in the skin. This "mother yaw" resembles the typical granulo-

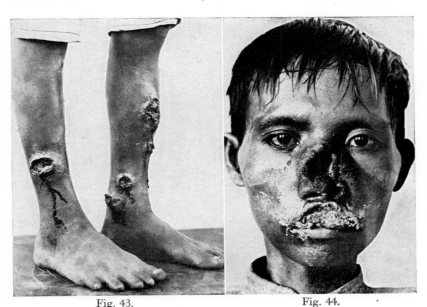

Fig. 43.                    Fig. 44.

Fig. 43. Yaws: chronic ulcers and periostitis.
Fig. 44. Gangosa.

matous secondary lesion except that it is often larger and spontaneous healing is less rapid. It is frequently present when the secondary eruption appears. When it is superimposed on a pre-existing ulcer a more extensive and ulcerating lesion is produced. The development of the primary yaw is accompanied by moderate systemic symptoms, aching of the limbs, joint pains, often by irregular fever, and there may be enlargement of the regional lymph nodes.

The secondary or generalized stage of the disease begins a few weeks to four months after the appearance of the initial lesion. It usually appears as elevated apparently granulomatous papules scattered over the surface of the body. These vary from a few millimeters to 50 mm. or more in diameter and tend to be round or oval. At first the surface is composed of greatly proliferated epithelium exuding clear serum which contains great numbers of spirochetes. Later a crust develops, yellow at first but becoming discolored by debris. In young children suffering from anemia or malnutrition the lesions may not be elevated but appear as erosions with bright pink borders and whitish centers. The eruption may involve the palms of the hands or the soles of the feet. The plantar lesions are painful and disabling.

Successive eruptions often appear before the preceding ones heal. The later lesions tend to be most numerous about the lips, axillae, genitalia and anus. Although typical generalized secondary lesions probably do not occur more than two to three years after the primary eruption, secondary lesions about the lips or on the soles of the feet may recur after many years (Figs. 45, 46).

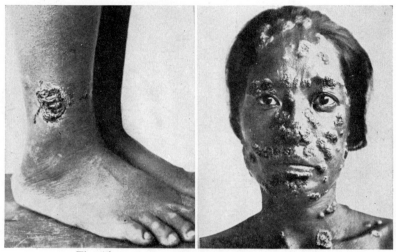

Fig. 45.                    Fig. 46.

Fig. 45. The primary lesion or mother yaw.
Fig. 46. Yaws: framboesiform lesions in a Filipino.

In cooler environments the skin lesions may be restricted to condyloma-like processes limited to the perianal, perineal and axillary regions.

Healing of the secondary lesions leaves only slight scarring and the scars are never permanently atrophic and pigmented.

Nondestructive lesions of the bones are frequent in the secondary stage. The characteristic changes are focal rarefactions—rarefying osteitis, and periostitis. These develop rapidly and usually resolve spontaneously in a few weeks or months. The rarefaction disappears but the periosteal reaction may lead to thickening of the bone. Goundou and sabre shin may be the result of this process (Fig. 47).

The tertiary stage of yaws commonly does not appear until after a relatively or completely symptom free interval of several years. A negative Kahn test during this quiescent period indicates termination of the infection. A positive reaction is an indication of latency.

The appearance of tertiary lesions is the only evidence of the beginning of the final stage. These destructive changes do not occur in the presence of the secondary eruption. Although they may develop within a few years after infection, they reach their highest incidence in the third and fourth decades of life. In this stage resolution and spontaneous cure may occur or the disease may again become latent with the subsequent appearance of relapsing tertiary lesions.

The lesions of the skin are characteristically of three types. There may be extensive, spreading superficial and relatively clean ulceration, ultimately healing from the center. Cutaneous and subcutaneous

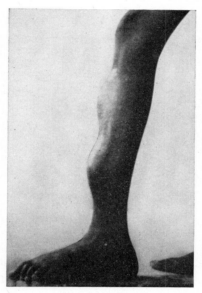

Fig. 47. Saber shin of late yaws. (Alan Fisher for the Office of the Coordinator of Inter-American Affairs.)

nodules develop which break down to form deep indolent ulcers with irregular bases. Spirochetes cannot usually be demonstrated. Healing proceeds from the margin and from isolated islands in the base, producing atrophic scars. These may be unpigmented in the early stages but later are often deeply pigmented and may cause severe contractures. Hyperkeratotic lesions of the soles of the feet and less commonly of the palms of the hands cause extensive thickening of the skin with fissuring and ulceration. These "crab yaws" are painful and the source of severe disability (Fig. 48). In different parts of the world they constitute from 40 to 90 per cent of all yaws cases. They are most common in young adults, particularly males, and develop especially during the rainy season and after trauma.

Destructive bone and periosteal lesions are frequent. They resemble the gumma of syphilis. They are usually single or few in number. They develop slowly and may extend through the subcutaneous tissues and the skin to produce chronic ulceration which responds only slowly to treatment. They are accompanied by local swelling, tenderness and pain. The tibia, other long bones and the bones of the hands are most commonly involved. Less frequently they occur in the tarsal and carpal bones, the skull, clavicles, scapulae and sternum. Involvement of the hard palate leads to perforation and the process may progress, causing extensive destruction of the structures of the nose to produce gangosa (Fig. 44). Joint lesions are not uncommon and fibromatous tumors in the vicinity of the appendicular joints— juxta-articular nodules—are often associated with the late lesions of yaws.

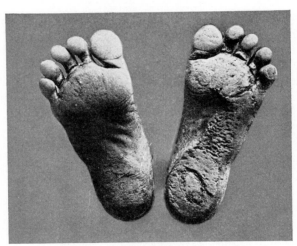

Fig. 48. Yaws: hyperkeratosis with fissuring of the soles of feet; "crab yaws."

**Diagnosis**  The diagnosis of yaws may often be made on clinical grounds and confirmed by the demonstration of spirochetes in a dark field examination of exudate from the lesion or by a smear stained by Giemsa's method. They may likewise be demonstrated by India ink preparations. The Wassermann and Kahn reactions of the blood are positive but such tests of the cerebrospinal fluid are usually negative.

The lesions of mucocutaneous leishmaniasis may be confused with the nasopharyngeal manifestations of yaws. Similarly ulcerating lesions of leprosy and tuberculosis may present differential diagnostic problems, the solution of which will depend upon demonstration of the specific etiologic agents.

The differential diagnosis between late lesions of yaws and syphilis, especially those affecting bony structures, may be extremely difficult if not impossible. The history and presence of a scar from a healed "mother yaw" are important.

**Treatment**  The response of early yaws to treatment by certain arsenicals and antibiotics is dramatic, and eradication of the disease has become practicable. Many authorities, however, believe that accomplishment of such an objective is not without hazard. Yaws, primarily a disease of childhood, confers partial immunity to syphilis. Eradication would therefore facilitate the introduction of syphilis or permit the subsequent re-appearance of yaws in epidemic form. The conservative objective of anti-yaws campaigns is reduction of the prevalence to low endemic levels.

PRIMARY AND SECONDARY YAWS. Neoarsphenamine, Mapharsen, chloramphenicol (Chloromycetin), aureomycin, oxytetracycline (Terramycin) and penicillin all exercise immediate and dramatic effects upon the primary and secondary lesions. They become noninfective within a day or two and even limited dosage frequently causes prompt healing. More intensive therapy is required to reverse the serologic reactions and to prevent relapses.

The reactions often met in primary arsenic therapy of syphilis do not occur in yaws. Penicillin appears to be less effective than the other antibiotics, and Chloromycetin, aureomycin and Terramycin have the advantage of oral administration.

TREATMENT SCHEDULES, MAPHARSEN AND NEOARSPHENAMINE. Four to six intravenous injections at weekly intervals as follows:

Mapharsen:
    Dose for adult males ................. 0.06 gm.
    Dose for adult females ................ 0.04 gm.
    Dose for children:
        Two to ten years of age ............ 0.03 gm.
        Under two years of age ............. 0.01 gm.

Neoarsphenamine:
    Dose for adult males ................. 0.75 to 0.9 gm.
    Dose for adult females ................ 0.6 gm.
    Dose for children:
        Two to ten years of age ............ 0.3 gm.
        Under two years of age ............. 0.1 gm.

TREATMENT SCHEDULES, ANTIBIOTICS. Chloromycetin 10-20 gm. in divided dosage in seven days; aureomycin 5-10 gm. in divided dosage in five days; Terramycin 10-14 gm. in divided dosage in seven days; penicillin up to 2,400,000 units in four days.

Serologic tests should be repeated three months and six months after treatment and additional therapy given if positive reactions are found.

TERTIARY YAWS. The late lesions of the disease are much more resistant to therapy and repeated courses may be required to accomplish healing and to render the patient serologically negative. Although bismuth is not recommended for primary and secondary yaws, it is a useful adjuvant in the late stages especially if plantar lesions are present. The antibiotics are much less effective in the late than in the early stages of the disease.

Mapharsen or neoarsphenamine should be given in two courses of six weekly intravenous injections, using the dosages recommended for primary and secondary yaws. Between the two courses six weekly injections of bismuth subsalicylate 0.2 gm. in oil should be given intramuscularly.

Treatment should be repeated if clinical relapse occurs or if the serologic test remains positive six months after the beginning of therapy.

Ulcerations of late yaws should be treated concomitantly with local antiseptic dressings. The hypertrophied nasal bones of goundou must be excised surgically. Other deformities such as contractures or chronic osteitis may also necessitate surgical relief, either plastic operations or amputation, although the response of such advanced lesions to chemotherapy alone is sometimes satisfactory if the pathologic process is still in an active stage.

**Yaws Control**    The primary objective of yaws control campaigns is to eliminate the infectious primary and secondary lesions from the population. It is not to effect radical cure of the disease. A single injection of penicillin has proved to be completely effective for such control operations.

Dose for children, 300,000 units.

Dose for adults, 600,000 units.

**Prophylaxis**    The prevention of yaws consists essentially in avoidance of contact with, and the adequate protection of open infectious lesions. In areas where the disease is endemic mass therapy constitutes an important control measure.

### Bejel

Bejel is a nonvenereal treponematosis occurring in Arabs on the deserts of Syria and Iraq (Fig. 40). There is much argument whether this disease is a form of syphilis or of yaws, since it resembles the former in its frequent exhibition of mucous patches and the latter in its affinity for children. The blood Wassermann reaction is positive. A condition resembling crab yaws is common and juxta-articular nodules have also been noted in many of the cases.

### 16    Pinta

**Synonyms**    Mal del pinto; carate; azul; boussarole.

**Definition**    Pinta is a treponematosis of the skin caused by *Treponema carateum*, in which depigmentation and hyperkeratosis are the outstanding manifestations. The disease is limited almost exclusively to dark-skinned races. The hands and wrists are involved most frequently, although other common sites are the feet and ankles.

**Distribution**    Pinta is a disease primarily of the Western Hemisphere, occurring in many parts of the American tropics. It is especially prevalent in Mexico and Colombia.

**Etiology**    Formerly thought to be a superficial mycosis, pinta is now known to be caused by a spirochete morphologically identical with that of syphilis. The organism, *Treponema carateum*, has not been cultivated or successfully inoculated into laboratory animals (Fig. 49).

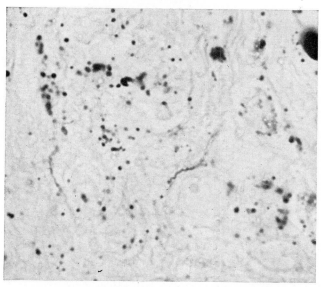

Fig. 49. Pinta: *Treponema carateum* in epidermis.

**Epidemiology**    The method of spread is unknown. *Treponema carateum* has been found in the fluid oozing from fissures in hyperkeratotic lesions of the disease, so that direct contact is suggested as the means of infection. Flies feeding on open sores are suspected of carrying the spirochetes from person to person.

No evidence of congenital transmission has been reported. The highest incidence of the disease is among young and middle-aged adults. It is most prevalent in hot humid areas.

**Pathology**    The epidermis and corium are both involved in a low-grade inflammation which results in (*a*) a disturbance of the melanophores and (*b*) a thickening of the corium. The causative spirochetes have been demonstrated in histologic sections of early lesions. Visceral lesions have not been proven.

**Clinical Characteristics**    Three stages have been described. The first is that of the initial papular lesion; the second is characterized by a spreading eruption of flat erythematous lesions known as pintids (Fig. 50). These two periods occupy about a year. In the tertiary stage pigmentary disturbances become manifest, often consisting first of variously colored patches and progressing finally to leukoderma (Fig. 51). Not infrequently these are symmetrically distributed. Hyperkeratoses appear simultaneously on the palms and soles, causing inconvenience if fissuring occurs.

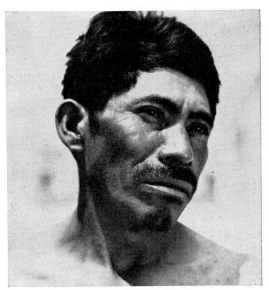

Fig. 50. Secondary lesion or pintid on right cheek.

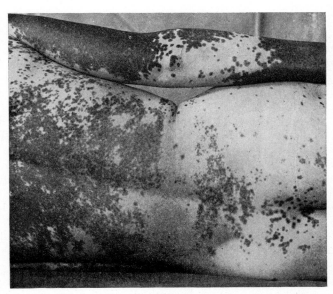

Fig. 51. Late pinta—areas of complete depigmentation of skin. (Courtesy of Dr. Howard Fox.)

Syphilis apparently does not confer immunity to pinta.

**Diagnosis** Symmetric vitiligo of the hands and possibly the feet in a dark-skinned native of tropical America is probably pinta. The blood Wassermann reaction is usually positive in the tertiary stage and an eosinophilia is often present.

**Treatment** Arsenical drugs, administered as in syphilis, are specific in the treatment of this disease. Penicillin is likewise effective.

**Prophylaxis** Although the epidemiology of pinta has not been fully studied it is probable that the measures applicable to yaws are efficient in the control and prevention of this disease.

# 17 The Leptospiral Diseases

The leptospiras causing disease in man are considered to be native to animal hosts, reaching man through contamination of food or water by the urine and feces of infected animals. These diseases are distributed throughout the world co-extensively with the geographic distribution of the normal mammalian hosts.

**Etiology** The genus *Leptospira* is comprised of two major groups of morphologically indistinguishable organisms. The saprophytic free-living leptospiras can be cultivated on Hindle's feces medium, while the pathogenic leptospiras require a substrate containing animal serum or tissue extracts.

The leptospiras range from 4 to 40 microns in length and are approximately 0.1 micron in diameter. An axial filament is uniformly coiled about the body of the organism. In fluid media they are actively motile and spin on their longitudinal axis; the ends are hooked and the body rigid (Fig. 52). In semisolid media the organisms move in a serpentine fashion. Leptospiras readily penetrate mucous membranes and the pores of Seitz-E-K filter pads. Because of their small size, they are usually demonstrable in the fresh state only by dark field examination. In tissue sections they are best shown by silver impregnation stains.

The pathogenic leptospiras are quite sensitive to heat, acids and alkalis. They are readily destroyed by pasteurization temperatures but will survive at $-50°$ C. for at least six months. The optimum $pH$ ranges are from $pH$ 6.8 to $pH$ 7.6.

No valid criteria exist for subdivision of the pathogenic members of the genus into species. Classification is based upon serologically demonstrable antigenic differences. At present nineteen closely related "serogroups" are recognized. These, in turn, are further subdivided into thirty-four serologically indistinguishable strains or "serotypes" (Table 5).

**Epidemiology** Leptospiral infections exhibit certain characteristic epidemiologic features which differ from those of bacterial and protozoan diseases. While any of the pathogenic members of the genus may cause disease in man, transmission from man to man is rare. The leptospiras persist in animal carriers in the tubules of the kidneys. The infected urine of these carriers contaminates water, food and moist soil. These organisms may survive outside the animal body in alkaline soil or water for varying periods of time up to approximately three weeks.

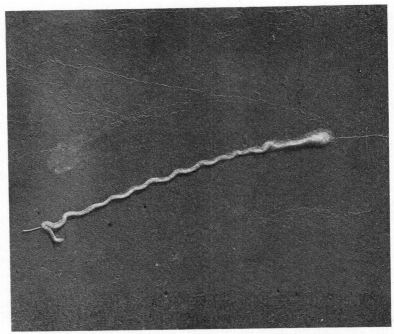

Fig. 52. Electron photomicrograph of *Leptospira hyos*, chromium shadowed, showing typical spiral shape and axial filament entwined along the central cell mass (10,600 ×). (Courtesy of Breese, Gochenour and Yager in Proc. Soc. Exper. Biol. & Med. *80:*185–188, 1952.)

The natural reservoirs of infection are rodents, small carnivores and certain domestic animals. In general, each leptospiral serotype has a primary mammalian host within a given geographic area; however, a single animal species may be the primary host of several serotypes and may be simultaneously infected with, and shed, two or more leptospiral serotypes. Development of the carrier state in the several animal species appears, in general, to be related to their position in the phylogenetic scale. Rodents, small carnivores and marsupials seem to be almost commensally related to the leptospiras, since virtually no apparent disease occurs following infection, and a lifelong renal carrier state is established.

Domestic animals are less adaptable. Clinical disease occurs frequently but the renal carrier state, when established, is of limited duration. Leptospiruria in cattle and horses probably does not persist for more than four months. The organisms, likewise, are present in the milk during the acute systemic phase of the disease in cattle. Despite the fact that they will survive in fluid raw milk for a number of hours and in diluted milk for several days, no proven case of milk-borne leptospirosis of man has been reported.

Arthropods have not been found naturally infected with leptospiras. At least one species of tick, *Ornithodorus moubata*, is capable

*Table 5    Reported Animal Hosts of Pathogenic Leptospiras*

| LEPTOSPIRAL SEROGROUP* | ANIMAL HOSTS |
|---|---|
| Icterohemorrhagiae | Rats, mice, mongooses, swine, dogs |
| Javanica | Rats, mice |
| Canicola | Dogs, swine, cattle |
| Ballum | Rats, mice, opossums |
| Pyrogenes | Rats, mice, mongooses |
| Autumnalis | Mice, voles |
| Australis A | Rats |
| Pomona | Swine, cattle, horses, dogs |
| Grippotyphosa | Rats, mice, voles, cattle, horses, sheep |
| Hebdomadis | Rats, mice, voles, cattle, dogs |
| Bataviae | Rats, mice, mongooses |
| Semeranga | Rats |
| Hyos | Swine, cattle |

* The names in this column are not to be confused with species names.

of transmitting leptospiras to a healthy guinea pig after having fed on an infected one.

Infections of man result from direct or indirect contact with the contaminated urine of an animal carrier. Infection may occur through the mucous membranes or through minute cuts or abrasions of the skin. Penetration of intact skin has not been conclusively proven. Although the acidity of the stomach is sufficient to destroy ingested leptospiras, infection may take place by penetration of the buccal, pharyngeal and esophageal mucous membranes.

The epidemiologic importance of particular animal carriers depends upon their collective mode of life. The population density and the rate of increase are important since the chain of infection can be maintained only when adequate numbers of susceptible animals are constantly available. Thus, in the serogroup Bataviae infections of man in the rice fields of northern Italy, the sudden increase of human cases in early July of each year corresponds with the appearance of large numbers of dwarfed mice and the resulting high degree of contamination of the fields.

Leptospirosis is often an occupational disease. The serogroup "Icterohemorrhagiae" infections are commonly found in miners, sailors, sewer workers and abattoir workers. "Canicola" infections are most frequently seen in animal caretakers, particularly the owners and breeders of dogs. "Grippotyphosa" infections occur in farmers, agricultural workers, pea pickers and flax workers. "Pomona" infections are seen in swineherds, creamery and cheese workers, swine slaughterers, veterinarians and animal husbandrymen.

Leptospirosis is primarily a disease of young adult males because of the greater opportunities for contact with infected environments. There is no difference in susceptibility between males and females or between different age groups. Epidemic outbreaks occur when groups of persons come into contact with a highly contaminated environment.

The leptospiroses of man are acute febrile diseases, protean in nature and presenting a wide variety of clinical syndromes which differ greatly in severity. They fall naturally into two groups: the classic leptospiral jaundice or Weil's disease, and the "benign" leptospiroses.

## Leptospiral Jaundice

**Synonyms** Weil's disease, spirochetal jaundice, mud fever, seven-day fever, swineherd's disease.

**Definition** Leptospiral jaundice is a febrile infection characterized, in severe cases, by fever, vomiting, jaundice, hemorrhage and enlargement and tenderness of the liver. The mortality has varied from 4 to 48 per cent in different outbreaks.

**Distribution** It has a world-wide distribution corresponding to that of the different natural reservoir hosts. The disease is most prevalent in regions where rodents are numerous, particularly in warm, moist, tropical areas.

**Etiology** The disease may be produced by any member of the pathogenic group of the genus *Leptospira.*

**Pathology** The principal pathologic changes are seen in the kidneys, the liver and the skeletal muscles. Hemorrhages are common in the skin, the mucosa, the viscera and the calf muscles.

The liver is usually somewhat enlarged and exhibits varying degrees of parenchymal degeneration and areas of focal necrosis. More rarely the lesions resemble those of acute yellow atrophy. Leptospiras are easily demonstrated in tissue sections by the Levaditi stain.

The kidneys are swollen and show degenerative changes and necrosis of the epithelial cells of the convoluted tubules. Between the tubules infiltration by lymphocytes and mononuclear cells occurs and hemorrhage is not uncommon; leptospiras may be numerous (Fig. 53).

**Clinical Characteristics** The incubation period is usually six to twelve days and the onset is abrupt, with high fever ranging from 102° to 104° F., headache, chills, prostration and myalgia. Anorexia, nausea and vomiting are not uncommon. Frequently there is a relative bradycardia. The face is flushed, the conjunctivae injected, and petechial hemorrhages are frequent. At times bronchopneumonia may be present and the sputum may contain blood. The muscles of the legs, especially the calf muscles, are tender and there are often signs of meningeal irritation. Leptospiras are present in the blood for the first three or four days. After two to five days the temperature tends to be lower and the pulse rate elevated. A polymorphonuclear leukocytosis of 10,000 to 50,000 is present from the onset, accompanied by an increase of immature forms.

The icteric stage occurs in about 50 per cent of cases. In the absence of icterus the patient enters upon convalescence.

In the more severe cases jaundice appears usually about the fifth day and may become intense, accompanied by enlargement and

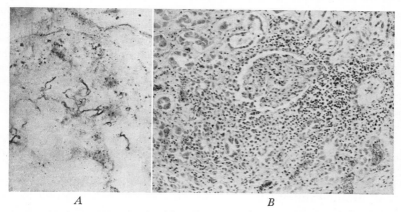

A                 B

Fig. 53. *A*. Levaditi stain: *Leptospira icterohaemorrhagiae* in kidney. *B*. Cellular infiltration, degeneration of epithelial cells of the convoluted tubules.

tenderness of the liver; the spleen is only rarely enlarged. At the same time evidence of impairment of renal function appears with oliguria of varying severity and nitrogen retention. The hemorrhagic tendency may be marked in this phase with petechial or purpuric spots in the skin and mucosae, and occasionally gastro-intestinal hemorrhage with hematemesis and melena. Meningism may be extreme, accompanied by increased spinal fluid pressure and pleocytosis composed principally of lymphocytes. Herpes is frequent and a varying skin rash (erythematous, papular, urticarial or purpuric) may be present. Leptospiras are present in the urine during this stage and are most numerous from the tenth to about the twentieth day. Death occurs in approximately 30 per cent of the jaundiced or severely ill patients, with fatal termination most commonly between the ninth and the sixteenth days.

In nonfatal cases improvement usually begins in the second or third week with increased urinary secretion and clearing of the jaundice. Convalescence may be prolonged.

For **Diagnosis, Treatment** and **Prophylaxis** see these headings under Benign Leptospirosis, pp. 124 and 125.

## Benign Leptospirosis

**Synonym**   Fort Bragg fever.

**Clinical Characteristics**   Benign leptospirosis is characterized by the absence of jaundice, a milder course and favorable outcome. The fever is of shorter duration, headache and myalgia are less intense, and hemorrhagic manifestations are far less common. Congestion of the conjunctival vessels remains a very characteristic sign in the early stage of the disease. Renal and vascular complications do not occur. Meningeal features, however, are often pronounced and may run a protracted although benign course. Occasionally the cutaneous manifestations may be the most characteristic feature of the disease. Toxicity disappears rapidly with defervescence.

**Diagnosis**   The severe forms of leptospirosis may be confused on clinical grounds with viral hepatitis, poisoning by certain toxic agents, or other severe diseases manifesting hepatic, renal and vascular derangements. The benign forms may simulate influenza or the viral meningitides. In either, laboratory confirmation of the clinical impression is essential for definitive diagnosis of leptospirosis and is usually made by demonstration of the organisms or by serologic methods.

Leptospiras are present in the blood and cerebrospinal fluid during the initial, febrile phase of the disease. They are more easily recovered by direct culture in Fletcher's or other suitable media (see p. 838) than by inoculation of laboratory animals. Multiple cultures using minimal quantities (ca. 0.03 ml.) of inoculum should be employed, and cultures should be incubated at 30° C. for at least twenty-eight days before discarding as negative. Direct dark field examination of blood or other fluids will rarely reveal the organisms and often yields confusing artefacts.

A four-fold rise of antibody titer of paired serum specimens demonstrated by complement fixation or by agglutination lysis may be accepted as diagnostic. The first specimen should be obtained early in the disease and the second two weeks later. Complement-fixing antibodies are usually first demonstrable about the eleventh day of disease and reach maximum levels in the third week. Agglutinating antibodies are first detectable about the twelfth day of disease, reach maximum levels in the third week, and may persist in high titer for many months or years.

Leptospiras may be demonstrated by biopsy or at autopsy in liver, calf muscle, or kidney. Silver impregnation techniques are most appropriate for this purpose.

**Treatment**   There is no specific therapy, treatment therefore is supportive and symptomatic. Antibiotics effective in vitro and in experimental infections in laboratory animals have given disappointing results in clinical trials so far. There is some evidence to suggest that oxytetracycline (Terramycin) may be useful if therapy is initiated not later than the second day of the disease.

**Prophylaxis** The great number of leptospiral serotypes, which fail to elicit cross immunity, makes prophylactic vaccination in man feasible only in cases of specific occupational hazards of infection with single serotypes. Preventive measures must at present be directed to control of wild-life reservoirs of infection and the prevention and therapy of leptospirosis in domestic animals.

# 18   Rat-Bite Fevers

The term "rat-bite fever" is employed to designate either of two febrile infections of man characterized by fever of sudden onset, myalgia, exanthemata, leukocytosis and frequent febrile relapses during the course of the disease. The micro-organisms, *Spirillum minus* causing Sodoku and *Streptobacillus moniliformis* which produces Haverhill Fever, are harbored in the nasopharynx of infected rats. The mortality in man is approximately 10 per cent.

## Sodoku

**Definition** Sodoku is a relapsing type of spirochetal infection transmitted by the bite of rats infected with *Spirillum minus*. It is characterized by a delayed local inflammatory reaction at the site of the wound accompanied by lymphangitis, regional lymphadenitis, rigors and fever of sudden onset. Numerous febrile relapses may occur.

**Distribution** The distribution of the disease is worldwide. It is to be anticipated that cases will be found wherever rats are prevalent and in close association with man. Proven cases have been reported from Great Britain, Holland, Germany, Italy, East Africa, French Equatorial Africa, the United States, the West Indies, South America, the Philippine Islands, Indonesia, Australia, and India.

**Etiology** *Spirillum minus* varies considerably in size usually ranging between 2 and 5 microns in length by about 0.2 micron in diameter. Much longer forms may be seen. The coils are uniformly spaced about 1 micron apart and vary in number with the length of the organism. The body is relatively rigid and one or more flagella originate from each extremity. Motility in dark field preparations differs from that of *Leptospira* and other spirochetes, resembling the movements of the vibrios. It is doubtful if it has been cultivated in artificial media (Fig. 54).

*Spirillum minus* is present in the blood of infected rodents during the first two weeks. Thereafter it localizes in connective tissue especially about the lips, tongue, and nose. It has not been found in the saliva but is reported to be present in the lachrymal secretions of infected experimental animals. Transmission by the bite may occur from this source or by escape of the organisms through breaks in the mucous membrane of the rat's tongue or lips.

**Epidemiology**  A number of rodents serve as the normal reservoirs of *S. minus* and the infection rate varies markedly in different areas. Thus in Japan infection rates of about 25 per cent and 3 per cent, respectively, have been reported in the rats, *Rattus norvegicus* and *R. rattus alexandrinus,* while in the vole, *Microtus montebelloi,* the rate is 12 to 54 per cent. In Bombay a rate of 11 per cent has been found in the bandicoot, *Nesokia bengalensis.* In other parts of the world rates up to 18 per cent have been reported in rats.

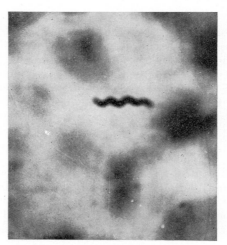

Fig. 54. *Spirillum minus* in blood film.

**Pathology**  The pathology in man has not been thoroughly studied. Degenerative changes in the liver and kidneys and hyperemia of the cerebral cortex have been reported. The spinal fluid pressure may be increased. The organisms are present at the site of the bite and may be recovered by animal inoculation of material aspirated from enlarged lymph nodes, or of blood taken in the early stages of the disease.

Inoculated guinea pigs or white rats may show lymphadenitis, enlargement of the spleen, and occasionally spirilla in the blood. The liver may be congested and contain scattered organisms. Most strains are fatal to guinea pigs within one to two months after inoculation.

**Clinical Characteristics**  After an incubation period which varies usually from five to ten days, rarely extending to five or six weeks, there is sudden onset of fever rising rapidly to 101° or 102° F., accompanied by headache, nausea, marked weakness, tachycardia, and often by chills. The site of the infecting bite, frequently healed, is inflamed, edematous, and may show vesiculation or necrosis with subsequent ulcer formation. This is accompanied by superficial lymphangitis and involvement of the regional lymph nodes. An eruption of purplish macules or papules is not uncommon, occurring chiefly on the chest and arms. Urticaria may be present. Joint pains, motor and sensory disturbances and indications of renal irritation may occur. During the febrile period there is an eosinophilia and a polymorphonuclear leukocytosis usually ranging from 15,000 to 20,000.

The initial fever commonly rises to about 104° F. by the second or third day and remains elevated for two or three days more, thereafter falling rapidly to normal. Local secondary infections of the wound may complicate the clinical picture.

Following the fall of temperature there is usually an apyrexial interval of several days during which the local manifestation at the site of infection and the lymphadenopathy subside. Successive febrile paroxysms of decreasing severity are common, the temperature curve resembling that of relapsing fever.

**Diagnosis**    A history of rat bite together with the clinical phenomena of the initial fever is suggestive. The Wassermann reaction may be positive or negative. Dark field examination of the blood or of material from an infected lymph node may reveal *S. minus* in early cases. Animal inoculation, however, is frequently necessary for recovery of the organisms.

**Treatment**    Aureomycin is the drug of choice for the treatment of infections by *S. minus*. Although penicillin and various arsenicals are useful, the results obtained with these preparations appear to be less uniformly satisfactory.

## Haverill Fever

**Synonym**    Erythema arthriticum epidemicum.

**Definition**    Haverhill fever is a febrile disease characterized by an exanthem and more or less severe generalized arthritis. It is caused by infection with *Streptobacillus moniliformis*, and is transmitted directly or indirectly by rats.

**Distribution**    The disease has been reported from the United States, the British Isles and Europe.

**Etiology**    *Streptobacillus moniliformis* is a gram-negative, nonmotile, pleomorphic bacillus which grows in irregular chains. It is best cultivated in media enriched with 10 to 30 per cent serum or ascitic fluid, incubated at 37° C. under aerobic conditions. Intraperitoneal inoculation of white mice causes a fatal infection terminating in twenty-four to forty-eight hours.

**Epidemiology**    Man usually acquires the infection from the bite of an infected rat or other rodent. One outbreak of milk-borne infection has been reported, presumably due to contamination of milk by infected rats.

**Clinical Characteristics**    A brief incubation period is followed by sudden onset of irregular fever which may persist for weeks or months in untreated cases. Early in the disease a reddish maculopapular rash appears on the hands, arms and feet which fades on pressure. Generalized arthritis of varying severity is common. Necrosis and ulceration at the site of inoculation rarely occur.

**Diagnosis** The diagnosis is established by recovery of the organism in culture from blood, synovial fluid or wound serum, or by demonstration of a specific agglutination titer of 1/80 or above in the patient's serum.

**Treatment** Penicillin and streptomycin are reported to be effective therapeutic agents.

**Prophylaxis** The general prophylaxis consists of effective rodent control. Wounds produced by rat bites should be promptly cauterized.

# 19    The Diarrheal Diseases—Introduction

The diarrheal diseases include the simple diarrheas and the dysenteries. They are widespread throughout the world and occur wherever local sanitary conditions permit the contamination of food and water with human feces. A polluted water supply, insanitary feces disposal, and the house fly are the most important means of transmission.

Clinically the simple diarrheas merge into the dysenteries. A variety of etiologic agents may be concerned and local clinical designations without reference either to the nature of the causative organism or to the response of the host are common in many parts of the world. Specific diagnosis is made in only a small proportion of cases.

Differentiation between the simple diarrheas and the dysenteries depends upon the reaction of the host rather than upon the classification of the infectious agent. It is based upon the presence or absence of an inflammatory reaction in the intestinal wall which is indicated by the microscopic characteristics of the stool. In the simple diarrheas there is no inflammatory reaction and consequently there is no inflammatory cellular exudate in the stool. In the dysenteries, on the other hand, inflammation is present and this is accompanied

**129**

by a characteristic exudate in the stool consisting of erythrocytes, polymorphonuclear leukocytes, and large mononuclear phagocytic cells, the macrophages.

**Etiologic Agents**    The etiologic agents include various bacteria, certain protozoa, and certain helminthic parasites. Only the bacterial diarrheas and dysenteries will be considered in this section. Typhoid, paratyphoid, and cholera infections are included in the classification of the diarrheal diseases because of their high endemicity in certain parts of the world and because they may require consideration in differential diagnosis especially in partially immunized individuals.

Most of these agents produce a true infection of the intestinal tract with an inflammatory reaction of greater or less severity. The paracolon organisms form a loose and indefinite group, some members of which seem closely related to *Salmonella* and others to *Escherichia*.

*Table  6    The  Bacterial  Diarrheas  and  Dysenteries*

| DISEASE | ORGANISM |
|---|---|
| Typhoid fever | *Salmonella typhosa* |
| Paratyphoid fever | *Salmonella paratyphi* A; *Salmonella paratyphi* B; *Salmonella typhimurium;* Other *Salmonella* species |
| Cholera | *Vibrio comma* (*cholera*) |
| Bacillary dysentery | *Shigella dysenteriae; Shigella flexneri; Shigella boydii; Shigella sonnei;* Alkalescens-Dispar group |
| Enteritis | *Salmonella paratyphi* C; *Salmonella oranienburg; Salmonella sendai;* Other *Salmonella* species; paracolon group |
| Food poisoning | *Salmonella* species (*Salmonella enteritidis* most common); *Staphylococcus* species (usually the hemolytic, salt-resistant, mannite-fermenting strains); *Streptococcus* species, particularly those strains of Lancefield's groups A, C, D and G |

Although their clinical importance has not been established, it is believed that they are factors in the etiology of enteritis. Certain others, notably the staphylococci, produce only an intoxication by an enterotoxin without true infection of the host.

**Differential Diagnostic Procedures**    Differentiation of simple diarrheas from the dysentery infections is of great importance in the clinical management and the prognosis since the therapeutic indications may be quite different. This differential diagnosis entails four essentials:

1. Microscopic examination of the fresh stool for the presence of exudate.

2. Character of the exudate (pus, mucus and blood).

3. Identification of protozoan and other parasites.

4. Bacteriologic examination for isolation and identification of enteric pathogens of the dysentery-enteritis-cholera group.

The bacteriologic examination is concerned principally with the isolation and identification of gram-negative intestinal bacilli of which there are three important genera:

1. GENUS *Salmonella*. The more important *Salmonella* types and the frequency of their isolation from man in the United States is shown in Table 7.

*Table 7   Frequency of* Salmonella *Types from Man in the United States*\*

| TYPES | GROUP | ANTIGENIC FORMULA | | | OLD NAME | PER CENT ISOLATED |
|---|---|---|---|---|---|---|
| *S. typhi-murium* | B | I, IV, V, XII | i | 1, 2, 3 | *B. pestis cavae* *S. aertrycke* Breslau bacillus | 30–35 |
| *S. paratyphi* B | B | I, IV, V, XII | b | 1, 2 | *B. paratyphosa* B *S. schottmuel-leri* Paratyphoid B bacillus | 20 |
| *S. typhosa* | D | IX, XII, (Vi) | d | — | *B. typhosa* *Eberthella typhcsa* Typhoid bacillus | 10–15 |
| *S. montevideo* | C–1 | VI, VII | g, m, s | | | |
| *S. oranienburg* | C–1 | VI, VII | m, t | | | |
| *S. choleraesuis* | C–1 | VI, VII | | 1, 5 | *B. suipester* *S. suipester* Hog cholera bacillus | 5–10 |
| *S. newport* | C–2 | VI, VIII | e, h | 1, 2, 3 | | |
| *S. derby* | B | I, VI, XII | f, g | — | | |
| *S. bareilly* | C–1 | VI, VII | y | 1, 5 | | |
| *S. enteritidis* | D | I, IX, XII | g, m | — | *B. enteritidis* Gaertner bacillus | |
| *S. panama* | D | I, IX, XII | e, v | 1, 5 or 1, 11 | | |
| *S. give* | E–1 | III, X | e, v | 1, 7 | | 1–5 |
| *S. anatum* | E–1 | III, X | e, h | 1, 6 | | |
| *S. senftenberg* | E–3 | I, III, XIX | g, s, t | z$_{27}$ | | |

\* Felsenfeld, Am. J. Clin. Path., *15:* 584, 1945.

2. GENUS *Shigella*. The dysentery bacilli of importance and most frequently encountered are:

    *S. dysenteriae* 1 (Shiga's bacillus)
    *S. dysenteriae* 2 (*Shigella's schmitzii, S. ambigua, etc.*)
    *S. flexneri* 2a (Andrews and Inman W)
    *S. flexneri* 3 (Andrews and Inman Z)
    *S. flexneri* 4a (Boyd 103)

*S. flexneri* 6 (Boyd 88, Newcastle and Manchester bacilli)
*S. boydii* 2 (Boyd P-288)
*S. boydii* 7 (*S. etousae*, "Lavington" Type T)
*S. sonnei* (*S. ceylonensis* A)

3. TRIBE ESCHERICHEAE (GENUS *Escherichia*). Certain other gram-negative bacilli of increasing importance in diarrheal disease are those coliform organisms that possess interrelationship with some of the *Shigella* types. These have recently been placed in the Alkalescens-Dispar group, and are no longer included in the genus *Shigella*. Classification is based on the antigenic relationship to *Escherichia coli* O groups as shown in Table 8.

*Table 8　The O Antigenic Schema for the*
*Alkalescens-Dispar Group\**

| O GROUPS | O ANTIGEN | RELATIONSHIP TO *E. coli* O GROUPS | EARLIER DESIGNATIONS |
|----------|-----------|-----------------------------------|----------------------|
| 1 | 1a<br>1a, 1b | Identical with<br>1a<br>1a, 1b | *B. alkalescens* or *Alkalescens*<br>Type I |
| 2 | 2 | Strong relationship with 25 and other groups | Alkalescens Type II or *S. tieté* |
| 3 | 3 | Strong relationship with 25 and other groups | *S. ceylonensis* B or *S. dispar* Type II or Alkalescens Type III (2–193) |
| 4 | 4 | Strong relationship with 4 | *S. madampensis* or *S. dispar* I |
| 5 | 5 | Identical with 2a | None |
| 6 | 6 | Identical with 9 | *S. dispar* Type III |
| 7 | 7 | Identical with 7 | None |
| 8 | 8 | Identical with 81 | None |

\* From Frantzen (1950), and Ewing, Taylor and Hucks (1950).

Differentiation of the pathogenic from the nonpathogenic enteric bacilli is based upon their behavior in lactose media. Pathogenic organisms usually do not attack lactose, and when they do, only after a considerable lapse of time. Definitive identification is dependent on good initial isolation and careful selection of suspect colonies for detailed biochemical and serologic study. Methods utilized for isolation and identification vary between laboratories. Although there are numerous acceptable variations of the method outlined in Table 9, it may be employed as an useful guide.

## Table 9 Outline of Procedure for Identification of Salmonella *and* Shigella *Cultures**

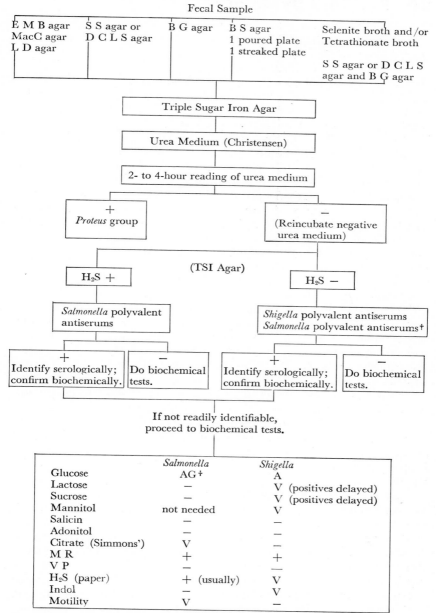

Fecal Sample

| E M B agar MacC agar L D agar | S S agar or D C L S agar | B G agar | B S agar 1 poured plate 1 streaked plate | Selenite broth and/or Tetrathionate broth |
| | | | | S S agar or D C L S agar and B G agar |

Triple Sugar Iron Agar

Urea Medium (Christensen)

2- to 4-hour reading of urea medium

| + *Proteus* group | — (Reincubate negative urea medium) |

(TSI Agar)

| H₂S + | H₂S — |

| *Salmonella* polyvalent antiserums | *Shigella* polyvalent antiserums *Salmonella* polyvalent antiserums† |

| + Identify serologically; confirm biochemically. | — Do biochemical tests. | + Identify serologically; confirm biochemically. | — Do biochemical tests. |

If not readily identifiable, proceed to biochemical tests.

| | *Salmonella* | *Shigella* |
| --- | --- | --- |
| Glucose | AG + | A |
| Lactose | — | V (positives delayed) |
| Sucrose | — | V (positives delayed) |
| Mannitol | not needed | V |
| Salicin | — | — |
| Adonitol | — | — |
| Citrate (Simmons') | V | — |
| M R | + | + |
| V P | — | — |
| H₂S (paper) | + (usually) | V |
| Indol | — | V |
| Motility | V | — |

\* From Edwards and Ewing, A Manual for Enteric Bacteriology, CDC, February, 1952.

† Occasional *Salmonella* cultures may fail to produce hydrogen sulfide in TSI agar. Also certain salmonellae and shigellae cross agglutinate (see text). *Salmonella typhosa* and *Salmonella gallinarum* are anaerogenic. Rarely anaerogenic cultures of other types appear.

# 20  Bacillary Dysentery

**Definition**  Bacillary dysentery is an acute or chronic inflammatory disease of the colon, occasionally involving the distal ileum, caused by members of the genus *Shigella*, the dysentery bacilli. It is characterized pathologically by inflammation and necrosis of the mucosa of the colon, most marked in the distal portions, and clinically by fever, abdominal pain, tenesmus and diarrhea with stools containing gross or microscopic blood and pus.

**Distribution**  The disease is widely distributed throughout the world; the virulent infections by *Shigella dysenteriae 1*, the Shiga bacillus, are more commonly seen in the tropics and the subtropics than in the temperate zone.

**Etiology**  The genus *Shigella* includes a variety of bacilli which vary among themselves in antigenicity and pathogenicity. *Shigella dysenteriae* 1, Shiga's bacillus, is highly toxic. It has been responsible for severe epidemic outbreaks and is more often present in the tropics and subtropics. The other members of the genus are not toxin producers and are generally somewhat less pathogenic, causing less serious disease and a lower incidence of chronic dysentery.

**Epidemiology**  The disease is most prevalent wherever local conditions permit the contamination of food and water by the feces of infected individuals. Carriers of the bacilli are not uncommon especially when the disease is prevalent. The most important means of transmission are contamination of food by infected foodhandlers, the transfer of the bacilli by house flies, and fecal pollution of water supply.

The organisms are easily killed by chemical agents and direct sunlight. They survive, however, for considerable periods in water, ice and the mucoid discharges of active cases. There are few diseases where the risk of infection to individuals caring for the patient is so great, since incontinence is common in severe cases and the soiled bedding and garments of the patient harbor great numbers of the bacilli.

Epidemic outbreaks of bacillary dysentery commonly follow upon the occurrence of mild "missed" cases. In the presence of an epidemic, positive cultures may be obtained from as many as 25 per cent of apparently healthy contacts. About 3 per cent of recovered cases become carriers of the organisms for shorter or longer periods of time. These individuals are often difficult to identify because the bacilli are present only irregularly in the feces. The agglutination reaction is not a dependable means for the identification of infected individuals since false positives and negatives and marked variations of titer in the same individual are common.

**Pathology**  The pathology of bacillary dysentery is essentially an acute diffuse inflammation of the mucosa of the colon with the formation of a diphtheritic membrane followed by necrosis and ulceration

134

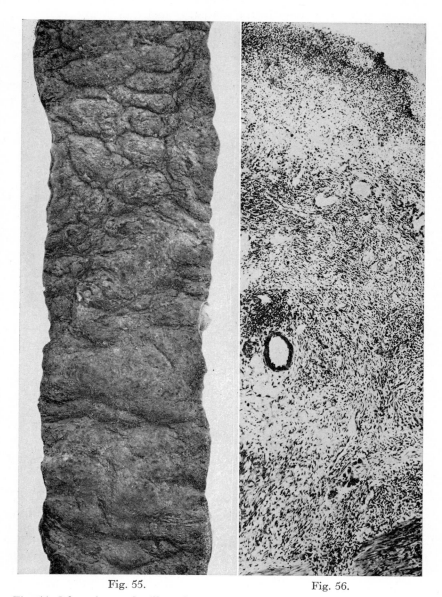

Fig. 55.                         Fig. 56.

Fig. 55. Colon of acute bacillary dysentery: diphtheritic membrane, thickening of
wall.
Fig. 56. Diphtheritic membrane on surface and phlegmonous thickening of the submucosa.

(Figs. 55, 56). This process is reflected by the presence of an inflammatory cellular exudate in the patient's stool.

In the early stage there is a rapidly spreading hyperemia of the mucosa often accentuated in the lymph nodules, followed by edema, hemorrhage, and infiltration with granular leukocytes and macrophages. This process frequently extends into the submucosa producing marked phlegmon-like thickening of the intestinal wall. The necrosis and desquamation of the epithelium with the formation of a diphtheritic type of membrane on the surface are followed by ulcera-

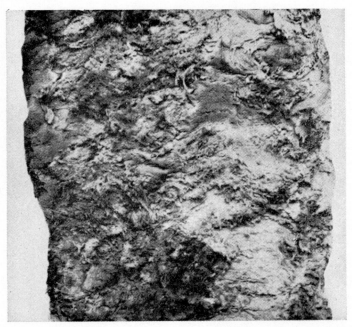

Fig. 57. Colon of acute bacillary dysentery: stage of sloughing and beginning ulceration.

tion beginning on the summits of the intestinal folds and often extending deep into the submucosa and sometimes into the muscularis (Fig. 57).

This process is usually not uniformly distributed throughout the colon, tending to be most acute in the distal portion. It may involve the lower ileum. Perforation is rare. With development of the ulcerated lesions secondary bacterial infection occurs which may participate importantly, especially in a subsequent chronic stage of the disease.

In cases of long duration adjacent ulcers may be connected by ulcerating channels beneath bridges of more or less hyperplastic mucosa. In chronic recurrent cases there is much fibrosis of the mucosa and submucosa, the epithelium losing its normal glandular structure. Epithelial cyst-like structures may be formed in the mucosa as the result of imperfect healing. These mucus retention cysts have been found to retain the bacilli and they may be responsible for the intermittent discharge of organisms so characteristic of the chronic carrier state (Fig. 58).

**Clinical Characteristics** The incubation period of the disease may vary from twenty-four hours to a week or more. In the early stages of an outbreak cases may appear to be mild and to be merely instances of simple diarrhea. Certain of these, however, may suddenly

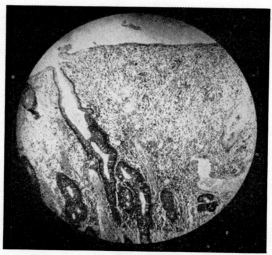

Fig. 58. Colon of chronic bacillary dysentery showing fibrosis and distortion of gland tubules.

be transformed into the acute or even fulminant types of the disease. Variations in severity have led to the classification of cases into the following *clinical types:*

1. Mild or catarrhal dysentery.
2. Acute dysentery.
3. Fulminant dysentery.
4. Relapsing dysentery.
5. Chronic dysentery.

In the usual case the onset is abrupt and accompanied by fever which may reach 104° F. Diarrhea appears promptly and the stools may number from twenty to forty in twenty-four hours. The evacuations, at first feculent, contain increasing amounts of blood and mucus and in the fully developed severe form of the disease may ultimately consist only of frequently evacuated small masses of sticky gelatinous bloodstained mucus which contain the characteristic cellular exudate and enormous numbers of the dysentery bacilli. Abdominal pain may be severe, the evacuations involuntary and accompanied by intense tenesmus.

Proctoscopic examination reveals a swollen diffusely inflamed mucosa often largely covered with muco-pus. When this exudate is removed the mucous membrane underlying it presents a somewhat granular surface which oozes blood freely. Gross ulceration may or

Fig. 59.

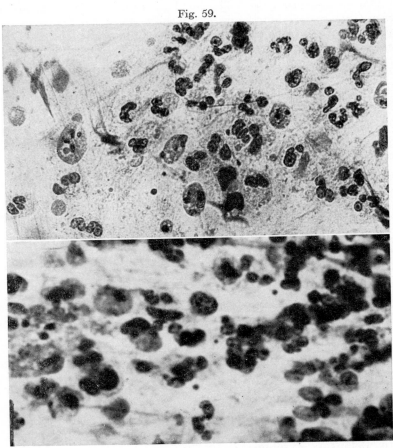

Fig. 60.

Fig. 59. Early exudate in stool showing polymorphonuclear leukocytes and macro-phage cells, one of which resembles an ameba with extruded pseudopod.
Fig. 60. Exudate in stage of ulceration: macrophage cells and many polymorpho-nuclear leukocytes, and erythrocytes.

may not be present. When present, the ulcers are usually shallow, irregular in size and shape, and covered with purulent exudate.

In the fulminating type of the disease collapse is not uncommon and the abrupt onset may be accompanied by chill, high fever and vomiting, followed shortly by falling temperature, profound toxemia and death.

In mild cases the stools may remain feculent throughout and may or may not contain gross blood and mucus. Even in the mildest cases, however, microscopic examination of the feces will reveal the characteristic cellular exudate composed of red corpuscles, many polymorphonuclear leukocytes and varying numbers of macrophage cells. The latter may contain erythrocytes and cell debris and be suggestive of nonmotile forms of *Endamoeba histolytica*. This possible confusion, however, is eliminated by the examination of stained smears, since the cell nuclei are usually degenerated and do not resemble those of the ameba (Figs. 59, 60).

Prior to the advent of sulfonamide therapy the average mortality from acute bacillary dysentery was from 4 to 5 per cent. Under epidemic conditions when the Shiga bacillus was the responsible organism the mortality has been as high as 50 per cent.

## Acute Bacillary Dysentery

*Diagnosis* The diagnosis of acute bacillary dysentery is based upon the demonstration of an inflammatory cellular exudate in the stools, the characteristic appearance of the mucous membrane as seen through the proctoscope, and recovery of the dysentery bacilli. The agglutination reaction is of no use for early diagnosis and is not dependable in later cases. The white blood count varies from normal to 15,000 or higher, with elevation of polymorphonuclear elements.

*Treatment* Experience with acute bacillary dysentery during World War II and more recently in Korea has led to material changes in treatment. These are the result of accumulated observations of the limitations of the sulfonamide drugs and evaluation of the antibiotics as specific therapeutic agents. There are three primary indications:

1. Early and intensive specific antibiotic or chemotherapy.
2. Correction and prevention of dehydration.
3. Control of toxemia.

1. SPECIFIC THERAPY. Recent experience with severe cases of acute bacillary dysentery in Korea has demonstrated that eradication of the *Shigella* infection is best accomplished by the use of oxytetracycline (Terramycin), aureomycin or chloramphenicol (Chloromycetin). Relatively small amounts administered within twenty-four hours have given as good results as larger doses administered over a longer period of time. These antibiotic agents appear to be equally effective against the various types of *Shigella,* and resistant strains have not been encountered. The recommended dosage of each of these antibiotics is as follows:

Initial dose, 2.0 gm.; subsequent doses, 1.0 gm. after twelve and twenty-four hours.

On this regimen almost all cases become bacteriologically negative before the seventh day. Sigmoidoscopic examination reveals that the active colitis is controlled within four to five days and symptoms are brought under control with equal rapidity.

Prior to the introduction of the antibiotic agents, sulfonamide therapy had been demonstrated to be the most effective method of treatment. However, certain strains of *Shigella*, notably of *S. sonnei*, showed relatively high initial resistance to these drugs. Furthermore, drug-resistant strains of various types were encountered with increasing frequency especially when large numbers of patients were treated with insufficient amounts and when these drugs were used for mass prophylaxis. These observations, together with the experience in Korea, have relegated the sulfonamide drugs to second place in the selection of therapeutic agents. When they are used, their effectiveness should be controlled by in vitro sensitivity tests and, in the presence of resistant strains, treatment with one of the antibiotics should be substituted.

Sulfonamide therapy must be instituted early and must be intensive if optimal results are to be obtained. It should be continued until clinical recovery has been achieved, the stools no longer contain an inflammatory exudate, stool cultures are negative, and until proctoscopic examination and x-ray examination of the colon demonstrate complete healing.

The soluble sulfonamides, sulfadiazine and sufathiazole, are considered to be more effective than the insoluble compounds sulfaguanidine and Sulfasuxidine. In the hot countries, however, the former must be used with caution and with strict attention to the urinary output because of the hazard of renal tubular obstruction. Fluid intake must be adjusted to yield a minimal urine output of 1500 ml. each twenty-four hours if renal complications are to be avoided. Maintenance of an alkaline urine during the period of sulfonamide therapy has been recommended as an auxiliary protective measure. However, it is doubtful if this is necessary if an adequate fluid balance is established and maintained. Furthermore, administration of alkalis may increase the rate of sulfonamide excretion and thereby reduce the effectiveness of the drug.

The sulfonamide drugs of choice in the order of effectiveness and the recommended dosages are as follows:

Sulfadiazine: initial dose, 2.0 gm.; 1.0 gm. every six hours thereafter.

Sulfathiazole: initial dose, 2.0 gm.; 1.0 gm. every six hours thereafter.

Sulfaguanidine: 5.0 gm. every six hours.

Sulfasuxidine: 5.0 gm. every six hours.

2. CONTROL OF DEHYDRATION. Dehydration and disturbance of electrolyte balance may occur rapidly in acute cases and may be severe, especially in infants and in the hot tropics. A large fluid intake should be instituted early and maintained at a level sufficient to insure a daily urine output in excess of 1500 ml. Electrolyte replacement therapy is frequently essential in the severe cases.

3. CONTROL OF TOXEMIA. In most instances the toxemia may be controlled by adequate administration of fluids.

Polyvalent antisera are of little if any value. In the rare severe cases of infection by *S. dysenteriae* 1 (Shiga's bacillus), specific monovalent antiserum may have a temporary beneficial effect. Such sera, however, are neither bactericidal nor bacteriostatic. It is doubtful if antisera have a place in the treatment of bacillary dysentery, especially when the rapidly acting antibiotic agents are immediately available.

If an antiserum is to be used, however, the patient must invariably be tested for sensitivity. The dose should be from 40 to 80 ml. diluted in 500 ml. of physiologic saline solution and given intravenously in severe cases, or intramuscularly in less fulminant cases, twice daily until the desired therapeutic effect is obtained. The antitoxic action of adequate dosage of serum usually becomes evident within a few hours.

The general measures of treatment include strict bed rest, an easily assimilated diet rich in protein and vitamins, and administration of sedatives as required. If sulfonamide therapy is to be used, daily administration in small dosage of a mild saline cathartic should be begun early in the acute stage of the disease and continued until the criteria of cure have been attained. This prevents injury to the inflamed mucous membrane by hard masses of fecal material. Sodium sulfate is the cathartic of choice, and for the average adult should be given in doses of approximately 4 gm. in 200 ml. of hot water each morning. This measure is unnecessary for cases which respond rapidly and completely to antibiotic therapy. However, if healing is incomplete and sigmoidoscopic examination reveals a persisting inflammatory reaction, it should be instituted to protect the mucosa from mechanical trauma.

## Chronic Bacillary Dysentery

*Pathology* Chronic bacillary dysentery is characterized pathologically by scarring of the colon, indolent ulceration, and continued subacute or chronic inflammation which periodically becomes acute. The dysentery bacilli in many instances are no longer demonstrable and there is extensive secondary infection by other intestinal bacteria which appear to play an important role in the maintenance of active pathology.

It is said that approximately 2½ per cent of the acute bacillary dysenteries among the British troops in the first World War became chronic with persisting disability. Although the extensive use of sulfonamide therapy during World War II greatly diminished the incidence of the chronic disease, it has not been eliminated. However, the greater effectiveness of the antibiotics and the rapid healing which accompanies their use should materially reduce the prevalence of chronic bacillary dysentery when specific treatment is instituted early.

*Clinical Characteristics* The chronic forms of the disease are usually characterized by successive periods of exacerbation and remission. Both clinically and pathologically they differ little if at all from certain types of so-called idiopathic ulcerative colitis. The periods of active disease are accompanied by fever and diarrhea with varying amounts of blood, mucus, and the characteristic cellular exudate in the stools. Macrophages, however, may be rare. Each period of activity contributes still further to the extensive scarring and fibrosis of the colon.

A variety of factors appears to contribute to the disease. In many instances there is disturbance of normal motor function with undue retention in the right half of the colon. Primary and secondary nutritional deficiencies are common and important. In many instances these are due to restriction of diet and in others to the inability of the patient to take sufficient amounts of protective foods. A significant proportion of these cases appear to develop sensitization of the colon to particular foodstuffs, notably milk, and inclusion of the particular food in the diet is followed by continued activity of the disease or even increased severity. It appears probable likewise that there is a similar sensitization to certain bacterial proteins. These factors together with the extensive and varied secondary bacterial infection complicate clinical management and greatly affect the prognosis.

**Treatment**    The treatment of chronic bacillary dysentery is commonly difficult and must be varied to meet the indications in the particular individual.

Dietary management is especially important. Possible harmful effects of roughage have been overemphasized and have led to dietary restriction of such nature as to produce serious secondary malnutrition.

Antibacterial therapy using the sulfonamides, Terramycin, aureomycin or Chloromycetin may be important. The antibiotics, however, should not be administered over long periods of time because of the effect on the normal intestinal bacterial flora and the hazard of establishing a secondary *Monilia* infection.

There is commonly functional disturbance of the colon with stasis on the right side which tends to increase symptoms. In most instances this is easily controlled by the daily administration of small amounts of sodium sulfate.

The possible role of sensitization to particular foods must be kept in mind. Skin tests are useless for the identification of this complication and reliance must be placed entirely on the use of test diets.

## Prophylaxis of Bacillary Dysentery

In the prophylaxis of bacillary dysentery particular precautions must be taken with respect to the isolation of patients and to the sterilization of bedding, clothing and other articles which have been in contact with them. Adequate disinfection and disposal of the stools are essential. Control of food handlers, the establishment of clean water and milk supplies, sanitary sewage disposal, and the elimination of flies are of fundamental importance. The sequence of feces to flies or fingers to mouth must be interrupted.

Ice manufactured from untreated water is an important factor in the transmission of the pathogenic intestinal bacteria.

In areas where a safe water supply is not available all drinking water should be boiled. Under field conditions chemical sterilization is reasonably effective for small quantities. For this purpose 1 drop of 7.5 per cent tincture of iodine should be added to each quart of water, or two or more tablets, 130 mg. each, of Halazone (*p*-sulfonedichloramido-benzoic acid) with thorough shaking to insure solution. Effective amounts of the latter impart a distinct odor and taste of chlorine to the water which after a contact period of thirty minutes may be removed by the addition of 35 mg. of sodium sulfite followed by thorough shaking.

Under special conditions and for brief periods when the disease is highly endemic or epidemic, sulfadiazine 0.5 gm. or sulfaguanidine 0.5 gm. every twelve hours may be used as a prophylactic agent. However, the possible prevalence of sulfonamide-resistant strains must be remembered. Similarly, if the antibiotics are used for prophylactic purposes, administration must be restricted to limited periods of time. There is no effective vaccine.

# 21 Food Poisoning

**Definition** Food poisoning is an inclusive term used to define a symptom complex. The usual types are characterized by acute gastro-enteritis with sudden onset of vomiting or diarrhea, or both, and abdominal pain, in some instances with fever, in others with prostration and shock. The duration is variable depending upon the etiology. An attack is frequently followed by instability and irritability of the gastro-intestinal tract in convalescence. The general mortality is approximately 1.5 per cent.

**Distribution** The disease is protean, occurring in epidemic outbreaks wherever groups of individuals are exposed to the factors responsible.

**Etiology** The causes of food poisoning fall into three categories:
1. Foods contaminated with metallic or other poisons.
2. Foods inherently toxic or poisonous.
3. Foods contaminated with certain bacteria.
    *a.* Infections, with or without intoxications.
    *b.* Intoxications without infection.

Foods contaminated with metallic poisons are relatively uncommon causes of food poisoning (Table 10).

A variety of substances used for human food may be inherently poisonous. These include certain plants, fruits, fish and shellfish. The more common causes of this type of food poisoning are listed in Table 11.

It is wise to consult with the native population before eating unfamiliar foods.

Contamination of food by bacteria, however, is the most important cause of food poisoning. Many of these become established in the in-

*Table 10   Metallic Poisons*

| CHEMICAL | FOOD | SYMPTOMS | ONSET |
|---|---|---|---|
| Antimony | Foods cooked in gray-enameled or galvanized utensils | Vomiting | Few minutes to 1 hour |
| Cadmium | Liquids prepared in cadmium plated refrigerator trays, pitchers and other utensils | Vomiting, abdominal cramps, diarrhea | 15–30 minutes |
| Sodium cyanide | Used in cleaning silver | Weakness, coma, respiratory failure | Few minutes |
| Sodium fluoride | Roach powder mistaken for baking powder or soda, or powdered milk | Vomiting, abdominal pain, diarrhea, convulsions, paresis | Few minutes to 2 hours |
| Zinc | Acid foods or drink (apples, lemonade) prepared in galvanized iron utensils | Astringent taste, pain in mouth and throat, gastric distress, vomiting, abdominal pain, diarrhea | Few minutes, or symptoms may be delayed as in food infections |

testinal tract causing true infections. Others in the course of proliferation within the food form toxic substances and the symptoms which result after ingestion are those of a true intoxication rather than infection. Ptomaines, which were formerly considered important in this latter group, are now recognized to be nontoxic when taken by mouth. The common groups of food poisoning due to bacterial agents appear in Table 12.

The bacterial type of food poisoning is the one most commonly encountered and will be the only one considered in detail.

**Botulism**   Botulism is a true intoxication produced by the exotoxin formed by *Clostridium botulinum* types A, B and E. These are anaerobic spore-bearing bacilli widely distributed in soil. A soluble toxin is produced which is inactivated by boiling for 10 minutes. The spores, however, are extremely resistant. The organisms are proteolytic, often but not invariably producing an offensive odor.

This type of poisoning is acquired by the ingestion of contaminated canned or preserved foods in which bacterial proliferation and toxin formation have occurred. Such foods exhibiting any indication of gas formation or change in appearance should be rejected without tasting, since severe effects may follow the ingestion of even minute amounts.

Botulism is characterized by an acute encephalitis, and interference with the parasympathetic system, leading particularly to cranial

### Table 11  Poisonous Foods

| FOOD | CAUSE | SYMPTOMS | ONSET |
|---|---|---|---|
| Fish | Unknown—occurs in many regions | Abdominal cramps and nervous symptoms | Few minutes |
| Shellfish (mussels and clams) | Dinoflagellates, Pacific coast U. S. A. | Numbness of lips, respiratory and motor paralysis | 5–30 minutes |
| Fava bean (or inhalation of pollen) | "Favism" | Fever, anemia, hematuria, jaundice | Within 1 hour |
| Milk from cows which have eaten snakeroot | Trematol or "alkali poisoning," not destroyed by pasteurization | Vomiting, colic, constipation | Variable, after repeated use |
| Mushrooms, toadstools, etc. | Alkaloids from 80 species | Vomiting, colic, diarrhea, convulsions | 6–15 hours |
| Rye | Ergot—a parasitic fungus | Gangrene of ears, toes, fingers; headache, convulsions, itching | Gradual after several meals |
| Water hemlock | Toxin from leaves and root | Vomiting, convulsions | 1–2 hours |
| Raw sprouted potatoes | Toxin (solanin?) | Vomiting, diarrhea, disturbed vision | ? |
| Rhubarb leaves | Oxalic acid | Vomiting, colic, diarrhea | 2 hours |

### Table 12  Bacterial Food Poisoning*

| DISEASE | AGENT | TYPE | SYMPTOMS | ONSET |
|---|---|---|---|---|
| Botulism | Exotoxin of *Clostridium botulinum* | Intoxication | Difficulty in swallowing, double vision, aphonia, respiratory paralysis | 18 hours to 3–4 days |
| Staphylococcus food poisoning | Enterotoxin from staphylococci | Intoxication | Vomiting, diarrhea, abdominal cramps, prostration | 1–6 hours |
| Salmonella food poisoning | *S. typhimurium, S. enteritidis, S. choleraesuis,* etc. | Infection, intoxication | Abdominal pain, chills, fever, diarrhea, vomiting | 7–72 hours |
| Streptococcus food poisoning | Lancefield's groups A, C, D, and G | Infection ? | Nausea, colic, diarrhea | 5–18 hours |

* Adapted from Dack, G. N.: Food Poisoning, Chicago, University of Chicago Press, 1943.

nerve palsies and respiratory paralysis. The *onset* may occur as early as eighteen hours after ingestion, and death may result in four to eight days, rarely earlier. Recovery is probable if the individual survives the ninth day. Aspiration pneumonia is frequent. The mortality rate is 60 to 70 per cent.

*Serum therapy* should be used if serum is available.

**Staphylococcus Food Poisoning** Varieties of *Staphylococcus*, usually hemolytic strains of *Staphylococcus aureus*, produce an enterotoxin which is an important cause of food poisoning. The toxin is thermostable and is not destroyed by boiling for thirty minutes nor by refrigeration for long periods. Certain of the strains will proliferate at icebox temperatures and others will grow in media having a salt content equivalent to that of the brine used in pickling hams (10 per cent sodium chloride plus 1 per cent potassium nitrate). Food contaminated with these organisms has no abnormal odor or taste.

*Epidemiology* The staphylococcus food poisonings in most instances are due to contamination of food by infected humans. This may be by droplet infection from foci in the respiratory tract or by direct inoculation with exudate from cutaneous staphylococcus infections such as furunculosis and impetigo. The foods most commonly involved in outbreaks of food poisoning due to these organisms are milk, custard and cream-filled pastries, minced meat, cured and "tenderized" hams, and sandwiches and salads containing mayonnaise or cream.

*Clinical Characteristics* The clinical response to this form of food poisoning is a true intoxication and not an infection. The onset is usually abrupt, acute and occurs within six hours after ingestion. The symptoms are characteristic, consisting of severe epigastric pain accompanied by continuous and even projectile vomiting and retching, in the severe cases with blood in the vomitus. Prostration, shock and syncope are not uncommon. Diarrhea may or may not occur. No inflammatory exudate has been found in the stools. Since this type of poisoning is the reaction to an enterotoxin which acts as a severe gastro-intestinal irritant, it is usually of short duration and terminates with elimination of the toxin and toxin-containing food.

*Treatment* Treatment is symptomatic. In severe cases the vomiting may produce marked dehydration and loss of chlorides which must be replaced by the intravenous administration of appropriate amounts of physiologic saline solution.

**Streptococcus Food Poisoning** Outbreaks of food poisoning rarely have been traced to contamination of food with species of *Streptococcus*, especially strains of Lancefield's groups A, C, D and G.

The epidemiology of these infections is similar to that of staphylococcus poisoning.

No true toxin is formed. The symptoms apparently are the result of actual infection of the intestinal tract. After a period of five to twelve hours there are nausea, occasionally vomiting, abdominal pain, cramps and diarrhea.

Treatment should include early purgation by repeated small doses of magnesium sulfate or sodium sulfate, rest and soft diet. If there is evidence of continuing infection, sulfonamide or antibiotic therapy should be considered.

**Salmonella Food Poisoning**  The most common form of bacterial food poisoning is that produced by certain members of the genus *Salmonella*. These organisms are commonly parasites of animals and birds, frequently infecting rats and mice. *Salmonella* food poisoning in man may be the expression of a true intoxication produced by food that contains products of the bacilli but no viable organisms. In other instances ingestion of food containing viable organisms is followed by actual infection of the intestinal tract. The resulting enteritis is usually of shorter duration than that produced by the *Shigella*. It is commonly self-limited and usually terminates without a prolonged carrier state. Occasionally, however, chronic infection occurs with persisting ulceration of the colon.

**Etiology**  The organisms most commonly encountered and their hosts are:

| Salmonella Species | Hosts |
|---|---|
| S. typhimurium (S. aertrycke) | Mice, rats, man |
| S. enteritidis (Gaertner's bacillus) | Cattle |
| S. choleraesuis (S. suipestifer) | Hogs |
| S. paratyphi B. (S. schottmülleri) | Man |
| S. paratyphi A | Man |

**Epidemiology**  Rats and mice are naturally subject to outbreaks of *Salmonella* infection and when these rodents have access to human food, contamination by their urine and feces may occur. Larger mammals are often infected with *S. enteritidis*, *S. typhimurium* or *S. choleraesuis*. Ingestion of meat from such infected animals is productive of disease in man. This is one of the important reasons for ante-mortem inspection of meat.

Unpasteurized milk and cheese are likewise common vehicles of this group of organisms, and the housefly having access to *Salmonella*-containing material may transmit them to human food. In other instances symptomless or relatively healthy human carriers working as food handlers may be responsible for outbreaks.

The foods most commonly found to be sources of outbreaks of *Salmonella* food poisoning have been made-up meats (*S. enteritidis*), sausage (*S. choleraesuis*), or salami, meat sandwiches, milk and milk products, mayonnaise and mixed salads, especially chicken salad (*S. typhimurium*), and smoked or pickled fish.

Outbreaks are usually explosive in character, affecting all or nearly all individuals who have partaken of the contaminated food. This characteristic is an important feature in the differentiation of food poisoning from infections by the *Shigella*.

**Clinical Characteristics**  The incubation period is variable, since the *Salmonella* may produce poisoning without infection, or may produce true infection of the intestinal tract. In the former instance symptoms occur within a few hours after ingestion of the contaminated food. When the syndrome is the expression of active infection, however, it is more prolonged and the clinical phenomena likewise are of longer duration.

In the majority of instances, after an interval of six to seventy-two hours violent diarrhea occurs, often with incontinence and accompanied by severe cramps and tenesmus. In the presence of active infection examination of the stools will yield, in most instances, the causative organism and microscopic study will demonstrate the presence of erythrocytes, polymorphonuclear leukocytes and macrophages. Nausea and vomiting may or may not occur. In the more acute forms fever may be present and there may be considerable prostration. The acute stage of food poisoning due to salmonella infection cannot be distinguished clinically from infections by the *Shigella*.

*Salmonella* food poisoning due to ingestion of bacterial products without infection may present the same symptoms. Both the incubation period and the duration of the clinical phenomena tend to be shorter, cultures are negative, and an inflammatory exudate has not been observed in the stools.

**Treatment**   Treatment should include purgation with magnesium sulfate or sodium sulfate, provided the patient is seen in the early stages of the attack. If, on the other hand, severe diarrhea has persisted for two or three days, purgation is of doubtful value. If the episode is accompanied by vomiting the administration of parenteral fluids may be necessary. In cases of established infection one of the sulfonamide drugs may be useful although they are less effective against *Salmonella* than against *Shigella*. The antibiotics, including aureomycin, Chloromycetin and Terramycin likewise frequently fail to modify significantly the course of the infection.

## Diagnosis and Prophylaxis of Food Poisoning

**Diagnosis**   The occurrence of food poisoning should be suspected when several individuals are seized with acute symptoms within a few hours or within a day or two of having had a meal in common. In the investigation of such outbreaks early study is of the utmost urgency.

A list must be prepared of all the foods served and specific information must be obtained from every individual as to which of the foods were taken. It is important to bear in mind, however, that such tabular investigation will often fail to identify clearly the offending food.

Foods which are under suspicion should be obtained for bacteriologic examination and, similarly, cultures should be made of the vomitus, stools and blood of each patient during the acute phase.

**Prophylaxis** The prevention of the bacterial types of food poisoning is dependent upon proper methods for the storage of food, satisfactory sanitation of the kitchen and icebox, sterilization of kitchen utensils and tableware, and inspection of food handlers. It is particularly important that rats, mice, and flies be prevented from gaining access to human food.

Such products as sausage and tenderized hams should be thoroughly cooked. Dishes prepared some hours in advance of the meal at which they are to be served must be stored at low temperatures in efficient iceboxes. Foods which are apt to become contaminated and have been frequently incriminated as causes of food poisoning, such as meat sandwiches or potato salad, should not be held at room temperature for more than three hours prior to consumption.

Kitchen personnel must be inspected for the presence of staphylococcus or streptococcus infections of the skin and be eliminated from the kitchen until the lesions have healed. Intestinal disturbances among food handlers must be reported and promptly investigated by appropriate bacteriologic techniques. Individuals infected with pathogenic organisms commonly transmitted by food or drink should not be employed in the preparation or serving of food. Proper attention to these measures will afford relatively great protection.

# 22 Cholera

**Synonyms** Asiatic cholera, Indian cholera.

**Definition** Asiatic cholera is an acute infectious disease caused by *Vibrio comma* and characterized by profuse and purging diarrhea, vomiting, extreme dehydration, muscle cramps, suppression of urine, collapse and, in a high proportion of untreated cases, death. The organism is present in the intestine and in the rice water stools during the acute stage. It multiplies especially in the small intestine and, undergoing lysis, liberates an endotoxin which is responsible for desquamation of the superficial epithelium of the mucosa and for other toxic manifestations of the disease.

**Distribution** The disease is widely endemic in Asia and the Far East. Most of the pandemics have originated in India, especially on the delta of the Ganges River which is the important persisting focus. There is scarcely a country of the world that has not at some time been visited by cholera. In recent years the most important outbreaks outside India and China have been in Russia and the Ukraine except for a severe epidemic in Egypt in 1947 with some 21,000 cases and a death rate of approximately 50 per cent.

The present major endemic centers are the Ganges Delta in lower

Bengal, and in China the Yuan River valley, Hunan in the upper Yangtze basin and areas adjacent to certain ports.

**Etiology**    *Vibrio comma* (*V. cholerae, Spirillum cholerae*), the comma bacillus, is a short curved organism often appearing S-shaped due to end-to-end attachment of two vibrios. It possesses a long terminal flagellum. It is gram-negative and actively motile.

**Cultural Characteristics**    The vibrio is strictly aerobic, growing readily on ordinary media having a *p*H from 7.0 to 9.0. Growth is inhibited by moderate acidity. A typical strain exhibits significant characteristics in culture. The more important include liquefaction of gelatin and coagulated blood serum, production of indole and reduction of nitrates to nitrites, which is responsible for the cholera red reaction. Glucose, maltose and saccharose are fermented without the formation of gas. Xylose and arabinose are not fermented and fermentation of lactose is absent or late.

*Vibrio comma* has little resistance to disinfecting agents or to drying. It is rapidly overgrown by other organisms and is not long demonstrable in water heavily contaminated with sewage. In ordinary river water, however, it will survive for one to two weeks and for as long as a month in spring water. The organisms remain viable in stools for one to two days in summer and up to a week in cold weather.

*Vibrio comma* produces a powerful endotoxin which is released when the vibrio undergoes disintegration. This appears to be responsible for the desquamation of intestinal epithelial cells and probably for some of the toxic phenomena of the disease. There is no proven exotoxin.

Different strains of the organism vary widely in colony morphology, in motility and in biochemical activity. Final identification depends, therefore, upon agglutination in specific monovalent "O" antigen serum.

Numerous other free-living vibrios inhabiting water have been found in man. These may exhibit the same staining and cultural characteristics as the true *V. comma*. Moreover, nonagglutinating strains are commonly found in man in endemic areas during interepidemic periods. Their significance is uncertain.

**Epidemiology**    Infection is acquired by ingestion of *V. comma* with food or drink. The reservoir consists of healthy carriers, infected individuals during the incubation period, and patients with mild or acute disease. In the presence of outbreaks 1 to 10 per cent of the healthy population of the area may be carriers. The period of excretion of vibrios by such individuals usually does not persist beyond seven to ten days but may continue for three weeks to two months. In general, it is said, 97 per cent of carriers become vibriofree within one month.

The organisms are rarely excreted in the feces of acute cases for more than seven to ten days and often for lesser periods.

Spread of the disease, as in the great pandemics, has always taken place along trade routes. Pilgrimages have frequently been intimately related to epidemic outbreaks and wide extension. Local dissemination down the river valleys commonly occurs in endemic areas, probably as a result of the contamination of water. Circumscribed outbreaks are associated with contaminated water supply and food and with exposure to fomites.

In the endemic regions climatic influences seem to be important. In India most epidemics have been preceded by failure of the rains. In Bengal the maximal incidence is in the hot dry months from March to June when the water supply is most limited and presumably most highly contaminated. In other areas epidemics not uncommonly follow sudden heavy rains and floods with their dispersal of human excreta.

In towns and cities two types of outbreak due to water transmission occur. When the general water supply is contaminated the outbreak is widespread and explosive. When, on the other hand, it originates from contamination of isolated wells, the cases are local or sporadic.

Contamination of food is an important factor in transmission. Food handled by infected persons is dangerous; so, also, is the ingestion of uncooked foods, vegetables and salads, especially lettuce and celery which have been fertilized with night soil or freshened with contaminated water. Milk is a common vehicle. The widespread practice in the Orient of eating uncooked or lightly cooked shellfish and fish also provides a ready means of transmission. Flies and cockroaches may be important vectors. Although the vibrios are usually rapidly destroyed in the fly's gut they may be recovered from the insect's feces for two to twelve hours.

**Pathology**   The pathology of cholera is essentially an acute intestinal intoxication leading to profound dehydration and chemical imbalance within the body. A severe or fatal toxic nephritis with little organic change may occur. In the intestinal tract there is desquamation of epithelial cells without ulcer formation and the vibrios are rarely found deeper than the superficial layer of epithelium.

In fatal cases the prominent findings are early rigor mortis and extreme shrinkage and dryness of the tissues evidenced particularly by the shrunken face and eyeballs and "washerwoman's" fingers. The subcutaneous tissue and muscles are dry; the peritoneum is dry, sticky and dull with the exception of the layer covering the ileum which is usually congested. The spleen is small and dry. The lumen of the intestine may be filled with the characteristic rice water transudate.

The serious manifestations of the disease are to be found in the field of clinical pathology. Loss of fluids is extreme and electrolytes are also depleted with relatively great loss of base and consequent diminution of the alkali reserve. The sodium chloride loss may exceed 50 gm. in twenty-four hours. The specific gravity of the blood may be increased from a normal of 1.056–1.058 to above 1.070. Concentration of the blood is further indicated by high values for the red cell count and hemoglobin percentage.

The degrees of salt and water depletion vary in different cases and at different stages of the disease. Although both exist in most cases and both are associated with dehydration, their effects are somewhat antagonistic.

In predominant water depletion thirst is prominent and urine output reduced. The sodium chloride and urea content of the blood are normal or elevated and the plasma volume normal until the late stages of dehydration.

When salt depletion predominates, thirst is absent, the urine output remains normal until late and sodium chloride is absent from the urine. The plasma chlorides are decreased, the blood urea elevated and plasma volume decreased. Vomiting and cramps occur, the blood pressure falls progressively, and shock develops from peripheral circulatory failure. These changes are accompanied by a pronounced and progressive acidosis which results from the accumulation of normal metabolic endproducts and the extreme loss of base. In severe cases there may be complete suppression of urine followed by uremia and death.

**Clinical Characteristics** The disease classically presents four clinical stages. The stage of incubation lasting one to three or four days is the least definite and may or may not be accompanied by mild or increasing diarrhea.

The incubation period is followed by the stage of evacuation. A typical attack as observed in epidemic outbreaks commonly presents an abrupt onset with the rapid development of progressive purging, vomiting and muscle cramps.

In severe infections this second phase is followed by an algid or collapse stage in which death commonly occurs. In the event of survival the fourth stage, that of reaction, appears accompanied by rise of temperature and progressive lessening of symptoms.

The stage of evacuation is dominated by purging, vomiting, muscle cramps and exhaustion. The stools, at first feculent, soon present the appearance of "rice water" and are passed without cramps or tenesmus. Several liters of fluid may be lost in twenty-four hours. Profuse, continuous vomiting and retching and often uncontrollable hiccough appear early in the second stage. The appearance of the patient changes rapidly owing to dehydration and progressive shrinking of the tissues, especially of the face and the extremities. The rectal temperature usually does not exceed 100° or 102° F.

In serious cases after a period of two to twelve hours the patient passes into the algid stage, or stage of collapse, which may persist for a few hours to several days. The purging and vomiting often cease and the clinical picture is essentially that of profound shock. Muscle cramps commonly continue and are severe, involving many muscle groups. This stage is dominated by failure of the circulation with increasing tachycardia, cyanosis and progressively falling blood pressure. The body as a whole is shrunken, the surface cold and the temperature usually below normal. There is oliguria with albuminuria and, in very severe cases, anuria. Consciousness is retained until the onset of terminal coma.

In the stage of reaction acute symptoms disappear, the stools become less liquid and their bile coloring returns. In favorable cases recovery may occur within a week. In others urinary secretion is not restored and progressive nephritis with rapidly increasing uremia may supervene. In other instances a typhoidal state develops.

In the presence of an epidemic of cholera a wide variety of clinical types may be encountered. These vary from ambulatory cases with only mild gastro-intestinal symptoms to the fulminating "cholera sicca" in which early death occurs without diarrhea or vomiting.

**Diagnosis** When cholera is prevalent in an area all intestinal disturbances, particularly those accompanied by diarrhea, must be considered as possible instances of the disease. The classic clinical picture is so characteristic that little difficulty should be encountered in its identification. Microscopic examination of the colorless albuminous fluid stools reveals epithelial and mononuclear cells and small flecks of mucus, but no true inflammatory exudate. The vibrios may likewise be seen.

Definitive diagnosis is based upon recovery of *V. comma:* selective media such as alkaline nutrient agar, Aronson's, a modified Wilson and Riley's solid media, or Read's modification of Wilson and Blair's fluid enrichment medium should be used for primary isolation. Final identification of the organism must be based upon agglutination in specific antisera containing the somatic or "O" agglutinins.

**Treatment** Replacement of fluids and electrolytes is the most essential feature of the treatment of cholera. Although certain sulfonamides, chloramphenicol (Chloromycetin) and oxytetracycline (Terramycin) cause rapid disappearance of the vibrios from the stools, they do not alter the clinical course nor significantly affect the mortality rate. Plasma and whole blood are seldom necessary and may be very harmful. They should be given only when specific indications exist.

The blood pressure, pulse rate and volume, color and consistency of the blood and the urine output are dependable clinical indications of the amounts of fluids required. Excess fluid is dangerous and is indicated clinically by palpitation, restlessness, chest pain, coughing and edema. As the blood specific gravity approaches normal, 1.056–1.058, administration must be reduced or discontinued.

Alkali deficit develops early and severe acidosis is frequent. Clinical appraisal is difficult. The type and rate of respiration are not dependable guides. Ketone bodies are not necessarily present in the urine in the acidosis of cholera. However, urine volume and acidity

are helpful within limits. The most accurate guides to the requirements for alkali are the *p*H, the carbon dioxide combining power
and the urea content of the blood.

Repeated determinations of blood specific gravity provide the most
accurate control of fluid administration. Roger's technique offers a
simple method. A series of solutions of glycerin and distilled water is
used. The specific gravities lie 0.002 apart, from 1.050 to 1.070 (i.e.,
1.050, 1.052, 1.054, etc.). Ten to 15 ml. of each solution is placed in
individual small bottles. A drop of blood is introduced into each container; the specific gravity of the blood is that of the solution in which
the drop neither rises to the top nor sinks to the bottom.

A newer method utilizes copper sulfate solutions; these expand
with changes in temperature at the same rate as does blood, thereby
eliminating errors inherent in the glycerin technique. The copper
sulfate is supplied by the U. S. Army in measured quantities with
instructions for preparing the appropriate dilutions.

Fluids should be administered intravenously during the active
stage and there should be no hesitation in cutting down on a vein and
inserting an indwelling cannula. Patients with cholera require relatively large amounts of fluid. Intravenous therapy may be required
for forty-eight hours. The following fluids are recommended:

1. Physiologic saline solution:
    In the less severe and uncomplicated cases and in the absence
    of severe acidosis and collapse physiologic saline solution
    may be adequate. It may be necessary to administer 1000
    ml. every four hours as determined by the criteria for fluid
    requirements.
2. Hypertonic saline solution:

    Sodium chloride ..................... 14.0 gm.
    Distilled water ..................... 1000 ml.

3. Alkaline saline solution:

    Sodium chloride ..................... 6.0 gm.
    Sodium bicarbonate ................. 18.0 gm.
    Distilled water ..................... 1000 ml.

This solution must not be sterilized by boiling or autoclaving since such procedures
change the bicarbonate to the caustic carbonate. The following technique may
be utilized: Dissolve the sodium chloride in distilled water and sterilize by boiling.
Remove from the heater and immediately add the sodium bicarbonate taken directly from the original container and weighed under sterile conditions. The solution should be cooled to body temperature or slightly higher and used immediately.

REPLACEMENT OF FLUIDS AND ELECTROLYTES. A total of 2000 ml.
of fluid should be given in the first two hours as follows:

500 ml. alkaline saline solution followed by 1500 ml. physiologic
saline solution. It is desirable but not essential to add to this solution
75 gm. glucose and 3 mg. thiamine hydrochloride.

Thereafter, physiologic saline solution should be administered in amounts as indicated up to 1000 ml. every three to four hours until the specific gravity of the blood approaches normal.

Additional alkaline saline solution may be required to control the acidosis. It must be given cautiously, however, with attention to avoidance of alkalosis. It should be discontinued immediately when the urine becomes alkaline.

Some clinicians consider that hypertonic saline solution in limited amounts is beneficial in early and more severe cases before marked dehydration has occurred.

SPECIFIC TREATMENT. Various of the sulfonamide drugs have been shown to eliminate the *V. comma* from the stools in relatively short periods of time. This does not appear to affect the clinical condition of the patient. Those preparations which are absorbed and produce measurable blood levels are contraindicated because of the depressed renal function.

The drug of choice is phthalylsulfacetimide (Thalamyd). Although this produces effective concentrations in the intestinal wall it is not absorbed into the blood stream. There are no toxic effects. *Dosage:* 5 gm. initially, thereafter 1 gm. every two hours for five days.

Chloromycetin and Terramycin likewise cause rapid disappearance of the vibrios but do not affect the course of the disease.

NONSPECIFIC TREATMENT. Absolute rest and quiet are essential. Food should be withheld. Even in the presence of thirst water should be given by mouth in only small amounts during the acute phase. Small doses of morphine or even light intermittent anesthesia may be necessary for the relief of muscle cramps, although these should not be used in the stage of collapse. Severe vomiting may be partially controlled by oral administration of dilute solutions of cocaine, 0.0075 gm. per dose.

Convalescence in severe cases may be delayed and after the acute stage there is usually a residual disturbance of the plasma proteins.

**Prognosis** The average mortality in virulent epidemics of cholera is 50 to 60 per cent. This may often be reduced to about 20 per cent in carefully treated patients.

**Prophylaxis** Effective prophylaxis against cholera entails proper isolation of cases, sterilization of bedding and other articles contaminated by the patient, and disinfection and sanitary disposal of fomites. Protection of water supply and sterilization of all water for human use, avoidance of all uncooked foods, and protection of food and drink against contamination by flies are essential.

In the presence of an epidemic outbreak mass immunization should be carried out if practicable. Individuals entering endemic or epidemic areas should be immunized with an approved cholera vaccine. The recommended dosage with an interval of seven to ten days between injections is: first dose, 0.5 ml.; second dose, 1 ml. A stimulating dose of 1 ml. should be administered every four to six months as long as danger of infection is present. When cholera is epidemic this procedure should be supplemented by a full course of vaccine prepared from strains of immunogenic potency.

Immunity is of short duration, not exceeding four to six months, and is much less effective than is the immunization against typhoid. It appears that maximal immunity is attained about the tenth day after immunization.

CHEMOPROPHYLAXIS. Preliminary observations with Thalamyd suggest that a daily dose of 0.2 gm. has significant protective value and that it may prove useful for both individual and mass protection in the presence of epidemic conditions.

## 23  Brucellosis

**Synonyms**  Undulant, Malta, Mediterranean, Gibraltar, rock, Neapolitan, or Cyprus fever. Mediterranean phthisis, melitensis septicemia, abortus fever, fièvre caprine, febris melitensis. In the southwest United States, Rio Grande fever, slow fever, goats' milk fever.

**Definition**  Brucellosis is a specific septicemia of man and animals produced by *Brucella melitensis*, *Br. abortus*, or *Br. suis*, characterized by prolonged disability, asthenia and varied symptomatology. It occurs as an acute or chronic disease characterized in its acute phase by remittent fever which may exhibit a series of relapses separated by brief apyrexial periods. The chronic form is often associated with little or no fever and may occur in the absence of an antecedent acute phase. The death rate of untreated or inadequately treated cases in different parts of the world varies from 2 to 5 per cent.

**Distribution**  The genus *Brucella* occurs in naturally infected animals in all parts of the world and human brucellosis in consequence has a cosmopolitan distribution. The clinical types and the severity of the disease will vary in different areas in accordance with the relative preponderance of the three species of the genus in these regions.

**Etiology**  Brucellosis is a disease primarily of animals, the caprine species *melitensis* occurring in goats, the bovine or *abortus* species in cattle, and the porcine or *suis* species in hogs. In these animals the infection is an important cause of abortion.

The members of the genus *Brucella* are small gram-negative, nonmotile, non–spore-forming coccobacilli. *Brucella melitensis* in culture exhibits coccoid and bacillary forms depending upon the strain, the age of the culture, and the medium for cultivation. *Brucella abortus* exhibits less variation and usually appears as a stumpy rod. *Brucella suis* commonly appears as a rodlike organism.

**Cultural Characteristics**  These organisms do not grow well on ordinary laboratory media. Primary blood stream isolations are not easily accomplished, probably owing to the paucity of organisms in the circulation. Furthermore, it has been demonstrated that certain peptones in the isolation media may be toxic to the brucella organisms. Once isolated, however, the various strains grow well on ordinary laboratory media. Trypticase-soy broth or agar, Albini *Brucella* media or liver infusion agar or liver infusion broth with a *p*H of 6.8 to 7.4 should be used, especially for primary isolation. Growth is slow, requiring up to fourteen days. On solid media the colonies are small, usually smooth and opaque. In liquid media they produce diffuse turbidity.

The *melitensis* and *suis* strains are aerobic. For primary isolation and a varying number of subsequent generations the *abortus* strains require a carbon dioxide content 10 per cent by volume over that of atmospheric air. Such increased carbon dioxide tension does not inhibit growth of *melitensis* or *suis*.

*Table 13  Differentiation of the Species of the Genus* Brucella

| | REQUIRE-MENT FOR CO$_2$ | PRODUCTION OF H$_2$S | | | | UTILIZATION OF GLUCOSE | GROWTH INHIBITED* | |
| | | DAYS | | | | | THIONIN 1/25,000 | BASIC FUCHSIN |
| | | 1 | 2 | 3 | 4 | | | |
|---|---|---|---|---|---|---|---|---|
| *Br. melitensis* | — | — | — | — | — | + | — | — |
| *Br. abortus* | +† | 3 + | 2 + | 1 + | 1 + | ± | + | — |
| *Br. suis* | — | 4 + | 4 + | 4 + | 4 + | + | — | + |

* Specified dilutions of dyes should be used to obtain differentiation. Using certified dyes and Bacto-tryptose, a 1:100,000 dilution, has been found optimal. This varies with different basic media.
† Laboratory strains that have become aerobic do not require CO$_2$ for isolation from inoculated animals.
Adapted from Smith, D. T., et al.: Zinsser's Textbook of Bacteriology, ed. 10, New York, Appleton-Century-Crofts, Inc., 1952.

Differentiation among the three species of the genus *Brucella* is difficult. Antigenic analysis by the agglutinin absorption test is not satisfactory. Small absorbing doses must be used and these in turn must be adjusted to the titer of the serum at hand. Furthermore, antigenic similarities are such that the test will serve to distinguish only between *melitensis* on the one hand and *abortus* and *suis* on the other. Serologic and cultural correlations are at times variable. Transitional types have been reported which do not conform to species identification by serologic methods.

Certain cultural characteristics, however, are useful for tentative identification. These are indicated in Table 13. *Brucella melitensis* does not require an increased carbon dioxide tension for primary isolation nor does it produce hydrogen sulfide. Glucose is utilized in the medium and growth is not inhibited by aniline dyes. *Brucella abortus*, on the other hand, requires increased carbon dioxide concentration. It produces varying amounts of hydrogen sulfide. Glucose utilization is variable and growth is inhibited by thionine but not by methyl violet, basic fuchsin or pyronine. *Brucella suis* is aerobic and is a strong producer of hydrogen sulfide. It utilizes glucose and growth is not inhibited by thionine but is inhibited by the other dyes.

**Epidemiology**   The genus *Brucella* is widely distributed throughout the world and produces natural infections in horses, fowl, dogs, sheep, cattle, goats, wild deer and wild buffalo as well as man. The human disease is acquired from direct or indirect contact with goats, cattle or hogs. The tissues and discharges of infected animals contain the organisms. The *Brucella* are commonly present in the milk of infected cattle and goats.

In animals which have aborted the organisms are present in large numbers in the vaginal discharges. They are less commonly present in the urine and feces. The frequent association of *Br. abortus* with both fistulous withers and abortion of horses provides a source of potential infection for individuals in contact with such animals.

The *Brucella* are not easily destroyed under natural conditions except by temperatures above 55° C. or by exposure to direct sunlight. They will survive in dry soil for forty to sixty days, in sterile tap water for forty-two days, in meat-curing brine for forty days, and in milk at 10° C. for ten days. They have been reported to remain viable in unpasteurized cheese for periods up to two months.

Man acquires the infection by ingestion of contaminated or infected food or drink, possibly by inhalation of dust containing the organisms, and by penetration of *Brucella* through the abraded or even unbroken skin and mucous membranes. Unpasteurized milk or milk products are the commonest vehicles of human infection. Since the disease in animals is a septicemia, slaughterhouse workers, meat handlers, animal husbandmen and veterinarians are particularly exposed.

In the past twenty-five years brucellosis has become an important public health problem. In the United States the prevalence of the disease varies directly with the extent of the hog-raising industry. In other highly endemic areas it is observed particularly in connection with goat raising or where goats' milk is commonly used as a beverage; elsewhere it is sporadic. In the United States it involves particularly young adult males and especially farmers, packing house workers and veterinarians. In Malta it is commonest in children under five years of age, in whom it is usually relatively mild and often unnoticed.

There is no evidence of transmission directly from man to man.

It is probable that infection, even subclinical infection, confers lasting immunity. Although artificial immunization has proved of value in animal husbandry it has not been successfully applied to man.

**Pathology.**   The organisms invade cells of the reticulo-endothelial system, producing granulomata which may undergo necrosis. There is little phagocytic action. These lesions occur in many tissues and organs, especially the liver, spleen and lymph nodes. Less frequently they are found in the meninges and brain, the male and female genitalia, and the skin, eyes and lungs. While there may be involvement of joints and long bones, the commonest lesion in the osseous system is spondylitis of the lumbar spine with destruction of the intervertebral disk and the adjacent vertebral bodies. Localization may occur on previously damaged heart valves, causing subacute bacterial endocarditis.

The blood shows a progressive microcytic anemia with leukopenia and relative lymphocytosis in which there may be an appreciable increase of immature small lymphocytes.

**Clinical Characteristics** Clinical, bacteriologic and epidemiologic studies indicate that there are significant differences in the clinical types and average severity of the disease produced by the different species. The prolonged relapsing type of fever which gave rise originally to the term "undulant fever" is much more commonly observed in *melitensis* infections (60 per cent of the cases in Malta) and the mortality rate in these infections is somewhat higher; the undulant type of fever, on the other hand, is only occasionally seen in *abortus* and *suis* infections. Three main types of disease are recognized on the basis of the temperature curves—the intermittent, the undulant and the malignant.

The incubation period varies from three to twenty-one days. The procedures recommended for establishing the diagnosis are:

1. Recovery of the organism by culture of blood, excreta, spinal fluid.

2. Agglutination reaction.

The onset is usually gradual and insidious with generalized aching, headache, anorexia, chilliness, insomnia, backache and stiffness or pain in the neck and various joints. Constipation is usual and there is commonly a slowly progressive loss of weight. As these symptoms develop, elevation of temperature occurs in the afternoon or evening, slowly increasing in degree and often accompanied by sensations of chilliness but rarely by frank chill. As the disease becomes established, cough productive of small amounts of mucoid or mucopurulent sputum is not uncommon. The fever appearing in the afternoon or evening commonly passes off during the night and is often accompanied by drenching sweats of such severity as to require change of bedclothing. In the fully established case the temperature may reach 104° F. or higher at night and be normal or under 100° F. in the morning. In most instances the febrile period persists for six weeks to several months, terminating slowly by lysis. There is often marked disparity between the subjective sensations of the patient and his appearance on the one hand, and the temperature record on the other.

Physical examination usually reveals little or nothing other than some degree of splenomegaly, hepatomegaly and lymphadenopathy, especially of the cervical and axillary lymph nodes. Even in the presence of considerable cough, physical signs over the lungs are usually absent. X-ray examination, however, may demonstrate small areas of confluent lobular pneumonia. Neurologic changes such as disturbances of reflex activity and gross tremors of the tongue and extended fingers are commonly noted.

In the undulant type of brucellosis after return of the temperature to normal and a varying afebrile period, a similar febrile phase recurs. These waves of fever may be numerous and extend over a prolonged period.

The malignant form of brucellosis is rare in the *Br. abortus* and *Br. suis* types of the disease. When it occurs it is characterized by sudden onset, an acute course of high sustained fever with great prostration, and is usually fatal.

During the acute phase there may be hydrarthrosis and transient periarticular swellings. Regional localizations are not unusual. Involvement of the central nervous system may produce the symptoms and signs of acute encephalitis, myelitis or meningitis. These may be very transitory.

Abdominal pain is common, especially in the early stages of the disease, and has frequently led to mistaken diagnosis and surgical intervention for a suspected acute appendicitis or acute cholecystitis. Less commonly there may be epididymitis, prostatitis, seminal vesiculitis or oophoritis. The infection may occasionally be a cause of abortion. In some instances there is a transient cutaneous eruption, usually papular, macular or maculopapular which may simulate the roseola of typhoid.

**Chronic Brucellosis** Chronic brucellosis is exceedingly protean in its phenomena. Its definitive diagnosis is frequently very difficult. Significant symptoms or signs may be entirely lacking, probably less than 10 per cent of such cases giving a history of antecedent acute disease. The individual suffering from this type of infection is often not entirely incapacitated. The most striking clinical phenomena are physical and nervous weakness and exhaustion which may or may not be accompanied by mild and usually unrecognized fever, the temperature often not exceeding 100° F. There are three cardinal features—weakness, low-grade fever and complete absence of other objective physical findings. Peripheral neuritis is a frequent complication.

Symptoms relating to the central nervous system are frequently observed and are usually evanescent. These include headache, vertigo, nuchal rigidity, aphasia, psychic disturbances and even transitory paralysis. In such instances the spinal fluid may exhibit increased pressure, a slight increase in the cell count and albumin, and a decrease of the globulin and sugar content.

**Diagnosis** The diagnosis of brucellosis on clinical grounds alone is undependable and hazardous. The protean manifestations of the disease often produce difficult problems of differential diagnosis. In many instances the clinical picture may resemble typhoid, tuberculosis, influenza or malaria. In other instances it may be confused with acute appendicitis, cholecystitis, bronchitis, pyelitis, and even with

Hodgkin's disease. The chronic form is commonly confused with neurasthenia or psychasthenia.

There are three important criteria for diagnosis:

1. Recovery of the organism.
2. An agglutination titer of 1/320 or higher.
3. Lower initial titer followed by a rising titer.

· Recovery of the organism constitutes the only absolute confirmation of diagnosis. Present techniques permit recovery of *Brucella* from venous blood in a high proportion of cases during the initial acute phase or during exacerbation. They are superior to guinea pig inoculation. However, repeated cultures may be necessary. It is recommended that no more than 2 to 3 ml. be used as inoculum because of the possible presence of inhibiting substances in the blood.

The initial culture should be made in tryticase-soy broth and Albini *Brucella* medium. Subcultures are made to trypticase-soy agar and Albini agar plates on the fourth day and thereafter at regular intervals unless growth occurs. All cultures should be incubated at 37° C. in closed jars containing an atmosphere with 10 per cent carbon dioxide. The initial cultures should be kept for at least one month unless growth appears earlier.

Cultures of sternal marrow or of an enlarged cervical lymph node may be positive when the blood is negative. These procedures may be useful particularly in long standing chronic cases.

The agglutination test when properly done is an invaluable aid in diagnosis. The reliability depends upon the use of a standardized antigen prepared from a completely smooth culture of any of the three species of *Brucella*. After growth on solid media and suspension in saline solution the organisms should be killed by heat, formaldehyde or phenol, and the suspension standardized by turbidimetric methods and tested against sera of known titer. The serial dilution test tube method should be used and the serum antigen mixture incubated at 37° C. for 18 to 24 hours before reading.

A titer of 1/320 or higher justifies a presumptive diagnosis of brucellosis, and a lower initial titer followed by a rising titer may have considerable significance.

Various other diagnostic procedures have been recommended. The complement fixation test has no advantages over the agglutination reaction. Dermal sensitivity tests have the same significance as the tuberculin test and consequently are of no assistance in diagnosis. Their use is often followed by a high titer of agglutinins which may confuse the interpretation of the agglutination reaction. The opsonocytophagic test is of little value and is not recommended.

**Treatment**   Aureomycin, chloramphenicol (Chloromycetin), oxytetracycline (Terramycin) and dihydro-streptomycin have proved to be effective therapeutic agents for both acute and chronic brucellosis. They have replaced all other forms of therapy.

Combined treatment using aureomycin or Terramycin and dihydrostreptomycin over a period of twelve to fourteen days is the preferred treatment for the acute disease. The recommended dosages for an adult are:

Aureomycin or Terramycin 3.0 gm. daily in divided dosage by mouth, and dihydrostreptomycin 1.0 gm. twice daily intramuscularly.

Aureomycin alone has given good results in the treatment of the acute stage and of relapses. The dosage recommended by the FAO/. WHO Expert Panel on Brucellosis is:

Aureomycin 2 to 4 gm. daily for fourteen to twenty-one days.

Chloromycetin is active against all three strains of *Brucella*. A total of 15 to 20 gm. over a period of six to ten days is advised for adults. This should be administered in accordance with the following schedule:

Fifty to 100 mg. per kilogram daily in divided dosage every three to four hours until the patient is afebrile, when the daily dose may be reduced to a total of 1.5 to 2.0 gm.

Cases of chronic brucellosis may require more protracted treatment.

**Prophylaxis**   Since there is no satisfactory method for artificial immunization, prevention depends upon avoidance of infection. The widespread geographic distribution, the occurrence of the *Brucella* in a variety of animals and the resistance of the organisms provide many opportunities for contact. Human infection, however, is probably in almost all instances acquired by the ingestion of the *Brucella* in food or drink or by direct contact with infected animal tissues or discharges. The most important factors in prophylaxis are a properly protected water supply and avoidance of unpasteurized milk and milk products.

# 24   Leprosy

**Synonyms**   Lepra; la lèpre; Aussatz; spedalskhed; Hansen's disease.

**Definition**   Leprosy is an infectious disease caused by *Mycobacterium leprae*, characterized by a prolonged latent period and a chronic course with conspicuous dermal and neural manifestations. Its several forms fall into two general groups, the *benign* and the *malign*. In the benign form resistance is indicated by paucity of bacilli in the lesions and the prognosis is relatively good. In the malign form there is little evidence of resistance, bacilli are abundant and the prognosis poor.

**Distribution**   The disease is widely distributed in tropical and subtropical regions. It occurs throughout most of Asia, with a high incidence in India, southern China and many of the Pacific islands.

It is widespread in equatorial Africa, and has become endemic in much of the Western Hemisphere, especially in certain South American countries. There are probably between three million and five million cases in the world.

**Etiology** *Mycobacterium leprae* is an acid-fast, gram-positive, non–spore-forming, nonmotile, pleomorphic bacillus. It has not been cultured successfully nor has infection been produced in experimental animals. Morphologically it may closely resemble the tubercle bacillus. Multiplication within the lesions is chiefly intracellular. Smears from lepromatous lesions are usually distinctive. Large numbers of lepra cells containing bacilli are commonly present and "globi", or groups or masses of bacilli in a semifluid matrix, are characteristic. The organism is less strongly acid fast than the tubercle bacillus and the results of culture and of animal inoculation readily differentiate the two.

**Epidemiology** The communicability of leprosy is low. Infection seems to depend upon prolonged and intimate contact with leprous persons. Susceptibility varies greatly among different individuals and probably, to some extent, among different races; it is much higher in childhood than in adult life. Among adults it is twice as common in men as in women. Although the conditions necessary for transmission cannot be defined, the skin, and to some extent the nasal mucous membranes, are believed to be the usual portals of entry. There is no definite incubation period. Ordinarily, several years elapse before manifestations appear and the latent period may be as long as thirty years.

The immunology of leprosy presents no known parallel with that of tuberculosis. There is no diagnostic skin test. There is evidently an innate factor of resistance, the presence or absence of which determines the course of the disease and the nature of the lesions. It is associated with the tissue reactivity or lack of reactivity, and with the results given by the Mitsuda or lepromin test. This is performed by intracutaneous injection of a suspension of heat-killed bacilli obtained from lepromas. A late (three weeks') papulonodular lesion constitutes a positive reaction. Cases of the benign forms of the disease generally react positively, whereas those with the malign forms are regularly nonreactive. The test therefore has significance for prognosis and for classification.

**Pathology** The lesions of leprosy are due to the presence of the causative organisms. In the benign forms, bacilli are so scanty that it is usually impossible to demonstrate them by the standard smear technique. The principal skin lesions are macules, infiltrations, nodules, and variations of the tuberculoid condition. The nonlepromatous lesions are referred to as *leprids*.

In lepromatous leprosy the superficial lymph nodes, the upper respiratory tract and the eyes are often conspicuously involved. The spleen, liver and testes are also affected but only in the latter is there disturbance of function. Bacilli may sometimes be demonstrable in the blood during the severe reactions of lepra fever. Involvement of the peripheral nerve trunks is important in all forms of the disease.

Histologically, the infiltrates in the skin, of whatever type, affect primarily the zones of vascular areolar tissue. Involvement of dermal nerve branches is unique among cutaneous infections. Lesions in other structures, including those in the nerve trunks, correspond to the different types occurring in the skin.

The only distinctive lesion of leprosy is the *leproma*. This is a granuloma composed mainly of massed macrophages, altered to form the lepra cells of Virchow, lying in a well vascularized supporting

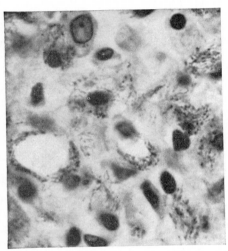

Fig. 61. Lepra cells in a skin lesion of lepromatous leprosy. Large mononuclear phagocytes loaded with *M. leprae*, some exhibiting different degrees of vacuolation due to globus formation.

stroma. These cells harbor but do not destroy the bacilli, and in the classic lesion they become vacuolated by the formation of globi (Fig. 61, top and center). "Giant globi" are often found within foreign body giant cells or ensheathed in a sort of syncytium (Fig. 61, left), and at times they constitute veritable microcolonies (Fig. 62). However, some lepromas may be composed of massed spindle-shaped cells loaded with bacilli in which globus formation is absent. As the lesions gradually age the lepra cells become foamy, multivacuolated and often multinucleated. They contain few bacilli but much acid-fast lipidic material.

As the infiltrate in the skin increases, it disrupts the normal architecture and seriously affects the accessory structures. These persist, however, even in massive lesions (Fig. 62), except in the tumorlike secondary nodules which are pure lepromas. The subcutis is commonly invaded and subcutaneous nodules may develop.

The lepromatous infiltrate in the peripheral nerve trunks involves the endoneurium, but despite its intensity, functional disturbance is long delayed unless reactional inflammation supervenes.

The tissue-reactive *tuberculoid* lesions are nonspecific in character, presenting focal masses of epithelioid cells with variable degrees of lymphoid cell accumulation and giant cell formation (Fig. 63). The epithelioid cells ingest and destroy the bacilli. When bacilli are demonstrable, they are usually in other cells or other structures, especially the nerves. The more marked lesions of the skin resemble

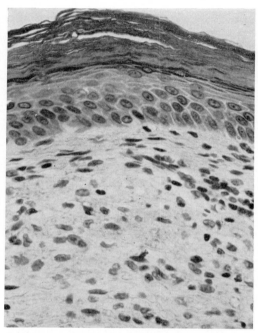

Fig. 62. A marked lepromatous infiltration, showing flattening of the epidermis with hyperkeratosis and the characteristic free zone below. The infiltrate is a solid mass of lepra cells, with many small globus spaces and beginning of change to the foamy condition.

noncaseating tuberculosis or Boeck's sarcoid, except for the involvement of the nerve branches. Extension of the process may be seen in the nerves of the subcutis, and caseation necrosis occasionally occurs.

In the lesser degrees of clinically tuberculoid lesions the epithelioid foci tend to be correspondingly smaller and more isolated. In their simplest form they appear as "pretuberculoid" groups of a few epithelioid cells which are often found in clinically simple flat macules. In reactional tuberculoid conditions the lesions are massive and less orderly. When such cases evolve to the borderline stage, the picture is even more atypical and confused. At times both tuberculoid and lepromatous changes may coexist.

Simple chronic inflammatory round cell infiltration is found in many pale, flat macules and often in the peripheral nerves in the classic neural leprosy. The cells are mostly lymphoid, but larger cells of the monocyte type may also be present. Bacilli are seldom demonstrable. The amount of infiltration in the nerve trunks is much less than in lepromatous leprosy, yet nerve fiber degeneration and fibrosis occur earlier.

In the past, leprosy cases were classed as lepromatous (nodular) or neural (maculoanesthetic). Present day classification recognizes four main forms based on clinicobacteriologic, immunologic and

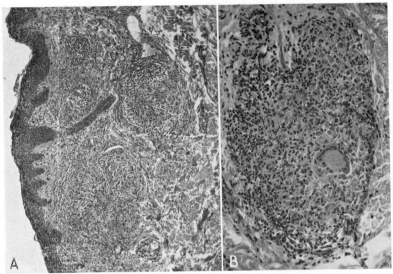

Fig. 63. Tuberculoid lesions of leprosy. *A,* Showing multiple epithelioid foci, in one place in contact with the epidermis, in a clinically minor tuberculoid lesion of moderate degree (80 ✕). *B,* A sarcoid-like focus, showing massed epithelioid cells and a Langhans giant cell, with lymphoid cell accumulation on one side (150 ✕). (Courtesy of Dr. H. W. Wade.)

histopathologic criteria. These are (1) lepromatous, (2) indeterminate (simple macular), (3) tuberculoid, and (4) borderline. However, the terms "neural" and "maculoanesthetic" are still applied informally in certain types of cases.

The tuberculoid and indeterminate forms belong in the benign category. Although they are usually bacteriologically negative and lepromin positive, numerous cases of the indeterminate type are nonreactive to lepromin. The lepromatous and borderline forms constitute the malign group. Many bacilli are present in the lesions and the lepromin reaction is negative. Borderline cases usually develop from the tuberculoid form as a result of repeated reactions. They occupy an intermediate position between tuberculoid and lepromatous, or are transitional to the latter form.

**Clinical Characteristics**   The onset of leprosy is usually insidious.

There are no definite prodromata although some patients may complain of early sensory disturbances or neuritic pain. Occasionally the disease appears abruptly, accompanied by more or less toxemia before the lesions develop.

Early leprosy is often difficult to recognize. Typically, there are one or a few small, well defined, simple, indeterminate macules. These are anesthetic and hypopigmented. Some cases, apparently lepromatous from the outset, present diffusely outlined, erythematous macules with little, if any, perceptible infiltration, no marginal thickening or differentiation between margin and center, little or no anesthesia but positive bacteriologic findings. These lesions may be found on the extremities, on the body, more commonly on the back than anteriorly, often on the buttocks, and not infrequently on the

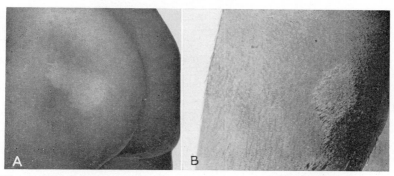

Fig. 64. Macular lesions of leprosy. *A*, Simple ("indeterminate") macule on the buttock; active progression indicated by the streaming outline. *B*, Minor tuberculoid lesion of the arm, superficial, with micropapulate elevated marginal zone of activity and healed center. (Courtesy of Dr. H. W. Wade.)

face (Fig. 64). In advanced cases, whatever the form, there are naturally immune areas: the cubital and popliteal fossae, the axillary and inguinal regions, the retroauricular area, and generally the scalp.

The evolution of the indeterminate cases is variable. Some clear up spontaneously; others persist and progress indefinitely as "maculoanesthetic"; in still others, increase of tissue reactivity leads to the development of the tuberculoid form, or conversely, loss of resistance results in transformation into the lepromatous type. Tuberculoid cases may persist as such for long periods. There may be wide extension of the lesions, but ultimately they tend to subside spontaneously. On the other hand they may change to the borderline type, and from that they occasionally become frankly lepromatous. Lepromatous cases seldom change in type and are usually progressive.

The color of the lesions may vary considerably, apart from the influence of racial characteristics. In the macular lesions there is dissociation of sensation. Discrimination between heat and cold is lost first, then sensitivity to pain and finally tactile sense. Perception of pressure remains intact. In most lesions there is little or no sweating and hairs are usually absent. Atrophy of the skin may occur in resolved lesions or parts of lesions; on the other hand the texture and even the color may return to normal. Ichthyosis of the legs is common and there may be marked thickening of the skin of the lower extremities in advanced lepromatous cases.

Frequently there is thickening and often tenderness of the peripheral nerve trunks at the points of flexure, the ulnars above the elbows, the external peroneals at the knees, and also the great auriculars. These are important diagnostic signs.

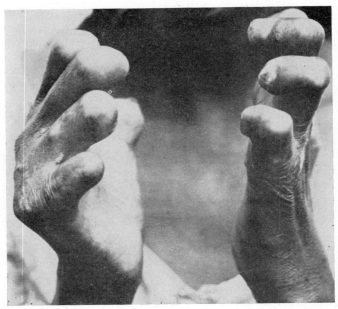

Fig. 65. Advanced trophic changes of the hands due to severe nerve damage, with muscular atrophy, contractures, and progressive absorption of the digits, on some of which residuae of the nails can be seen.

Degeneration of the trunk nerves leads to anesthetic, paralytic and trophic changes of the extremities, followed by mutilations often aggravated by trauma. Muscle atrophy of the hands becomes conspicuous, contractures slowly develop, and the bones of the phalanges gradually undergo absorption, or become necrotic or infected and are extruded (Fig. 65). The soft tissues of the fingers are absorbed, leaving distorted residua of the nails on the stumps of the hands. Wristdrop is occasionally seen. Similar changes occur in the feet and troublesome trophic ulcers develop on the plantar surfaces. There are seemingly "pure neural" or "polyneuritic" cases which present only such changes.

In its ordinary course leprosy is a nontoxic disease despite the immense numbers of bacilli in the lepromatous lesions. The ultimate deterioration of such cases, producing indolent bacillus-discharging ulcerations and other changes, comes on very gradually. However, acute episodes of "lepra reaction," with or without fever, apparently allergic in nature, occur in many cases. These reactions, which differ greatly in the different types, may or may not be harmful.

Death from leprosy itself is infrequent. Pulmonary tuberculosis and nephritis are common terminal events. Amyloidosis is often found at autopsy.

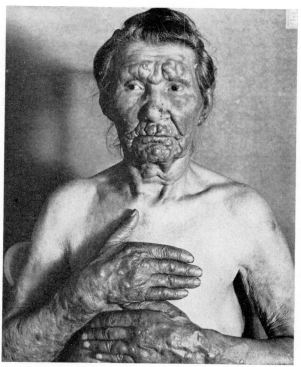

Fig. 66. An advanced lepromatous case with leonine face, both furrowed and nodulate, and with marked involvement of the forearms and hands, less of the upper arms and still less of the body.

LEPROMATOUS LEPROSY. Symmetric distribution of the lesions is typical. The brownish red macules often appear first on the face but may be on any part of the body. Thickening of the earlobes is sometimes an early development. As the disease progresses, the lesions increase in numbers, size and thickness, the infiltrations appearing smooth and tense, and discrete nodulations or the leonine furrowing of the face may appear (Fig. 66). The loss of eyebrows is often helpful in type diagnosis.

In advanced cases, ulceration of the nasal mucosa may lead to perforation of the cartilaginous septum and to falling of the nose.

Infiltration of the vocal cords causes the characteristic raucous voice, and occasionally leads to severe stenosis. The eyes may be involved either by extension of infiltration from the conjunctiva to the cornea or by involvement of the uveal tract.

Mild lepra reactions in this type of the disease are often beneficial, leading to recession of the lesions. If they are severe and repeated, however, they are harmful; ulcerations of the skin may occur, especially on the extremities, and acute neuritis, iridocyclitis, or orchitis. Also in this type, usually in cases improving under treatment, an erythema nodosum–like reaction occurs, with the appearance of small acute nodules which typically are tender, often bacteriologically negative in smears, and usually of short duration although this condition may become chronic, producing dense indurations on the extremities.

The peripheral nerve trunks are usually much more thickened than in "neural" cases because of the amount of specific lepra cell infiltration. When nerve damage finally occurs the resulting sequelae produce the picture of "complete leprosy" (Leloir), a stage often but unfortunately called "mixed" leprosy.

MACULOANESTHETIC LEPROSY. This benign group comprises most of the cases having simple macules and, in the older sense, many of those of the lesser tuberculoid type. In these cases the skin lesions persist, increase in numbers and spread centrifugally, at times with fusion of adjacent lesions.

If the process is not arrested, involvement of peripheral nerves becomes evident sooner or later. Typically, there is less thickening of the nerve trunks than occurs in lepromatous leprosy. In some instances attacks of acute neuritis hasten and intensify the nerve damage. In many cases the skin lesions will disappear spontaneously and neural manifestations, if present, may be so slight that the recovered patients appear practically normal. Often, however, they are crippled and deformed (Fig. 66).

Paralysis of the lower eyelids results in lagophthalmos, and traumatic corneal damage is apt to follow. There may be paralysis of the orbicularis oris muscles and even of the masseters. Occasionally nasal ulcers develop, in which case the bacilli can be demonstrated in this lesion but not elsewhere.

TUBERCULOID LEPROSY. This variety of the benign form is characterized primarily by distinctive skin lesions presenting more or less elevation. In spite of this, they are still called macules (Fig. 68). In the common minor variety the elevation, which usually has an irregular or micropapulate surface, occurs only in the outer advancing margin of the lesion or in a part of it. In the less common major form there is more marked thickening and elevation of the marginal zone, which is broader, and the process tends to show deeper extension. Recent lesions of this sort may show incomplete central resolution, and those of reactional origin may be solid plaques. Hyperesthesia is often found in the active outer zones of the tuberculoid macules, with anesthesia in the central areas.

Thickening of the cutaneous nerve cephalad to a lesion, especially of the major variety, is sometimes found. It may extend to, and involve, the corresponding nerve trunk. This condition is typically asymmetric and unilateral, which is distinctive. Massive thickening, especially if it is irregular, signifies caseation necrosis which may undergo liquefaction to produce a nerve abscess.

The reactional lesions of the skin in this type are often spectacular. They may easily be mistaken for lepromatous lesions, especially

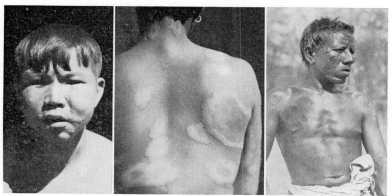

Fig. 67.                Fig. 68.                Fig. 69.

Fig. 67. Major tuberculoid plaque of face, of reactional origin, in a Chinese patient. Isolated nodules on chin and other cheek are of the same nature, reactional dissemination. (The grossly thickened right great auricular nerve in relation to the plaque is not demonstrated.) (Courtesy of Dr. H. W. Wade.)

Fig. 68. Multiple broad-margined tuberculoid macules of back, spreading and fusing, in a South African patient. Note central healing with recovery of normal color and texture in the largest one. (Courtesy of Dr. H. W. Wade.)

Fig. 69. A borderline case, in febrile reaction, an Indian patient. Modified tuberculoid lesions on chest and shoulder, abruptly outlined plaques on face, but with ear of lepromatous aspect. (Courtesy of Dr. H. W. Wade.)

when there are disseminated metastatic nodules. With repeated severe reactions, change to the atypical borderline type of disease is apt to occur.

BORDERLINE CASES. These cases belong to the malign group and they may progress to become truly lepromatous. In the past they have usually been classed as lepromatous, sometimes called atypical because of the asymmetry of the lesions and other peculiarities (Figs. 67, 68, 69). However, if not too far advanced, they may regress to the original tuberculoid form. In general they respond better to treatment.

**Diagnosis**    The cardinal diagnostic signs are the finding of bacilli, anesthetic lesions, or thickening and tenderness of peripheral nerve trunks. Search should be made for suspicious macules or infiltrations of the skin and for thickening of the earlobes and the eyebrows. The peripheral nerves should be palpated carefully.

Smears for bacilli should be made from several sites, skin lesions, earlobes and the nasal septum. Since bacilli are usually obtainable only from lepromatous lesions, many cases must be diagnosed on the basis of anesthesia in simple macular or tuberculoid leprids. In such lesions, loss of sensitivity to light touch and absence of pain on pinprick justify the diagnosis. Tests for histamine flare and for sweating afford confirmatory evidence. In the absence of skin lesions, muscular

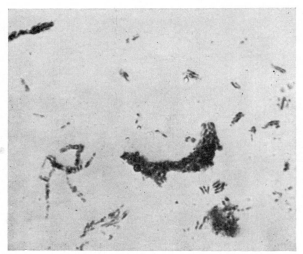

Fig. 70. *Mycobacterium leprae* in stained smear from the nasal septum of an advanced lepromatous case, with typical grouping but without globi or lepra cells.

weakness of the face or areas of numbness on the extremities should be regarded as suspicious. Polyneuritic anesthesias, stocking and glove distribution, will almost certainly be due to leprosy, especially if the nerve trunks are thickened.

The histamine flare test is performed by making a needle puncture into the skin through a drop of 1/1000 histamine acid phosphate solution. The test is positive if there is no erythema flare when the puncture is made within the lesion area, or if the flare stops at the margin of the lesion when the puncture is made a little to the outside of it. The sweating tests are seldom used.

Smears for bacteriologic examination from the skin should be obtained by the scraped incision method, performed at any point in the lepromas and at the active marginal zone of leprids. A fold of skin is compressed between thumb and forefinger, an incision is made well into the corium, and material is scraped from the cut surface with as little blood as possible. Smears from the nasal mucosa should be made under direct observation using a speculum, searching the septum for infiltrations or ulcers. In lepromatous cases bacilli may be very numerous (Fig. 70). Puncture and aspiration of an enlarged lymph node or thickened ulnar nerve is rarely called for.

DIFFERENTIAL DIAGNOSIS. The lesions of leprosy are protean in character and resemble those of many other conditions. Simple macular leprids must be distinguished from such conditions as tinea versicolor, leukoderma (vitiligo), hypochromia of yaws, pale birthmarks and scars, and certain lichenoid lesions. In these conditions anesthesia is absent and the histamine and sweating tests are negative. Syringomyelia, Raynaud's disease, Bernhardt's syndrome and other peripheral neuritic conditions may be confused with neural (polyneuritic) leprosy without skin lesions.

Various lesions of tuberculoid leprosy, which is often misdiagnosed, must be distinguished from Boeck's sarcoid, granuloma annulare, lupus vulgaris, lupus erythematosus, tinea circinata, psoriasis, and certain lesions of secondary syphilis and yaws. With respect to the first two, the confusion may even extend to the histologic findings.

In lepromatous leprosy, infiltrations and nodules may have to be distinguished from such conditions as dermal leishmaniasis, mycosis fungoides, leukemia cutis and neurofibromatosis. Smears of such lepromas will always be found positive. If bacilli are not obtained from the reactional lesions of the erythema nodosum type, they should be demonstrable elsewhere.

**Treatment** General treatment, including personal and environmental hygiene, an ample well balanced diet, and the correction of concomitant conditions is important. With such measures even severe lepromatous cases often show more or less amelioration, at least for a time.

The sulfones have almost entirely displaced the preparations of chaulmoogra (hydnocarpus) oil in the field of specific therapy. The effectiveness of these drugs is most striking in lepromatous leprosy in which their proper use is followed by rapid healing of skin ulcers and lesions of the respiratory mucosa, and in most cases gradual recession of cutaneous lepromata. Bacteriologic improvement and disappearance of the bacilli is slower, frequently requiring two years or more of treatment. The sulfones are also effective in the other forms of the disease. They do not alleviate the effects of nerve destruction.

For the most part, because of the toxicity of the parent substance, 4-4'-diaminodiphenyl sulfone (DDS), derivatives of it have been used. Most of them are disubstituted and apparently have to be broken down in the body to be effective. These include glucosulfone sodium (Promin, etc.), which is given intravenously, and sulfoxone sodium (Diasone, etc.) and Sulphetrone, which are usually given by mouth. Certain monosubstituted sulfones (Promacetin) seem to exert their effect without necessarily being broken down.

These drugs must be employed in doses based on the degree of absorption of those which are given by mouth, and on the DDS content of that portion which becomes available to the tissues. Recently, however, the inexpensive parent substance itself has been used extensively with good results, even in outpatient clinics. Three dosage schedules are used:

1. 100 mg. daily by mouth, or
2. 300 to 400 mg. twice a week by mouth, or
3. Larger doses given by injection once a week or even once in two weeks.

**Prognosis**  The prognosis of untreated leprosy is generally unfavorable. In the self-healing benign cases, crippling deformities often develop before the disease is overcome. Lepromatous cases almost always deteriorate intermittently. With modern treatment many benign cases are cleared up before the development of neural sequelae, and many of the lepromatous type are rendered bacteriologically negative. It must always be assumed, however, that deep-seated bacilli still persist and that relapse may occur after treatment is suspended. With modern treatment of secondary or concurrent conditions the death rates in leprosy institutions have decreased greatly.

**Prophylaxis and Control**  The control of leprosy depends upon the discovery and treatment of early cases, with special attention to contacts and some form of effective isolation of bacteriologically positive "open" cases. Prevention of contact with children is especially important. In most areas it is not considered necessary to segregate "closed" cases. These are treated in dispensaries, but they cannot be regarded as entirely noninfectious and appropriate precautions must be taken in the home.

It is possible but not proved that BCG inoculation of persons nonreactive to lepromin may be of value in prophylaxis by rendering such individuals reactive.

# 25  Plague

**Synonyms**  Oriental plague, pest, black death.

**Definition**  Plague is an acute, febrile, infectious, highly fatal disease which is characterized by inflammation of the lymphatics, septicemia, and by petechial and diffuse hemorrhages into the skin, subcutaneous tissues and viscera. It is frequently characterized by buboes, less often by secondary plague pneumonia and rarely by primary pneumonia.

**Distribution**  In the course of the last pandemic, which is believed to have originated in Yunan on the Tibetan border of China, nearly every important country in the world was invaded. The more important present endemic centers appear in Table 14 and Figure 71.

**Etiology**   *Pasteurella pestis* (Yersin and Kitasato 1894) is a member of the group producing hemorrhagic septicemias (pasteurellosis) in animals. It is a short, nonmotile, gram-negative, bipolar-staining bacillus which exhibits marked pleomorphism and is often encapsulated. Three general forms may be seen:

1. Short, rounded or oval, often appearing as diplococci.
2. Longer rods.
3. Large, oval or pear-shaped, or club-shaped involution forms.

Specific identification is based upon the morphology, staining reactions, the cultural characteristics, and the results of animal inoculation.

*Table 14   Principal Endemic Foci of Plague in Rodents*

| TYPE | LOCALITY |
|---|---|
| Murine plague: (domestic rodents) | India China, Manchuria, Mongolia Burma Indonesia East Africa Madagascar West Africa South America: Brazil, Bolivia, Peru, Ecuador |
| Sylvatic plague: (wild rodents) | [United States: western states China, Mongolia Transcaucasia South Africa Argentina |

**Cultural Characteristics**   *Pasteurella pestis* grows equally well at 30° to 37° C. This is of value for its isolation in pure culture and for identification. On alkaline agar small translucent dewdrop colonies appear in eighteen to twenty-four hours. Acid without gas is formed from glucose, maltose, mannite and salicin. Lactose is not fermented. Milk is not coagulated. There is no indole production. In bouillon under oil there is a characteristic stalactite growth extending downward from the surface. Salt agar, 2.5 to 3.5 per cent, is useful for the production of involution forms which are of value in diagnosis.

ANIMAL INOCULATION. The guinea pig is the best laboratory animal for the recovery of these organisms since a single virulent bacillus produces fatal infection. Inoculation should be made by rubbing into the shaved scarified skin of the abdomen. If the inoculum contains plague bacilli death results in three to five days with the following characteristic findings:

1. Marked subcutaneous edema, congestion and hemorrhage about the site of inoculation.
2. Buboes in one or both inguinal regions.

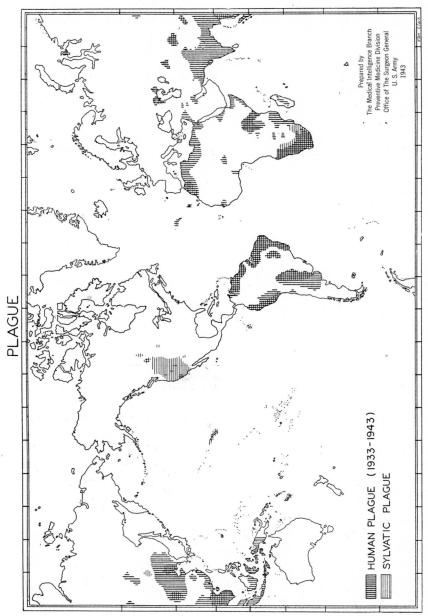

Fig. 71. Geographical distribution of plague.

3. Numerous yellowish white necrotic foci in the spleen and at times in the liver.

4. Hemorrhages in the lungs and other tissues and occasionally in the heart muscle.

5. Smears from the lesions and from the heart blood revealing large numbers of typical bipolar-staining bacilli.

*Pasteurella pestis* is easily killed by drying in sunlight and by ordinary disinfectants. Its viability varies greatly in different environments; in putrefying animal matter, four days; in buried bodies, three to thirty days, depending upon the temperature; in the

*Table 15    Cultural Characteristics of* Pasteurella *Species**

| | P. pestis | P. pseudotuberculosis | P. avicada |
|---|---|---|---|
| Motility in 18-hour cultures at 22° C. | — | + | — |
| Litmus milk | — or slight acid | Alkaline | — |
| Sugars | Acid in glucose, maltose, mannitol and salicin | Acid in glucose, maltose, mannitol and salicin, sometimes in sucrose | Acid in glucose, mannitol and sucrose, sometimes in maltose |
| Indole | — | — | + |
| Methyl red | + | + | — |
| Methylene blue reduction † | — | + | + |
| Growth on MacConkey's agar | + | + | — |
| Pathogenicity to white rats | + | — | + |

* From Topley, W. W. C., and Wilson, G. S.: Principles of Bacteriology and Immunity, ed. 3, William Wood & Company, 1946.

† Personal observations on a relatively few strains.

cowdung floors of houses in India, forty-eight hours; in grain and meal if there is sufficient moisture, thirteen days; and in dried flea feces, four weeks. In frozen sputum or in frozen corpses the bacilli remain viable for prolonged periods.

Rodents may not infrequently be found infected with bipolar-staining bacilli which are difficult to differentiate from *P. pestis*. The more important of these are *P. pseudotuberculosis rodentium*, and *P. avicada* (Table 15).

**Epidemiology**    Although plague is a disease primarily of rats and other rodents, in man it is one of the most fatal of all infectious diseases. It occurs in three forms—bubonic, primary septicemic and primary pneumonic. Age, sex, race and occupation play no role in susceptibility. Epidemics are usually bubonic but always include a small number of primary septicemic cases and cases of secondary plague pneumonia.

The reservoirs of infection are rats and other rodents in which the disease occurs in acute, subacute and chronic or latent forms. Domestic rodents belonging to the family MURIDAE are primarily concerned in the infection of man. Plague infection among the rat population is referred to as murine or rat plague, and among wild rodents as sylvatic or wild rodent plague.

Meteorologic conditions exert an important influence upon the epidemiology of the disease. The gross climate is important in determining the survival of plague bacilli and the types of disease which they may produce in man. Primary pneumonic plague epidemics rarely if ever occur in the absence of constantly low temperatures and high relative humidity. Microclimate, that is, the immediate environment of the flea, is of extreme importance in determining the life of the vector.

Extreme heat and dryness are inimical to the spread of plague. The disease is more commonly seen in the temperate zone in the summer and autumn months when fleas are most numerous and human disease in consequence often takes the bubonic form. In India and other parts of the tropics the plague season frequently prevails during the cooler months of the year.

Dissemination from one area to another may occur in a variety of ways but usually by the transportation of infected rats in ships. Occasionally it may be by the importation of fleas in bales of material containing the infected and living insects. Occasionally an ambulatory or more severe human case may be responsible. In areas where sylvatic plague is present migrations of the rodent population may extend the endemic area.

Murine or rat plague is disseminated primarily by the brown sewer rat, *Rattus norvegicus*, to the smaller domestic black house rat, *R. rattus rattus*. The infected sewer rat not infrequently will enter the lower parts of buildings and die. Immediately after its death the fleas leave the carcass in search of a new host to whom the infection is transmitted.

*Rattus r. rattus* is rare in Europe today but widespread and common in the tropics in close association with man. *Rattus norvegicus* has a world-wide distribution. *Rattus r. alexandrinus* has been important in the epidemiology of plague in Egypt in the past and has been reported to be present in the South Pacific islands. *Rattus hawaiiensis* is the reservoir in the Hawaiian Islands. Rats in different areas apparently possess varying degrees of resistance to infection by the plague bacillus. The disease is transmitted from rat to rat and from rat to man by fleas.

SYLVATIC PLAGUE. Some seventy-two other rodents, of which the ground squirrel (Western United States) and the gerbille and the multimammate mouse (South Africa) are the most important, may act as reservoirs of the infection. Sylvatic plague in wild rodents occurs in areas sparsely inhabited by man. The rarity of human infections in the United States, even in the presence of marked epizootics, implies a weakness in the flea link of the transmission chain, since man is rarely infected unless directly exposed to fleas from rodent burrows or, more often, to contamination by handling infected animals. The spread to a domestic rodent population, that is to say translation from sylvatic to murine plague, is most apt to occur when uncontrolled rodent populations come into contact and freely exchange their ectoparasites (Fig. 72).

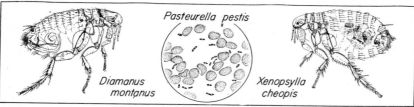

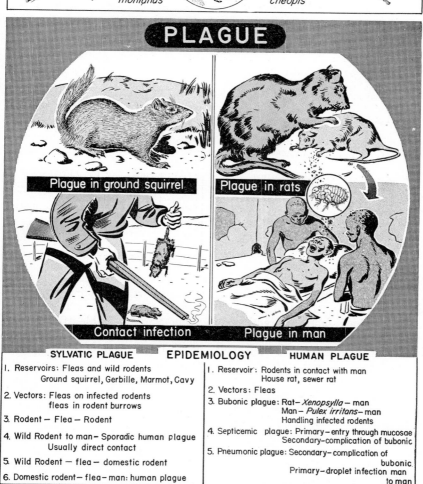

|  SYLVATIC PLAGUE | EPIDEMIOLOGY | HUMAN PLAGUE |

| SYLVATIC PLAGUE | HUMAN PLAGUE |
|---|---|
| 1. Reservoirs: Fleas and wild rodents<br>    Ground squirrel, Gerbille, Marmot, Cavy | 1. Reservoir: Rodents in contact with man<br>    House rat, sewer rat |
| 2. Vectors: Fleas on infected rodents<br>    fleas in rodent burrows | 2. Vectors: Fleas |
| 3. Rodent — Flea — Rodent | 3. Bubonic plague: Rat– *Xenopsylla* – man<br>    Man– *Pulex irritans* – man<br>    Handling infected rodents |
| 4. Wild Rodent to man– Sporadic human plague<br>    Usually direct contact | 4. Septicemic plague: Primary–entry through mucosae<br>    Secondary–complication of bubonic |
| 5. Wild Rodent — flea — domestic rodent | 5. Pneumonic plague: Secondary–complication of<br>    bubonic.<br>    Primary–droplet infection man<br>    to man |
| 6. Domestic rodent– flea – man: human plague | |

Fig. 72. Epidemiology of plague.

THE VECTOR. Various fleas are immediately responsible for transmission of the infection from the reservoir to man. These insects may live for one to two years under favorable conditions of temperature and moisture. They survive several months without food in cool and moist environments but die quickly in a hot dry climate. In moderate temperatures they may remain infective for prolonged periods.

A flea feeding upon its infected rodent host ingests the plague bacilli which then multiply in its gut, sometimes becoming so numerous as to block the lumen. Man may be infected by the bite of such an insect since *P. pestis* is regurgitated from the esophagus and proventriculus as the flea attempts to feed. The organisms are likewise passed in the feces of the flea and may infect man either through

*Table 16   Some Important Flea Vectors of* Pasteurella pestis

| FLEA | DISTRIBUTION | RESERVOIR-HOSTS | TRANSMITS PRIMARILY TO: |
|---|---|---|---|
| *Xenopsylla cheopis* . . . . . | Widely disseminated | *Rattus rattus* *R. norvegicus* | Rats and man |
| *X. brasiliensis* . . . . . . . | Uganda Kenya, Nigeria | Rats | Rats and man |
| *X. astia* . . . . . . . . . . . | India, Ceylon, Burma, Mesopotamia, Mombasa | Rats | Rats |
| *X. nubicus* . . . . . . . . . | Tropical East and West Africa | Rats | Rats |
| *X. eridos* . . . . . . . . . . | South Africa | Wild rodents | Wild rodents |
| *Pulex irritans* | Nearly cosmopolitan | Man, swine, rodents | Man, rodents |
| *Nosopsyllus fasciatus* . . . | Temperate zone | *R. norvegicus* | Rats |
| *Diamanus montanus* . . . | Western United States | Ground squirrels | Ground squirrels |
| *Rhopalopsyllus cavicola* . | South America | Cavies | Cavies |
| *Ceratophyllus tesquorum* . | Russian steppes | Ground squirrels | Ground squirrels |
| *Oropsylla silantiewi* . . . . | Manchuria | Rodents | Rodents |

the bite wound or through a minute abrasion of the skin. It is possible that the body louse, *Pediculus humanus* var. *corporis*, and, more remotely, the bedbug, *Cimex lectularius*, may occasionally transmit the infection directly from man to man (Table 16).

OTHER MEANS OF TRANSMISSION. Transmission of plague to man by other means is less common. A small proportion of cases of bubonic plague may be traced to entry of the bacilli through abraded skin of the feet as in cowdung-floored houses in India, or of the hands in the performance of an autopsy or in the handling or skinning of infected animals.

Primary septicemic plague may result from the entry of the bacilli through mucous membranes, especially those of the mouth, throat and conjunctiva.

PREDISPOSING FACTORS. Bubonic plague is commonly acquired through the bite of an infected human flea or rat flea. Important contributory factors are an overcrowded human population housed in unsanitary buildings which provide adequate food and harborage for an uncontrolled rodent population. Epidemics of bubonic plague are associated with a high incidence of the disease in rats with great mortality among them. When the rodent population is sufficiently reduced, many of the infected fleas migrate to man.

A few severe epidemics of plague have been of the *primary pneumonic type* which is transmitted directly from man to man by droplet infection from the cough. Meteorologic conditions, particularly temperature, are exceedingly important factors in determining the spread or failure to spread of the pneumonic type of the disease.

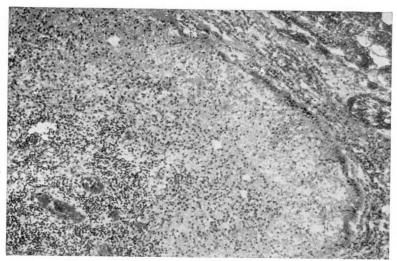

Fif. 73. Section through plague bubo showing necrosis and beginning abscess formation, capsule of lymph node and surrounding edema and infiltration.

Freezing temperatures with high relative humidity favor transmission, since pulverized and frozen sputum and cough droplets retain infective and virulent bacilli for long periods of time. Communities in which there is overcrowding of the population with close contact between sick and well and in which unsanitary conditions and practices are usual, provide a fertile field for this type of the disease. Isolated cases of secondary plague pneumonia occurring as a complication of bubonic or of primary septicemic plague often constitute the immediate origin of such an outbreak. Such secondary pneumonia, however, is not as infectious as is primary pneumonic plague and unless the conditions for respiratory transmission are wholly suitable it is less apt to initiate large epidemics.

**Pathology** The pathology of plague is essentially that of lymphangitis, lymphadenitis or bubo formation and bacteremia with metastatic localization.

In bubonic plague the lymph nodes draining the site of infection are swollen, edematous, congested and hemorrhagic, forming the primary bubo which often undergoes necrosis. Adjacent nodes are matted together and there is much edema and hemorrhage in the surrounding tissues (Fig. 73).

There are often secondary inflammatory changes, similar in character, in other lymph nodes in the body. There is extensive

Fig. 74A.

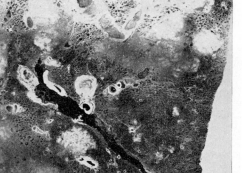

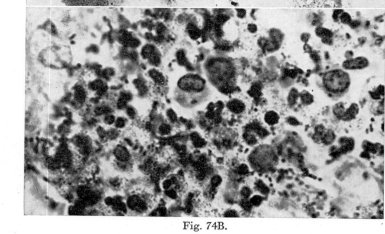

Fig. 74B.

Fig. 74. Primary pneumonic plague. *A*, Confluent lobular pneumonia. *B*, Bacilli and exudate in alveolus.

damage to vascular and lymphatic endothelium which contributes to this process and to the development of cutaneous petechiae and hemorrhages in many parts of the body.

There is marked visceral congestion, involving the brain and the meninges as well as other organs. The spleen is frequently enlarged two or three times its normal size.

PNEUMONIC PLAGUE. The pneumonia of plague is lobular in character, extending to involve entire lobes. There is intense congestion of the air passages with hemorrhagic exudate in the alveoli and bronchi but with little or no fibrin formation. Great numbers of *P. pestis* are present. The bronchial and hilar nodes are involved and ecchymoses and fibrinous pleurisy may be present over the affected portion of the lung (Fig. 74).

**Clinical Characteristics**  The incubation period of bubonic plague is usually two to four days, less often up to ten days. In primary pneumonic plague it may not exceed two to three days.

BUBONIC PLAGUE. Usually there is no prodromal period in bubonic plague although occasionally there may be a day or two of malaise and headache. In the majority of instances the onset is abrupt with chill, rapidly rising temperature to 103° or 104° F., accompanied by rapid pulse and accelerated respiration. A severe attack is usually attended by mental dullness which is followed by anxiety or excitement. The eyes are injected, the face congested, the tongue coated and nausea and vomiting may be present. Constipation is usual and the urine scanty with moderate albuminuria. An expression of intense anxiety is very characteristic of the disease. In some instances maniacal delirium may occur, in others lethargy or coma; convulsions are common in children. The acute stage with high fever commonly lasts two to five days following which, in favorable cases, the temperature falls by slow lysis reaching normal in about two weeks.

Definite bubo formation occurs in 75 per cent of cases, usually appearing from the second to the fifth day and preceded by local pain. When fully developed the bubo may be the size of an egg and is hard and tender. In fatal cases it remains indurated; in others suppuration is common. Incision, especially prior to the appearance of definite fluctuation, is hazardous because of the risk of initiating blood stream infection. The common sites of the bubo are as follows:

Inguinal .................... 65 to 75 per cent
Axillary .................... 15 to 20 per cent
Cervical .................... 5 to 10 per cent

The acute stage is accompanied by a high leukocytosis which may reach 40,000 with a corresponding increase in the polymorphonuclear cells. Positive blood culture is obtained in 45 per cent of cases. Death may occur within five days.

PESTIS MINOR. Mild ambulatory cases of plague with little or no fever or toxemia may be encountered. Frequently there is a bubo in one groin, less commonly on one side of the neck or in one axilla. These may suppurate or be gradually resorbed (Fig. 75).

PRIMARY PNEUMONIC PLAGUE. The onset of primary pneumonic plague is usually abrupt with fever rising to 103° or 104° F. within twenty-four to thirty-six hours. True rigor is rare. Painless cough and dyspnea appear within the first twenty-four hours. The sputum at first is mucoid, becoming blood-tinged but not tenacious; in the fully developed case it is thin, bright red in color, and contains enormous numbers of *P. pestis*. Physical signs are often not marked even in advanced cases. There is usually a high leukocytosis.

PRIMARY SEPTICEMIC PLAGUE. Septicemic plague can occur as a form of primary infection. However, a secondary septicemia occurs invariably in primary pneumonic cases and may occur in the course of bubonic plague. In primary septicemia cerebral symptoms fre-

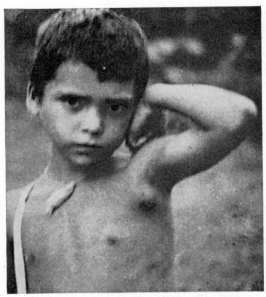

Fig. 75. Pestis minor; case of ambulatory plague showing axillary bubo. (Courtesy of Dr. A. Macchiavello.)

quently develop with great rapidity and intensity, rapidly progressing to coma. This form of the disease, if untreated, is fatal, death occurring usually within three days of onset and frequently before there is demonstrable enlargement of superficial lymph nodes.

**Diagnosis** The clinical picture of sudden onset of high fever, marked toxemia, lymphadenitis, extreme anxiety and high leukocytosis is suggestive. The appearance of a bubo is important supporting evidence. However, in primary septicemic plague there may be no significant clinical signs and in primary pneumonic plague physical signs over the chest may be trivial even in the presence of enormous numbers of bacilli in the sputum.

The definitive diagnosis depends upon the demonstration and identification of *P. pestis*. In bubonic cases, material aspirated from the bubo should be stained by Gram's method and examined for the characteristic bipolar pleomorphic bacilli. In septic and pneumonic cases, smears of blood and sputum should be similarly examined. The results of culture and animal inoculation are too delayed to permit the early diagnosis essential for effective treatment.

All material suspected of containing *P. pestis* must be handled with extreme care. Inoculated animals must be free from fleas and maintained under strict quarantine in insect-free cages. All individuals handling infected material such as cultures, inoculated animals, or cages, should wear gowns, rubber gloves and masks. All procedures must be carried out with the strictest possible aseptic technique.

DIFFERENTIAL DIAGNOSIS. In the early stages of the disease certain of the clinical types may be confused with typhus fever, relapsing fever, malaria, dengue, tularemia and rarely with typhoid.

**Prognosis** Untreated, or inadequately treated, primary pneumonic and septicemic plague are generally fatal diseases. In the past, the mortality from bubonic plague has varied from 60 to 90 per cent. Since the introduction of the sulfa drugs and the antibiotics in recent years, the mortality has been reduced remarkably. In India, streptomycin has lowered the fatality rate of bubonic and septicemic plague to 10 per cent.

**Treatment** Streptomycin is the drug of choice for the treatment of all forms of plague. It should be administered intramuscularly in the following dosage: 0.5 gm. every three or four hours until the temperature becomes normal, thereafter 1.0 gm. daily in divided doses until a total of 15.0 gm. has been given.

In severe cases, aureomycin, oxytetracycline (Terramycin) or chloramphenicol (Chloromycetin) should be used in addition to streptomycin.

Sulfadiazine and sulfamerazine are also recommended for use in large outbreaks or when the antibiotics are not available. The following dosages are advised: sulfadiazine initial dose 4.0 gm. followed by doses of 1.5 to 2.0 gm. every four hours for ten days.

SURGICAL TREATMENT OF BUBO. Hot wet applications may hasten localization. Incision should be avoided until frank fluctuation occurs.

**Prophylaxis** Prophylaxis against plague is accomplished (1) by strict isolation of the sick, (2) by appropriate sanitary measures, and (3) by protection of the individual.

1. ISOLATION OF THE SICK. Strict isolation of the patient in a separate insect-proof room is essential. All waste articles possibly contaminated and all discharges from the patient should be burned or otherwise satisfactorily disinfected. Bodies of humans and animals dead from plague should be disposed of with extreme sanitary precautions. A room previously occupied by a patient with plague must be completely and thoroughly cleaned and treated with DDT residual spray or powder (see Table 69, p. 750).

In the presence of pneumonic or suspected pneumonic plague, physicians, nurses, and any others in contact with the patient or entering the patient's room must be protected by complete coveralls, gloves, and hoods equipped with goggles or plastic face pieces. Contacts, or suspected contacts, should be treated with DDT dusting powder, segregated, and have daily temperatures recorded. Sulfadiazine or sulfamerazine, 3.0 gm. daily, should be given for at least five days after the last exposure. Streptomycin is not recommended for prophylactic purposes because of the rapid excretion and the difficulties of repeated dosage. It should, however, be given immediately if suggestive symptoms develop.

2. SANITARY MEASURES. The general sanitary measures directed to the prevention or control of plague are concerned primarily with rat and rat flea eradication.

Importation of rats from an endemic area should be guarded against by rat-proofing of ships, application of measures to prevent rats from leaving ships, and appropriate fumigation by cyanide gas.

In towns and cities buildings should be rat-proofed and natural harborages, especially rubbish, refuse and garbage, eliminated. Trained personnel should be utilized in well organized programs to distribute the highly effective rodenticides sodium fluoroacetate ("1080") and dicoumarin (Warfarin). Other poison baits using red squill, thallium sulfate, zinc phosphide, or barium carbonate may be used, but these are generally considered less effective than "1080" or Warfarin.

All rats obtained should be systematically examined for the presence of *P. pestis* in their ectoparasites and in their viscera. Examination of rats found dead is of great importance, since rodent epizootics commonly precede the appearance of plague in man.

In the control of outbreaks or epidemics of human plague, the destruction of rat fleas is of major importance. DDT (5 per cent in kaolin powder) has proved highly effective for this purpose. The powder should be dusted extensively in and around houses, as well as in clothing, bedding and house furnishings. "Cyanogas" is also effective, particularly in nests and burrows, but is used to a lesser extent since the advent of DDT.

The eradication program must be energetic and promptly activated, and must be directed by personnel who are familiar with current epidemiologic control measures. A continuous program should be instituted to maintain the flea index under 2.

Clothing and personal effects of passengers at ports of departure from an active plague area, and departing vehicles and aircraft, should be thoroughly dusted with DDT dusting powder.

3. PERSONAL PROPHYLAXIS. In the presence of an outbreak, all possible exposed persons should be vaccinated. Vaccination confers immunity for four to six months, the degree of which is still uncertain. The two-dose heat-killed vaccine has been used extensively. However, the single-dose vaccine composed of living avirulent plague bacilli has been observed to reduce the attack rate markedly.

The use of DDT dusting powder and the sulfa drugs after contact with septicemic or pneumonic cases has been discussed above.

Personnel engaged in rat control programs should be immunized and should wear flea-proof DDT-dusted clothing with particular emphasis on high boots, tight wristbands and tight collars. This insures maximum protection against fleas found on the rodents and present abundantly in their burrows and nests.

# 26 Tularemia

**Synonyms**   Plague-like disease of rodents; deer fly fever; rabbit fever.

**Definition**   Tularemia is a bacteremic plague-like disease of various small mammals, especially rabbits and hares, caused by *Pasteurella tularensis* (*Bacterium tularense*). It is highly infectious. In man it is characterized by an ulcer at the site of inoculation, regional lymphadenitis, and severe constitutional symptoms.

**Distribution**   The disease occurs in the United States, Canada, Alaska, Norway, Sweden, Germany, Austria, Czechoslovakia, Turkey, Russia and Japan.

**Etiology**   *Pasteurella tularensis* is a small pheomorphic, gram-negative, nonmotile, non–spore-bearing aerobic bacillus. Stained smears exhibit coccoid bacilli and bipolar- stained bacillary forms. It grows well on blood-dextrose-cystine agar, and coagulated egg yolk media, but not on plain agar or other ordinary media.

**Epidemiology**   *Pasteurella tularensis* is widely distributed in nature in a variety of animal hosts, the more important of which are wild rabbits and hares. Among these it is transmitted by blood-sucking arthropods such as ticks, fleas, lice and flies. Other animals infected include ground squirrels, wild rats, meadow mice, the opossum, beaver and water rats. Less frequently it occurs as an epizootic in certain game birds, particularly quail and grouse.

Ticks belonging to the genera *Haemaphysalis* and *Dermacentor* are most important vectors of the disease among mammals and birds. In these arthropods the infection is transmitted transovarially from one generation to another. Species of *Ixodes* are likewise active in transmission among rabbits. Passage of the infection through the ova, however, has not been demonstrated for this genus.

The infection reaches man by a variety of means which may be loosely classified as contaminative, inoculative, and ingestive. Infection by contamination may occur through minor abrasions of the skin or even the unbroken skin and mucous membranes by the handling, skinning, and dressing of diseased animals or birds, and by contact with the feces of infected ticks which contain the organisms.

Infection by inoculation is acquired by the bite of infected ticks, particularly *D. andersoni* and *D. variabilis*, the deer fly *Chrysops discalis*, and other blood-sucking arthropods. Bites or scratches by diseased animals may likewise cause infection.

Tularemia may also be acquired by the ingestion of insufficiently cooked meat and, rarely, through contaminated water.

Although *P. tularensis* has been demonstrated in the sputum from human cases of the disease there is no record of direct spread from man to man.

**Pathology**   In the acute form of the disease a primary ulcer develops at the site of inoculation, accompanied by lymphangitis and regional lymphadenitis. The affected lymph nodes may become considerably enlarged, closely resembling the bubo of plague, and often undergo necrosis and suppuration. Focal necroses occur in the spleen, liver and lungs with infiltration by polymorphonuclear leukocytes and large mononuclear cells. In some instances there is a lobular pneumonia with an exudate containing many monocytes. The organisms rarely can be demonstrated in the tissues.

The subacute form of the disease is characterized by tuberculoid lesions in various organs. These present a central zone of focal necrosis enclosed by epithelioid cells and fibroblasts, surrounded by small lymphocytes. Occasional giant cells are present.

**Clinical Characteristics**    The various clinical phenomena of tularemia tend to divide the disease into four distinct clinical types:

1. The ulceroglandular type.
2. The oculoglandular type.
3. The glandular type.
4. The typhoidal type.

These have much in common, being distinguished one from the other by certain particularly prominent features.

The *incubation period* in the majority of cases varies from three to five days and is terminated by abrupt onset of acute disease without antecedent prodromal symptoms, frequently accompanied by severe headache, sharp chill and rapid rise of fever to 103° or 104° F. There is frequently a one to three day remission of fever accompanied by amelioration of constitutional symptoms in the first week of the disease followed by return of the pyrexia and other phenemona. The acute phase is self-limited with a usual duration of two to three weeks. During this period recurring chills, drenching sweats, marked prostration, aching pains in the back and extremities, severe headache and vomiting are often prominent features. There is a moderate leukocytosis, seldom exceeding 15,000. Various types of skin eruption may occur. Defervescence is by lysis.

1. ULCEROGLANDULAR TYPE. This includes about 84 per cent of cases. The primary lesion commonly occurs on the hands or fingers. Usually within forty-eight hours of the onset a painful regional lymphadenitis develops preceding the appearance of an inflamed papule at the site of inoculation (Fig. 76). This progresses to pustule formation and subsequently to the development of a punched-out ulcer which heals with considerable scarring. A superficial lymphangitis between the primary lesion and the enlarged regional lymph nodes is common, and nodular swellings along the course of the inflamed lymphatics may be suggestive of sporotrichosis. The epitrochlear and axillary lymph nodes are most frequently involved. Suppuration occurs in about 50 per cent of cases; in the others resolution is slow and may require several months.

2. OCULOGLANDULAR TYPE. This type includes about 6 per cent of cases.

3. GLANDULAR TYPE. This form of tularemia comprises about 4 per

cent of cases. It is characterized by a regional lymphadenitis, but there is no lesion at the site of infection.

4. TYPHOIDAL TYPE. This type includes about 5 per cent of cases.

COMPLICATIONS. Bronchopneumonia, bronchitis and pleurisy with or without effusion may occur as complications. In the presence of pulmonary involvement *P. tularensis* may be recovered from the sputum. Other serious complications are blindness following the oculoglandular type, *P. tularensis* septicemia and meningitis.

**Prognosis** Without adequate treatment the mortality is approximately 7.4 per cent.

**Diagnosis** The clinical picture and a history of contact with wild rabbits or other rodents, or of bites by ticks or deerflies should

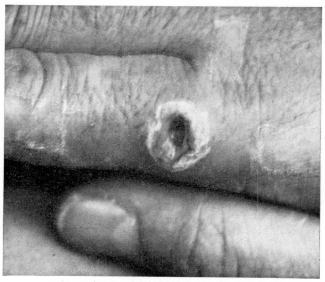

Fig. 76. Tularemia: primary lesion on hand.

be suggestive of tularemia. The fever rises sharply, with a temporary remission followed by a febrile period of two to three weeks' duration. Local lesions such as ulcer, enlarged lymph nodes or conjunctivitis may not be present during the first few days. Definitive diagnosis is reached by recovery of the organism. Blood cultures should be made on dextrose-cystine agar or thioglycolate blood agar. Positive cultures may likewise be obtained from primary lesions, material aspirated from softened lymph nodes, or the sputum (Fig. 76). Inoculation of suspected material into guinea pigs is a useful diagnostic procedure, since these animals are susceptible and usually die within a week. The gross lesions closely resemble those of plague but are distinguishable by histopathologic examination and by culture. The failure of *P. tularensis* to grow on plain agar and the characteristic morphologic variants of *P. pestis* on salt agar permit easy differentiation. Inoculated animals can also be used for agglutination tests.

Demonstration of a rising agglutinin titer in the patient's serum during the course of the disease is significant. Antibiotic treatment does not affect the rise of titer sufficiently to interfere with diagnosis.

The diagnosis of the typhoidal or pneumonic type may be difficult. Suspected cases, particularly in endemic areas or among laboratory workers exposed to infection, should be treated promptly.

DIFFERENTIAL DIAGNOSIS. Inflammatory nodules along the superficial lymphatics in the ulcerograndular type may suggest sporotrichosis. The glandular type particularly may be confused with plague and in the presence of inguinal lymphadenitis, pyogenic infections, venereal bubo and climatic bubo must be considered as well. The frequent cross agglutination with *Br. abortus* and *Br. melitensis* may be misleading. However, as the disease progresses the agglutinin titer for *P. tularensis* far exceeds the titer for the *Brucella* group.

**Treatment**    Streptomycin or dihydrostreptomycin are the drugs of choice for the treatment of tularemia. Although good results have been reported with aureomycin and chloramphenicol (Chloromycetin), relapses are said to be more common following their use.

Streptomycin or dihydrostreptomycin should be administered intramuscularly. A total of 2.0 to 4.0 gm. given in individual doses of 0.5 gm. every eight hours is usually sufficient to effect a cure, except in the typhoidal type of the disease. Other recommended regimes are: 0.5 gm. daily for two days followed by 0.25 gm. daily for four days; or, 0.5 gm. daily for six days.

In the typhoidal type of tularemia the antibiotic should be continued until the patient is afebrile.

Defervescence usually occurs within three days except in the typhoidal type of the disease. Antibiotic therapy early in the clinical course may inhibit natural immunity, so subsequent reinfection may occur.

**Prophylaxis**    The essential feature of the prophylaxis of tularemia is avoidance of the reservoir hosts. In heavily endemic areas rabbits and other rodents should be handled with caution, since *P. tularensis* may be present not only in the animal itself but in tick feces in its fur. When ticks are prevalent suitable precautions should be taken, including the wearing of protective clothing and the prompt removal of ticks before their attachment. Trouser legs should be tucked into boots and insect repellent (612 or dimethyl phthallate) applied generously to the boot tops and trousers below the knees. Gloves and shirt sleeves may be similarly treated (Table 69, p. 751). It is highly important that the body be carefully inspected at the end of the day and all ticks removed.

Prophylactic vaccination has proved effective for the prevention of tularemia among laboratory workers exposed to these organisms. It is to be recommended for those exposed to tularemia as an occupational hazard if precautions are taken to exclude hypersensitive persons.

Wild birds and game used for food must be thoroughly cooked. The usual methods for water purification confer protection against the rare water-borne infections.

# 27  Introduction

The superficial and the systemic mycoses comprise a group of diseases resulting from infection of the skin or the viscera by pathogenic fungi. Although many of these agents are widely spread geographically, they have greatest importance in the tropics where the conditions of climate and of sanitation provide an especially favorable environment.

The fungi belong to a subdivision of the plant kingdom known as the THALLOPHYTA. These are characterized by a simple filamentous structure without differentiation into roots, stems and leaves. The THALLOPHYTA in turn are subdivided into the ALGAE, which contain chlorophyll, and the FUNGI, which lack chlorophyll and which are, therefore, parasitic or saprophytic in character. These latter include the SCHIZOMYCETES, or bacteria, the MYXOMYCETES, or slime moulds, and the EUMYCETES, or true fungi (Fig. 77).

The majority of those organisms which are pathogenic for man belong within the FUNGI IMPERFECTI, a group comprising those true fungi which lack a sexual stage in their life cycles. They are characterized by a vegetative body composed of filamentous elements or hyphae, and reproductive organs or spores of various types produced in various ways. Final identification of the fungi requires cultivation on artificial media and study of the gross colony, the hyphae, the method of spore formation, and the type of spores produced.

**191**

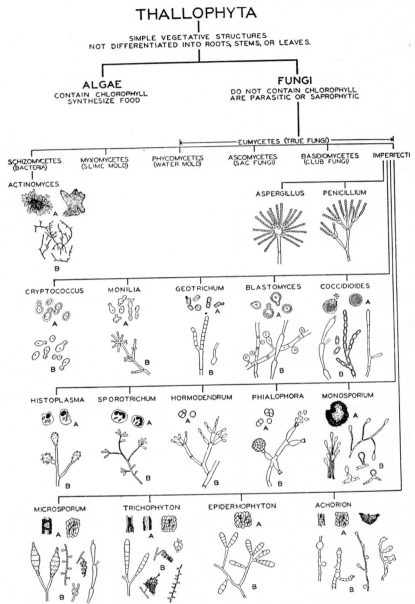

Fig. 77. Classification of the THALLOPHYTA. Forms labelled *A*—forms occurring in the pathologic lesion; forms labelled *B*—forms occurring in culture. (After Musser, Internal Medicine, Its Theory and Practice, ed. 3. Lea & Febiger, 1938.)

# 28    Cutaneous Mycoses

The dermatomycoses are superficial infections of the skin or its appendages, caused principally by members of three closely related genera of the FUNGI IMPERFECTI—*Trichophyton, Microsporum* and *Epidermophyton*. They do not invade the deeper tissues or the internal organs. Members of the genus *Trichophyton* attack the hair, the skin, and the nails. The fungus may be confined to the cortex of the hair, appearing as chains of spores arranged in parallel rows, or it may be on the surface of the hair in chains of small (microspore type) or large (macrospore type) spores. In the skin and the nails these fungi present segmented, branching, mycelial elements with or without chains of spores and are distinguishable from *Microsporum* and *Epidermophyton*.

The genus *Microsporum* attacks the hair and the skin. Infected hairs from the scalp commonly present a characteristic appearance produced by a sheath of small spores surrounding the shaft of the hair and tending to be in a mosaic arrangement rather than in parallel rows as in *Trichophyton* infections. In the skin, species of *Microsporum* form segmented mycelial elements which are identical in appearance with those of *Trichophyton* and *Epidermophyton*.

The genus *Epidermophyton* attacks the skin and nails, forming segmented branching mycelial elements which are indistinguishable from those of *Microsporum* and *Trichophyton* (Table 17).

**Diagnosis of Dermatomycoses**    A diagnosis of dermatomycosis may be made by direct microscopic examination of an infected hair or of scrapings from the margins of lesions of the skin or nails. Although a clue to the particular genus may be obtained by such examination in the case of *Trichophyton* or *Microsporum* infections of the hair, definitive diagnosis can be made only by examination of the growth characteristics in artificial culture media. Since the morphology of all three genera in infected skin and nails is identical, differentiation and species identification must be based entirely upon the cultural characteristics.

MICROSCOPIC EXAMINATION. For the microscopic examination of scrapings from the skin or nails, or fragments of hair, the material should be placed in a drop of 10–40 per cent potassium hydroxide on a clean glass slide, covered with a cover slip and heated gently. If clearing is not adequate, additional potassium hydroxide may be run in under the cover slip and the preparation reheated. Following such treatment the mycelia and spores are easily distinguished (see p. 817).

CULTURES. Similiar material should be used for culture. Hair or scrapings collected should be placed between two slides previously wrapped in paper and sterilized. After rewrapping the material may be transported to the laboratory for immediate inoculation on Sabouraud's glucose agar to which has been added ten units of penicillin and thirty units of streptomycin per milliliter of agar. Such a medium will inhibit bacterial growth. Also, actidione may be added (0.1 mg./ml.) to the above medium to inhibit saprophytic fungus growth. All cultures should be maintained at room temperature for two to three weeks. Differentiation of the genera and identification

*Table 17   Mycotic Infections of the Skin and Appendages*

| DISEASE | ETIOLOGIC AGENTS |
| --- | --- |
| Tinea capitis | *Microsporum audouini*<br>*M. canis*<br>*M. gypseum*<br>*Trichophyton mentagrophytes*<br>*T. violaceum*<br>*T. schoenleini*<br>*T. sulfureum*<br>*T. tonsurans* |
| Tinea favosa | *T. schoenleini*<br>*T. violaceum*<br>*M. gypseum* |
| Tinea barbae | *M. canis*<br>*T. rubrum*<br>*T. mentagrophytes*<br>*T. album* |
| Dermatophytosis | *Trichophyton* species<br>*Epidermophyton floccosum*<br>*Candida albicans* |
| Tinea cruris | *E. floccosum*<br>*Trichophyton* species |
| Tinea circinata (corporis) | *Trichophyton* species |
| Tinea imbricata | *T. concentricum* |
| Tinea versicolor (pityriasis versicolor) | *Malassezia furfur* |
| Otomycosis | *Aspergillus* species<br>*Penicillium* species<br>*Monilia* species |

of the species are based upon the gross and microscopic characteristics of the colonies and their elements.

## Tinea Capitis

**Synonyms**   Tinea tonsurans; herpes tonsurans; tinea of the scalp.

**Definition**   A fungus infection of the stratum corneum of the scalp and the hair, most common in children, characterized by scaling, occasionally dermatitis, and breaking of infected hairs. It usually disappears spontaneously at puberty.

**Distribution**   This infection is widespread without geographic limitations and may occur epidemically in schools and among crowded populations.

**Etiology** Tinea capitis is produced by several species of *Microsporum* and *Trichophyton*.

**Pathology** The fungus first invades the stratum corneum of the scalp, producing a minute rounded scaling patch or a reddish papule from which a hair projects. Subsequently there is invasion of the hair follicle and then the deeper or superficial portions of the shaft of the hair. More severe reactions lead to kerion formation, and an edematous pustular infection of the scalp.

**Clinical Characteristics** The infected hairs become lusterless and brittle and finally break, leaving short stubs projecting from the lesion. Temporary or permanent alopecia may result. The more severe infection or kerion is a painful, weeping, pustular infection with crusting.

**Diagnosis** Microscopic examination of a potassium hydroxide preparation of scrapings from the scalp or of the hair. Cultures should be made and the etiologic agent specifically identified.

**Treatment** Treatment is difficult and often unsatisfactory but spontaneous recovery usually follows an inflammatory reaction to the infection. The scalp should be shampooed daily with soap and water to remove all crusts and scales, after which local agents such as propionate-caprylate compound ointment (Sopronol), 5 per cent undecylenic acid ointment (Desenex), salicylanilide ointment or 5 per cent ammoniated mercury ointment should be rubbed into the scalp. X-ray epilation, although considered the most direct method of treatment, should not be attempted in the presence of inflammation or until a trial of three to four months of local treatment has proven unsatisfactory. Manual epilation of infected hairs and crusts is helpful. If secondary infection is present, warm saline compresses may be necessary. Three per cent sulfur and 3 per cent salicylic acid in petrolatum may be substituted for the ammoniated mercury as an adjunct. Personal effects such as combs and hair brushes, caps or hats must be sterilized and should not be used by others.

## Tinea Favosa

**Synonym** Favus.

**Definition** A fungus infection of the scalp, of the non-hairy skin of the body or of the nails commonly seen in children; it may extend into adult life. It is characterized by the formation of yellowish crusts overlying shallow ulcers.

**Distribution** Classic favus is common in China and Central Asia. It is not uncommon in North Africa, the Balkan region, Germany and Mexico. The disease is rare in other areas. As is the case with tinea capitis, it may occur epidemically.

**Etiology** This condition is usually caused by *Trichophyton schoenleini* (Fig. 78).

**Clinical Characteristics** The initial lesions appear as minute, whitish, scaly patches; subsequently sulfur-colored crusts are produced, piling up to form an elevated mass with raised edges. These crusts are very adherent. Removal reveals a superficial ulcer oozing serum or blood-tinged exudate. This infection may cause permanent alopecia.

**Diagnosis** Microscopic examination of a potassium hydroxide preparation of scrapings from the early lesions and identification of the fungus by culture.

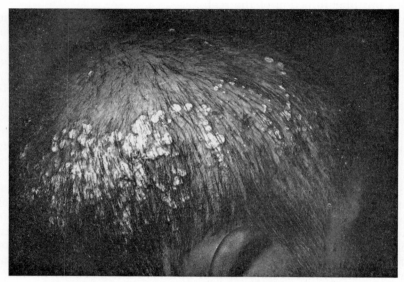

Fig. 78. Favus, showing alopecia and crusted lesions of scalp.

**Treatment** The methods advised for tinea capitis should be used. Roentgen epilation is almost always necessary.

## Tinea Barbae

**Synonyms** Tinea sycosis; barber's itch; ringworm of beard.

**Definition** A fungus infection of the bearded area and neck of men, involving the skin, hair and hair follicles, usually resulting in a chronic, deep suppurative lesion.

**Distribution** This infection is widespread without geographic limitations but may occur in small epidemics as a result of contact with infected cattle.

**Etiology** Tinea barbae is produced by *Trichophyton mentagrophytes*, *T. rubrum*, *T. violaceum* and *Microsporum canis*. Infection from cattle can be caused by *T. mentagrophytes* or *T. verrucosum*. The latter is difficult to isolate on standard media.

**Pathology** Superficial infection of the skin produces scaling circular lesions with a vesiculopustular border. Deep infection of the skin produces suppurative lesions with follicular pustules, kerion formation and extensive abscess formation.

**Clinical Characteristics** The superficial lesions resemble those of tinea circinata of the glabrous skin (Fig. 86). Progressive infection may lead to a suppurative folliculitis, forming large nodular crusted lesions which extrude pus on slight pressure. The infected hairs are brittle, easily removed and few are seen in older lesions.

**Diagnosis** Microscopic examination of potassium hydroxide preparations of skin and hair should reveal fungus elements. Cultures of such material are necessary to determine the exact etiologic agent of a given case.

**Treatment** Early superficial lesions may be treated successfully with 3 per cent ammoniated mercury or tincture of iodine. Treatment of chronic suppurative lesions is difficult. Compresses with Burow's solution (1:15), Vleminck's solution (1:33) or hypertonic saline solution. Hairs in the affected area should be manually epilated. Potassium iodide by mouth may be necessary in recalcitrant cases. Antibiotics and/or sulfonamides should be used to control secondary bacterial infections.

## Dermatophytosis

**Synonyms** Trichophytosis, epidermophytosis, ringworm of hands and feet, Hong Kong foot, athlete's foot.

**Definition** Dermatophytosis is a chronic superficial infection of the skin, especially of that between the toes, with maceration and cracking, occasionally extending to involve adjacent skin areas. Less commonly it may affect the hands, groins, axillae and other regions. It is accompanied by intense itching (Fig. 79).

**Distribution** The infection is widespread and may be particularly troublesome in the moist tropics and subtropics.

**Etiology** It is usually due to a species of *Trichophyton,* or less commonly *Epidermophyton floccosum,* or *Candida albicans.*

**Epidemiology** This infection is extremely common and widespread. The fungi are resistant and persist indefinitely in shoes and other contaminated leather objects. They may be transmitted by towels and clothing unless these are sterilized in washing. They frequently contaminate the floors of baths and washrooms. The infection is acquired directly from contact with an infected individual or indirectly from contaminated floors and articles of clothing. A hot, humid climate and wet feet are predisposing factors.

**Pathology** The infection is limited to the cornified layer of the skin, producing acute, chronic, and hyperkeratotic lesions. The acute stage is accompanied by erythema, scaling and cracking of the affected skin. Secondary infection is common. Invasion of the nails (onychomycosis) is frequent.

Remote skin sensitization may occur and be accompanied by eruptions, dermatophytids, on various parts of the body. These do not contain the fungi and subside with control of the active focus.

**Clinical Characteristics**   The interdigital areas, especially between the third and fourth and fourth and fifth toes, are the usual sites of infection. The lesion may consist of simple erythema with scaling. Fissuring between the toes is common and the process may be complicated by secondary bacterial infection. In chronic infections the skin is thickened, white and macerated. Not infrequently deep, shotty vesicles appear on the soles of the feet and the palms of the hands. These are accompanied by pruritus and contain clear mucoid ma-

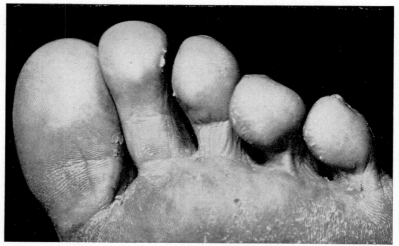

Fig. 79. Dermatophytosis of foot: early lesions, scaling of skin of toes. (Courtesy Dr. Ray O. Noojin, Duke University.)

terial. In severe cases eczematoid lesions may occur involving the foot, ankle, groin, axilla, hand, and other areas. These may present an acute inflammatory process with edema and cellulitis due to secondary bacterial invasion (Figs. 80, 81).

Less commonly there may be involvement of the perianal skin with severe pruritus.

Involvement of the nails, especially the toenails, is frequent and characteristically one or more escape invasion. The affected nail becomes deformed, discolored, opaque and friable. Onychomycosis is resistant to therapy and consequently constitutes an important reservoir for reinfection (Fig. 82).

The remote skin rashes or dermatophytids are considered to be an allergic reaction following upon cutaneous sensitization to the fungus. The lesions are not distinctive and may be acute, chronic or eczematoid in nature. They usually appear immediately following a flare-up of the infection between the toes (Fig. 83).

**Diagnosis**   It is extremely important to make a careful examination of the skin between and beneath the toes. Scrapings should be made from the margin of the lesion with a sharp scalpel. Microscopic examination of the potassium hydroxide preparation of this material or of the epithelial covering of vesicles will reveal the mycelia of the fungus. Cultures should be made for specific identification of the fungus.

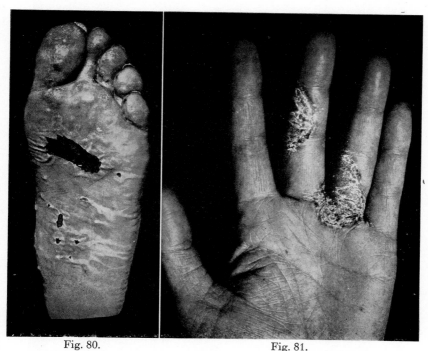

Fig. 80.                    Fig. 81.

Fig. 80. Dermatophytosis of foot: advanced lesions showing undermining, bullous response with vesicles and pustules. (Courtesy Dr. Ray O. Noojin, Duke University.)
Fig. 81. Dermatophytosis of hand. (Courtesy Dr. J. Lamar Callaway, Duke University.)

**Treatment** The commonest error in the therapy of both acute and chronic dermatophytosis is *overtreatment* which frequently produces severe dermatitis. There is no standardized or universally successful method of management. Treatment must be individualized for each case. Roentgen therapy is not fungicidal but is useful in the control of the eczmatoid complications.

Chronic Stages. For the chronic stages the recommended measures are as follows:

1. Daily 1:4000 potassium permanganate soaks for one-half hour followed by mechanical débridement of all of the crusts, scales, and dead skin.

2. One-half strength Whitfield's ointment, propionate-caprylate

Fig. 82.

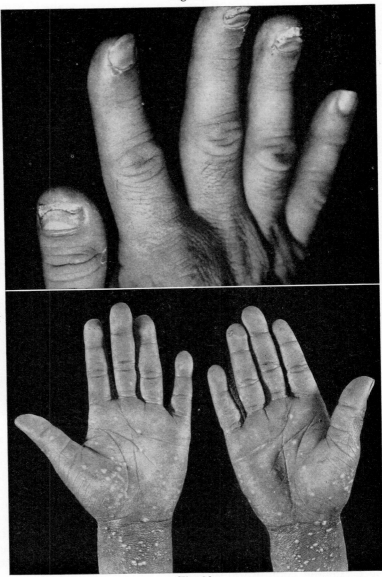

Fig. 83.

Fig. 82. Onychomycosis invasion of the nails. (Courtesy Dr. J. Lamar Callaway, Duke University.)

Fig. 83. Dermatophytid of hands. (Courtesy Dr. J. Lamar Callaway, Duke University.)

compound ointment (Sopronol), 5 per cent undecylenic acid ointment (Desenex), or salicylanilide ointment should be applied overnight. The excess should be removed the following morning, followed by the application of:

3. Fifteen per cent calcium propionate talcum powder (Sopronol) or Desenex powder for daytime use.

4. One per cent iodine and 3 per cent salicylic acid in 70 per cent alcohol may be used at night instead of one-half strength Whitfield's ointment.

5. Castellani's paint may be used at night instead of the one-half strength Whitfield's ointment.

SEVERE CASES WITH ECZEMATOID LESIONS. None of these fungicidal preparations should be used in the presence of acute eczematoid lesions or with secondary bacterial infections. They should be treated by bed rest, elevation of the affected parts, and wet dressings of saturated boric acid solution or Burow's solution diluted 1:20. After the acute process has been controlled, the treatment regimen outlined above may be started cautiously beginning with greatly reduced concentrations.

ONYCHOMYCOSIS. Treatment of onychomycosis is exceedingly unsatisfactory and surgical avulsion is not recommended. Daily filing of the nails to tissue paper thinness followed by 1:4000 potassium permanganate soaks for one-half hour, after which 10 per cent sulfur and 10 per cent salicylic acid in petrolatum is rubbed in, will sometimes effect a cure. Filtered roentgen therapy in fractional doses (75 r.) at weekly intervals for four to six weeks may help further with the control of the onychomycosis.

DERMATOPHYTIDS. The treatment of dermatophytids is symptomatic but eventual cure depends on control of the active fungus focus.

**Prophylaxis** The prophylaxis of dermatophytosis consists of careful drying of the skin, especially between the toes, the use of slippers in public baths and washrooms, the avoidance of borrowed clothing, and proper sterilization of clothing, including socks and towels. The regular use of a foot powder consisting of calcium propionate 15 per cent in a talc base is a highly efficient prophylactic measure.

## Tinea Cruris

**Synonyms** Dhobie itch, eczema marginatum, ringworm of the groin, crotch itch, jock itch.

**Definition** Tinea cruris is a superficial fungus infection of the skin, primarily of the upper and inner aspects of the thighs. In severe cases it may extend to involve adjacent skin areas and the axillae.

**Distribution** The infection is widespread without particular geographic limitation.

**Etiology** It is commonly due to infection by *Epidermophyton floccosum*, less commonly by species of *Trichophyton*.

**Epidemiology** Heat, humidity, excessive perspiration and friction from clothing are predisposing causes. Indirect transmission occurs through the use of unsterilized towels and borrowed clothing.

**Clinical Characteristics** Tinea cruris is characterized by brownish or reddish lesions having a scaly surface and presenting a papular or finely vesicular border. These spread peripherally and tend to clear in the center. Small satellite lesions are not infrequent. The in-

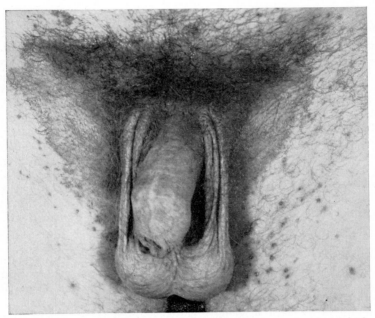

Fig. 84. Tinea cruris, showing margination and scattered active foci which may later coalesce. (Courtesy Dr. J. Lamar Callaway, Duke University.)

fection may extend to adjacent areas, particularly the scrotum, perineum and lower abdomen, and in severe cases the axillae may be involved (Figs. 84, 85).

**Diagnosis** The diagnosis of tinea cruris is based in part upon the appearance and distribution of the lesions and in part upon the microscopic examination of potassium hydroxide preparations of scrapings from the margin of an active lesion. Such examination will reveal the mycelia of the fungus. Specific identification requires examination of cultures. (*See Diagnostic Methods*, p. 838.)

**Treatment** The recommended measures are as follows:

1. 1:4000 potassium permanganate sitz baths or compresses at night, followed by:

2. Castellani's paint or one-fourth to one-half strength Whitfield's ointment or sodium propionate ointment.

3. Pragmatar ointment may be used instead of No. 2.

4. Fifteen per cent calcium propionate in talcum should be used during the daytime.

5. Extreme cleanliness is absolutely necessary.

6. The affected areas should be kept as dry as possible during the daytime. Cool loose-fitting clothing is helpful.

It is important to remember that strong fungicidal preparations should not be used on the scrotum or in the vicinity of the anus. In the presence of an active inflammatory process fungicidal prepara-

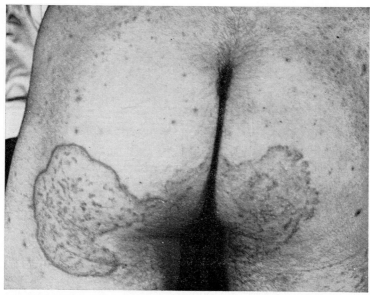

Fig. 85. Tinea cruris, active serpiginous border sharply marginated. (Courtesy Dr. J. Lamar Callaway, Duke University.)

tions should not be used until the inflammation has been completely controlled by wet boric acid or 1:20 Burow's solution dressings.

**Prophylaxis**  The prophylaxis of tinea cruris consists of the avoidance of borrowed clothing, the proper sterilization of towels and laundry, and the use of dusting powder consisting of calcium propionate 15 per cent in a talc base.

## Tinea Circinata

**Synonyms**  Tinea corporis, tinea glabrosa, trichophytosis, or "ringworm" of the body.

**Distribution**  This infection has a widespread distribution but is more common in the tropics and subtropics than in the temperate zones.

**Etiology**  It is due to infection of the skin by species of *Microsporum* and *Trichophyton*.

**Clinical Characteristics**   The early lesions of tinea circinata appear as flattened, reddish papules having a marked tendency to peripheral spread and central healing. The margins of the lesion are sharply defined and scaly or vesicular. The infection may be accompanied by a varying degree of inflammatory response, or an eczematoid reaction as well as other variations (Fig. 86).

**Diagnosis**   Examination of potassium hydroxide preparations of scrapings from the lesions reveals the fungus etiology (see p. 817). Cultures should be made for specific identification.

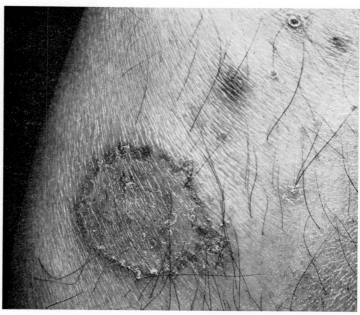

Fig. 86. Tinea circinata: active vesicular border and scaling of center of lesion. (Courtesy Dr. J. Lamar Callaway, Duke University.)

**Treatment**   In the presence of an acute inflammatory reaction initial treatment should consist of wet dressings of boric acid solution. Burow's solution diluted 1:20, aqueous solution of potassium permanganate 1:5000, or calamine lotion. When the acute process has subsided the following preparations are recommended:

1. Whitfield's ointment one-half strength may be rubbed into the lesions two or three times daily.

2. Five per cent ammoniated mercury ointment may be rubbed in two or three times daily or 3 per cent precipitated sulfur and 3 per cent salicylic acid in petrolatum should be rubbed in two or three times daily, or

3. One-fourth to one-half strength tincture of iodine may be painted on two or three times daily.

# Tinea Imbricata

**Synonyms** Tokelau, Burmese ringworm, Malabar itch.

**Distribution** Tinea imbricata is restricted to the tropics, chiefly the islands of the South Pacific, and the Malay Archipelago. It also occurs in southern China, southern India, Ceylon and Central Africa. It has been reported from Colombia, Brazil and Guatemala.

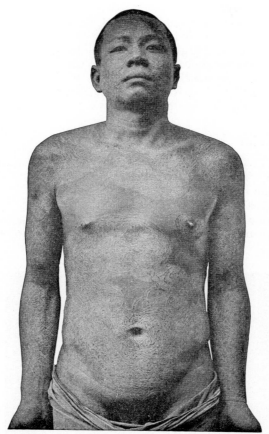

Fig. 87. Tinea imbricata showing scaling rosette-like lesions (After Henggeler in Strong Stitt's Diagnosis, Prevention and Treatment of Tropical Diseases. The Blakiston Co.)

**Etiology** It is due to infection of the skin by *Trichophyton concentricum.*

**Clinical Characteristics** The early lesion of tinea imbricata appears as a raised brownish or reddish plaque which gradually extends peripherally. The superficial epithelium desquamates, producing a scaling margin with the free inner edges of the scales turned up and directed toward the center of the lesion. Peripheral extension of the process leaves a smooth central area in which a new and similar lesion appears, producing a further circle of scales within the peripheral circle. These scaled circles following one another may be one-eighth to one-half inch apart, producing rosette-like lesions (Fig. 87). There is no accompanying inflammatory reaction. The axillae, groins, face, palms of the hands and soles of the feet are much less often affected than in the other cutaneous mycoses. The scalp is not involved. Itching is frequently intense.

**Diagnosis**    The clinical appearance of the lesions is characteristic and microscopic examination of a potassium hydroxide preparation of scrapings from the margin will reveal the mycelia of the fungus (see p. 838). Cultures should be made and identified.

**Treatment**    1. Chrysarobin ointment 5 to 10 per cent.

2. Resorcinol 12 to 25 per cent in compound tincture of benzoin applied daily or twice daily to the lesions.

## Tinea Versicolor

**Synonym**    Pityriasis versicolor.

**Distribution**    This is a very common though unimportant mycotic infection of the skin.

**Etiology**    It is due to infection by *Malassezia furfur*.

**Clinical Characteristics**    Tinea versicolor is characterized by yellowish or brownish irregular macular patches which occur especially

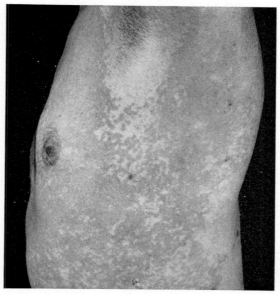

Fig. 88. Tinea versicolor: brownish pigmented eruption. (Courtesy Dr. J. Lamar Callaway, Duke University.)

on the skin over the shoulders, chest, upper back, axillae and upper abdomen. The individual lesions show fine scaling. Healing is frequently followed by partial depigmentation which may persist for a number of weeks or months (Fig. 88).

**Diagnosis** Potassium hydroxide preparations of scrapings from the lesion will reveal the characteristic clumping of round bodies and mycelial fragments.

**Treatment** The following preparations are recommended:

1. Fifteen per cent solution of sodium hyposulfite should be sponged on twice daily, or:

2. Pragmatar ointment may be applied to the lesions twice daily, or:

3. Three per cent sulfur and 3 per cent salicylic acid in petrolatum ointment may be applied each night.

4. Daily baths with removal of all scales are necessary and are rendered somewhat more efficacious by the use of vinegar, which tends to loosen the scales.

## Otomycosis

**Synonyms** Singapore ear, myringomycosis.

**Distribution** It is common in the moist tropics and likewise is frequently observed in regions of high wind and dust.

**Etiology** Many different saprophytic fungi have been isolated from this infection but the disease is primarily one of bacterial etiology.

**Clinical Characteristics** Otomycosis is rarely a mycotic infection of the skin of the external auditory canal and may present variable clinical phenomena. In mild cases the skin of the canal is reddened and scaly, producing an appearance often confused with seborrhea. In other instances the canal may be packed with a grayish mass of mycelia having an appearance of wet grayish blotting paper. Complications involving deeper structures are exceedingly rare. Infection of the canal by bacteria may result in mild symptoms or in pustule formation, cellulitis, edema and occasionally intense pain (Fig. 89).

**Diagnosis** Microscopic examination of a potassium hydroxide preparation of scrapings from the lesion or of a portion of the mycelial mass reveals the mycelia and spores of *Monilia* or the mycelia and so-called fruit-heads of *Aspergillus* or *Penicillium*. The bacterial flora should be cultured and identified.

**Treatment** If cellulitis with bacterial infection is present the condition must be treated with compresses of saline or boric acid solution for one hour three times daily followed by local application of chemotherapeutic agents selected by sensitivity tests against the cultured bacteria.

If there is no bacterial infection, as much of the mycelial mass, cerumen, and other debris as possible should be removed with a curette, after thorough soaking with hydrogen peroxide. After this, one of the following regimens is recommended:

1. The external canal is packed for twelve hours with a pledget of wool saturated with 1 per cent thymol in Cresatin. The patient should be instructed to remove this if it produces severe burning. Thereafter 1 per cent thymol in Cresatin drops are placed in the ear night and morning.

2. Three per cent salicylic acid in 70 per cent alcohol may be swabbed in the external auditory canal and on the affected part of the ear twice daily.

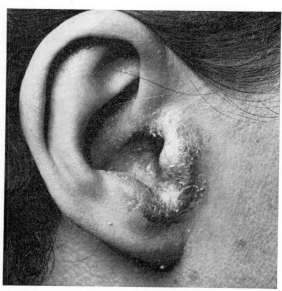

Fig. 89. Otomycosis. (Courtesy Dr. J. Lamar Callaway, Duke University.)

3. After cleansing the canal and drying with warm air it is packed for twelve hours with wool saturated with Cresatin. Thereafter for eight days the canal is packed daily for nine minutes, using a 1 per cent solution of thymol in alcohol. For three days thereafter thymol iodide is dusted into the canal three times daily. Concurrently the patient should take potassium iodide 1.8 gm. by mouth daily for three days.

4. After cleansing the canal with hydrogen peroxide solution, it should be swabbed out with 12 per cent silver nitrate. Alcohol drops should be introduced three times daily.

5. Soap and water should be avoided locally and the patient should not be allowed to go swimming.

**Prophylaxis** The prophylaxis of this infection is not satisfactory. The use of plugs in the canal does not confer protection. Precautions should be taken to keep the canal dry and against trauma with the finger or objects small enough to enter the canal.

# 29  Systemic Mycoses

Unlike the dermatomycoses the systemic or deep mycotic infections are produced by members of many genera of the fungi including representatives from the SCHIZOMYCETES, or true bacteria, as well as the FUNGI IMPERFECTI. Many tissues may be invaded and the clinical picture in consequence may be extremely variable. Identification of the genera concerned may not be difficult as is seen from

*Table 18    The Systemic Mycoses*

| DISEASE | ETIOLOGIC AGENTS |
|---|---|
| Actinomycosis | *Actinomyces bovis* |
| Maduromycosis | *Monosporium apiospermum* *Madurella* species *Indiella* species *Allescheria boydii* *Aspergillus* species *Penicillium* species *Cephalosporium* species |
| Nocardiosis (Mycetoma) | *Nocardia asteroides* *N. brasiliensis* *N. madurae* *N. pelletieri* |
| Cryptococcosis | *Cryptococcus neoformans* |
| Moniliasis | *Candida albicans* |
| Blastomycosis—North American Blastomycosis—South American | *Blastomyces dermatitidis* *B. brasiliensis* |
| Coccidioidomycosis | *Coccidioides immitis* |
| Histoplasmosis | *Histoplasma capsulatum* |
| Sporotrichosis | *Sporotrichum schenckii* |
| Chromoblastomycosis | *Phialophora verrucosa* *Hormodendrum pedrosoi* *H. compactum* |

the accompanying table. Identification of species within the genera, however, may require specialized experience and training. (See pp. 817, 838.)

An important feature of systemic mycotic infections is the common development of sensitization to the fungus and its products. This reaction probably plays a significant part in the progress of the disease and likewise constitutes a factor of great importance in the planning of therapy. In a sensitive individual or in an anergic individual with active infection, the use of roentgen therapy or the exhibition of iodides may be followed by rapid and grave extension of the infection. Sensitivity should invariably be evaluated by the intracutaneous injection of stock or autogenous vaccines. In the presence of a positive skin test desensitization should be carried out by repeated graduated doses of vaccine prior to the use of iodides. The prognosis is bad in anergic patients who give negative skin tests in the presence of active infection, since this indicates that they have little or no resistance.

*Table 19*   *Key to Microscopic Appearance of Pathogenic Fungi Found in Scrapings, Sputum, Pus, Etc.*

(Does not apply to appearance in culture)

| | | | |
|---|---|---|---|
| 1 | (2) | Mycelia present ........................................................... | 3 |
| 2 | (1) | Without mycelia ........................................... | 7 |
| 3 | (4) | Mycelia of bacterial narrowness ................................. | 5 |
| 4 | (3) | Mycelia broader than bacteria (yeastlike forms also present) Moniliasis: *Candida* | |
| 5 | (6) | Mycelia like branching strings of bacteria .............. *Actinomyces* | |
| 6 | (5) | Mycelia like long branching tubercle bacilli (some of them acid-fast) *Nocardia* | |
| 7 | (8) | Yeastlike; budding forms ....................................... | 9 |
| 8 | (7) | Saclike or sporelike; no budding ............................ | 13 |
| 9 | (10) | Within enormous gelatinous capsule ................... *Cryptococcus* | |
| 10 | (9) | Without capsule ......................................... | 11 |
| 11 | (12) | Thick double-contoured wall; single buds ...... *Blastomyces dermatitidis* | |
| 12 | (11) | Thick double-contoured wall; multiple buds .... *Blastomyces brasiliensis* | |
| 13 | (14) | Extracellular; large ........................................ | 15 |
| 14 | (13) | Usually intracellular; small .............................. | 17 |
| 15 | (16) | Sacs filled with endospores ........................... *Coccidioides* | |
| 16 | (15) | Spherical, dark brown spores showing equatorial splitting *Phialophora, Hormodendrum* | |
| 17 | (18) | Cigar-shaped, in polymorphonuclears (rarely seen) ...... *Sporotrichum* | |
| 18 | (17) | Like Leishman-Donovan bodies, packed in WBC's ........ *Histoplasma* | |

In such cases vaccine therapy is contraindicated because of the already excessive amount of antigen present. X-ray and iodides must be administered to these patients with extreme caution. Roentgen therapy may be given in doses of 75 to 100 roentgens filtered through 1 mm. of aluminum at weekly intervals until not more than 1200 roentgen units have been administered. The area should be carefully screened with lead and the roentgen therapy should be given by one especially trained in its use.

## Actinomycosis

**Definition**   A chronic, suppurating, granulomatous infection characterized by multiple abscesses and fistula formation, in the drainage from which the characteristic granules of the fungus are present. It is produced by various species of *Actinomyces bovis.*

**Distribution**   The causative organism is an obligate parasite of man and animals. In humans it is found in the absence of disease on the mucous membranes of the mouth, around carious teeth and in tonsillar crypts. Because of this association, the disease has a worldwide distribution.

**Etiology**   In Bergey's "Determinative Bacteriology," 1948, the family ACTINOMYCETACEAE is classified among the SCHIZOMYCETES, or true bacteria. The pathogenic members of this family are the

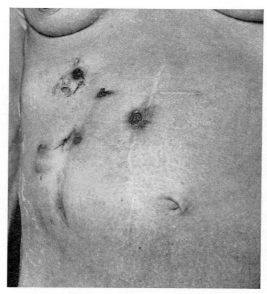

Fig. 90. Actinomycosis of chest wall with draining sinuses. Ribs involved and sinus tracts extending through abdominal wall. (Courtesy Dr. D. T. Smith, Duke University.)

anaerobic *Actinomyces bovis,* and various species of aerobic *Nocardia.* They are nonmotile, gram-positive, in certain instances acid-fast, aerobic or microaerophilic organisms having branching threadlike mycelia seldom exceeding 1 micron in diameter. In tissues, sputum or pus the fungus is visible to the naked eye as the characteristic "sulfur granules" composed of a mass of tangled, branching mycelial threads which at the periphery of the granule may or may not show radially arranged, club-shaped swellings, giving rise to the term "ray fungus."

**Pathology**   The fundamental lesion is a granulomatous process in which the colonies of the fungus, or granules, of the *Actinomyces* are surrounded by mononuclear cells, with occasional giant cells, and numerous polymorphonuclear leukocytes in the areas of necrosis. There is marked new connective tissue formation and fibrosis, producing hard tumor-like masses or indurations. In these are multiple abscesses interconnected by sinus tracts, often with multiple external fistula formation, which discharge sanguinopurulent material containing the granules. Extension of the infection is by continuity, rarely by the blood stream or lymphatics (Fig. 90).

**Clinical Characteristics** The clinical types of actinomycosis fall into three general groups:

1. Cervicofacial .............. 50 per cent of cases
2. Abdominal ................ 20 to 30 per cent of cases
3. Pulmonary ............... 15 per cent of cases

In the *cervicofacial type* the portal of entry appears to be the mucous membrane of the mouth or pharynx. Marked induration is

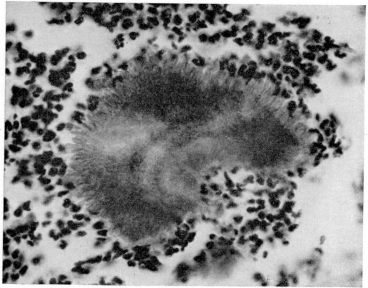

Fig. 91. Actinomycosis. Sulfur granule in pus from sinus tract.

produced and direct extension may lead to involvement of the bones of the skull, or to the skin with the formation of multiple fistulous tracts. Pain is not marked and there may be little or no systemic reaction.

The *abdominal or intestinal type* usually originates in the region of the appendix and cecum with the formation of a gradually increasing mass in the right lower quadrant, followed by internal and external sinus formation. Extension occurs to adjacent structures, often with involvement of the liver and spleen and subsequently the lung. Abdominal actinomycosis may be accompanied by toxemia, fever, chills and other evidence of an intra-abdominal inflammatory process.

The *pulmonary type* may be primary, or secondary to a cervico-facial lesion with extension through the mediastinum. It is characterized by cough, sputum, hemoptysis, fever, dyspnea, and night sweats. Invasion of the pleura is accompanied by pain, and empyema is not unusual. This is frequently followed by invasion of the chest wall with the development of areas of induration, abscess formation, and multiple external sinuses. Involvement of the mediastinum may be followed by invasion of the esophagus or pericardium.

**Diagnosis**    The combination of the clinical picture and demonstration of the characteristic sulfur granules in the tissues, or in pus, is characteristic. Microscopic examination of a granule crushed beneath a cover slip revealing the characteristic structure, and the presence of branching mycelial threads, permit specific diagnosis of infection by a member of the family ACTINOMYCETACEAE. Identification of the particular organism, *A. bovis* or *Nocardia* species, depends upon cultural characteristics. The material should be cultured on suitable media under both anaerobic and aerobic conditions (Fig. 91).

**Treatment**    Penicillin, aureomycin and chloramphenicol (Chloromycetin) have been used successfully. Penicillin, however, is the drug of choice. Associated organisms may necessitate concurrent treatment with sulfonamides and/or streptomycin.

## Maduromycosis

**Synonym**    Madura foot.

**Definition**    The term madura foot is used to define a clinical entity characterized by a chronic granulomatous process usually limited to the lower extremities, producing extensive destruction of the soft tissues and the bony structures, particularly of the feet. It is caused by many different filamentous fungi.

**Distribution**    Maduromycosis is widespread in India, especially in the Madras Presidency, and in Africa, Ceylon, Cochin China, Indonesia and Madagascar. Sporadic cases have been reported from Italy, Greece, the West Indies, Cuba, Argentina and occasionally the United States.

**Etiology**    The disease is produced by several different fungi: *Monosporium apiospermum*, *Allescheria boydii*, *Cephalosporium* sp., etc.

**Pathology**    There is extensive invasion by the fungus. The early lesion is granulomatous in character, with the fungus granules or colonies in edematous granulation tissue infiltrated with mononuclear cells and polymorphonuclear leukocytes. As the lesion progresses it is surrounded by a dense fibrous capsule and often intersected by fibrous trabeculae. There is extensive necrosis of tissue and thrombosis of vessels. In advanced cases the foot becomes a mass of cystlike areas with intercommunicating sinus tracts and multiple externally draining sinuses. In these instances there is complete destruction of muscles, bones, and tendons (Fig. 92).

**Clinical Characteristics**    The initial lesion usually appears on the sole of the foot as a superficial or deep cutaneous nodule. The overlying skin becomes discolored, breaks down and a persistent sinus tract develops. In other instances the process may begin as a deep abscess, ultimately opening externally. As extension occurs the foot becomes enlarged, presenting a convex sole and swollen dorsum. Nodules appear in uninvolved areas of the skin, breaking down to form new sinuses. Ultimately the foot may be enlarged to three or four times the normal size.

There is little or no systemic reaction and in uncomplicated cases little or no lymphangitis or lymphadenitis.

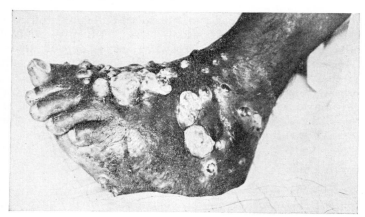

Fig. 92. Madura foot.

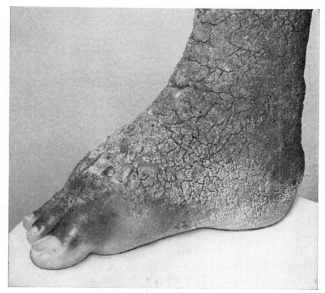

Fig. 93. Mossy foot: a superficial verrucous dermatitis of varied bacterial etiology. (Alan Fisher for the Office of the Coordinator of Inter-American Affairs.)

**Diagnosis**  The clinical picture, together with demonstration of the characteristic granules composed of wide, septate branching mycelia and the development of a typical mold in culture, is diagnostic. Mossy foot should not be confused with this condition (Fig. 93).

**Treatment**  Early diagnosis may allow successful treatment by surgical intervention, penicillin and sulfonamides. The usual case of maduromycosis, however, cannot be treated successfully and amputation is required.

## Nocardiosis

**Synonyms**  Actinomycotic mycetoma, systemic nocardiosis.

**Definition**  A subacute or chronic infection of the subcutaneous tissues characterized by tumorlike lesions often discharging through multiple draining sinuses; and, a systemic infection with protean symptoms such as pseudotuberculosis, meningitis, brain abscesses, etc., caused by species of *Nocardia*.

**Distribution**  The causative organisms are widely distributed in nature and therefore there is no particular geographic distribution of the disease although certain clinical types are encountered more frequently in the tropics.

**Etiology**  Species of *Nocardia* are aerobic members of the ACTINO-MYCETACEAE which have gram-positive branching threadlike mycelia 1 micron in diameter. One species, *N. asteroides*, is also acid-fast. In tissue and from draining sinuses the fungus may be organized into granules, with or without clubs, which cannot be distinguished microscopically from granules of *A. bovis*. In sputum or spinal fluid, granules usually are not seen but the organism appears as branching gram-positive or acid-fast filaments.

**Pathology**  In subcutaneous tissues multiple abscess formation with resulting chronic inflammatory response leads to granulomatous processes with large cell infiltration, giant cells and fibrosis. The organism is usually seen in the areas of necrosis as granules of varying size. Systemic nocardiosis is the result of hematogenous spread from a primary pulmonary infection, resulting in generalized pyemia with abscesses and granulomatous lesions found in many organs.

**Clinical Characteristics**  Subcutaneous tissues are inoculated with the organism by trauma to establish a slowly evolving chronic suppurative disease characterized by swelling and multiple fistulae. Spread through tissue by contiguity, with fibrosis, and bone destruction and tumefaction result in a mycetoma (Fig. 94).

Systemic infection follows a primary pulmonary disease which may simulate tuberculosis or malignancy. Hematogenous spread resulting in abscess formation in many organs, including the brain, causes protean symptoms which makes a differential diagnosis difficult (Fig. 95).

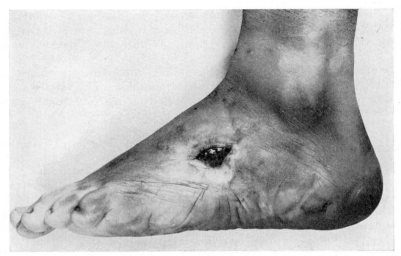

Fig. 94. Nocardiosis: actinomycotic mycetoma caused by *Nocardia asteroides*. (Courtesy Dr. Norman F. Conant, Duke University.)

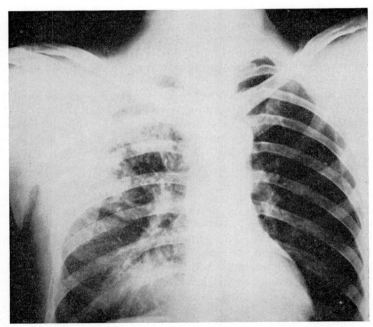

Fig. 95. Nocardiosis: pulmonary nocardiosis caused by *Nocardia asteroides*. (Courtesy Dr. Norman F. Conant, Duke University.)

**Diagnosis** The clinical picture of mycetoma is identical with that of subcutaneous infection caused by *A. bovis* and with maduromycosis caused by a variety of filamentous fungi. Microscopic appearance of the whole and crushed granules of *Nocardia* and *Actinomyces* is identical; either may be seen as tangled masses of delicate mycelia which break up into branching gram-positive bacillary elements 1 micron in diameter. Differentiation by cultures is essential: *A. bovis* is anaerobic while *Nocardia* species grow well aerobically on Sabouraud's glucose medium at room or incubator temperatures. The granules of actinomycetic mycetoma and those of maduromycosis may be distinguished microscopically or by culture. Microscopically the granules of *Nocardia* are composed of delicate hyphae 1 micron in diameter while those of the filamentous fungi are composed of wide septate hyphae 2 to 2.5 microns in diameter. In culture *Nocardia* species appear similiar to cultures of saprophytic acid-fast organisms while the filamentous fungi develop as typical molds.

**Treatment** The sulfonamides offer specific therapy for infections caused by *Nocardia*. Treatment with sulfadiazine alone or with sulfamerazine, to obtain higher serum concentrations, has proven effective.

## Cryptococcosis

**Synonyms** European blastomycosis, Busse-Buschke's disease, torula meningitis.

**Definition** A subacute or chronic infection by a yeastlike fungus which has a predilection for invasion of the central nervous system. Two clinical types are recognized: the *cutaneous form*, characterized by acneform lesions and subcutaneous nodules, may precede or follow the *generalized form*, in which a primary pulmonary infection is followed by invasion of the body, especially the central nervous system. The prognosis is grave in both forms and central nervous system infections are almost invariably fatal.

**Distribution** The fungus is widely distributed in nature and has been isolated from the soil, plants and animals. Human infections have been reported from Europe, India, Australia, Japan, Canada, the United States, and Central and South America.

**Etiology** *Cryptococcosis* is produced by *Cryptococcus neoformans* (*Torula histolytica*), a budding yeastlike organism. In tissue and in exudates it appears as an ovoid or spherical body measuring 5 to 20 micra in diameter; it has single buds and is surrounded by a characteristic wide, refractile, gelatinous capsule. In culture it presents a brownish, mucoid, yeastlike growth, with the budding cells exhibiting the characteristic capsule.

**Pathology** The cutaneous form may produce acneform lesions, granulomatous ulcers, and deep nodules or tumor-like masses which are filled with gelatinous material. There is commonly little acute inflammatory reaction but there is infiltration with giant cells, "foam" cells, plasma cells and lymphocytes together with fibroblasts and newly formed connective tissue. At times typical tubercles are produced.

In the central nervous system a variety of pathologic changes may be seen including diffuse meningitis, granulomas in the meninges, endarteritis, infarcts, areas of softening, increase in neuroglia, and extensive destruction of nerve tissue (Fig. 96).

The organisms are present singly or in groups in the lesions.

**Clinical Characteristics**   The *cutaneous type* (European blastomycosis) may precede or follow systemic infection. It is characterized by

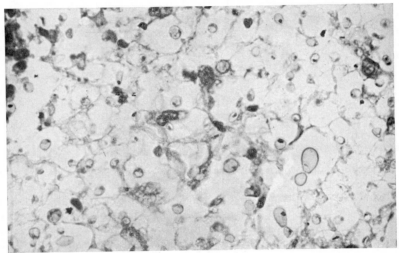

Fig. 96. Cryptococcosis. Torula meningitis, H & E stain showing numerous organisms.

pustule formation, granulomatous ulcers of the skin or subcutaneous tumors.

The *generalized type* (torula meningitis) is usually characterized by symptoms and signs of extensive and progressive involvement of the central nervous system. In this form the onset is usually insidious, although occasionally sudden, with fever, headache and vomiting. Death usually occurs after the onset of coma with signs of increased intracranial pressure. The spinal fluid is usually under increased pressure and the cell count increased to 200 to 800 per cubic millimeter; the cells are chiefly mononuclears. The organisms may be present in small numbers and may be mistaken for erythrocytes or small lymphocytes. This form of the disease is often mistaken for tuberculous meningitis.

Involvement of the lungs is accompanied by cough and signs of chronic bronchitis with peribronchial involvement which may be confused with pulmonary tuberculosis. A low grade intermittent fever may or may not be present.

Rarely invasion of the liver, spleen and joints occurs; among the latter the knees are most commonly affected.

**Diagnosis**   The fungi appear in infected tissue, spinal fluid, sputum, or the gelatinous content of subcutaneous nodules, as characteristic round or ovoid, single-budding, yeastlike bodies with heavy capsules. Satisfactory demonstration of the capsule requires smears

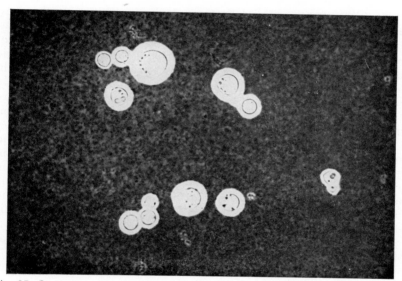

Fig. 97. *Cryptococcus neoformans* in pus. (Courtesy Dr. Donald S. Martin, Communicable Disease Center, U.S.P.H.S.)

in India ink of the sediment from centrifuged spinal fluid or of pus (Fig. 97).

**Treatment**   A local lesion may be treated by excision and roentgen therapy. When the infection has extended with multiple cutaneous lesions or primary pulmonary infection, sulfadiazine therapy has proven effective, but there is no effective treatment for infection of the central nervous system. Occasionally, patients develop low grade chronic infections which persist for years.

## Moniliasis

**Definition**   An infection by a yeastlike fungus, *Candida albicans*, which occasionally involves the skin and deeper tissues, particularly the lungs and meninges.

**Etiology**   *Candida albicans* is an ubiquitous fungus for which there are over a hundred synonyms. It produces small, round, budding forms in the lesions with occasional mycelia. On Sabouraud's medium white, yeastlike colonies having a yeasty odor are formed.

**Clinical Characteristics**   *Candida albicans* is widespread in nature and has frequently been recovered from the normal mouth, throat and gastro-intestinal tract. It is commonly present in the sputum of patients with pulmonary tuberculosis or carcinoma of the lung. It is likewise frequently present in the stools in cases of pernicious anemia, sprue and various other gastro-intestinal diseases. It is usually difficult to ascribe definite etiologic significance to the presence of this fungus.

*Candida albicans* has been shown to be capable occasionally of producing a primary bronchitis, infections of the skin and systemic infections. The most common conditions attributed to it are thrush, onychia, paronychia and dermatitis in moist skin areas, particularly the axillae, beneath the breasts and in the intergluteal folds. The rare systemic infections, which are highly fatal, include abscess formation and meningitis.

**Diagnosis**   The ubiquity of this fungus necessitates extreme caution in etiologic diagnosis. Examination of scrapings from the skin or nails, or of sputum or other material in 10 per cent potassium hydroxide preparations demonstrates the round, single or budding yeast forms and occasionally mycelia. The appearance in culture and the lesions produced after injection into rabbits are characteristic (see p. 818).

**Treatment**   Cutaneous infections by *C. albicans* may be treated as follows:

1. Soaking twice daily for thirty minutes with 1:1500 potassium permanganate solution.

2. Daily application of 1 per cent solution of gentian violet.

Oral lesions should be treated with alkaline mouthwashes or by irrigations with gentian violet 1:10,000. For vaginitis, douches of potassium permanganate 1:1500 or gentian violet 1:10,000, also, propionate vaginal jelly, are recommended.

The pulmonary are the more important of the systemic infections. Skin test for sensitivity should be performed and, if positive, iodides should be avoided until the patient has been desensitized. Following desensitization iodides should be initiated with caution. Intravenous gentian violet in dosage of 5 mg. per kilogram of body weight given daily or every other day for four to six doses has proved useful.


## Blastomycosis

**Synonyms**   (1) North American blastomycosis; Gilchrist's disease. (2) South American blastomycosis; Lutz-Splendore-Almeida's disease.

## North American Blastomycosis

**Definition**  An infection due to *Blastomyces dermatitidis* characterized in the cutaneous type by granulomatous ulcerating lesions,
and in the systemic type by a close resemblance to tuberculosis with
involvement of the lungs and less often the abdominal viscera, the
skeletal system and the central nervous system.

**Distribution**  North American blastomycosis is a relatively uncommon disease, recognized at present only in North America.

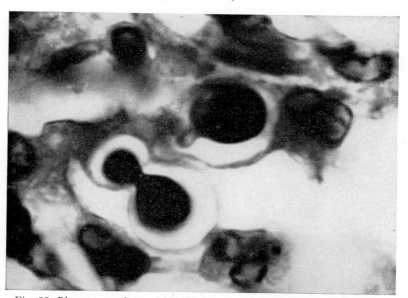

Fig. 98. *Blastomyces dermatitidis.* Budding yeastlike cells in tissue section.

**Etiology**  *Blastomyces dermatitidis* appears in tissue and pus as
single, budding, round or ovoid yeastlike cells 8 to 15 microns in
diameter. They have a thick refractile outer wall, often giving a
double-contoured appearance. Mycelia are not present (Fig. 98).

Growth in culture at 37° C. is yeastlike, and at room temperature
moldlike with cottony growth of branched aerial mycelia.

**Pathology**  The initial cutaneous lesion usually appears on an
exposed skin surface, developing into a verrucous, peripherally extending, crater-like ulcer with raised, irregular, undermined edges
and a granulation tissue base. The visceral type closely simulates
tuberculosis but numerous small abscesses with polymorphonuclear
leukocytic infiltration are produced (Fig. 99).

**Clinical Characteristics**  The cutaneous lesions of North American
blastomycosis usually occur on the face, neck, hands, wrists, arms,
feet or legs, appearing first as papules or pustules, extending to form
the chronic ulcers. There is usually little pain, tenderness or systemic
reaction and commonly no lymphadenitis (Figs. 100, 101).

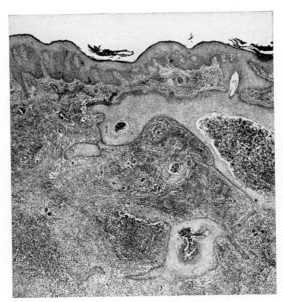

Fig. 99. North American blastomycosis. Granulomatous lesion in subcutaneous tissues.

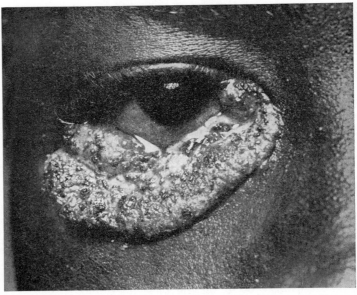

Fig. 100. North American blastomycosis. (Courtesy Dr. J. Lamar Callaway, Duke University.)

Systemic infections usually start in the lungs, frequently producing a clinical picture that is confused with tuberculosis or malignancy.

**Diagnosis** The characteristic budding organisms are found within giant cells in granulation tissue and in necrotic material from the lesion. They may be demonstrated in the sputum in cases of pulmonary infection.

**Treatment** Excision of the cutaneous lesion is not recommended. In a sensitive individual or in an anergic individual with active infection the use of roentgen therapy or the exhibition of iodides may

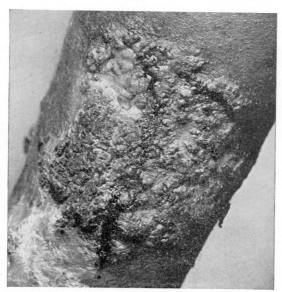

Fig. 101. North American blastomycosis. (Courtesy Dr. J. Lamar Callaway, Duke University.)

be followed by rapid and grave extension of the infection. Evaluation of sensitivity should invariably be performed with an intracutaneous injection of stock or autogenous vaccine. In the presence of a positive skin test desensitization should be carried out by repeated graduated doses of vaccine prior to the administration of iodides.

The *prognosis* is unfavorable in anergic patients who give negative skin tests in the presence of active infection, since the negative tests indicate that the patient has little or no resistance. In such cases vaccine therapy is contraindicated because of the already excessive amount of antigen present. Roentgen therapy and iodides must be used with extreme caution for these patients.

After desensitization, administration of a saturated solution of potassium iodide may be started with a daily dose of 3 drops after meals, three times daily, increasing the dose 1 to 3 drops each day until a total of 30 drops three times a day is reached. Roentgen therapy of the skin lesions is sometimes a useful supplement.

Stilbamidine has been used in a few cases of cutaneous and systemic infection with excellent results. This drug is toxic, however, and the patient should be closely watched for signs of neuropathy, especially of the fifth nerve.

### South American Blastomycosis

**Definition**    An infection by *B. brasiliensis* which has a predilection for lymphatic tissue. The disease appears in two forms: a cutaneous type usually starting about the mouth, and a lymphaticovisceral type with involvement of the lymphatics, liver and spleen. The lungs are seldom affected.

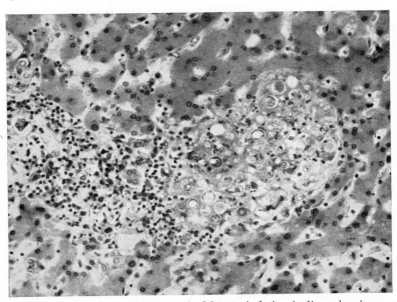

Fig. 102. South American blastomycosis. Metastatic lesion in liver showing many round and ovoid forms of *B. brasiliensis*.

**Distribution**    South America, principally Brazil.

**Etiology**    *Blastomyces brasiliensis* (*Paracoccidioides brasiliensis*) appears in the lesions as thick-walled, round or ovoid yeast cells resembling *B. dermatitidis* except that they are characteristically larger, reaching diameters of 60 microns. Multiple-budding forms are likewise characteristic.

**Clinical Characteristics**    The portal of entry is usually the buccal cavity. A slowly extending ulcer is produced. This has a granular base presenting numerous pinpoint yellowish-white areas in which the fungus is particularly abundant. The infection may extend to adjacent skin areas, producing lesions similar to those of the North American disease. The primary lesion may extend directly to the tonsils and secondarily to lymphoid follicles in the gastro-intestinal tract, producing nodules and follicular ulceration. This may be followed by involvement of the regional lymphatics and invasion of the spleen and the liver (Fig. 102).

**Diagnosis**   Diagnosis is based upon demonstration of the large multiple-budding yeastlike forms.

**Treatment**   The sulfonamides are specific for this disease.

## Coccidioidomycosis

**Synonyms**   Coccidioidal granuloma, San Joaquin fever, valley fever.

**Definition**   An acute, subacute or chronic infection of the lungs produced by *Coccidioides immitis*, usually acquired by inhalation. Clinically it resembles acute bronchitis or pulmonary tuberculosis. Occasionally there is involvement of the skin, bones, joints, lymph nodes, larynx, meninges and other visceral structures. Multiple cold abscesses are not uncommon.

**Distribution**   The disease is endemic in the southwestern United States and sporadic cases have been reported from the Hawaiian Islands, Italy and southeastern Europe. Many cases which have been reported from Brazil have been confused with paracoccidioides infections (*B. brasiliensis*).

**Etiology**   *Coccidioides immitis* appear in tissue and exudates as round, non-budding, thick-walled spores measuring 20 to 80 microns in diameter and containing numerous endospores. Culture on Sabouraud's medium at room temperature produces a cottony white growth, becoming brownish in color, with branching septate filamentous hyphae.

**Epidemiology**   *Coccidioides immitis* has been recovered from pulmonary lesions in various wild rodents in the endemic areas in the southwestern United States and it has been suggested that it is primarily a rodent disease. It has also been reported to produce infection in cattle, sheep, and dogs. Infection of man occurs by inhalation of dust containing the highly infectious chlamydospores. There is no evidence of direct animal to man or man to man transmission.

Primary infections have a definite seasonal incidence occurring predominantly in the hot dusty autumn months.

**Pathology**   The fundamental pathology is that of a granulomatous process, acute, subacute or chronic in nature, accompanied by varying degrees of fibrosis, with or without central necrosis of the lesion (Fig. 103).

In chronic lesions of the lung, cavity formation or pleurisy with effusion may occur. The organisms are surrounded by giant cells, epithelioid cells, lymphocytes and plasma cells.

Occasional granulomatous masses may reach considerable size without necrosis. Abscess formation, however, is more frequent than in tuberculosis.

**Clinical Characteristics** Primary pulmonary infection produces the clinical picture of pneumonia or acute bronchitis with or without sputum and is occasionally accompanied by pleurisy with effusion. Physical signs may be absent. In the majority of cases recovery occurs in two to three weeks without sequelae. Sensitivity to the organism frequently develops and may be manifested by erythema multiforme or erythema nodosum. It is accompanied by a positive skin test to coccidioidin. This form of the disease is known as "San Joaquin fever" or "valley fever." These infections are accompanied

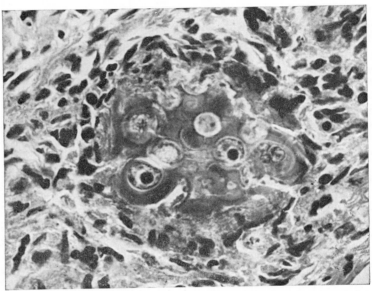

Fig. 103. *Coccidioides immitis.* Round, non-budding spores in section of granulomatous lesion.

by an initial leukocytosis with a normal differential count. Later there is lymphocytosis with an increase in large mononuclear cells.

The secondary or chronic phase of the disease, coccidioidal granuloma, develops by dissemination of the infection from the primary focus either in the course of the acute attack or subsequently. Lesions may occur anywhere in the body, producing a variety of signs and symptoms.

**Diagnosis** Diagnosis is based upon demonstration of the large non-budding, thick-walled spores containing numerous endospores in clinical materials and the development of a cottony culture with typical arthrospores on Sabouraud's glucose agar. Intratesticular injection of infected material into guinea pigs produces lesions containing the typical spores.

A positive skin test to coccidioidin has the same significance as the tuberculin test in tuberculosis.

Precipitins are present in primary cases and complement-fixing antibodies increase in titer as the disease progresses.

*Differential diagnosis* entails differentiation from tuberculosis, syphilis, bacterial osteomyelitis, malignancy and other mycotic infections.

**Treatment** Most primary infections heal without specific treatment. There is no specific treatment for progressive coccidioidomycosis.

## Histoplasmosis

**Definition** A disease of the reticulo-endothelial system produced by infection with *Histoplasma capsulatum.*

**Distribution** The majority of reported cases have been from the United States. There are isolated reports of cases from the Panama Canal Zone, Philippine Islands, Honduras, Argentina, Brazil, Java and England.

**Etiology** *Histoplasma capsulatum* appears as a small encapsulated organism, 1 to 5 microns in diameter, in mononuclear cells in the blood and in the reticulo-endothelial cells of the internal organs and bone marrow.

Cultivation on blood agar at 37° C. produces a yeastlike growth of small oval budding cells. On Sabouraud's medium at room temperature growth is moldlike, at first cottony and white, later becoming brown.

**Epidemiology** *Histoplasma capsulatum* has been isolated from the soil and from numerous animals. Infection in man probably occurs by inhalation. There is no evidence of animal to man transmission.

**Pathology** Histoplasmosis is a disease essentially of the reticulo-endothelial system. Grayish or white nodules, or more or less extensive areas of necrosis surrounded by granulomatous tissue, are produced. The organisms multiply in the reticulo-endothelial cells and may be seen in phagocytic cells in the lesions (Fig. 104).

**Clinical Characteristics** Primary pulmonary infection may be asymptomatic or simulate a mild cold, bronchitis, influenza or tuberculosis. Such an infection results in sensitivity to histoplasmin and spontaneous recovery usually results in miliary calcification which may be detected months or years later by routine x-ray. In many areas of the United States large population groups have been found to have nontuberculous pulmonary calcifications with a positive histoplasmin skin test and a negative tuberculin skin test. Such individuals are thought to have had primary histoplasmosis as described above.

Systemic progressive infection may result in nasopharyngeal ulcerations resembling carcinoma, pulmonary infection with diffuse or localized consolidation, abscess or cavitation resembling tuberculosis or visceral infection resembling leishmaniasis. Not infrequently lymphadenopathy suggests lymphosarcoma, Hodgkin's disease or leukemia.

**Diagnosis**   The organisms stain well with Wright's stain and in infected cells may be confused with Leishman-Donovan bodies or *Toxoplasma*. They may be demonstrated in blood films, or in smears

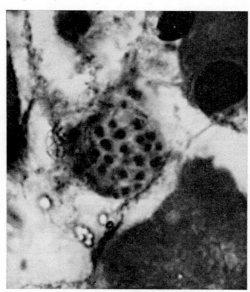

Fig. 104. *Histoplasma* in Kupffer cell of liver. (Courtesy Dr. Norman F. Conant, Duke University.)

of the sternal marrow or splenic pulp. Final identification is based on culture.

**Treatment**   None.

## Sporotrichosis

**Definition**   A subacute or chronic granulomatous fungus infection producing gumma-like nodules, ulcers and abscesses, usually confined to the skin and superficial lymph nodes.

**Distribution**   World-wide.

**Etiology**   Sporotrichosis is produced by infection with *Sporotrichum schenckii*, which is widely distributed in nature. In infected experimental animals this organism produces gram-positive, cigar-shaped spores which are readily seen in polymorphonuclear leukocytes. They are rarely seen in man.

**Pathology**   The gumma-like nodules usually show a central necrotic area surrounded by granulation tissue, epithelioid cells and giant cells with a peripheral zone of connective tissue.

**Clinical Characteristics**   The initial lesion usually appears as a hard, movable, elastic nodule beneath the skin. This enlarges and becomes attached to the skin, which becomes red, inflamed and then necrotic with the formation of a chronic ulcer. Similar nodules develop along the superficial lymphatics draining the area, resulting in the formation of secondary ulcers. The lymphatic channels between the lesions are frequently palpable, thickened and cordlike (Fig. 105).

Rarely other structures including mucous membranes, muscles, the skeletal system and the viscera may be involved.

When untreated the lesions may persist for years.

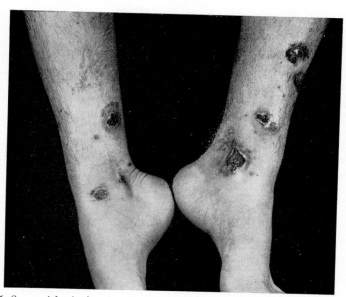

Fig. 105. Sporotrichosis showing active and healed lesions. (Courtesy Dr. J. Lamar Callaway, Duke University.)

**Diagnosis**  *Sporotrichum schenckii* is rarely demonstrable in material from the lesions in man. Diagnosis is based upon the cultural characteristics after inoculation of infected material on Sabouraud's medium (see p. 838) and inoculation into laboratory animals—rats, mice or guinea pigs.

**Treatment**  Potassium iodide is a specific for this infection and should be administered from the outset in massive dosage.

## Chromoblastomycosis

**Definition**  A fungus infection of the skin, producing verrucous, wartlike nodules or papillomata which may or may not ulcerate.

**Distribution**  This disease occurs sporadically in many areas of the world.

**Etiology**  Chromoblastomycosis is produced by any of three fungi

—*Phialophora verrucosa, Hormodendrum pedrosoi* or *H. compactum*. All of these present an identical appearance in pus or in tissue sections from the lesions. They appear as clusters of large, spherical, dark brown spores which reproduce by equatorial splitting and not by budding. Specific identification is based upon the characteristics in culture on Sabouraud's medium at room temperature.

**Pathology** The pathology is essentially that of an infectious granuloma with numerous giant cells, mononuclears, phagocytes, epithelioid cells and plasma cells. The organisms may be seen lying free within the tissues or within giant cells.

**Clinical Characteristics** Chromoblastomycosis is a very chronic infection, usually occurring on the extremities, appearing first as pustules which subsequently develop into elevated, scaling, warty nodules or papillomata. The infected extremities gradually become covered with these lesions. When infection occurs on the face, neck or buttocks the lesions are often atypical.

**Diagnosis** Diagnosis is based upon demonstration of the characteristic spores in smears of exudate or in potassium hydroxide preparations of scrapings from the lesions.

**Treatment** When the infection is superficial and not too extensive surgical excision is recommended. Iodides have no effect. Iontophoresis with copper sulfate is said to be useful.

## 30   The Intestinal Protozoa

Infection of the human intestine by certain members of the Protozoa is common in many parts of the world. Five different amebae, three or more flagellates, one ciliate and one sporozoan which are of direct or indirect medical importance may be encountered. Of these, the ameba, *Endamoeba histolytica*, and the ciliate, *Balantidium coli*, are recognized pathogens for man. The ameba, *Dientamoeba fragilis*, the flagellate, *Giardia lamblia*, and the sporozoan, *Isospora hominis*, are of doubtful pathogenicity. The remaining organisms are of importance partly because of diagnostic problems which they may present and partly for the evidence they furnish as to the environment in which their host has previously resided. Those organisms whose modes of transmission are known are spread from one individual to another by contamination of food or drink with human feces. In the case of *B. coli* it is probable that infection of man originates from the pig as well as from infected humans.

The flagellate, *Trichomonas vaginalis*, is included in this section because of its morphologic resemblance to *T. hominis*, a resident of the human intestinal tract. A yeast, *Blastocystis hominis*, is likewise

**231**

described because of its common occurrence in stools and the frequency with which it may be confused with encysted forms of certain of the intestinal protozoa.

Most of the intestinal protozoa of man pass through two stages, an active trophozoite stage and a resting nonmotile or encysted stage. The trophozoites are motile; they feed actively and undergo multiplication by binary fission. Subsequently certain of the trophozoites cease feeding, lose their motility and secrete a surrounding resistant cyst wall. These encysted forms, or cysts, are much less susceptible to changes of environment than are the trophozoites, and they are

*Table 20    The Important Intestinal Protozoa of Man*

| ORGANISM | PATHOGENIC | NON-PATHOGENIC | STAGES OF ORGANISM | |
| --- | --- | --- | --- | --- |
| | | | TROPHOZOITE | CYST |
| Amebas: | | | | |
| *Endamoeba histolytica* | + | − | + | + |
| *E. coli* | − | + | + | + |
| *Iodamoeba bütschlii* | − | + | + | + |
| *Endolimax nana* | − | + | + | + |
| *Dientamoeba fragilis* | ? | ? | + | − |
| Flagellates: | | | | |
| *Chilomastix mesnili* | −− | + | + | + |
| *Trichomonas hominis* | − | + | + | − |
| *T. vaginalis* | ± | ± | + | − |
| *Giardia lamblia* | ? | ? | + | + |
| *Embadomonas intestinalis* | − | + | + | + |
| Ciliate: | | | | |
| *Balantidium coli* | + | − | + | + |
| Sporozoan: | | | | |
| *Isospora hominis* | ± | ± | ?* | + |

* A sporozoite

responsible for transmission of the infection (Table 20). Trophozoites do not long survive outside the favorable environment of the intestinal tract.

Identification of the individual protozoan is based upon certain specific characteristics of the trophozoite and of the cyst. These distinguishing features include the type of motility of the trophozoite, food inclusions, contained glycogen, the number and structure of the nuclei and other morphologic details. Similarly the encysted forms may be distinguished by differences in size and shape, by the number and structure of the nuclei, the characteristics of chromatoid bodies when these are present, the amount and distribution of contained glycogen and by other details of the internal morphology (Figs. 106, 107). To demonstrate all of these features it is frequently necessary to examine not only unstained fresh preparations but films stained by iodine and fixed smears stained by Heidenhain's or other iron-hematoxylin methods. The latter techniques are essential for demonstration of the finer morphologic details upon which specific identification is based. These methods are described on pp. 826–828.

Certain of the intestinal protozoa may be isolated and maintained in artificial culture media.

The important differential features of the trophozoites and the cysts are indicated in Tables 21 and 22.

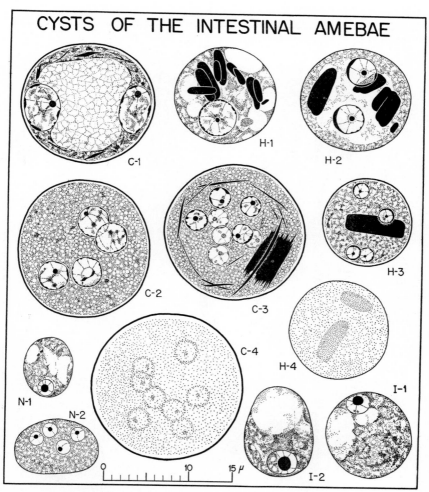

Fig. 106. C1: Iron-hematoxylin stained binucleate cyst of *Endamoeba coli*. C2: Iron-hematoxylin stained quadrinucleate cyst of *E. coli*. C3: Iron-hematoxylin stained mature cyst of *E. coli*. H1: Iron-hematoxylin stained uninucleate cyst of *E. histolytica*. H2: Iron-hematoxylin stained binucleate cyst of *E. histolytica*. H3: Iron-hematoxylin stained mature cyst of *E. histolytica*. N1: Iron-hematoxylin stained uninucleate cyst of *Endolimax nana*. N2: Iron-hematoxylin stained mature cysts of *E. nana*. I1, I2: Iron-hematoxylin stained mature cysts of *Iodamoeba bütschlii*. C4: Unstained mature cyst of *E. coli*. H4: Unstained mature cyst of *E. histolytica*.

## Endamoeba histolytica

*Endamoeba histolytica* (Schaudinn 1903) Hickson 1909 is an important pathogenic parasite of man. It localizes principally in the colon and only rarely invades the terminal ileum. Metastatic lesions, particularly of the liver, follow invasion of the blood stream. The life cycle includes both trophozoite and encysted stages.

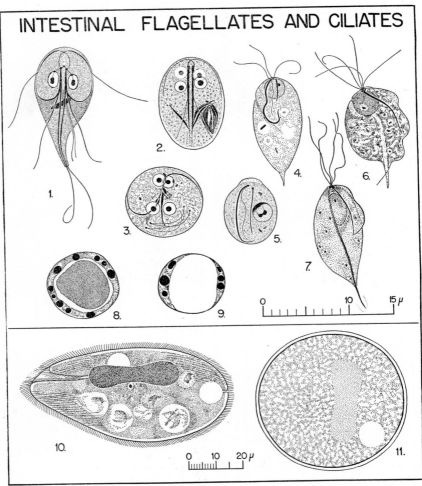

Fig. 107. Iron-hematoxylin stained trophozoite of *Giardia lamblia*. 2. Iron-hematoxylin stained cyst of *G. lamblia*. 3. Iron-hematoxylin stained cyst of *G. lamblia* end-view. 4. Iron-hematoxylin stained trophozoite of *Chilomastix mesnili*. 5. Iron-hematoxylin stained cyst of *C. mesnili*. 6. Iron-hematoxylin stained trophozoite of *Trichomonas hominis*. 7. Iron-hematoxylin stained trophozoite of *T. vaginalis*. 8. Iron-hematoxylin stained *Blastocystis hominis*. 9. Unstained *B. hominis*. 10. Trophozoite of *Balantidium coli*. 11. Unstained cyst of *B. coli*.

*Table 21   Salient Features of Trophozoites of Common Intestinal Protozoa of Man*

| PARASITE | SIZE (μ) LIVING | NORMAL MOTILITY | MOTILITY AFTER COOLING | STAINED NUCLEUS | OTHER CHARACTERISTICS |
|---|---|---|---|---|---|
| Endamoeba histolytica | 10–25 (Rounded forms) | Active, progressive, "limax" streaming | Rapidly emitted, clear pseudopods | Round; minute central karyosome; fine chromatic lining of membrane | Living nucleus indistinct; cytoplasm clear save for red cells |
| E. coli | 20–30 (Rounded forms) | Like E. histolytica, but more sluggish | Slowly protruded, granular pseudopods | Round; coarse eccentric karyosome; coarse chromatic lining of membrane | Living nucleus visible; cytoplasm coarsely alveolar, containing bacteria, yeasts, etc. |
| Iodamoeba bütschlii | 9–13 (Rounded forms) | Like E. coli | Like E. coli | Round; huge central karyosome surrounded by small clear granules | Cytoplasm contains bacteria, yeast, etc. |
| Endolimax nana | 8–12 (Rounded forms) | Like small E. histolytica | Very slight activity | Round; large irregular karyosome, single or connected with 1 or 2 smaller masses | Cytoplasm quite clear, contains bacteria, yeast, etc. |
| Dientamoeba fragilis | 8–10 (Rounded forms) | Active; clear indented pseudopods in front of granular mass | Inactive, round | 2 (or 1) nuclei, with mass of chromatin granules embedded in clear matrix | Very sensitive to cooling; ingests bacteria, yeasts, etc. |
| Chilomastix mesnili | 13–24 × 6–11 | Flagellate; jerky, spiral; body rigid | Slowed activity | Round; small, eccentric or central karyosome | Body pear-shaped; buccal structures prominent; spiral twist in body; ingests bacteria. |
| Trichomonas hominis | 10–15 × 5–8 | Flagellate; continuous, wobbly; body plastic | Slowed activity; body often ameboid | Round or oval; karyosome more or less central | 3–5 anterior flagella; undulating membrane and axostyle present; ingests bacteria. |
| T. vaginalis | 10–30 × 5–15 | Similar to T. hominis | Same as T. hominis, but much more sensitive to cooling | Elongate oval; chromatin grains small and uniformly distributed | 4 anterior flagella; undulating membrane short; few food inclusions |
| Giardia lamblia | 11–18 × 6–9 | Active; tumbling and turning like falling leaves | Marked slowing or inactivity | Right and left nuclei; ovoid with prominent irregular karyosomes | Has sucking disc, 8 flagella, etc. |
| Embadomonas intestinalis | 4–9 × 3–4 | Flagellate; jerky and progressive | Slowed activity | Round; membrane delicate; karyosome eccentric | 2 anterior flagella and 2 blepharoplasts near nucleus. |
| Balantidium coli | 50–70 × 30–60 | Ciliary; strong progressive swimmer | Becomes rounded; sluggish | Macronucleus sausage-shape; micronucleus, ovoid or round | V-shaped peristome; anus at posterior end |

*Table 22  Salient Features of Cysts of Cyst-forming Intestinal Protozoa of Man*

| PARASITE | USUAL SHAPE | USUAL SIZE (μ) | NUMBER NUCLEI | NUCLEAR KARYOSOME | GLYCOGEN MASS (IN IODINE) | CHROMATOID BODIES | OTHER CHARACTERISTICS |
|---|---|---|---|---|---|---|---|
| Endamoeba histolytica | Round | 4–20 | 1–4 | Punctiform, typically central | Diffuse, brown. In young cysts | Rod-shaped or thick bars | In fresh unstained cyst: nuclei not visible; chromatoids conspicuous |
| E. coli | Round | 15–20 | 1–8 | Coarser than in E. hist. Eccentric | Large, deep brown. In young cysts | Splinter-like, or filamentous | Nuclei usually visible in unstained cyst; cyst wall heavy |
| Iodamoeba bütschlii | Ovoid Round | 6–15 | 1 | Bulky, often eccentric | Large or small, sharply delimited, deep brown | None | Usually granular mass next to karyosome |
| Endolimax nana | Ovoid Round | 7–10 × 6–7 | 1–4 | Eccentric mass connected with smaller masses | Occasionally present in young cysts | None | Often cytoplasmic volutin grains confusable with karyosomes |
| Chilomastix mesnili | Lemon-shaped | 7–9 × 4.5–6 | 1 | Mass at one pole | Sometimes present | None | Oral apparatus beside nucleus |
| Giardia lamblia | Ovoid | 8–12 × 6–10 | 4 | Punctiform, central | None | None | Nuclei at anterior pole; fibrils in cytoplasm |
| Embadomonas intestinalis | Pear-shaped | 4–7 × 3–5 | 1 | Slightly eccentric | None | None | Cyst wall appears double in fresh preparations; margin of cytosome may show when stained |
| Balantidium coli | Round | 50–65 | 1 macronucleus 1 micronucleus | — | None | None | Macronucleus kidney-shaped, large, conspicuous; contractile vacuole present |
| Isospora hominis | Ovoid | 22–33 × 11–18 | 1 granular mass, or 2 sporoblasts | — | None | None | Smooth, colorless cyst wall appears to be composed of two layers |
| Blastocystis hominis (A yeast, not a protozoon) | Round | 10–15 | 1–8 | — | None | None | Nuclei marginal, between inner and outer wall |

**The Trophozoite**  Iron-hematoxylin stained specimens are usually 15 to 25 microns in diameter. There is a single spherical nucleus with a delicate nuclear membrane the inner surface of which is lightly encrusted with a layer of minute chromatin granules. Within the nucleus and classically central in position there is a punctiform karyosome; occasionally it may be eccentrically placed. Ingested erythrocytes may be present in the cytoplasm.

The living unstained organism exhibits active progressive motility which is characteristic of this species. The ameba usually assumes a ribbon-like form and moves across the microscope field by continuous flowing of cytoplasm into the leading element. This "anterior" portion or pseudopod of ectoplasm is clear and glasslike, often contrasting sharply with the less hyaline or finely granular endoplasm of the ameba. The nucleus is usually not visible. Ingested erythrocytes are frequently present. Motility is rapidly lost as the trophozoite is cooled below the temperature of the human body, at which time the distinction between the glasslike pseudopodia and the more granular endoplasm becomes more marked.

**The Cyst**  The cysts are spherical bodies varying from 4 to 20 microns in diameter. Young cysts are uninucleate, possessing a large rather coarse nucleus which may be one-third the diameter of the cyst in size. As nuclear division occurs, binucleate as well as the fully developed quadrinucleate forms are produced, the size of the individual nuclei decreasing as they increase in number.

In iron-hematoxylin stained preparations the hyaline single wall of the mature cyst is unstained and the cytoplasm appears grayish white. The delicately beaded nuclear membranes and the centrally placed karyosomes are deep black, and blunt-ended black-stained bodies, the chromatoid bodies, are frequently but not invariably present in the cytoplasm.

In unstained fresh smears the colorless cytoplasm has a finely granular appearance and the nuclei can only rarely be seen as delicate rings of fine refractile granules. In young or immature cysts chromatoid bars are commonly observed. These appear as blunt-ended rods or rounded bodies having a different refractive index from the rest of the cyst. They are distinctive and diagnostic.

In iodine stained preparations the cysts of *E. histolytica* can usually be differentiated from the cysts of the other intestinal protozoa. The cytoplasm appears yellowish in color and frequently contains a diffuse mass of glycogen staining mahogany brown. The nuclei are readily seen and although the chromatoid bodies may be visible they are more easily seen in the unstained or hematoxylin stained smears.

## Endamoeba coli

*Endamoeba coli* (Grassi 1879) Hickson 1909 is a common nonpathogenic ameba of the human colon. Its importance lies in possible confusion with *E. histolytica*. Its presence in the stool provides evidence concerning the sanitary environment to which the host has been exposed. The life cycle includes both trophozoite and encysted stages.

**The Trophozoite** The motile ameba averages 20 to 30 microns in diameter. In iron-hematoxylin stained smears the single nucleus is relatively large and coarse. The nuclear membrane is thicker and the chromatin granules larger than in *E. histolytica*, while the karyosome is coarser and occupies an eccentric position. The cytoplasm is more coarsely granular and typically contains many food inclusions such as bacteria, yeasts and detritus.

The living unstained organism is sluggishly motile, extending and withdrawing pseudopodia with little progressive motion. The pseudopodia are less hyaline or glasslike and are shorter and more blunt than those of *E. histolytica*. The nucleus is frequently visible, appearing as a large refractile ring containing a small eccentric hyaline mass representing the karyosome. This ameba rarely ingests red blood cells.

**The Cyst** The cysts of *E. coli* are spherical or ovoid bodies ranging between 15 and 20 microns in diameter. The younger forms are uni- or binucleate. Successive nuclear divisions occur to produce the characteristic eight nuclei of the mature cyst; rarely there may be sixteen to thirty-two. The individual nucleus decreases in size and becomes more delicate with each division.

In iron-hematoxylin stained smears the cyst wall is unstained. The nuclei are larger than those of *E. histolytica*, the nuclear membrane is heavier and the chromatin granules are coarser. The karyosome is relatively large and eccentrically placed. Chromatoid bodies are commonly present in immature cysts and characteristically appear as black-staining splinter-like bars with jagged ends.

In unstained fresh smears the nuclei are often visible and the large eccentric karyosomes are easily seen. The chromatoid bodies likewise may be seen when present. The contour of the latter and the visibility of the nuclei in unstained preparations have diagnostic significance.

The structure of the nuclei is clearly shown in iodine stained smears and the glycogen mass stains a deep mahogany brown. The splinter-like chromatoid bars usually do not appear.

## Endolimax nana

*Endolimax nana* (Wenyon and O'Connor 1917) Brug 1918 is a small nonpathogenic ameba of man occurring as a commensal in 10 to 30 or more per cent of normal individuals throughout the world. Both trophozoite and encysted stages are known.

**The Trophozoite** The motile ameba averages 8 to 10 microns in diameter. The structure of the spherical nucleus is characteristic and diagnostic in iron-hematoxylin stained smears. The nuclear membrane is relatively thick and lacks chromatin beading. The karyosome is large, irregular or lobulated in shape and may be central or eccentric in position. The cytoplasm is granular, vacuolated and contains bacteria, yeasts and other food inclusions. Red blood cells are not ingested.

In fresh unstained preparations the trophozoite is sluggishly motile, extruding and withdrawing short blunt hyaline pseudopodia but exhibiting little progressive motion. The nucleus and its large karyosome may be visible. The trophozoites of *E. nana* are approximately one half the size of those of *E. histolytica* (except the small race), and *E. coli*. This difference has diagnostic value.

**The Cyst**　The cysts are thin-walled, oval or spherical bodies varying from 7 to 10 microns in diameter. The single nucleus of the young form undergoes division to produce the mature four-nucleate cyst.

The characteristic structure of the nucleus is clearly shown in iron-hematoxylin stained preparations. The absence of chromatin beads on the coarse nuclear membrane and the large irregular eccentric karyosome are diagnostic.

The nuclei are usually not visible in fresh preparations and chromatoid bars are absent. The nuclear membrane and the karyosome are readily seen in iodine stained smears.

## Iodamoeba bütschlii

*Iodamoeba bütschlii* (v. Prowazek 1911) Dodell 1919 is a nonpathogenic intestinal ameba of man. It is found in a considerable number of normal individuals especially in the tropics and the subtropics. Both trophozoite and encysted stages occur in its life cycle. The trophozoite, however, is rarely seen.

**The Trophozoite**　In iron-hematoxylin stained preparations the trophozoite averages 9 to 13 microns in diameter. The large spherical nucleus consists of an achromatic nuclear membrane and a very large centrally placed, deeply stained karyosome. The cytoplasm contains bacteria, yeasts and other inclusions. This ameba never ingests red blood cells.

In unstained warm smears from freshly passed stools the ameba exhibits sluggish progressive motility, protruding broad hyaline pseudopodia. The nucleus may be visible if not obscured by ingested bacteria and other particles. Motility ceases as the organism is cooled.

**The Cyst**　The cysts are very irregular in shape, a distinctive characteristic, and vary from 6 to 15 microns in diameter. The cysts are relatively thick-walled, usually uninucleate, and characteristically contain a large round or oval, sharply demarcated glycogen mass.

In iron-hematoxylin stained preparations the single nucleus presents a thin unbeaded nuclear membrane. The large deeply stained karyosome is often eccentrically placed and in contact with the nuclear membrane. The position of the glycogen mass is indicated by a large vacuole.

In unstained smears the nucleus is usually not visible and the glycogen mass appears as a vacuole.

In iodine stained preparations the large sharply defined deep-mahogany colored glycogen body is the most striking feature of the cyst. The single nucleus is visible if not obscured by the glycogen mass.

## Dientamoeba fragilis

*Dientamoeba fragilis* Jepps and Dobell 1918 is a relatively uncommon and probably nonpathogenic ameba. The life cycle of this organism has not been determined. An encysted stage has not been identified and the exact means of transmission are in doubt.

**The Trophozoite**  This ameba varies from 8 to 10 microns in diameter. About four-fifths of the specimens seen are binucleate. The structure is characteristic in iron-hematoxylin stained preparations. The nuclear membranes of the two nuclei are very delicate and often invisible. The centrally placed coarse, lobulated karyosome is composed of a group of chromatin granules. The two nuclei may be connected by a dark-staining thread. The cytoplasm is granular and contains a variety of food inclusions. Red blood cells are not ingested.

In warm smears from freshly passed stools these amebae at first appear as immobile spherical bodies. After a variable period of time active progressive motility begins.

The pseudopodia are clear, glasslike, sharply differentiated from the endoplasm and characteristically clover-leaf in outline. The nuclei are rarely visible. Motility ceases promptly on cooling and the ameba rounds up into a spherical body.

## Giardia lamblia

The flagellate, *Giardia lamblia* Stiles 1915, inhabits the duodenum, the upper jejunum and occasionally the gallbladder of man. Despite the fact that it is one of the most common of the intestinal protozoa, there is controversy concerning its pathogenicity. The life cycle comprises both trophozoite and encysted stages.

**The Trophozoite**  This flagellate resembles a longitudinally cut pear in shape and measures 11 to 18 microns in length by 6 to 9 microns in width. It is convex dorsally and concave ventrally, with an ovoid sucking disc occupying the anterior ventral surface. There are eight flagella. Multiplication occurs by longitudinal fission.

The detailed morphology is visible only in iron-hematoxylin preparations. A pair of axostyles, originating anteriorly from a pair of blepharoplasts, are continued backward to extend posteriorly as flagella. The two anteriorly situated nuclei lie on either side of the axostyles. Three additional pairs of flagella, an anterolateral, a posterolateral and a ventral, originate from the blepharoplasts. The cytoplasm does not contain food inclusions or red blood cells.

In fresh unstained preparations the trophozoite is actively motile, combining irregular progression, rotation and rocking movements.

The eight flagella become visible only as motility almost ceases. The cytoplasm is hyaline or finely granular in appearance.

**The Cyst** The cysts of *G. lamblia* are ovoid in contour. They measure 8 to 12 microns in length and 6 to 10 microns in width. They contain two to four nuclei usually situated near one pole.

In iron-hematoxylin stained preparations the individual nucleus is seen to consist of a delicate nuclear membrane and a small central or eccentrically placed karyosome. The axostyles appear as two longitudinally placed curved rods, and the flagella as groups of stained fibrils.

In unstained smears the cysts appear as ovoid colorless hyaline bodies in which refractile structures representing the nuclei may sometimes be seen.

In iodine stained smears the four nuclei and their karyosomes may be identified and the distorted sucking disc, the longitudinal axostyles and fibrils representing the flagella may be seen. The cytoplasm stains a brownish color and may contain diffuse glycogen.

## Embadomonas intestinalis

*Embadomonas intestinalis* Wenyon and O'Connor 1917 is a non-pathogenic, relatively uncommon intestinal flagellate of man. It has been reported from the United States, Brazil, Egypt, Malaya, the Philippines, China and Japan. Because of its small size it is possible that it is sometimes overlooked. Both trophozoite and encysted stages occur in its life cycle.

A larger, closely allied species, *E. sinensis* Faust and Wassell 1921, has been reported twice from man in China. A third species, *E. hominis* da Fonseca 1915, may be distinguished from *E. intestinalis* by the presence of three flagella in the trophozoite and of two nuclei in the ovoid or rounded cysts.

**The Trophozoite** In hematoxylin stained specimens the ovoid trophozoite measures 4 to 9 microns in length and 3 to 4 microns in breadth. The nucleus lies forward of the mouth (cytosome) at the anterior end; it has a fine membrane and a central karyosome. Near the nucleus are two small dots (blepharoplasts) from which two flagella arise.

In unstained warm smears from freshly passed stools the trophozoites appear rounded or ovoid, are colorless and progress in an irregular, jerky fashion. The finely granular cytoplasm may contain vacuoles; the flagella are rarely visible.

**The Cyst** In hematoxylin stained specimens the cysts appear as small, pear-shaped bodies and measure between 4 and 6 microns in greatest diameter. The single nucleus with its delicate membrane and central karyosome are characteristic.

The unstained cysts may appear to be slightly larger and to have a double cyst wall; other details of their morphology are difficult to see.

## Chilomastix mesnili

*Chilomastix mesnili* (Wenyon 1910) Alexeiff 1912 is a nonpathogenic flagellate inhabiting the large intestine of man. It is frequently found in normal individuals in many parts of the world. Both trophozoite and encysted stages occur in its life cycle.

**The Trophozoite** This flagellate measures 13 to 24 microns in length and 6 to 11 microns in breadth. Occasionally, minute, almost spherical forms less than five microns in length are observed. The typical specimen has a rigid pear-shaped body with a spiral groove and is pointed at the posterior end. Multiplication occurs by binary fission.

In iron-hematoxylin stained preparations the spiral groove is clearly visible. The cytoplasm is finely granular. A mouthlike cytostome, appearing as a cleft, originates anteriorly and extends posteriorly for nearly one-half the length of the body. The nucleus, situated anteriorly near the point of origin of the cytostome, has a well defined nuclear membrane and a small round centrally or eccentrically placed karyosome. Three free anterior flagella and one oral flagellum originate from a blepharoplast complex in the anterior portion of the organism.

In warm smears from freshly passed stools the trophozoites are actively motile, progressing in a jerky, spiral fashion. The cytoplasm is colorless or faintly greenish. In sluggishly motile specimens the three anterior flagella, the cytostome and the spiral groove may be visible.

**The Cyst** The cysts of *C. mesnili* are ovoid in shape averaging 7 to 9 microns in length by 4.5 to 6 microns in breadth. A blunt protuberance at one pole gives them a lemon-shaped appearance. There is a single spherical nucleus.

In iron-hematoxylin stained smears the nuclear membrane is distinct and the karyosome may be central or eccentric and in contact with the nuclear membrane. The condensed cytostome is longitudinally placed in close proximity to the nucleus. The flagella may appear as dark-stained fibrils.

In unstained preparations the cysts are colorless and the internal structures are not visible.

In iodine preparations they are stained yellowish brown and the nucleus and cytostome may sometimes be faintly seen. One or more small glycogen masses may rarely be demonstrated.

## Trichomonas hominis

The flagellate, *Trichomonas hominis* (Davaine 1860) Leuckart 1879, is an inhabitant of the lower ileum and the cecum or colon of man. It is probably nonpathogenic and is widely distributed throughout the world. It is known only in the trophozoite stage.

One other species, *T. tenax* (O. F. Müller 1773) Dobell 1939, has been found only in the human mouth where it occurs in dental cavities, alveolar pus pockets and in the tartar on the teeth. It is the only flagellate known to inhabit the human mouth.

**The Trophozoite**  *Trichomonas hominis* is a pear-shaped flagellate possessing three to five anterior flagella and a distinct undulating membrane. It averages 10 to 14 microns in length. Reproduction is by longitudinal fission.

In iron-hematoxylin stained preparations the single ovoid nucleus with central karyosome and delicate nuclear membrane is visible near the anterior or blunt end. A blepharoplast complex just anterior to the nucleus provides the origin of (1) the anterior flagella, (2) a marginal flagellum which shortly leaves the body to form the edge of the undulating membrane, and (3) an axostyle which is continued longitudinally through the body and protrudes posteriorly for a variable distance.

In fresh unstained preparations it exhibits active wobbly progressive motion due to the activity of the flagella and the undulating membrane. Red cells may be ingested occasionally if blood is present in the stool. The nucleus and other internal structures are not visible in the colorless finely granular cytoplasm.

## Trichomonas vaginalis

*Trichomonas vaginalis* Donné 1873 is closely related to *T. hominis* and occurs in the human vagina and urethra. It may be pathogenic and is associated particularly with a form of vaginitis. It is widely distributed throughout the world. Multiplication occurs by longitudinal fission. This organism is known only in the trophozoite stage.

**The Trophozoite**  *Trichomonas vaginalis* closely resembles *T. hominis* although there are certain morphological differences. It is larger, measuring 10 to 30 microns in length, there are four anterior flagella and the undulating membrane is shorter than that of *T. hominis*, extending only about one-half the length of the body where its marginal flagellum terminates. There is no free posterior flagellum.

## Balantidium coli

*Balantidium coli* (Malmsten 1857) Stein 1862 is the only ciliate pathogenic for man. It inhabits the large intestine and less commonly the lower portion of the ileum. *Balantidium coli* is widely distributed throughout the world and parasitizes the pig, various species of monkeys and man. Both trophozoite and encysted stages occur in its life cycle.

**The Trophozoite**  *Balantidium coli* is the largest of the protozoan parasites of man, measuring 50 to 70 microns in length by 30 to 60 microns in breadth. It is ovoid in shape and actively motile. Multiplication occurs by transverse binary fission and by conjugation of two trophozoites.

In iron-hematoxylin stained preparations the external surface is seen to be covered with cilia arranged in longitudinal rows. The oral apparatus or peristome is a V-shaped groove or depression at the anterior end lined by somewhat larger cilia. The mouth lies at the base of this structure, opening into the gullet. A large kidney-shaped macronucleus and a smaller micronucleus, usually in apposition to the concave surface of the former, are situated in approximately the central portion of the body. There are two contractile vacuoles, one anterior and one posterior. The cytoplasm contains a variety of food inclusions including red blood cells, leukocytes, starch granules and bacteria.

In unstained fresh smears the trophozoite moves actively with a smooth gliding motion. The rapidly beating cilia cannot be seen. The two nuclei are sometimes faintly visible.

**The Cyst** The cysts of *B. coli* are oval, measuring 50 to 65 microns in greatest diameter, and the cyst wall appears to have a double outline. They stain poorly with either iodine or hematoxylin although the nuclei and the unstained contractile vacuoles are easily seen.

In unstained preparations the organism may show motility within the cyst wall. The cytoplasm has a faintly greenish tinge. The nuclei and the contractile vacuoles may be faintly visible.

## Isospora hominis

*Isospora hominis* (Rivolta 1878) is a relatively uncommon parasite of man. It is believed to inhabit the ileum. This protozoan is the

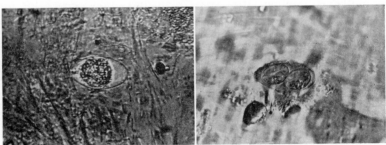

Fig. 108.                    Fig. 109.

Fig. 108. Immature oocyst of *Isospora hominis* from freshly passed feces (1000 ×). (Courtesy Dr. T. B. Magath, Mayo Clinic.)
Fig. 109. Older oocyst of *Isospora hominis* showing two sporoblasts (1000 ×). (Courtesy Dr. T. B. Magath, Mayo Clinic.)

only known member of the Sporozoa (Coccidia) to infect the intestine of man.

**The Oocysts** Only the oocysts of *I. hominis* are known from man. These are ovoid, somewhat elongated and measure 22 to 33 microns in length by 11 to 18 microns in breadth. In freshly passed feces only the immature oocyst is usually seen. This is unsegmented and contains a single spherical mass of granular material (Fig. 108). A small, obscure micropyle at the narrower end has been reported by some observers. Development of the oocyst occurs as the inner granular mass divides to form two sporoblasts (Fig. 109). Each of these in turn secretes a cyst wall and so eventually becomes a spore. The nuclear material within each spore divides twice to produce four crescent-shaped sporozoites. In unstained fresh smears only oocysts with one or two granular masses are seen.

The development of sporoblasts, spores and sporozoites has been observed. Although details of schizogonic development of *I. hominis* are unknown, they are presumed to resemble those of other coccidia such as *I. felis*, in which case the intracellular forms would occur in the epithelial cells of the small intestine.

## Blastocystis hominis

The yeast, *Blastocystis hominis*, although a nonpathogenic commensal in the digestive tract of man, is included because it may be mistaken for encysted forms of intestinal protozoa.

It is ovoid or spherical in shape, averaging 10 to 15 microns in greatest diameter, and occasionally reaching considerably larger size. The hyaline refractive cytoplasm is included within a membrane resembling a cyst wall. The outer layer of cytoplasm immediately adjacent to the membrane is frequently differentiated, creating the appearance of a double-walled cyst. This outer layer contains refractile granules and one or more nuclei which are visible in unstained preparations. The central portion is structureless and resembles a large vacuole. Dividing forms are common and exhibit marked variation in size and shape.

In iron-hematoxylin stained preparations the central cytoplasmic mass appears grayish in color while the peripheral band is unstained except for the nuclei and their large centrally placed karyosomes. Iodine likewise stains the nuclei and the central cytoplasm may appear brownish in color.

## 31   Amebiasis and Related Infections

### Amebiasis

**Synonyms**   Amebic dysentery, amebic enteritis, amebic colitis.

**Definition**   Amebiasis is an infection of the colon by the pathogenic ameba, *Endamoeba histolytica*, characterized by acute or chronic phases, or both, and by a variable clinical picture. The so-called chronic cyst-passer may exhibit few or no significant symptoms. In other instances infection may be characterized by intermittent episodes of constipation and diarrhea; in still others the diarrhea may be relatively severe and the stools contain varying amounts of blood and mucus. Acute amebic dysentery is not infrequent in the tropics but is less common in the temperate zone. Any of the clinical types of this infection may be followed promptly or after prolonged periods by the serious complications, acute amebic hepatitis, or acute or chronic amebic abscess of the liver. Less frequently metastatic abscesses occur in other organs.

**Distribution**  Amebiasis has a cosmopolitan distribution and is not restricted to the tropics. The incidence in any population is determined by the level of sanitation existing in the particular area, varying from an average of 8.1 per cent in the United States to considerably over 50 per cent in some areas of the tropics and subtropics.

**Etiology**  *Endamoeba histolytica* is the most important of the intestinal protozoa of man. The motile vegetative forms (trophozoites) are invasive and are responsible for the pathologic changes. After a period of activity and multiplication certain of these trophozoites round up, secrete a resistant capsule and are discharged in the feces of the host. These cysts are not found within the tissues of the host.

**Epidemiology**  The actively motile trophozoites present in the freshly passed feces of patients suffering from amebic diarrhea or dysentery are short-lived outside the body. It is unlikely that they can survive exposure to the hydrochloric acid and digestive enzymes of the stomach and upper intestinal tract. They are therefore of little, if any, importance in the epidemiology of the disease.

The encysted forms, however, are resistant to marked changes in their environment and are responsible for transmission. The infection is acquired by the ingestion of these encysted forms in food or drink contaminated by the feces of infected individuals.

The cysts of *E. histolytica* are readily destroyed by drying; they are also killed rapidly at 55° C. They will survive as long as one month in water at about 10° C. The cysts are relatively resistant to chlorine and are not destroyed by concentrations customarily used for water purification. If dependence is to be placed upon chlorination alone, the concentration and contact time must be adjusted in accordance with the temperature and hydrogen ion concentration of the water.

Dilute disinfectants as ordinarily used are not markedly effective in destroying the encysted forms. In moist feces survival time is reduced to approximately twelve days and is controlled by the rate of putrefaction and the temperature. At 4° C. cysts remain viable for at least sixty days in both sewage and natural surface waters.

Man is the principal reservoir of infection. However, amebae which are morphologically identical with *E. histolytica* have been recovered from the dog, cat, rat, pig and various types of monkeys.

*Transmission* of the infection from one individual to another may be accomplished by a variety of mechanisms. The house fly and the cockroach feed upon human feces when available and cysts of *E. histolytica* have been recovered from the intestinal tracts of these insects, apparently undamaged, after periods as long as forty-eight hours. It is highly probable that one of the most important factors in the spread of infection is transmission of cysts by flies. Flies breed in,

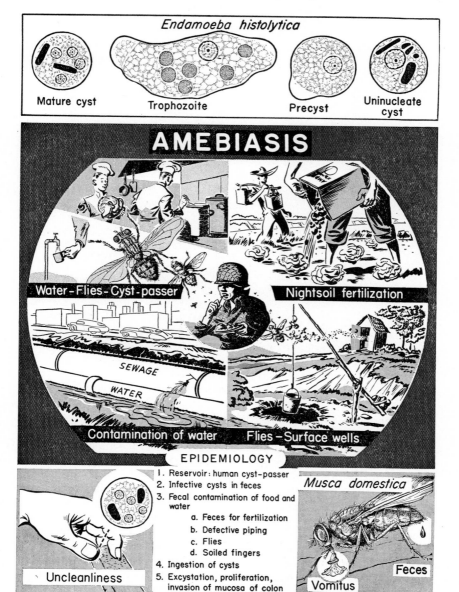

Fig. 110. Epidemiology of amebiasis.

and feed upon, human excreta as well as other waste products. In the course of a subsequent feeding the fly evacuates its gut and contaminates food with bacteria, cysts of the intestinal protozoa and perhaps at times even helminth eggs (Fig. 110).

Polluted water may likewise be an important vehicle of infection. Fecal contamination of water commonly occurs by surface run-off into springs, unprotected shallow wells and streams, or by discharge of crude sewage into streams and rivers. Less frequently cross seepage between water and sewer pipes laid in the same ditch, or direct cross connections with siphonage of sewage into the water supply system

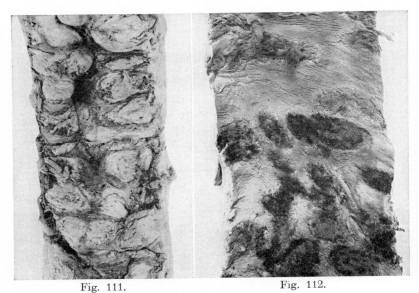

Fig. 111.    Fig. 112.

Fig. 111. "Sea anemone" ulcers of colon.
Fig. 112. "Dyak hair" ulcers of colon showing superficial and deep ulceration.

are responsible for outbreaks of infection. The freshening of vegetables in contaminated water or even in crude sewage, before sale is widely practiced in many parts of the world. Ice made from polluted water may likewise be an important source of infection.

In many regions human excreta, night soil, are widely used as garden fertilizer. In other areas sludge from sewage disposal plants is similarly utilized. Either practice may be responsible for heavy contamination of root and leafy vegetables which customarily are eaten raw.

The infected individual passing large numbers of cysts in his stools is an important potential source of infection, especially if engaged in the preparation and handling of food. There are numerous instances, especially in family outbreaks, which indicate the hazard of such employment of the cyst-passer.

Epidemic outbreaks of amebiasis are uncommon and all reported instances have been traced to a heavily contaminated water supply or to fly transmission. The disease occurs characteristically in endemic form. The *infection rate* is low in young children but in the school age group the incidence reaches that of the general population of the area in which they live. There is no recognized immunity.

**Pathology**   The fundamental pathology of amebiasis is characterized by penetration of the host's tissues by *E. histolytica*, necrosis of tissue cells, and absence of inflammatory reaction.

Lesions are most commonly found in the cecum, ascending colon, sigmoid and rectum. In the early stage lysis of the epithelium and the underlying stroma produces superficial erosions of the mucosa. Macroscopically these appear as shallow ulcers having a necrotic base and a narrow surrounding zone of hyperemia with normal mucosa intervening. Extension occurs peripherally and downward into the submucosa. In other instances small amebic abscesses are found in the submucosa eventually opening through the surface to produce the characteristic flask or bottle-neck ulcer. Both the superficial and the deeper lesions may form the "sea anemone" ulcer with deep crater and partly necrotic undermined edges which are raised above the level of the surrounding mucosa (Fig. 111).

Initially there is little edema and no leukocytic response (Figs. 113, 114, 116). Secondary bacterial infection of the ulcers occurs rapidly, however, producing a varyingly severe inflammatory reaction. Occasionally bacillary dysentery is superimposed; rarely secondary infection by *Cl. perfringens* may produce a rapidly spreading and fatal gangrene of the colon. In some instances, extensive and rapid invasion of the colonic wall by the amebae may lead to severe or fatal hemorrhage or perforation. The resulting ulcer, the so-called "Dyak hair" ulcer, is sharply circumscribed and the base is formed by fringelike projections of the more resistant supporting tissues (Fig. 112).

The characteristics of the stool mirror the pathology in the colon. In the presence of the Dyak hair type of ulceration hemorrhage is usual. In less severe cases of dysentery the stools are foul and usually bloody. In milder infections there may be little abnormality, or small flecks of blood-stained mucus intimately mixed with liquid feces produce the so-called "sago-grain" stools.

On microscopic examination of the particles of mucus the cellular exudate is characteristic. Pyknotic bodies, the nuclear remnants of tissue cells and leukocytes, form 60 to 90 per cent of the cellular elements apart from erythrocytes. The latter are often clumped when present only in small numbers. Leukocytes appear and increase in numbers as secondary bacterial infection of the ulcers occurs and extends. Macrophages are not seen in the absence of infection by a member of the genus *Shigella*, except after arsenical therapy.

Invasion of the submucosa may be followed by entry of *E. histolytica* into radicles of the portal vein and metastasis of the infection to the liver. This is followed by amebic hepatitis or amebic abscess of the liver. Such abscesses may be single or multiple, acute or chronic. Multiple foci of necrosis may coalesce to form a single large abscess. Leukocytic infiltration of the wall occurs even in the absence of secondary bacterial infection. Right lobe abscesses of the liver

Fig. 113.                                    Fig. 114.

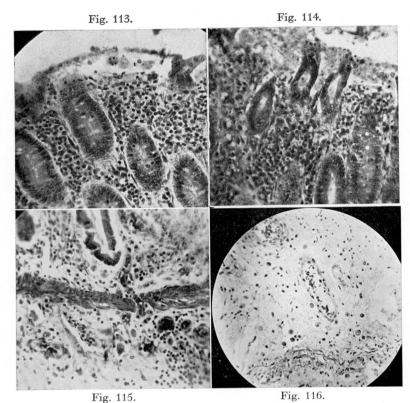

Fig. 115.                                    Fig. 116.

Fig. 113. Early lesion; trophozoites of *E. histolytica* under superficial epithelial layer. (Courtesy Dr. R. W. Nauss, Cornell University Medical College.)

Fig. 114. Superficial ulceration of the mucosa. (Courtesy Dr. R. W. Nauss, Cornell University Medical College.)

Fig. 115. Invasion of submucosa along vessel penetrating muscularis mucosae.

Fig. 116. Trophozoites in submucosa: note absence of inflammation.

commonly extend upward and may penetrate the diaphragm and rupture into the lung (Figs. 115, 117).

Amebic abscess of the brain and other organs occurs rarely; secondary amebic infections of the skin and subcutaneous tissues, the bladder, uterus and vagina have been reported.

**Clinical Characteristics**    The clinical response to infection by *E. histolytica* is exceedingly variable and depends upon the localization of the amebae, the intensity of the infection, and possibly variations

in virulence of different strains. There is little exact knowledge concerning the prevalence of amebic disease in relation to the incidence of asymptomatic infection. Surveys indicate, however, that the ratios of amebic abscess of the liver, acute dysentery, and diarrhea to the known prevalence of amebic infection in the population are low.

The factors determining the wide variations in the clinical response to this infection have not been evaluated. It is generally recognized that frank amebic dysentery is more common in the tropics and subtropics than elsewhere and that in the temperate zones it is more prevalent in the warmer months of the year. Large and small races of *E. histolytica* have been identified which differ one

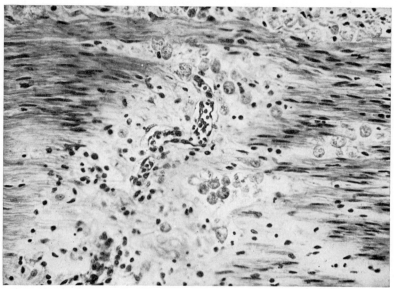

Fig. 117. Invasion of muscularis along penetrating vessel. (Collection of Dr. W. M. James and Dr. Lawrence Getz.)

from the other clinically, pathologically and immunologically both in experimental animals and man. The small races tend to be less pathogenic. It appears, however, that virulence may be augmented by repeated serial passage.

Infection by this parasite may persist for many years, running a protracted course that is frequently characterized by periodic exacerbation of intestinal symptoms, and by remissions during which the patient may be largely if not entirely symptom-free.

THE CYST-PASSER. The cyst-passer is the commonest clinical type. Two classes are recognized: convalescents who, following acute dysentery or amebic diarrhea, retain a chronic infection and more or less continuously show encysted forms in their stools, and those who have acquired the infection but have not experienced active clinical disease.

The relationship between the asymptomatic carrier state and active disease is controversial. Some authorities state that not more than 10 per cent of cyst-passers suffer damage from the infection. Others hold that at least 50 per cent exhibit symptoms attributable to *E. histolytica*. The problem is complicated by the fact that symptoms when present may be extremely variable and many of them cannot be considered as specific responses to the infection. Careful study of human autopsy material, however, supports the contention that *E. histolytica* invariably attacks the intestinal wall of the host even though significant symptoms may not result. It is known also that infected individuals may be essentially symptom-free for periods of years only to develop without warning acute involvement of the liver with hepatitis or actual abscess formation. It appears, therefore, desirable to regard the infected individual not only as a source for potential spread to others but also as a person who may at any time develop acute symptoms and serious disease.

The clinical picture of the chronic cyst-passer characteristically lacks specificity and is extremely variable. Some individuals are often apparently healthy, while in others the most striking features are chronicity, mildness and recurrence of symptoms. The onset is usually insidious and frequently there are alternating periods of ill health and relative well-being. During the former, abdominal distention and flatulence accompanied by constipation are common complaints. Anorexia and poor nutrition together with loss of weight or inability to gain weight are usual, and there is often intolerance to fats in the diet. These symptoms are commonly accompanied by vague abdominal discomfort and sense of abnormal fullness of the abdomen, particularly on the right side. Many such individuals are irritable, unduly susceptible to fatigue, and exhibit the lassitude and other phenomena associated with neurasthenia. Although the constipation may be interrupted by occasional brief periods of loose stools, these ordinarily do not attract attention, especially since gross blood and mucus are not present in the feces. Chronic microcytic anemia is not unusual.

When these patients seek medical advice a common tentative diagnosis is chronic cholecystitis. Frequently, however, negative roentgenologic studies ultimately lead to the erroneous diagnosis of psychoneurosis or menopause accompanied by emotional instability.

AMEBIC DIARRHEA. When the host-parasite balance is less exact, periodic bouts of diarrhea occur with four to six loose or liquid stools a day. Abdominal discomfort and cramps may be present. Tenesmus does not occur and fever is usually absent. There is usually little change in the white blood count although there may be a slight leukocytosis and some increase in monocytes. Careful examination of the stools will commonly reveal small flecks of blood-tinged mucus in which there are large numbers of trophozoites. The spontaneous cessation of diarrhea is usually followed by a variable period of constipation during which the vague symptoms of the cyst-passer dominate the clinical picture.

ACUTE AMEBIC DYSENTERY. Acute amebic dysentery is one of the less common clinical manifestations of intestinal amebiasis. The incubation period may be as short as eight to ten days and in approximately 50 per cent of cases the onset is sudden. This is especially true of mixed infections with *Shigella*. In other instances acute dysentery may occur in the previously healthy cyst-passer who has carried his infection for long periods of time.

When the onset is acute it may be accompanied by headache, nausea, chills, fever, severe abdominal cramps and, if there are lesions of the descending colon, by tenesmus. Some degree of enlargement of the liver with tenderness on palpation occurs in approximately 25 per cent of cases. The stools usually average fifteen to twenty in each twenty-four hours and consist of liquid fecal matter containing pinhead flecks of bloody mucus, the so-called "sago-grain stools." The white blood count may vary from 5000 to 15,000 with a polymorphonuclear leukocytosis as high as 85 per cent. The fever tends to be lower and the leukocytosis slightly higher in acute amebic dysentery than in acute bacillary dysentery.

In very severe cases extensive involvement of the colon may lead to massive destruction of the mucosa and the formation of a pseudo-diphtheritic membrane which may be passed intact, or actual gangrene of large portions of the colonic wall may occur. In severe cases the deeply penetrating ulceration may produce serious or even fatal hemorrhage. Usually, however, death, when it occurs, is due to cardiac failure and exhaustion, or to perforation of the colon and peritonitis.

CHRONIC AMEBIC DYSENTERY. Repeated and inadequately treated attacks of acute dysentery or of amebic diarrhea may be followed by chronic dysentery. This is the result of long continued mixed infection of the colonic wall by *E. histolytica* and by bacteria. It is associated with progressive scarring and deformity of the colon and clinically differs little from chronic bacillary dysentery or so-called idiopathic ulcerative colitis. It is characterized by recurrent acute attacks of fever and by diarrhea with blood and pus in the stools. It is frequently difficult to demonstrate the amebae. In the intervals between acute attacks the stools are generally loose, increased in number and mixed with variable amounts of blood, mucus and pus. Chronic dysentery is commonly accompanied by malnutrition and cachexia.

AMEBIC APPENDICITIS. Infection of the appendix by *E. histolytica* may occur and with secondary bacterial invasion the clinical picture of subacute appendicitis may be encountered. In instances when the appendix occupies a retrocecal position the clinical picture may be exceedingly confusing. Demonstration of *E. histolytica* in the patient's stools, however, should be regarded as potentially significant evidence and in the absence of imperative indications for operation anti-amebic therapy should be given before laparotomy is decided upon.

AMEBIC TYPHLITIS. In certain individuals the localization of the amebae remains principally restricted to its primary site in the cecum and ascending colon and the pathology is limited principally to this area. Under such conditions, and in the presence of a progressive infection, the clinical picture may be that of an acute or chronic typhlitis rather than acute dysentery and may arouse grave suspicion of a surgical lesion in the right lower quadrant. Operative procedure upon such infected tissue will almost invariably result in the breakdown of suture lines causing fatal peritonitis.

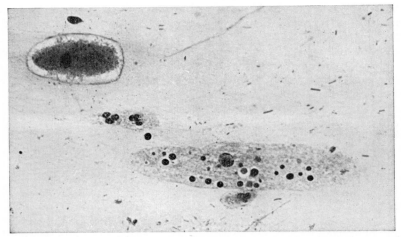

Fig. 118. Early exudate in stool: young and old trophozoites of *E. histolytica* in stool; scanty exudate. Note ingested red blood corpuscles in this stained preparation.

AMEBIC GRANULOMA. In certain instances intestinal amebiasis is accompanied by the formation of granulomatous lesions of the colon which are commonly misdiagnosed as carcinoma. They may occur in any area from the cecum to the rectum. Those that can be visualized through the sigmoidoscope may present many of the characteristics af adenocarcinoma. In other instances roentgen examination following a barium enema may reveal a picture characteristic of an annular carcinoma producing partial or even complete obstruction of the colon.

**Diagnosis** The diagnosis of intestinal amebiasis depends upon demonstration of *E. histolytica* in the feces of the infected person. If the individual is passing formed stools, ordinarily only cysts will be found. In the rare instances of active ulceration predominantly confined to the rectum, however, trophozoites may be found in flecks of blood-stained mucus adherent to the surface of the stool. If there is active diarrhea or acute dysentery, on the other hand, only the trophozoites are to be expected (Fig. 118). These do not survive long after passage from the body and, especially when exposed to chilling, rapidly lose the motility and normal morphologic characteristics upon which identification must be based. The detailed morphology is described on page 237. In contrast to the lack of need for haste in examining a formed specimen a diarrheal stool must be kept warm and examined at the earliest possible moment unless the PVA or MIF technique is employed (see pp. 819, 828).

EXAMINATION OF FORMED STOOL. A small portion of the fecal matter should be emulsified in tap water or saline solution on a glass slide

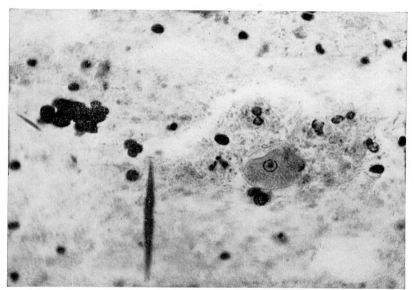

Fig. 119. Early exudate in stool (iron-hematoxylin stain) showing trophozoite, clumped erythrocytes, pyknotic bodies and Charcot-Leyden crystals.

and covered with a coverslip. The preparation should be of a density that just permits the reading of news print through it. A similar fecal emulsion should be made with Lugol's, D'Antoni's or other iodine solution.

In the unstained suspension the cysts of *E. histolytica* appear as round refractile bodies in which no nuclei are visible or in which the nuclei can barely be distinguished. When the condenser of the microscope is racked down the characteristic and diagnostic blunt-ended chromatoid bar may often be seen in some cysts.

In the iodine suspension the nuclei are easily visible. These are four in number in the mature cysts but it is not unusual to observe younger forms which are uni- or binucleate. Chromatoid bars are usually less frequently seen than in a water or saline suspension.

In light infections demonstration of the cysts is facilitated by concentration methods. These techniques are described in the section on Diagnostic Methods, pp. 821–824.

EXAMINATION OF DIARRHEAL STOOL. The freshly passed stool should be kept at body temperature by immersion of the container in warm water unless examination can be carried out immediately after evacuation. A small quantity of liquid feces should be poured into a petri dish and should be carefully scrutinized for small flecks of blood-stained mucus. Such a particle of mucus should be placed on a slide, covered with a coverglass and immediately examined, prefer-

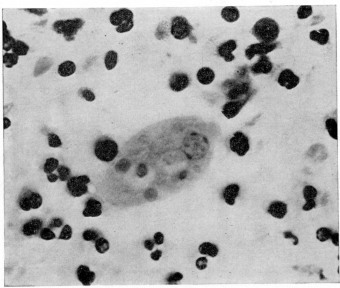

Fig. 120. Exudate in stool in stage of secondary bacterial infection (H & E): trophozoite, pyknotic bodies, erythrocytes, round cells and polymorphonuclear leukocytes with pyknotic nuclei.

ably on a warm stage. In the presence of an active amebic infection many of the flecks of bloody mucus contain large numbers of motile trophozoites which appear as elongated ribbon-like amebae exhibiting progressive motion across the microscopic field. The presence of ingested red blood cells within the trophozoite, the glasslike pseudopodia and the characteristic progressive motion are diagnostic. It is to be emphasized that the amebae are much more numerous in the flecks of mucus than in the fecal material of the stools (Figs. 119, 120, 121). *Endamoeba histolytica* may be isolated in culture (p. 833).

Charcot-Leyden crystals are frequently present in the stools. Although suggestive, they are not pathognomonic of infection by *E. histolytica* since they occur in association with other parasitic infections and with any chronic ulcerative condition of the colon.

PROCTOSCOPIC EXAMINATION. Proctoscopic examination of the chronic cyst-passer rarely yields information of value. In the more active clinical types of infection, however, lesions may be observed which are characteristic. These are small, discrete, inflamed areas scattered about an otherwise entirely normal mucous membrane. Characteristically they appear as minute, pinpoint, yellowish spots surrounded by a narrow band of hyperemia. Each of these represents a minute amebic abscess of the mucosa. Immediate microscopic examination of the contents expressed with a spatula will reveal enormous numbers of trophozoites.

X-ray Examination. Roentgen examination of the colon is not a dependable aid in diagnosis since demonstrable lesions are by no

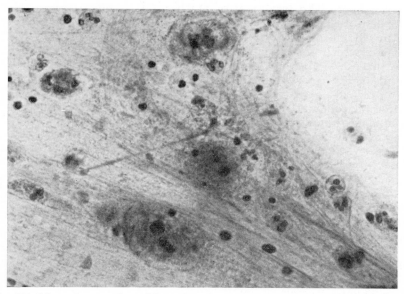

Fig. 121. Mucus from surface of formed stool: exudate, trophozoites, pyknotic bodies (H & E stain).

*Table 23    Diagnostic Characteristics of* Endamoeba histolytica

|  | FORM | WHERE FOUND | MORPHOLOGY |
|---|---|---|---|
| Liquid stools | Trophozoites | Blood-stained mucus | Progressive motion; glasslike pseudopodia; may contain red blood cells |
| Formed stools | Cysts | In the fecal mass | Saline preparation: Blunt-ended chromatoid visible; nuclei not visible<br>Iodine preparation: 4 nuclei paired at different levels usually with centrally placed karyosome; chromatoid not always visible |

means always present. However, in acute cases, the barium enema may reveal spasm and evidence of ulceration particularly in the proximal colon, and some degree of deformity of the cecum is not unusual in long-standing chronic infections. In the presence of amebic granuloma a filling defect suggestive of carcinoma may be seen.

COMPLEMENT FIXATION. A reliable complement fixation test has not been developed. When performed under optimal conditions, however, it may be of assistance in cases of extra-intestinal amebiasis. It does not give dependable results when infection is limited to the intestine.

**Treatment** The treatment of amebiasis is frequently unsatisfactory and unsuccessful. The basis of the therapeutic problem is the nature of the pathology and the anatomic situation of the amebae, some of which are in the intestinal contents, some on the surface of the mucosa, and others at various depths within the tissues. It is necessary, therefore, to deliver an active amebacidal agent in effective concentration to the sites of localization in the tissues and to the intestinal contents. The ideal amebacide to meet these two fundamental requirements is not yet available, consequently combined treatment using two or more of the recommended drugs is usually necessary. Since they differ with respect to their pharmacology and their sites of action, these factors are extremely important in the selection of the individual preparations.

The problem of therapy is further complicated in the long-standing chronic case in which repeated ineffective treatment may develop a drug-refractory strain of *E. histolytica*, or in which extensive secondary bacterial infection has altered the pathogenesis of the disease, or in which the administration of antibiotics has affected the normal flora.

DRUGS. The recommended drugs fall into five groups based upon their chemical composition:

1. COMPOUNDS OF ARSENIC. *Carbarsone,* *p*-carbamido-benzene-arsonic acid, is a pentavalent arsenical containing approximately 28 per cent arsenic. It is readily absorbed, excreted rather slowly in the urine and is the least toxic of the arsenic group, rarely producing ill effects at therapeutic levels. It is active against the amebae in the lumen of the colon and in the tissues. It is contraindicated in the presence of disease of the liver or kidneys and for arsenic-intolerant patients.

The recommended dosage for adults is 0.25 gm. by mouth two or three times a day for ten days. Following a rest period of equal length, the course may be repeated. The dosage for children should be reduced as follows:

Age 2– 4 years, 2.0 gm. total in ten days
Age 5– 8 years, 3.0 gm. total in ten days
Age 9–12 years, 4.0 gm. total in ten days
The drug may likewise be administered by rectum for the treat-

*Table 24   Treatment of Amebiasis*

| DRUG | AMEBACIDAL POWER | SITE OF ACTION | CONTRAINDICATIONS | RECOMMENDED DAILY DOSAGE | APPROXIMATE DURATION OF THERAPY |
|---|---|---|---|---|---|
| 1. Pentavalent arsenic: | | | | | |
| Carbarsone | Good | Tissues and intestinal contents | Hepatic and renal disease | 0.75 gm. | 7–10 |
| Milibis | Good | Intestinal contents only | Hepatic and renal disease | 1.5 gm. | 7–10 |
| Trivalent arsenic: | | | | | |
| Thiocarbarsone | Good | Tissues and intestinal contents | Hepatic and renal disease | 0.3 gm. | 10 |
| 2. Halogenated hydroxyquinolines: | | | | | |
| Diodoquin | Good | Intestinal contents | Hyperthyroidism | 1.95 gm. | 21 |
| Vioform | Good | Intestinal contents | Hyperthyroidism | 1.5–3.0 gm. | 7–10 |
| Chiniofon | Good | Intestinal contents | Hyperthyroidism | 0.75 gm. | 8–10 |
| 3. Chloroquine | Good | Tissues only | None | (a) 0.9 gm. base | (a) 2 |
| (a) 4-Aminoquinoline | | | | (b) 0.3 gm. base | (b) 14–21 |
| (b) Chloroquine base | | | | | |
| 4. Ipecac: | | | | | |
| Emetine hydrochloride | Good | Tissues only | Myocardial disease | 1 mg./kg.* | * |
| 5. Antibiotics: | | | | | |
| Oxytetracycline (Terramycin) | Good | Intestinal contents | None | 1.5–2.0 gm. | 10 |
| Aureomycin | Good | Intestinal contents | None | 2.0 gm. | 10 |
| Fumagillin (Fumidil) | Good | Intestinal contents | None | 30–60 mg. | 10–14 |

* Total dosage not to exceed 10 mg./Kg.

ment of lesions in the lower colon, 2.0 gm. dissolved in 200 ml. of 2 per cent solution of sodium bicarbonate, given as a retention enema every other day to a total of five treatments. Oral carbarsone should be omitted during the period of rectal therapy.

*Milibis,* bismuth glycolylarsanilate, contains approximately 15 per cent arsenic and 42 per cent bismuth. It is absorbed to only a slight degree. It is active against the amebae in the lumen of the intestine, but, because of lack of absorption, has little if any activity against the organisms in the tissues. The contraindications are similar to those of carbarsone. The recommended dosage for adults is 0.5 gm. three times daily for seven days.

*Thiocarbarsone,* 4-carbamidophenyl di-(carboxymethylthio) arsenite, provides 19.1 per cent of available trivalent arsenic. It is supplied in enteric coated capsules which minimize gastric irritation. However, in some cases abdominal discomfort, vomiting and diarrhea may require cessation of therapy, although in most instances these symptoms, when they occur, can be controlled by sedation. It is contraindicated in the presence of impaired hepatic or renal function, amebic hepatitis and for arsenic-sensitive individuals. It is effective against the amebae both in the lumen of the colon and in the tissues. It is said to be particularly useful for the treatment of chronic intestinal infections.

Recommended dosage: for adults, 100 mg. three times a day for ten days; for children, 4–6 mg. per kilogram of body weight in divided doses daily for ten days. The treatment may be repeated after a rest period of ten to fourteen days.

Thiocarbarsone may likewise be given as a retention enema, 0.5–1.0 gm. in 200 ml. of 2 per cent sodium bicarbonate solution for not more than six days. During this period oral administration must be discontinued. The amount of the drug should be reduced proportionately for children.

2. HALOGENATED HYDROXYQUINOLINES. *Diodoquin,* 5,7-diiodo-8-hydroxyquinoline, contains 63.9 per cent iodine. Although this compound is relatively insoluble, administration is accompanied by elevation of the blood iodine and excretion of iodine in the urine. It is contraindicated for iodine-sensitive persons and should be used with caution, if at all, in the presence of hyperthyroidism.

Diodoquin is an efficient amebacide for the treatment of intestinal amebiasis but it is not effective for the treatment of amebic hepatitis or abscess of the liver. Recommended dosage: 0.65 gm. three times daily for three weeks. Because of insolubility, this drug cannot be used for rectal therapy.

*Vioform,* 5-chloro-7-iodo-8-hydroxyquinoline, contains 41 per cent iodine and 12 per cent chlorine. It is the most readily absorbed of the hydroxyquinoline drugs, producing high blood iodine levels which reach a peak about the seventh day of treatment. It is somewhat irritating to the gastro-intestinal tract, tending to cause diarrhea, and should not be used for rectal therapy. The drug is contraindicated for iodine-sensitive patients and in the presence of hyperthyroidism. Recommended dosage: 1.5 gm. to 3.0 gm. by mouth in divided dosage daily for seven to ten days.

*Chiniofon.* Synonyms: Anayodin, Quinoxyl, Yatren. This is 5-iodo-8-hydroxyquinoline and contains 26 to 29 per cent iodine.

Chiniofon is relatively nonabsorbable and consequently elevation of blood iodine levels of clinical importance does not occur. Despite this, it probably should not be used in the presence of hyperthyroidism, and it is contraindicated for iodine-sensitive individuals.

It is effective only against the amebae in the lumen of the colon. Recommended dosage: 0.25 gm. three times daily for eight to ten days. It may likewise be given rectally as a retention enema, 1.0 gm. to 5.0 gm. dissolved in 200 ml. of water.

3. *4-Aminoquinoline, Chloroquine Base.* Synonyms: Aralen, Nivaquine, Alvochlor. Absorption is rapid, relatively complete and excretion is slow. The drug is stored in the tissues and, usually, is well tolerated. However, in certain persons it may cause transient headache, visual disturbances, pruritus, mild gastro-intestinal symptoms and psychic stimulation.

It is active against the amebae in the tissues but is ineffective against the intestinal infections. It has proved to be a satisfactory substitute for emetine in the treatment of amebic hepatitis and abscess of the liver.

The drug is supplied as chloroquine diphosphate in tablet form. Each 0.5 gm. of the salt is equivalent to 0.3 gm. of the base. Recommended dosage: 0.5 gm. (0.3 gm. base) by mouth three times daily for two days followed by 0.25 gm. (0.15 gm. base) twice daily for two to three weeks. The dihydrochloride may be administered intramuscularly or intravenously.

4. *Ipecac; Emetine Hydrochloride.* The active principle, an alkaloid of ipecacuanha, historically has been the single most valuable drug for the treatment of amebiasis despite the fact that, when used alone, it will not eliminate the infection from more than 15 per cent of cases.

Emetine is a general protoplasmic poison which is eliminated from the body slowly and consequently may produce cumulative effects. In overdosage it produces focal necrosis of cardiac muscle and may cause cardiac failure and sudden death. Even in a dosage which is generally considered safe, toxic effects on the myocardium are frequently demonstrable during a standard treatment course. These danger signs include elevation of pulse rate, fall of systolic blood pressure, and electrocardiographic changes including depression or inversion of the "T" waves. When they appear, these changes in the electrocardiogram may persist for prolonged periods of time. Emetine should not be used for patients with myocardial disease or marked hypertension. It should never be administered to ambulatory patients.

Dosage: The *maximum safe dose* is 1 mg. per kilogram of body weight per day. The maximum safe total dose in any single course of therapy is 10 mg. per kilogram of body weight. When repetition of therapy is indicated, at least two weeks should intervene before further administration of this drug.

Emetine is prepared as the hydrochloride for parenteral injection. It should be given intramuscularly. When administered subcutaneously it is extremely irritating and produces painful indurations which may persist for considerable periods of time. It should not be given intravenously.

Other salts, especially emetine bismuth iodide, have been recommended for oral administration. They are not more effective than the hydrochloride and have the additional drawback of powerful emetic action unless accompanied by heavy sedation. These preparations are seldom necessary or desirable.

Since the demonstration of the value of chloroquine base against *E. histolytica* situated within the tissues of the host, emetine is no longer the drug of choice even for the treatment of amebic hepatitis and abscess of the liver.

5. ANTIBIOTICS. Many of the antibiotic agents have been investigated to determine their potential value in the treatment of amebiasis. The majority of these preparations showing activity against the amebae act indirectly through their bacteriostatic activity rather than directly against the parasite, and consequently have not proven to be efficient amebacides. Two, however, oxytetracycline and fumagillin, appear to act directly against the amebae and give promise of being important additions to the list of effective drugs.

*Oxytetracycline (Terramycin)* has proved to be the most effective of the antibiotics. When used alone for the treatment of enteric infections, oral administration is followed by prompt cessation of diarrhea and dysentery, and general clinical improvement. However, relapses occur in a proportion of cases and the development of amebic hepatitis has been observed during Terramycin treatment. The best results have been obtained when it is used in combination with standard amebacidal drugs.

Recommended dosage: 2.0 gm. initial dose by mouth followed by 0.5 gm. three or four times daily for ten days.

*Aureomycin* acts primarily though its bacteriostatic activity against the associated bacteria in the colon. It does not exert a direct amebacidal effect. When used alone for the treatment of intestinal amebiasis, cure of the infection can be anticipated in only approximately 60 per cent of cases. It has proved to be more effective when used in combination with other standard amebacidal drugs.

Unlike Terramycin, aureomycin therapy is frequently associated with evidence of gastro-intestinal irritation. Recommended dosage: 2.0 gm. initial dose by mouth followed by 0.5 gm. four times daily for ten days.

*Fumagillin (Fumidil)* has not been fully evaluated but gives promise of being an important addition to the therapeutic agents for intestinal amebiasis. It is a crystalline substance, derived from *Asper-*

*gillus* sp., which is an active amebacide in extremely high dilutions in vitro. Unlike most of the antibiotics it acts directly against *E. histolytica*. It has proved very effective against experimental infections in young rats and rabbits, and in limited clinical trials in man. Recommended dosage: 20 mg. three times daily for ten consecutive days. When used alone at this dosage level it has eliminated the infection in over 90 per cent of cases. No serious toxic or side effects have been reported, although lower abdominal discomfort and cramps, nausea without vomiting, and vertigo occur not infrequently during the treatment period.

Although fumagillin is at least relatively inactive against the normal intestinal bacterial flora, in general the antibiotic agents should be used with caution. With too prolonged administration the bacteriostatic action may be followed by overgrowth of yeasts and fungi and the development of clinical candidiasis (moniliasis).

TREATMENT OF THE CYST-PASSER. The therapeutic problem presented by the chronic cyst-passer differs only in degree from that of the patient with acute or chronic dysentery. The essential differences between clinical types are the extent of infection and the number of infecting organisms. In all cases it must be remembered that many of the amebae are present within the tissues of the host and consequently are not accessible to the action of drugs not absorbed or incompletely absorbed from the intestinal contents. The prevalence of encysted forms as opposed to trophozoites in the stools is not of itself an indication for a different type of therapy.

The symptomless or relatively asymptomatic cyst-passer may be satisfactorily treated as an ambulatory patient using Terramycin, aureomycin, Fumidil, thiocarbarsone, carbarsone, Milibis, or one of the hydroxyquinoline series. The best results may be anticipated from concurrent therapy using Terramycin and carbarsone, thiocarbarsone, or one of the hydroxyquinolines. The daily dosages are shown in Table 24.

TREATMENT OF ACUTE AMEBIC DYSENTERY. The patient suffering from acute amebic dysentery or acute amebic diarrhea should be confined strictly to bed. The diet should be high in protein and low in carbohydrate and be supplemented by ample sources of vitamins, especially of the vitamin B complex. Although dehydration and toxemia are much less frequent and less severe than in acute bacillary dysentery, adequate fluid balance must be maintained.

Combined anti-amebic therapy is essential. In planning the details of the therapeutic program it is necessary to select a combination of drugs which will exert maximal amebacidal activity simultaneously against the amebae in the colon and against those deep within the tissues. The first indication is met by the arsenicals, the halogenated hydroxyquinolines and the antibiotics. Maximal effect within the tissues of the host can be obtained only by emetine or chloroquine base.

The Joint Dysentery Unit sponsored by the Commission on Enteric Infections of the Armed Forces Epidemiological Board in 1953 evaluated the treatment of acute amebic dysentery among prisoners of war in Korea with particular emphasis on the antibiotics. The most favorable immediate clinical results and the lowest relapse rates were obtained with one or other of three regimes:

1. *Terramycin*, initial dose 2 gm., thereafter 0.5 gm. three times daily for ten days administered concurrently with one of the standard amebacidal drugs.

2. *Terramycin*, initial dose 2 gm., followed by 0.5 gm. every six hours for five days and chloroquine 0.3 gm. twice daily for two days followed by 0.3 gm. daily for three days.

3. *Aureomycin*, initial dose 2 gm., thereafter 0.5 gm. every six hours for ten days and chloroquine 0.3 gm. twice daily for two days followed by 0.3 gm. daily for three days.

An additional regimen which was not included but which meets the theoretical requirements and has given excellent clinical results should be considered:

4. *Emetine hydrochloride* or *chloroquine* given in combination with Diodoquin for a period of seven days.

The daily doses of the various drugs are listed in Table 24, page 259.

In severe cases which are associated with extensive secondary bacterial infection of the colon wall eradication of *E. histolytica* may not be followed by cessation of symptoms. The stools may continue to be loose and to contain pus, mucus and blood. In such instances anti-amebic therapy should be followed by intensive sulfonamide treatment, preferably with sulfadiazine, until symptoms are controlled and microscopic pus and blood are no longer present in the feces.

TREATMENT OF CHRONIC AMEBIC DYSENTERY. The indications for treatment of chronic amebic dysentery differ from those of simple acute dysentery since the problem is complicated by extensive and mixed secondary bacterial infection and frequently by fibrosis and permanent anatomic damage to the colon. It is not unusual, therefore, to find that anti-amebic therapy alone is ineffective. Specific therapy should be followed by intensive sulfonamide treatment. The prognosis will depend upon the extent of the bacterial infection and the degree of permanent damage to the colon. Advanced cases differ little if at all clinically or pathologically from chronic bacillary dysentery or chronic ulcerative colitis.

**Complications** Amebic hepatitis and abscess of the liver are grave complications of intestinal amebiasis. They may occur relatively early in the course of the disease or only after a prolonged period of chronic and often clinically latent infection. During World War II numbers of cases of amebic abscess of the liver occurred among British troops within a few months after their arrival in India or Burma. In New Guinea hepatomegaly and liver tenderness were observed in 25 per cent of military personnel treated for dysentery of varying severity. More recently, hepatomegaly was reported in 18 per cent of cases of acute amebic dysentery of short duration among prisoners of war in Korea, and in 68 per cent of a clinically mixed group of persons with intestinal amebiasis in South America. Hepatic involvement results from metastasis of the infection in the wall of the colon to the liver by the portal blood stream. A history of dysentery or of symptoms suggestive of antecedent amebic disease can be obtained in 60 to 90 per cent of cases of hepatic infection. These complications are proportionately rare in native races.

Amebic Hepatitis. Amebic hepatitis may develop during an acute stage of the intestinal infection or during a remission. Less commonly it occurs in the absence of definite history of amebic disease. The clinical picture may be extremely variable. In the mild and subacute forms slight enlargement of the liver with moderate tenderness on palpation may be the only significant signs. On the other hand, acute amebic hepatitis is characterized by severe pain in the hepatic region, toxemia, marked pyrexia and an enlarged and markedly tender liver. The fever usually is irregularly remittent, reaching 103° to 104° F., and in severe cases may closely simulate the Charcot type of curve observed in suppurative cholangitis. The marked variations in temperature, often accompanied by chills and profuse sweats, may suggest malaria.

There is diffuse but variable enlargement of the liver. Palpation and even light percussion over the lower ribs produce extreme pain. The white blood count is commonly elevated to 25,000 or 30,000 with a polymorphonuclear leukocytosis of 70 to 80 per cent.

diagnosis. The diagnosis must be based primarily on clinical evidence. A history suggestive of antecedent intestinal amebiasis or demonstration of *E. histolytica* in the patient's stools together with remittent fever, high leukocytosis, and right upper quadrant pain associated with enlargement and tenderness of the liver should immediately arouse suspicion. Definitive diagnosis, however, depends upon the response to the therapeutic test with full dosage of chloroquine, or emetine hydrochloride. Diagnostic aspiration of the liver should never be attempted since it may be followed by severe or fatal hemorrhage. Amebic hepatitis may be confused with malaria, suppurative cholangitis or suppurative cholecystitis.

treatment. *Chloroquine* and *emetine hydrochloride* have a specific amebacidal action against amebae within the tissues of the host. The temperature, pain, tenderness, enlargement of the liver and leukocytosis all show marked diminution within forty-eight to seventy-two hours after the initiation of specific therapy. The recommended dosages are:

1. *Chloroquine diphosphate* 0.5 gm. (0.3 gm. base) by mouth three times daily for two days followed by 0.5 gm. daily for twelve to fourteen days.

2. *Emetine hydrochloride* 0.1 mg. per kilogram of body weight per day by intramuscular injection daily for five to seven days.

Whichever drug is selected should be supplemented by concurrent administration of *Terramycin* or one of the halogenated *hydroxy-quinolines*.

AMEBIC ABSCESS OF THE LIVER. Amebic abscess of the liver is commonly a late complication of amebiasis; occasionally, however, it may develop within a relatively few months after the initial infection. When it occurs as a complication of active dysentery the abscess is commonly acute and often multiple. Abscesses which develop as late complications of longstanding intestinal infection are frequently large, single and chronic.

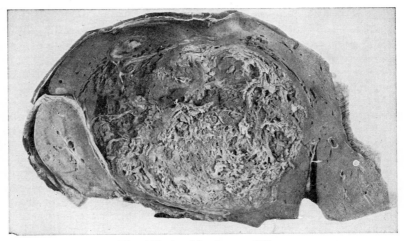

Fig. 122. Amebic abscess of liver.

The great majority of amebic abscesses of the liver occur in the right lobe; approximately 16 per cent are in the left lobe. In about 70 per cent of cases the cavity is large and single while in approximately 30 per cent two to four abscesses are present (Fig. 122).

The clinical picture of acute amebic abscess is exceedingly difficult to distinguish from that of acute amebic hepatitis, particularly if the abscesses are multiple and involve both the right and left lobes. Under such conditions the clinical phenomena will closely, if not exactly, resemble those of hepatitis without abscess and again the response to specific therapy provides the most satisfactory means of differential diagnosis. Whereas the response to chloroquine and emetine is rapid and complete in cases of hepatitis, commonly it is only partially effective in cases of abscess. The fever may not be wholly controlled; pain, tenderness and enlargement of the liver may persist, and disproportionate residual leukocytosis may continue.

Chronic abscess is more commonly observed in the right lobe than in the left. The symptoms are very variable depending upon the size of the lesion, its situation with relation to other structures and the activity of the infection. In many instances there is a history of gradual and progressive weight loss extending over a considerable period of time, with or without periods of low grade fever. Variable and irregular pain referred to the right upper quadrant is often present and a variety of digestive complaints which may arouse suspicion of chronic cholecystitis or even appendicitis are usual. Right lobe abscesses commonly extend upward to involve the diaphragm. In such cases irritation of the basal pleura frequently causes unproductive cough and pain on respiration. Pain referred to the right shoulder is a not infrequent complaint and may be the presenting symptom.

With further involvement of the pleura there may be signs of consolidation in the right lower lobe, with or without pleural effusion, leading to an erroneous diagnosis of pneumonia, empyema or tuberculosis. If the process remains unrecognized, spontaneous rupture into the right lower lobe with evacuation of the abscess contents through the bronchial tree may occur.

DIAGNOSIS. Careful physical examination of the patient suffering from large single abscess of the liver should immediately arouse suspicion of the true nature of the pathology. Enlargement of the liver is asymmetric. The edge of the right lobe is usually easily palpable and palpation elicits deep pain. If the process is in the left lobe, that portion of the liver is similarly affected. When the abscess is on the right the diaphragm is commonly elevated; this may be demonstrable on physical examination as well as by roentgen examination. Heavy percussion of the chest wall in the region of an abscess elicits deep pain. As peripheral extension occurs toward the capsule of the liver a small area of intercostal tenderness may be noted. When present it is the site of election for diagnostic aspiration.

The white blood count is variable. In cases with small abscesses there is almost always an increased percentage of polymorphonuclear leukocytes but the total white count may be little elevated. In the presence of a very large chronic abscess there may be no leukocytosis, absolute or relative. Generally speaking, the larger the abscess the lower the count and the smaller and more numerous the abscesses the higher the count.

In those instances when it is impossible accurately to differentiate between acute abscess and hepatitis, the therapeutic test with chloroquine or emetine should invariably be performed before attempting aspiration. In the presence of actual abscess formation specific drug therapy frequently fails adequately to control the fever, leukocytosis, pain and hepatic enlargement.

Diagnostic aspiration of the left lobe should never be attempted. For aspiration of the right lobe a large calibre needle attached to a syringe should be used and equipped with a stop so that the point cannot be introduced for a distance greater than $2\frac{1}{2}$ inches from the skin. In the absence of finger-point intercostal tenderness the site of election is in the anterior axillary line in the ninth interspace. After novocain anesthesia of the skin and deep infiltration the aspiration needle should be introduced medially and cephalad.

The contents of an amebic abscess of the liver are usually semifluid and chocolate brown in color although in old chronic abscesses they may be yellowish or even white. Amebae are not present in the necrotic contents of the cavity and therefore cannot be demonstrated in liver abscess. They are present, however, in enormous numbers in the advancing border of the abscess wall. Culture of the contents of such an abscess is usually bacteriologically sterile but may on occasion reveal slight growth of avirulent bacteria (Fig. 123).

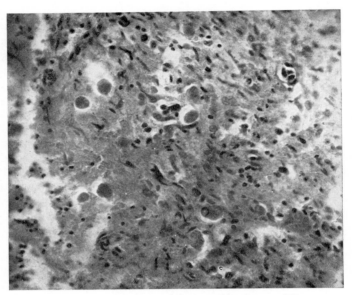

Fig. 123. Trophozoites in wall of amebic abscess of liver.

*Differential diagnosis* is frequently difficult. An acute abscess may be confused with acute hepatitis, acute cholecystitis, subphrenic abscess and malaria. In the presence of chronic liver abscess the clinical picture may simulate carcinoma of the liver, cirrhosis of the liver, pleurisy with effusion, atypical pulmonary tuberculosis, arthritis of the cervical spine or shoulder, and chronic cholecystitis or appendicitis.

TREATMENT. The high mortality previously associated with abscess of the liver was in large part due to the universal use of open drainage and the great difficulty in preventing secondary infection. With the advent of emetine and the use of repeated aspiration of the cavity, the mortality has been reduced to 2 per cent.

In cases of right lobe abscess a full course of *chloroquine* or of *emetine hydrochloride* should be given. The contents of the abscess cavity should be emptied as completely as possible by closed aspiration. This is followed by prompt drop of fever and leukocytosis and by marked diminution in liver pain and tenderness. In patients with large abscesses, fever, pain and leukocytosis may recur or increase a few days after the primary aspiration. This constitutes an imperative indication for further drainage of the cavity. It does not indicate failure of specific therapy. Such repeated closed drainage should be continued as indications require. Such conservative treatment is attended by a lower mortality rate and a very much shorter period of disability than is open surgical drainage.

Laparotomy is required, however, for drainage of a left lobe abscess because of the proximity of the pericardium. It should not be used for treatment of right lobe abscesses unless failure to respond to chloroquine or emetine and to aspiration indicates the presence of another cavity which cannot be drained by the aspirating needle.

## Dientamoeba Diarrhea

**Synonyms** None.

**Distribution** Worldwide.

**Clinical Characteristics** *Dientamoeba fragilis* has been considered to be a cause of chronic though mild intestinal symptoms. There is controversy, however, concerning its actual pathogenicity and it has not been shown to be a true parasite with ability to invade the tissues of the host. Infection is not associated with pathologic changes in the colon.

The syndrome commonly ascribed to this organism consists of recurring episodes of flatulence associated with the evacuation of two or three loose "mushy" stools each day. There is no mucus, blood, or inflammatory exudate in the feces. Symptoms are absent in the intervals between attacks.

**Diagnosis** Microscopic examination of a fresh loose stool will reveal the motile trophozoites with characteristic pseudopodia (p. 240). Red cells are not ingested and no encysted stage is known. *Dientamoeba fragilis* may likewise be isolated in culture (p. 833).

**Treatment** Little exact information on therapy is available. Carbarsone is recommended by some and it is possible that certain of the newer amebacides will prove effective.

## Giardiasis

**Synonyms** None.

**Distribution** Worldwide.

**Etiology** There is controversy concerning the pathogenicity of *Giardia lamblia*. Although it has been recovered from both the duodenum and the gallbladder and has been associated with symptoms referable to the biliary system and the intestinal tract, it has not been clearly demonstrated to be a true parasite invading the tissues of the host. There is no characteristic pathology.

*Clinical Characteristics* The biliary symptoms associated with this infection are those of a mild but chronic catarrhal cholecystitis. Heavy infections of the intestinal tract are not infrequently accompanied by chronic recurring diarrhea and variable degrees of flatulence and distention. There is no blood or inflammatory exudate in the stools. Constipation is usual in the intervals between attacks.

*Diagnosis* Large numbers of actively motile trophozoites are commonly present in the liquid feces. In the absence of diarrhea only encysted forms are found. The detailed morphology is described on page 240. This flagellate has not been isolated in culture.

*Treatment* Atabrine is a highly effective drug against *G. lamblia*. It should be given by mouth three times daily after meals for five to seven days. The recommended individual dose is 0.1 gm. Two or more courses may be required to eliminate the infection.

## Trichomonas Vaginalis Infection

*Synonyms* None.

*Distribution* Worldwide.

*Etiology* *Trichomonas vaginalis* is a flagellate often associated with a specific vaginitis or urethritis. Infection becomes established when the acidity of the vaginal secretions is reduced. *T. vaginalis* will not survive at the normal vaginal acidity of $pH$ 3.8 to 4.4 which is maintained by the conversion of glycogen in the epithelium to lactic acid by the normal bacterial flora and, indirectly, by activity of the sex hormones.

Although invasion of the flagellates into inflamed, eroded areas occasionally occurs, it is probable that this is a secondary phenomenon.

The means of transmission have not been established.

*Clinical Characteristics* Trichomonas vaginitis is accompanied by vulval pruritus, often intense, and a more or less profuse and irritating vaginal discharge which, in untreated cases, may lead to actual excoriation of the vulva and dermatitis of the adjacent skin of the thighs. The vaginal mucosa is usually diffusely congested and inflamed. A chronic urethritis may be seen in the male.

*Diagnosis* Diagnosis depends upon demonstration of the flagellates in the vaginal or urethral secretions. The detailed morphology of *T. vaginalis* is described on page 243. It may be isolated in culture (p. 837).

*Treatment* Successful treatment of trichomonas vaginitis is difficult and time consuming, and requires persistence and complete cooperation by the patient. The basic principles are cleanliness, restoration of normal vaginal epithelium and secretions, and destruction of the trichomonads by chemotherapeutic agents. Patients who have passed the menopause may require estrogen therapy and lesions of the cervix must be corrected.

Various chemotherapeutic agents, including arsenicals, sulfonamides, and oxyquinoline derivatives, used locally in the form of powders, vaginal tablets and jellies have been recommended. They are used in conjunction with measures for maintaining vaginal acidity.

A compound containing diiodohydroxyquinoline, dextrose, lactose and boric acid (Floraquin) has given good results. It is recommended that two vaginal tablets be inserted into the fornices daily, or that 4 to 8 gm. of the powder be insufflated into the vagina three or more times a week. Treatment should be continued until three monthly vaginal smears are negative.

## Balantidiasis

**Synonyms**   Balantidial dysentery.
**Distribution**   Worldwide.

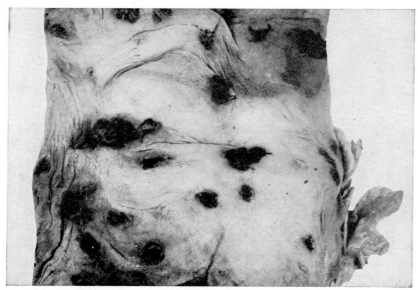

Fig. 124. Balantidial dysentery. Ulcerations of colon with intervening normal mucosa.

**Etiology**   *Balantidium coli* is a pathogenic ciliate which occasionally infects the colon and distal ileum of man, producing diarrhea and dysentery (Fig. 124).

**Pathology**   *Balantidium coli* penetrates the mucosa mechanically, producing necrosis and ulceration. There is no leukocytic infiltration until secondary bacterial infection occurs. Occasionally masses of balantidia are found in the submucosa in a collagenous stroma without an accompanying inflammatory reaction (Fig. 125).

As the ciliates invade the mucosa, secondary infection rapidly occurs. Superficial erosions are produced which extend laterally and

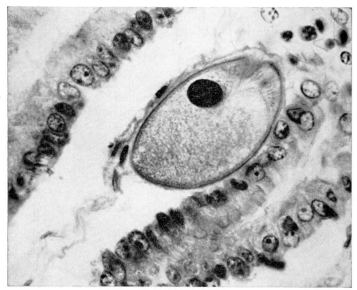

Fig. 125. *B. coli* entering mucosa between basement membrane and epithelium.

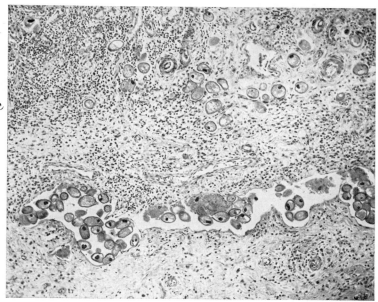

Fig. 126. Chronic balantidial dysentery. *B. coli* in submucosa, inflammation and fibrosis.

penetrate into the deeper layers of the intestinal wall. These are often hemorrhagic and in their gross appearance resemble the "Dyak hair" ulcers of amebic dysentery. The lesions are discrete and the intervening mucosa is normal. An inflammatory exudate is present in the stool (Fig. 126).

**Clinical Characteristics**  Balantidiasis may be asymptomatic or may be associated with diarrhea or acute dysentery.

**Diagnosis**  Diagnosis depends upon demonstration of *B. coli* in the feces. The motile trophozoites will be found when the stools are liquid or semiliquid, and the cysts in semiformed or formed stools. The detailed morphology of the ciliate is described on page 243. It may be isolated in culture (p. 837).

**Treatment**  Several of the anti-amebic drugs have been used with varying success for the treatment of balantidiasis. The most favorable results have been obtained with diiodohydroxyquinoline (Diodoquin) and carbarsone.

The recommended dosage of Diodoquin is as follows: adults and children over nine years of age, 0.63 gm. three times daily for three weeks; for children from one to four years the individual doses are 0.21 gm. and for children from five to nine years 0.42 gm., likewise three times daily for three weeks.

If carbarsone is used, two courses each of ten days duration are recommended, with daily doses of 0.5 gm. for adults and 0.25 gm. for children under nine years of age.

Recently both aureomycin and oxytetracycline (Terramycin) have been reported to eliminate the parasites within four days. The dosage of aureomycin was 2.0 gm. daily, and that of Terramycin 2.0 gm. the first day and 1.5 gm. daily thereafter.

## Isosporiasis

**Synonyms**  None.

**Distribution**  Widely distributed, especially in the Southwest Pacific and Philippines. Infection has been reported from man also in southern Europe, the Middle East, Africa, Indo-China, Manchuria, South and Central America and parts of the West Indies.

**Etiology**  *Isospora hominis* is a relatively nonpathogenic, coccidial parasite of the alimentary canal (ileum) of man.

**Clinical Characteristics and Pathology**  *Isospora hominis* has been alleged to cause lassitude, nausea, abdominal pain and mild diarrhea. Although no lesions have been demonstrated at autopsy it is believed that transient microscopic lesions must be produced in the epithelial cells. Infections are self limited. In experimental infections in man symptoms developed in a week, oocysts were recovered 9 to 15 days after ingestion and persisted for less than a month.

**Diagnosis**  Diagnosis depends upon demonstrating the unstained oocysts in the stool (see p. 244).

**Treatment**  None, as the infection is self limited.

## Prophylaxis Against Intestinal Protozoal Infections

Infection by the intestinal protozoa does not produce a protective immunity and artificial immunization has not been accomplished. Prophylaxis, therefore, depends upon avoidance of infection. These organisms reach man through water or food polluted by human feces, and foods contaminated by the droppings and vomitus of flies or by the soiled hands of infected foodhandlers. Ice may be a vehicle of infection and should not be used in beverages or placed in contact with food. In heavily endemic areas all water for human consumption should be chemically treated or preferably boiled before use. Raw vegetables must be scrupulously avoided and fruits should be scalded before consumption. Whenever practicable foodhandlers should be examined and treated if infected. Latrines must be fly-proofed and kitchens and dining-rooms adequately screened.

## 32 Malaria

**Synonyms** The synonyms of malaria in general are ague, jungle fever, paludism. Synonyms of malaria due to *Plasmodium vivax:* Benign tertian, *vivax* malaria. Synonyms of malaria due to *Plasmodium falciparum:* Malignant tertian, subtertian, estivo-autumnal, E-A, *falciparum* malaria. Malaria due to *Plasmodium malariae* is designated quartan malaria. Malaria due to *Plasmodium ovale* is designated *ovale* malaria.

**Definition** Malaria is an acute and chronic infection characterized by fever, anemia, splenomegaly and often serious or fatal complications. It is caused by protozoa of the genus *Plasmodium.* Four species are pathogenic for man—*P. vivax, P. falciparum, P. malariae* and *P. ovale.*

**Distribution** Malarial infections are prevalent between 45° north and 40° south latitude. In certain areas these limits are wider (Fig. 127). Malaria due to *P. vivax* is more widely distributed than the other types. It is the prevalent infection in most areas within the temperate zones, but is widespread throughout the tropics as well. *Plasmodium malariae* is comparatively rare; it is observed most commonly in temperate areas and in the subtropics. *Plasmodium falciparum* tends to predominate throughout all tropical regions. *Plasmodium ovale* is relatively uncommon, the majority of cases of this infection being reported from East Africa and recently, in isolated instances, from South America.

**Etiology** The parasites causing malaria are protozoa belonging to the genus *Plasmodium.* The *life cycle* of the parasites consists of an exogenous sexual phase, termed sporogony, with multiplication in

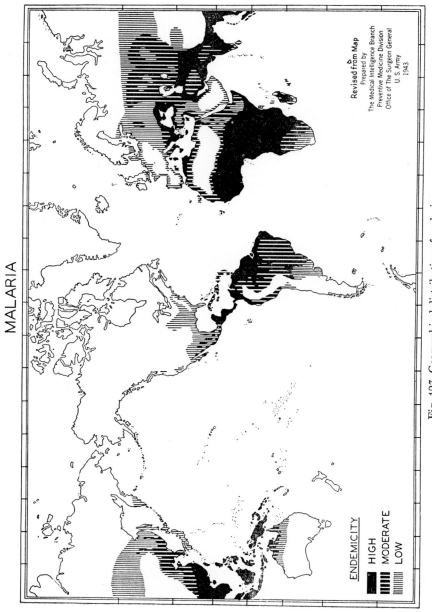

MALARIA

ENDEMICITY

◼ HIGH

▦ MODERATE

▤ LOW

Revised from Map
Prepared by
The Medical Intelligence Branch
Preventive Medicine Division
Office of The Surgeon General
U. S. Army
1943

Fig. 127. Geographical distribution of malaria.

certain anopheline mosquitoes, and an endogenous asexual phase, termed schizogony, with multiplication in man.

The *exogenous, or anopheline phase* of the cycle, begins when a suitable anopheline mosquito ingests blood containing the mature sexual forms, the gametocytes. Within a few minutes after reaching the insect's stomach the male cell or microgametocyte extends actively motile flagellum-like structures each of which contains a portion of the nuclear chromatin of the parent cell. These flagella shortly become detached to form microgametes which migrate to the

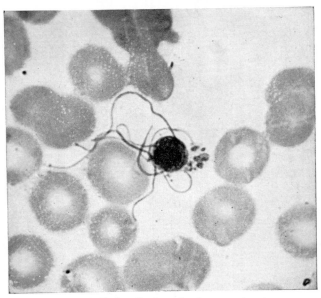

Fig. 128. Exflagellation of microgametocyte.

female cell or macrogametocyte. Meanwhile the latter has undergone reduction division of its nuclear chromatin by extruding a polar body in preparation for fertilization. Completion of these changes marks the end of gametogony, while subsequent fertilization of the macrogamete by a microgamete initiates the processes of sporogony (Fig. 128).

When a microgamete enters the female cell, fusion of the nuclear chromatin from each parent occurs, and shortly thereafter the fertilized cell elongates and becomes motile, forming the ookinete or traveling vermicule. This actively penetrates the wall of the mosquito's stomach, finally lodging beneath the outer layer.

It then undergoes progressive vacuolization to form a growing oocyst (Fig. 129). The nuclear chromatin subdivides repeatedly, its particles becoming arranged along cytoplasmic strands bordering the vacuoles. From each particle of chromatin in the protoplasmic mesh a filamentous structure extends into the lumen of a vacuole. The chromatin particles become incorporated in these filaments to form sporozoites. At maturity the oocyst consists of a spongelike spherical body that projects into the body cavity of the insect. In a suitable in-

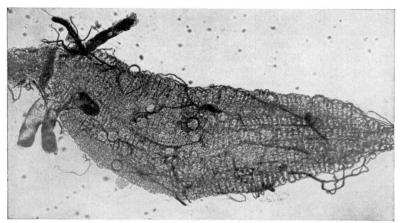

Fig. 129. Fresh unstained preparation showing oocysts on wall of mosquito's stomach.

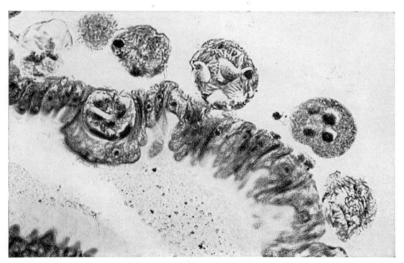

Fig. 130. Various stages in development of oocysts—showing sporozoite formation and pigment masses. (Courtesy Mr. P. G. Shute, F.R.E.S., Ministry of Health, Epsom, England.)

fected vector several hundred oocysts may be found on the stomach wall, although as a rule they are scarce (Fig. 130).

Spontaneous rupture of the oocyst finally occurs (Fig. 131). Liberated motile sporozoites, which may number several hundred to several thousand, migrate throughout the body cavity of the mosquito, certain ones reaching and entering the salivary glands. Here they lose their motility and remain dormant until injected into man.

The duration of the exogenous phase of the cycle, termed the extrinsic incubation period, varies with the species of *Plasmodium*, with the vectors, and with conditions of temperature and humidity. Under optimal conditions *P. vivax* and *P. falciparum* complete their development within the mosquito in seven to ten days. *Plasmodium malariae* develops more slowly (Fig. 132).

The *endogenous or human phase* of the cycle begins with the injection of sporozoites by an infected anopheline mosquito. The sporozoites of *P. vivax*, *P. falciparum* and probably *P. malariae* and *P. ovale* disappear from the peripheral blood after about a half hour and undergo an exo-erythrocytic stage. They penetrate into the parenchymal cells of the liver where they undergo a period of multi-

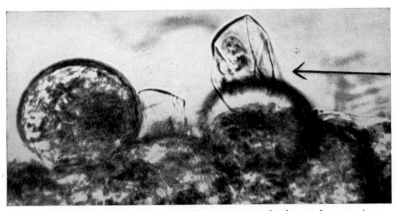

Fig. 131. Empty capsule of oocyst after rupture and release of sporozoites.

plication and development (schizogony), with the production of merozoites which enter the blood stream, invade erythrocytes, and initiate the parasitemia. This primary development constitutes the pre-erythrocytic stage of the endogenous cycle.

MORPHOLOGY. All forms which occur in the blood, stain well with Romanowsky stains; the cytoplasm is blue and the chromatin or nuclear substance is bright red. Pigment produced by the parasite in its growth appears as brownish or blackish granules. The earliest form seen in erythrocytes consists of a small ring of blue-stained cytoplasm with one or two dots of chromatin, giving rise to the descriptive term, "signet ring." In the course of a few hours the ring develops into an actively motile ameboid form, the trophozoite. This term is applied to all the more mature intermediate stages in which the chromatin still appears as a single mass. Later in development the chromatin undergoes repeated division. Stages which exhibit cleavage of the chromatin without segmentation of the cytoplasm are referred to as presegmenting schizonts. When division of both the chromatin and cytoplasm has been completed the form is termed a mature schizont, each member of the resulting new generation of parasites being called a merozoite.

After several generations of schizogony gametocyte formation occurs. The ring stage of this form tends to be thicker, intermediate stages are less motile and pigment formation is greater.

In *vivax*, *ovale* and *malariae* infections all forms from the early ring to the mature schizont and gametocyte are found in the peripheral blood. In *falciparum* infections, on the other hand, only rings and gametocytes are usually demonstrable. The intermediate development of this species occurs in the capillaries of the viscera and

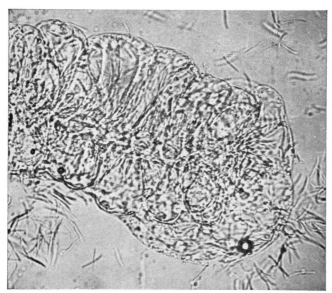

Fig. 132. Sporozoites in salivary gland of mosquito and in surrounding fluid.

the intermediate stages are seen in the peripheral blood only as an agonal phenomenon.

*Plasmodium vivax.* The young plasmodia appear in stained blood films as delicate rings of blue cytoplasm each with a red bead of chromatin, the so-called "signet ring." They are approximately one-third the diameter of a normal red blood cell. The chromatin dots are usually but not invariably single, and usually not more than one parasite is observed within a single red cell. The ring undergoes rapid growth and development, the cytoplasm becomes heavier and thicker and the chromatin mass enlarges. Within five or six hours yellowish brown pigment granules appear within the substance of the parasite which now develops into an actively motile trophozoite with bizarre outlines in the stained film. The infected red cell gradually becomes swollen; it stains less deeply and presents a diffuse bright red stippling, the Schüffner's dots. At about forty hours the parasite fills or nearly fills a considerably enlarged and decolorized red cell. At this stage motility ceases and the chromatin undergoes successive divisions into twelve to twenty-four fragments with an average of sixteen. The cytoplasm then undergoes similar subdivision, each portion including one of the chromatin masses. This mature schizont contains the new generation of asexual parasites, called merozoites, and also the pigment formed during the period of growth clumped into one or two loose masses (Figs. 133 and 134).

The mature microgametocyte or male gametocyte is often about the size of a normal red cell and lies within an enlarged decolorized erythrocyte; its cytoplasm stains a light grayish or pinkish blue and the chromatin appears as granules loosely aggregated in the center or distributed as a transverse band. The pigment is darker than in the schizont and is uniformly distributed. The macrogametocyte may be almost twice the size of a normal erythrocyte; its cytoplasm takes a deep blue stain, and the chromatin is compact, usually situated near the periphery.

*Plasmodium falciparum.* The young rings are smaller and more delicate than those of *P. vivax;* they are often hairlike and may show single or double chromatin dots. Multiple infection of erythrocytes is common. The frequently seen accolé or appliqué form appears as a fine blue line with a delicate chromatin dot, apparently applied to the margin of a red cell. *Plasmodium falciparum* remains in the ring stage longer than most species of *Plasmodium.* The rings increase only slightly in size and remain smaller and more delicate. After a few hours ring forms disappear from the peripheral circulation to undergo further development in the capillaries of the viscera. There intermediate and mature forms appear as small masses of light-stained cytoplasm containing a chromatin granule which is only slightly larger than that of the ring and a small mass of almost black pigment. The mature stages of the parasite are only about two-thirds the size of a normal red blood cell.

Parasitized cells of the peripheral blood may show cleftlike or comma-like red markings, Maurer's dots. These are larger and less numerous than the Schüffner's dots. The infected red blood cells

Fig. 133. *Plasmodium vivax.* (Courtesy National Institute of Health, U.S.P.H.S.). 1. Normal sized red cell with marginal ring form trophozoite. 2. Young signet ring form trophozoite in a macrocyte. 3. Slightly older ring form trophozoite in red cell showing basophilic stippling. 4. Polychromatophilic red cell containing young tertian parasite with pseudopodia. 5. Ring form trophozoite showing pigment in cytoplasm, in an enlarged cell containing Schüffner's stippling. (Schüffner's stippling does not appear in all cells containing the growing and older forms of *P. vivax* as would be indicated by these pictures, but it can be found with any stage from the fairly young ring form onward.) 6, 7. Very tenuous medium trophozoite forms. 8. Three ameboid trophozoites with fused cytoplasm. 9, 11, 12, 13. Older ameboid trophozoites in process of development. 10. Two ameboid trophozoites in one cell. 14. Mature trophozoite. 15. Mature trophozoite with chromatin apparently in process of division. 16, 17, 18, 19. Schizonts showing progressive steps in division ("presegmenting schizonts"). 20. Mature schizont. 21, 22. Developing gametocytes. 23. Mature microgametocyte. 24. Mature macrogametocyte.

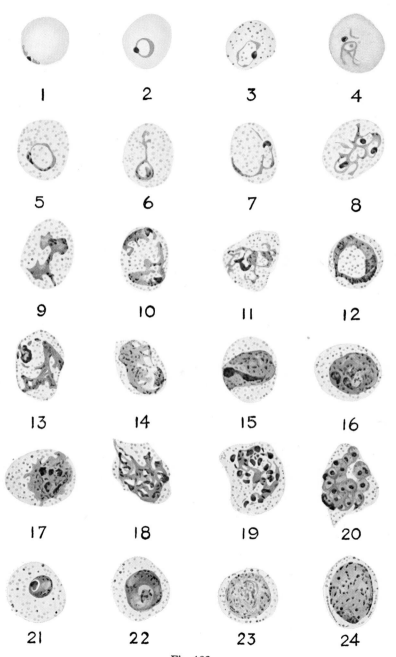

1  2  3  4

5  6  7  8

9  10  11  12

13  14  15  16

17  18  19  20

21  22  23  24

Fig. 133.

Fig. 134.

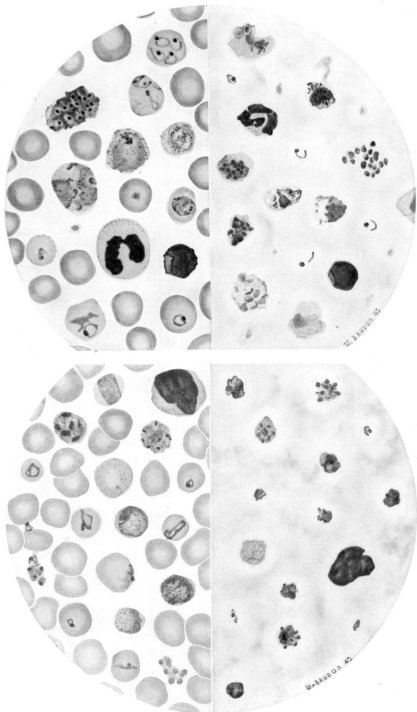

Fig. 135.

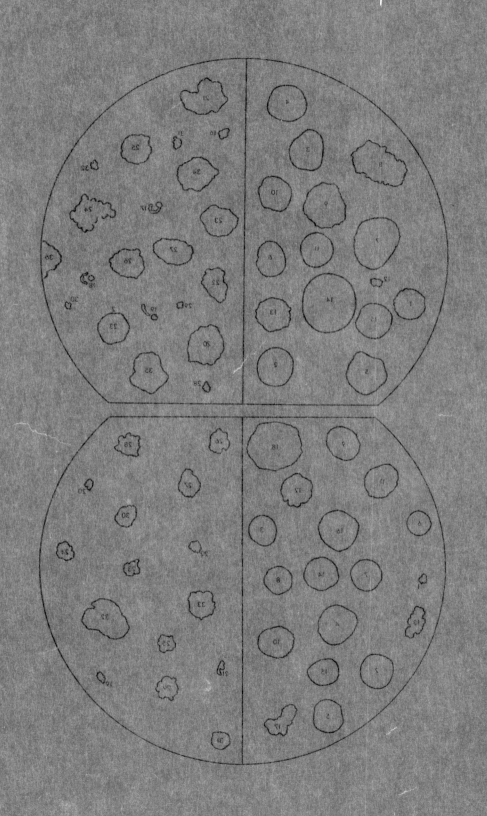

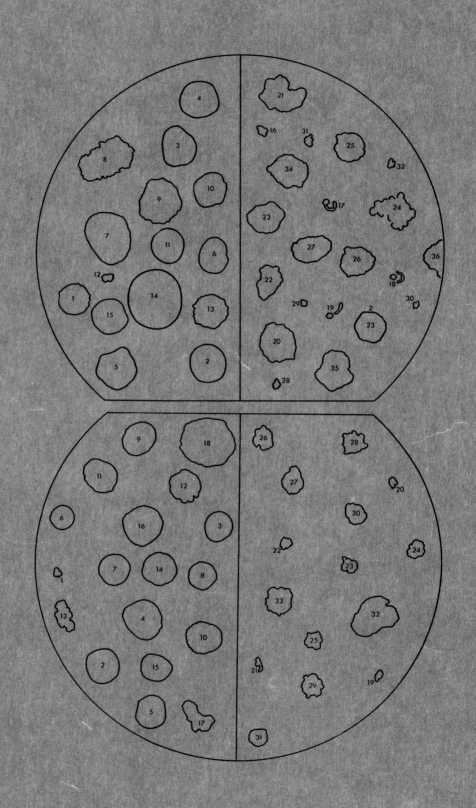

Fig. 134. *Plasmodium vivax. Left:* Thin smear (Giemsa-stained) 650 ×. *1*, Very young trophozoite, with a few Schüffner's dots already in evidence (these may appear very early). *2*, Ring stage, with host cell somewhat enlarged, but not yet stippled. *3*, *4*, Erythrocytes with 3 and 4 ring stages (respectively). In part *3*, two of these forms are marginal, simulating somewhat *P. falciparum*. *5*, Trophozoite, exhibiting characteristic ameboid form. *6*, Trophozoite (probably a young gametocyte). *7*, Schizont with two nuclei. *8*, Segmenter, with sixteen massed merozoites. *9*, Macrogametocyte. *10*, Microgametocyte (somewhat smaller than usual). *11*, Erythrocyte, with superimposed platelet. (These are not infrequently mistaken for parasitized cells by the inexperienced. Compare with part *1*.) *12*, Platelet. *13*, Lymphocyte. *14*, Polymorphonuclear neutrophil leukocyte. *15*, Normal red cell (compare these cells with those containing parasites. The increased size of the latter is very noticeable.) *Right:* Thick smear (Giemsa-stained) 2000 ×. *16*, Young trophozoite. *17*, *18*, *19*, Ring stages (note the detached chromatin). *20*, Trophozoite (note the characteristic ameboid form). *21*, Trophozoite (note the reddish halo or shadow about the parasite—when seen this is diagnostic of *P. vivax*. It may represent the remains of the reticulum of the host cell, or of the Schüffner's dots, or both). *22*, Presegmenter. *23*, Nearly mature segmenter, with the "shadow" or "halo" noted in *21*. *24*, Group of merozoites, with mass of pigment. *25*, *26*, Large trophozoites, or macrogametocytes (these may be difficult to tell apart in thick smears). *27*, Remains of a microgametocyte. *28*–*32*, Platelets. *33*, Lymphocyte. *34*, Polymorphonuclear leukocyte (usually only the nuclear remains of leukocytes are visible). *35*, *36*, "Blue clouds," sometimes mistaken for parasites. These represent (probably) the reticulum of young erythrocytes, often numerous in malaria. (From Russell, West and Manwell, Practical Malariology.)

Fig. 135. *Plasmodium malariae. Left:* Thin smear (Giemsa-stained) 650 ×. *1*, A young merozoite, which gives the impression (probably by accident) of being just about to enter an erythrocyte. *2*, An erythrocyte containing a very young parasite. *3*, A young ring. Though rings of this species are small and grow rather slowly, they are often described as having an especially "solid" appearance. *4*, A trophozoite simulating the marginal or appliqué forms so often seen in *falciparum* malaria. *5*, This trophozoite is assuming the band form which is especially characteristic of *P. malariae*. *6*, Here is a moderately advanced trophozoite. Note particularly the small size of the host cell (not only does *P. malariae* cause no hypertrophy of the invaded cell, but it often appears either to cause shrinkage of the erythrocyte, or to have a predilection for the smaller, and perhaps senescent, red cells), and the absence of pseudopodial processes. *7*, A slightly older trophozoite. *8*, The trophozoite shown here illustrates the typical band, or straplike form so often assumed by the younger stages of this plasmodium. *9*, An older parasite, still exhibiting the band form. *10*, A schizont, with the chromatin already divided more than once, but the pigment still scattered. *11*, A more advanced schizont. *12*, A segmenter with the eight merozoites (still not quite separated) typical of this species. *13*, A group of five free merozoites. *14*, A macrogametocyte. Note that it virtually fills the host cell, takes a rather strong blue stain, and has a sharply stained marginal mass of chromatin. Pigment (in both sexual and asexual forms) is relatively dark and abundant. *15*, A microgametocyte. Pigment is abundant, rather coarse, and the cytoplasm takes a lighter stain than in the female. The chromatin stains lightly, and is quite diffuse. *16*, An erythrocyte exhibiting basophilic stippling. Such cells are often abundant in the blood of malarious persons. When invaded by parasites they may give an erroneous impression of containing Schüffner's (or Maurer's) dots. *17*, A mass of platelets, sometimes mistaken for a group of free merozoites. *18*, A large monocyte. *Right:* Thick smear (Giemsa-stained) 650 ×. *19*, *20*, *21*, Ring forms. In the thick smear, however, the ring shape is often lost, and the chromatin and cytoplasm are likely to appear slightly separated. *22*, A young parasite. *23*, *24*, *25*, Somewhat older trophozoites. In the thick smear little structure is likely to be visible, and the parasite has a somewhat condensed appearance which, together with the pigment, causes it to appear very dark. *26*, A schizont, with two masses of chromatin and conspicuous pigment. *27*, A segmenter. *28*, *29*, A still more advanced segmenter. The eight merozoites so characteristic of this species of malaria are almost diagnostic. *30*, *31*, These forms are probably macrogametocytes, but in the thick smear it is not always easy to distinguish the sexual stages from the large trophozoites. Their small size and heavily stained appearance, however, should make them recognizable as quartan malaria parasites. *32*, The nucleus of a leukocyte—probably a monocyte. *33*, A "blue cloud." These are believed to represent the remains of reticulocytes, and often appear in smears of malarial blood. They are occasionally mistaken for parasites. (From Russell, West and Manwell, Practical Malariology.)

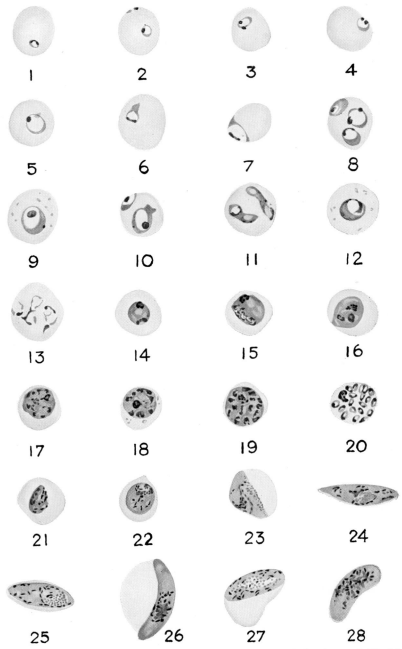

Fig. 136. *Plasmodium falciparum.* (Courtesy National Institute of Health, U.S.P.H.S.) 1. Very young ring form trophozoite. 2. Double infection of single cell with young trophozites, one a "marginal form," the other "signet ring" form. 3, 4. Young trophozoites showing double chromatin dots. 5, 6, 7. Developing trophozoite

are not enlarged or decolorized. The time required by *P. falciparum* for completion of one generation of schizogony is more variable than that for *P. vivax* and the period of release of merozoites more protracted. From eight to twenty-four merozoites are formed (Figs. 136 and 138).

The gametocytes are elongate, usually curved, sausage-shaped bodies. The male, or microgametocyte, stains lightly. Its chromatin is loose and scattered and abundant granular brownish pigment is dispersed through the cytoplasm. The female, or macrogametocyte, is often more slender, longer, and stains more deeply blue. Its chromatin tends to appear as a compact mass in or near the center and the pigment is usually closely approximated to the chromatin.

The gametocytes or "crescents" first appear after several generations of schizogony and subsequently recur in successive waves alternating with waves of trophozoites.

*Plasmodium malariae.* The ring forms of *P. malariae* are about the size of those of *P. vivax*. Trophozoites are more compact, less ameboid and tend to assume round or ovoid shapes. Band forms are common, the parasite extending as a band across the infected cell. The pigment is darker brown, coarser, and appears in greater quantity and earlier than with *P. vivax*. The mature schizont fills or nearly fills an unenlarged and normally stained red cell. Six to twelve merozoites are formed; the usual number is eight. These are arranged about the centrally collected pigment mass, giving rise to a "daisy head" or rosette appearance.

Gametocytes are fewer than with the other plasmodia and closely resemble trophozoites. They present the same differences between the sexes with respect to staining qualities and arrangement of chromatin granules (Figs. 135 and 137).

*Plasmodium ovale.* This relatively uncommon species resembles *P. vivax* in many respects. Infected cells very early show large numbers of coarse Schüffner's dots. The growing trophozoites exhibit relatively little ameboid activity and consequently are more compact and more regular in outline than *P. vivax*. Band forms are noted frequently. The mature schizonts form six to twelve merozoites with an average of eight. The gametocytes resemble those of *P. vivax* and are difficult to distinguish from them. The infected red cells are less enlarged than in *P. vivax* infections but are decolorized. The margin of

forms. 8. Three medium trophozoites in one cell. 9. Trophozoite showing pigment, in a cell containing Maurer's dots. 10, 11. Two trophozoites in each of two cells, showing variation of forms which parasites may assume. 12. Almost mature trophozoite showing haze of pigment throughout cytoplasm. Maurer's dots in the cell. 13. Estivo-autumnal "slender forms." 14. Mature trophozoite, showing clumped pigment. 15. Parasite in the process of initial chromatin division. 16, 17, 18, 19. Various phases of the development of the schizont ("presegmenting schizonts"). 20. Mature schizont. 21, 22, 23, 24. Successive forms in the development of the gametocyte—usually not found in the peripheral circulation. 25. Immature macrogametocyte. 26. Mature macrogametocyte. 27. Immature microgametocyte. 28. Mature microgametocyte.

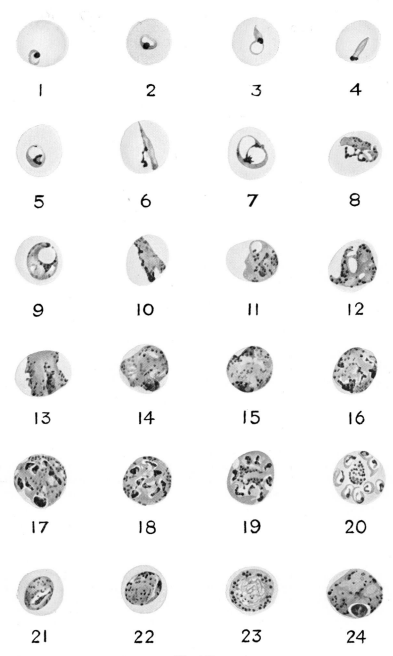

Fig. 137.

the infected cell is often crenated or fimbriated and the cell tends to be oval in shape (Fig. 139).

**Host-Parasite Relationships**   Following the injection of sporozoites by an infected anopheline mosquito at the end of the extrinsic incubation period, the pre-erythrocytic stage is initiated during which parasites are absent from the peripheral blood. In infections by *P. vivax* invasion of erythrocytes begins about the sixth day and in infections by *P. falciparum* about the seventh to the ninth day. The parasites are demonstrable by microscopic examination of the blood after a period which averages about eight to fifteen days following infection.

The Prepatent Period. This period is considerably longer in infections by *P. malariae*, averaging about twenty-three days. The first possible microscopic finding of plasmodia corresponds to a density of approximately ten parasites per cubic millimeter of blood. The development of parasitemia usually antedates the onset of clinical symptoms by two or three days.

The interval between the infective bite and the first elevation of temperature to 100° F. is termed *the intrinsic incubation period*. It averages eleven to thirteen days in infections by *P. vivax* and *P. falciparum* and four to five weeks or even longer in infections by *P. malariae*.

There are fundamental differences in the invasive characteristics of these three species of *Plasmodium*. These differences are to a considerable extent responsible for the marked variations in severity of the disease produced by them.

*Plasmodium vivax* attacks almost exclusively the reticulocytes and appears incapable of invading mature erythrocytes. This imposes a limit on the magnitude of the parasitemia, which usually ranges from 8000 to 20,000 per cubic millimeter and only rarely exceeds 50,000 per cubic millimeter.

*Plasmodium falciparum*, however, invades all the red cells irrespective of age. There is consequently no limiting factor to prevent progressively increasing parasitemia. Very high densities may therefore be encountered in *falciparum* infections. A parasitemia of 500,-000 parasites per cubic millimeter carries a grave prognosis and even low parasite densities should be considered dangerous. Unlike *P. vivax* and *P. malariae*, *P. falciparum* induces physical changes in the infected red blood cells which contribute importantly to the pathology

Fig. 137. *Plasmodium malariae.* (Courtesy National Institute of Health, U.S. P.H.S.) 1. Young ring form trophozoite of quartan malaria. 2, 3, 4. Young trophozoite forms of the parasite showing gradual increase of chromatin and cytoplasm. 5. Developing ring form trophozoite showing pigment granule. 6. Early band form trophozoite—elongated chromatin, some pigment apparent. 7. 8, 9, 10, 11, 12. Some forms which the developing trophozoite of quartan may take. 13, 14. Mature trophozoites—one a band form. 15, 16, 17, 18, 19. Phases in the development of the schizont ("presegmenting schizonts"). 20. Mature schizont. 21. Immature microgametocyte. 22. Immature macrogametocyte. 23. Mature microgametocyte. 24. Mature macrogametocyte.

Fig. 138.

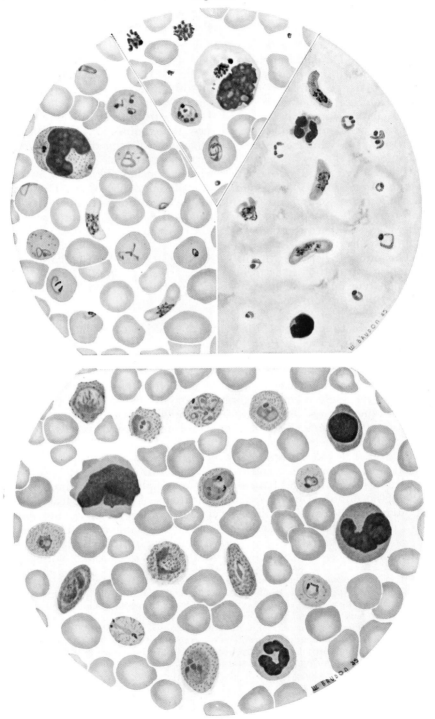

Fig. 139.

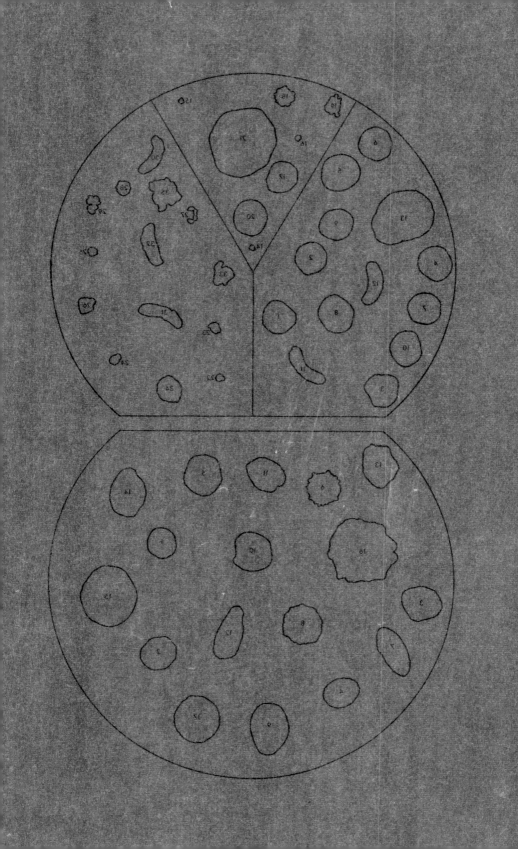

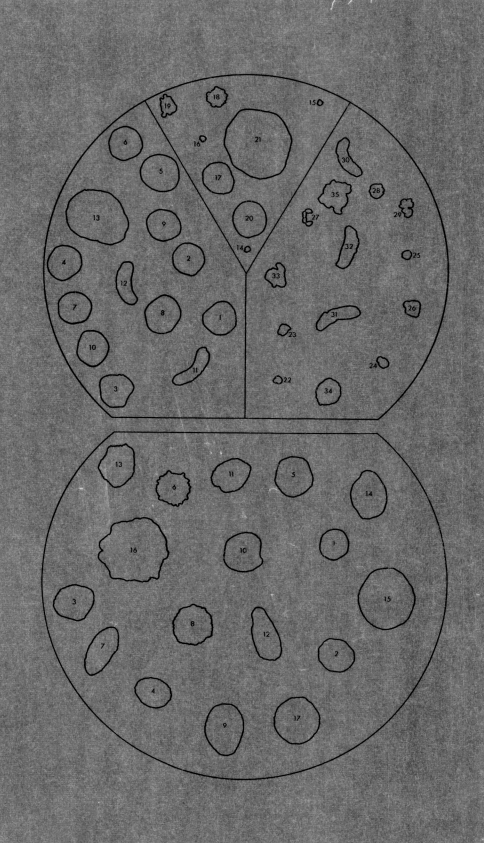

Fig. 138. *Plasmodium falciparum. Left:* Thin smear (Giemsa-stained) 650 ×. *1,* A young ring in an erythrocyte containing a trace of basophilic stippling. *2,* A ring of slightly greater age in the marginal position so frequently assumed by young parasites of this species. *3,* A ring similar to that in (*2*) above, but perhaps a little older. *4,* The so-called "*accolé*" form characteristic of this species. *5,* Multiple infection of the erythrocyte is very frequent in *falciparum* malaria (though it may also occur in the other types). This erythrocyte contains three young parasites; four or five, or even more, may be observed. *6,* A young trophozoite, marginal in position, but not of the "*accolé*" type. *7,* A more than usually ameboid trophozoite. In certain cases such forms have been so frequent that they have been described as new species, or subspecies. The erythrocyte also exhibits Maurer's dots. *8,* Another very ameboid trophozoite, but one which has not caused the stippling of the host cell. *9,* This shows a slightly older parasite than in (*8*) above. It is even more ameboid, and the Maurer's dots are very conspicuous. Note that they are rather coarse, stain almost brick-red, are not numerous, and that several of them resemble clefts more than points (for which reason they are called not only "Maurer's dots" but also "Stephens and Christopher's clefts"). *10,* This trophozoite exhibits the two chromatin masses which are often seen in the rings of *P. falciparum. 11,* A macrogametocyte. It is characteristically sausage-shaped, with both chromatin and pigment condensed near the center. It takes a bluer stain than the male cell. *12,* A microgametocyte, showing the relatively dispersed chromatin and pigment, the greater breadth and more blunt ends, as compared to the female (above). *13,* A large mononuclear leukocyte containing malarial pigment. *Upper center:* Thin smear of placental blood (Giemsa-stained 650 ×. *14, 15, 16,* Young parasites lying free in blood (probably just liberated from some ripe segmenter). *17,* A schizont. *18, 19,* Two segmenters. No trace remains of the host cell. *20,* A half-grown crescent. Such forms (which may also appear in the peripheral blood in severe cases) may simulate the band forms of *P. malariae. 21,* A mononuclear which has ingested a segmenter. *Right:* Thick smear (Giemsa-stained) 650 ×. *22, 23, 24, 25,* Four very small rings. They are characteristically of delicate appearance, and generally smaller than the corresponding stages of the other species. *26,* Not all *falciparum* rings are small, since they grow considerably before becoming concentrated in the visceral blood. Here is a moderately large one. *27, 28,* Two rings, each with a double chromatin dot. *29,* Although there is, of course, nothing left of the host cell in the thick smear, one may see indications of the multiple infection so frequent in this species. These two rings were no doubt contained in the same red cell. *30, 31,* The crescents are not greatly changed in the thick smear. Here are two macrogametocytes. *32,* This is (apparently) a microgametocyte. *33,* Some crescents may be considerably altered in the making of a thick drop preparation, but they are usually recognizable as crescents nevertheless, as in this case. *34,* The nucleus of a leukocyte (lymphocyte?). *35,* The nucleus of a granulocyte. (From Russell, West and Manwell, Practical Malariology.)

Fig. 139. *Plasmodium ovale*—Thin smear (Leishman-stained) 650 ×. *1,* A young trophozoite. Note that it has already produced some stippling in the host cell. *2,* A slightly older stage, in which the parasite has assumed a ring form. *3,* A parasite of about the same age as that in part *2,* but with a smaller central vacuole. The stippling is more prominent and the erythrocyte appears somewhat enlarged. *4,* Sometimes the smaller stages of *P. ovale* assume a strap of band form, just as do the corresponding stages of *P. malariae.* One such parasite is shown here. *5,* This trophozoite may have started to divide somewhat precociously. The lack of any pseudopodial processes is characteristic of this species. In this it resembles *P. malariae.* 6, The stage shown here is similar to that depicted in the preceding figure, but the invaded erythrocyte exhibits the fimbriated edges which are often characteristic of *P. ovale. 7,* This parasite appears to be a schizont. It is figured because it shows the oval distortion of the host cell which gives this species its name. *8,* A stage which probably corresponds to that just described, although the pale tint of the cytoplasm suggests that it may be a somewhat distorted microgametocyte. The host cell shows the intense stippling and the fimbriated edge, both of which are more or less characteristic of the species. *9,* A schizont with four masses of chromatin. Note that the host cell has a somewhat oval shape. *10,* A presegmenter, with six chromatin dots. This stage resembles *P. malariae* more than *P. vivax.* 11, A segmenter with six merozoites. The usual number is eight, but the actual number is variable, as in nearly all other species of plasmodia. *12,* A macrogametocyte, which has produced the typical oval distortion of the host erythrocyte. But this distortion is by no means constant, appearing in only a fraction of the invaded cells. *13,* A microgametocyte, with the typical large, marginal chromatin mass. *14,* A lymphocyte. 15, A mononuclear leukocyte. *16,* Also a mononuclear. *17,* A neutrophil polymorphonuclear leukocyte. (From Russell, West and Manwell, Practical Malariology.)

of the infection. The infected cells agglutinate, forming thrombi and emboli. They likewise adhere to the capillary endothelium. These effects produce capillary obstruction and severe ischemia in many tissues of the body.

*Plasmodium malariae* attacks predominantly the aging erythrocytes which are about to be removed from the circulation by the normal process of blood destruction. The inability of this species to attack younger forms provides a limit to the parasitemia and accounts for the fact that densities in excess of 10,000 per cubic millimeter are uncommon.

CHARACTERISTICS OF *P. vivax* INFECTIONS. In the early stages of infection by *P. vivax* two groups of parasites undergo schizogony concurrently, maturing on alternate days. This results in the release of a new generation of merozoites each day and a corresponding quotidian febrile reaction. Gradually or suddenly one group may drop out. Maturation of the parasites then occurs approximately every forty-eight hours and the accompanying febrile curve becomes characteristically tertian. In an untreated case the dropped group ultimately may reappear, its members gradually increasing in numbers as the others decrease and the fever again becomes quotidian. The naturally evolving *vivax* infection, therefore, consists of a series of such alternating and overlapping groups with corresponding periods of tertian and quotidian fever. The latter type of curve depends upon this phenomenon and not, as has been said in the past, upon double infection acquired on different days.

Gametocytes appear in the peripheral blood within a few days after the end of the prepatent period. They become infective for mosquitoes shortly thereafter.

CHARACTERISTICS OF *P. falciparum* INFECTIONS. Infections by *P. falciparum* differ in certain important respects from those by *P. vivax*. The period required for maturation of the parasites is approximately forty-eight hours and schizogony is less synchronized. Release of the new generation of parasites is continued over a longer period. As a result the febrile episodes are less regular and more prolonged in duration. In severe infections the fever is frequently continuous.

Gametocytes do not appear in the peripheral blood until about ten days after the onset of the primary parasitemia. They become infective for mosquitoes about four days later. In naturally evolving infections, as the gametocyte count rises the trophozoite count diminishes and clinical improvement or remission of symptoms frequently occurs. The primary parasitemia is characterized by such a series of successive trophozoite-gametocyte waves.

Parasite counts in *falciparum* malaria characteristically fluctuate much more markedly than do those of *vivax*.

CHARACTERISTICS OF *P. malariae* INFECTIONS. In the early stages of infections by *P. malariae* there is usually only one group of parasites undergoing schizogony. The febrile episodes, therefore, recur at intervals of approximately seventy-two hours. Subsequently one or two additional groups may appear producing a double quartan fever or even quotidian fever. Gametocytes are usually scanty.

CHARACTERISTICS OF MIXED *P. vivax* AND *P. falciparum* INFECTIONS. When infection by both *P. vivax* and *P. falciparum* occurs the latter plasmodia appear first and the initial clinical activity is due to the *falciparum* infection. Subsequently the *vivax* parasitemia increases and the *falciparum* falls, producing alternate periods of dominance. Clinically this may be expressed by continuous clinical disease, at one time the expression of *P. falciparum* infection and at another *P. vivax* infection.

THE PRIMARY ATTACK AND RELAPSES. Study of naturally induced mosquito-transmitted *vivax* infection indicates that in wholly susceptible persons the patent primary parasitemia may persist for as long as 100 to 130 days. In the course of this period, however, there may be transitory intervals when the parasite densities are depressed. Such depressions are frequently accompanied by clinical remissions. The duration of clinical symptoms is considerably shorter than the total period of primary parasitemia and it may be continuous or interrupted by one or more remissions. Any clinical activity occurring within this period is considered part of the primary attack of malaria. The term recrudescence is applied to secondary clinical episodes following the initial attack but occurring within 130 days after infection or within eight weeks after cessation of the initial clinical phenomena.

The relapse appears to depend upon a different biologic mechanism. It is known that a residual exo-erythrocytic infection persists in the liver of the rhesus monkey infected with *P. cynomolgi*. There is strong inferential evidence that a similar mechanism in man may account for the late relapses of *vivax* malaria.

Furthermore, strains of *P. vivax* obtained in the temperate zone and in the tropics appear to behave differently. Temperate zone malaria characteristically has a long latent interval between the primary attack and the first relapse. Tropical strains, on the other hand, do not exhibit the long latent interval and activity tends to be continuous.

The natural duration of *P. vivax* infections is variable. Although the majority are terminated within two to three years, certain strains encountered in the Southwest Pacific during World War II persisted for considerably longer periods. *Plasmodium falciparum* infections are of shorter duration seldom exceeding one year. *Plasmodium malariae*, however, may remain latent for many years even in the absence of demonstrable parasitemia or clinical evidence of infection.

**Immunity**  The colored race has a relative racial immunity to malaria which is particularly effective against *P. vivax*. It exists, however, in lesser degree against *P. falciparum* which, in the Negro, usually causes milder clinical episodes of shorter duration than those usually encountered in the white race.

Experimental studies have indicated that infections by *P. vivax* and *P. falciparum* produce an homologous immunity. This is strictly strain-specific, the individual becoming refractory to subsequent reinfection by the strain previously used. He is not immune, however, to other strains of the same species although the severity of the infection produced by them is frequently modified. There is no cross immunity between species; thus infection by *P. vivax* confers no immunity against *P. falciparum*, and the clinical disease produced by the latter is unmitigated in severity.

The development of immunity is first characterized by the acquisition of *tolerance* to the infection. This is expressed by cessation of clinical phenomena despite persistence of a parasitemia considerably in excess of that which accompanied the onset of the initial clinical activity. It represents apparently a form of immunity depending upon a persisting latent infection. Agglutinins, precipitins and complement-fixing antibodies are produced. The defense mechanism, however, is probably largely cellular in nature.

This immunity, expressed as tolerance and premunition, is of great importance in the epidemiology of malaria.

**Epidemiology**    Malaria has a higher morbidity rate and is responsible for more deaths per year than any other transmissible disease. The health organization of the League of Nations in 1932 estimated that 17,750,000 cases were treated annually and considered an annual incidence of 300,000,000 cases a conservative estimate. The great importance of malaria as a military problem was first clearly demonstrated in World War I when, in the course of campaigns in Macedonia, the British, French and German armies were immobilized by this disease. In World War II it constituted the major problem of military medicine throughout the tropical and subtropical theaters, particularly the Mediterranean, India, Burma, China, the Philippines and the south and southwest Pacific. In the latter area malaria had a profound effect upon the development and the progress of military operations. In this region also a peculiarly resistant strain of *P. vivax* was encountered which was characterized by repeated relapses over an unusually long period of time. More recently, experience in Korea has demonstrated that malaria may be a problem for armies in the field even in the temperate zone.

The degree of endemicity or the level of transmission of malaria in any region is determined by a variety of interrelated factors. The most important of these are:

1. The prevalence of infection in man—the reservoir.
2. The species of indigenous anopheline mosquitoes, their relative abundance, their feeding and resting behaviors and their individual suitability as hosts for plasmodia—the vector.
3. The presence of a susceptible human population—the new host.
4. Local climatic conditions.
5. Local geographic and hydrographic conditions which determine anopheline breeding areas (Fig. 140, Table 25).

It is apparent, however, that there must be other controlling influences for in areas in which the disease is endemic the incidence of malaria over long periods of time exhibits cyclic increases and recessions, the causes of which are not understood.

In many parts of the world there is a definite annual fluctuation and a usual sequence in the times of appearance of the different types of the disease. These are probably dependent upon seasonal variations

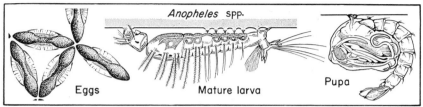

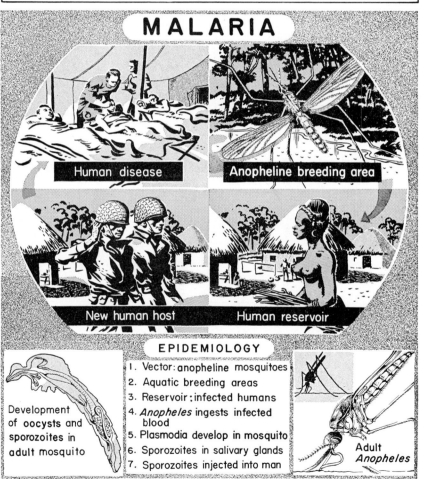

Fig. 140. Epidemiology of malaria.

*Table 25   Principal Vectors of Human Malaria*

| REGION | AREA | SPECIES | TYPE OF BREEDING PLACE | | ADULT BEHAVIOR | EFFICIENCY AS VECTOR |
|---|---|---|---|---|---|---|
| | | | LIGHT REQUIREMENTS | WATER, VEGETATION, ETC. | | |
| Nearctic | United States (and bordering areas): Drier portions of Rocky Mountain and Pacific area and N.W. Mexico | Anopheles freeborni | Sun | Fresh, clear seepage from ditches, rice fields, edges of slow streams; irrigation water | Enters houses; feeds readily on man | Dangerous in interior valleys of west coast of U. S. |
| | Coastal Mexico to New Hampshire and Ontario west to Minnesota | A. quadrimaculatus | Sun usually, sometimes in partial shade | Fresh pools, ponds, lakes, lagoons, swamps, slow flowing rivers, in dense aquatic vegetation | Active at night; feeds on human or animal blood; may remain in houses all day | Most important carrier in the eastern U. S. |
| Neotropical (Largely) | Mexico, Central America (and bordering areas): S.E. Texas, through Mexico and West Indies, south to Colombia and Ecuador; east through northern Venezuela | A. albimanus | Sun or partial shade | Fresh or brackish fairly pure, stagnant water; matted vegetation favorable in large lakes; swamps; lagoons; hoof prints | Nocturnal; prefers man, but also bites animals; enters houses, usually leaves at dawn after feeding | Most important vector in C. A. and Caribbean, especially in rainy season |
| | See South America, etc., for: South Central U.S., south to Chile and Argentina; Grenada | A. darlingi · A. pseudopunctipennis pseudopunctipennis | ........... · Sun | Clear pools, streams and springs rich in algae, in dry season | Enters houses and feeds readily on man in certain areas only | .......... in mountain valleys of South America, Central America and Mexico, but not in Panama |
| | Mexico, through Central America and Trinidad to Peru, Brazil | A. punctimacula | Shade preferred | Shaded pools, swamps, sluggish streams | Abundant in undrained jungle; strong flier; enters dwellings; feeds on man | Vector in parts of Panama; proved vector in parts of W. Colombia |
| | Caribbean area: See Mexico, Central America for: Panama, Trinidad, Lesser Antilles, south to Brazil | A. albimanus (tarsimaculatus of certain authors) · A. aquasalis | ....... or shade · Sun | Brackish tidal swamps; rarely in fresh water of rice fields (inland Trinidad) | May fly three miles; enters houses, feeds on man (less true in Panama?) | Important in many localities: Trinidad, Coastal Brazil |
| | Trinidad and Venezuela to So. Brazil | A. bellator | Partial shade | Leaf bases of bromeliads (epiphytic on *Erythrina* and other trees) | Prefers man; bites at night or in shade (day time); enters dwellings occasionally, returns to forest | Important in cocoa-growing areas of Trinidad, and in coastal states of So. Brazil |

| Region | Distribution | Species | Light | Water | Habits | Remarks |
|---|---|---|---|---|---|---|
| Neotropical | South America (and bordering areas): See Mexico, C. A. for: So. Brazil | A. albimanus / A. cruzii | Partial shade | Leaf bases of bromeliads | Bites man readily; enters houses | Important in coastal states of So. Brazil |
| | Guatemala to N.E. Argentina and Paraguay; Trinidad | A. albitarsis | Some shade (not extreme) | Among mats of aquatic vegetation in large ponds, marshes, overflows near rivers; hoof prints; artificial containers | Enters houses and shows preference for human blood in some areas | Important in Brazil and probably N.E. Argentina |
| | Central America (British Honduras and Guatemala); South America (Venezuela to Argentina) | A. darlingi | Shade | Clear, fresh lagoons, overflows, etc., among debris, surface vegetation; avoids brackish water | Invades houses; prefers human blood. A domestic species | Most dangerous vector in tropical S. America from Venezuela, the Guianas to S. Brazil |
| | See Mexico, C. A. for: | A. pseudopunctipennis pseudopunctipennis | . . . . . . . . . . | . . . . . . . . . . | . . . . . . . . . . | . . . . . . . . . . |
| Palaearctic | Europe: S. Palaearctic, North of Mediterranean; from England to Japan; from Sweden and Siberia to Portugal, Spain, Italy, Mongolia | A. labranchiae atroparvus | Sun | Brackish water along coast; fresh water inland | Frequents houses; feeds readily on man, also stabled animals | Carries "house malaria," of winter months, especially in Netherlands |
| | N.W. Africa, Spain, Sicily, Sardinia, Corsica, Italy, Dalmatian Coast, islands of central Mediterranean | A. labranchiae labranchiae | Sun to partial shade | Brackish, coastal marshes; fresh water of rice fields, upland streams; other situations | Prefers human blood; enters houses in large numbers | Important vector |
| | Norway and Sweden to Italy; England to Black Sea; eastern Mediterranean | A. messeae | Sun | Cool, fresh standing water; lakes, marshes | Prefers animal to human blood; hibernates in barns, houses | Vector in Hungary and Albania |
| | N.E. and central Italy, Sardinia, Balkans, Russia to W. China | A. sacharovi (= elutus) | Sun | Open inland marshes and coastal marshes even if brackish | Feeds without preference on man, animals; enters houses (bedrooms); hibernates in cold weather, but feeds on cattle in lowlands during winter | Important in Balkans, Palestine; preference for cattle reduces its importance as vector in other areas |
| | See Persian Gulf etc. for: | A. superpictus | . . . . . . . . . . | . . . . . . . . . . | . . . . . . . . . . | . . . . . . . . . . |
| | North Africa, Middle East: Europe, N. Africa, Asia Minor, Turkestan | A. claviger (= bifurcatus) | Sun or shade | Marshes, rock pools, wells, cisterns | Domestic in Palestine; enters houses, bites man freely (wild in some regions) | Most important urban vector in Palestine, Syria |
| | See Europe for: N. Africa, Egypt, A–E Sudan, Cyprus, Anatolia, Palestine, E. Persia, Baluchistan | A. labranchiae labranchiae / A. multicolor | Sun | Stagnant or flowing drains, pools, shallow wells; tolerates salinity (desert) up to 5.96 per cent | Enters houses readily; bites freely; travels with wind up to 8 miles | Evidence epidemiological only |

*Table 25   Principal Vectors of Human Malaria (Continued)*

| REGION | AREA | SPECIES | TYPE OF BREEDING PLACE | | ADULT BEHAVIOR | EFFICIENCY AS VECTOR |
|---|---|---|---|---|---|---|
| | | | LIGHT REQUIREMENTS | WATER, VEGETATION, ETC. | | |
| Palaearctic (cont'd) | See Central and South Africa for: See Europe for: Canaries, Algeria, Tunisia, Egypt, Palestine, Syria, N.W. India | A. pharoensis A. sacharoni A. sergenti | .......... Sun to partial shade | .......... Rice fields, borrow pits, slow irrigation flows (dense vegetation); seepage, neglected drains | .......... Enters houses readily; bites mostly after dark; may migrate 2 miles | .......... Vector in Egypt and Palestine |
| | Persian Gulf and Caucasian area See Europe for: E. Arabia, S. Iraq; Iran, India, Burma | A. sacharoni A. stephensi stephensi | .......... Relative shade | .......... Wells, cisterns, flower pots, cans, roof-gutters | .......... Feeds readily on man; rests in barracks, houses, cowsheds | .......... Important in urban areas |
| | Spain, Italy, Balkans to southeast Asia | A. superpictus | Sun | Fresh-water pools, streams, drains, seepages, especially in hill districts | Prefers human blood; readily enters houses, tents, barracks; strong fliers | Important in Europe, Mesopotamia, Baluchistan |
| | Japan, North and Northeast China, Korea, South Ukraine See Burma, etc. for: China (not south of 30° N. lat.) | A. hyrcanus sinensis A. pattoni | .......... Sun | .......... Among algae along stream margins; rain pools, small pools of stream beds in hills | .......... Bites man | .......... Important vector |
| Ethiopian | Central and South Africa: Tropical Africa, north to Ethiopia | A. funestus funestus | Partial shade | Clear water of swamps, weedy banks of streams, rivers, ditches; margins of lakes, ponds; underground seepages | Enters houses in large numbers; feeds freely on human blood; a few migrate up to 4½ miles | Always important (also carries filariasis) |
| | Tropical Africa, Arabia, Madagascar, Reunion, Mauritius; other points | A. gambiae | Sun or slight shade | Puddles, shallow ponds, borrow pits, hoof prints, ditches, overflows; rarely rain barrels, cisterns | Prefers human blood; abundant in huts and houses; a few migrate up to 3½ miles | Always important (also carries filariasis) |
| | Sierra Leone, Liberia, Cameroons, Uganda, Belgian Congo | A. hancocki | Sun to slight shade | Clear water in grassy holes, native wells, streams, swamps | Found commonly in human dwellings | Important where prevalent |

| | Species | Light | Breeding places | Habits | Importance |
|---|---|---|---|---|---|
| Sierra Leone, Liberia, S. Nigeria, Gaboon, Belgian Congo | A. hargreavesi | More or less shade | Among *Pistia* in open jungle; swamps, stream margins (vegetation) | Abundant in huts in Nigeria; bites at midnight or later | Important where common |
| Belgian Congo, Uganda, Cameroons | A. moucheti moucheti | Sun to slight shade | Among vegetation on margins of pools, streams, permanent swamps | Often found indoors | Rather important where common |
| Belgian Congo | A. dureni | Shady | Small, sandy, well vegetated | Bites readily near breeding places | Incriminated as vector |
| Southern Nigeria | A. moucheti nigeriensis | Sun, largely | Clear water, in swamps (*Pistia* and other vegetation) | Found in native huts | Rather important where common |
| Sierra Leone, Liberia, Gold Coast, Nigeria, Cameroons—eastward to Mozambique | A. nili | Heavy shade | Among vegetation along sides of running streams | Common in huts and camps, but rare in houses | Possibly important where prevalent |
| Sierra Leone, Gold Coast | A. melas | Shade | Breeding associated with black mangrove trees (*Avicennia* sp.) in brackish water, coastal streams and tidal swamps | Feeds more on dark nights; most remain in huts after feeding | Important in some coastal areas of West Africa |
| Many parts of Africa; Madagascar, Palestine | A. pharoensis | Sun to partial shade | Swamps and rice fields; vegetation essential | Enters houses in large numbers; bites man readily but prefers animal blood | Important in upper Nile Province, Sudan, Fr. W. Africa |
| Gold Coast, N. Nigeria, E. Belgian Congo, Uganda, Natal, Transvaal, Kenya, Mozambique; other areas | A. pretoriensis | Sun | Rock pools, semi-stagnant pools in streams and ditches, hoof marks (no vegetation) | Frequents houses in some areas only | Of secondary importance |
| E. Central and S. Africa, N. and S. Rhodesia, Sudan | A. rufipes | Sun | Pools, marshes, hoof-marks, artificial containers | Rests in crevices and outdoor haunts near breeding places; occasionally found in large numbers indoors | S. Rhodesia, Fr. W. Africa, Sudan; usually of secondary importance |
| Angola, Belgian Congo, N and S. Nigeria, Gold Coast, Sierra Leone | A. brumpti | Sun to partial shade | Slowly flowing water or fresh-water pools | Rests principally in human habitations | May be a vector during colder months, when other vectors not active |
| **Oriental** Afghanistan, Baluchistan, India, Ceylon; India, S. China, Formosa, entire Malay region and Philippines | A. annularis (= *fuliginosus*) | Sun to partial shade | Large tanks or fresh-water ponds, slowly moving streams, lake margins (with aquatic vegetation) | Prefers cattle to man; flies great distances; occurs up to 7000 ft. | Of doubtful importance |

*Table 25   Principal Vectors of Human Malaria (Continued)*

| REGION | AREA | SPECIES | TYPE OF BREEDING PLACE | | ADULT BEHAVIOR | EFFICIENCY AS VECTOR |
|---|---|---|---|---|---|---|
| | | | LIGHT REQUIREMENTS | WATER, VEGETATION, ETC. | | |
| Oriental (cont'd) | Baluchistan to Burma; Ceylon; Siam, Tonkin Prov., S. Arabia | A. culicifacies | Sun to partial shade | Wide variety of places; prefers fresh, clean water in pools but can survive in brackish | Prefers cattle but bites man freely; rests in cow sheds and houses during day | Most important vector in India; only vector in Ceylon |
| | In foothills from Baluchistan to Burma; South India, Ceylon (?), Turkestan, Thailand, Tonkin Prov. | A. fluviatilis (= listoni) | Sun | Stream edges, stream pools, springs, irrigation channels; more rarely swamps, lakes | Prefers human to animal blood; found in houses, cow sheds | Important vector in rural foothills (1000–5000 ft.) |
| | Eastern India; Indo-China (?) | A. jeyporiensis jeyporiensis | Sun to slight shade | Flowing water and marshy edges of lakes, ponds, streams | Feeds on man; found in houses, cow sheds | Found infected in nature but not considered important |
| | E. and S India, Ceylon, Burma, Thailand, Indo-China, S. China, Formosa | A. minimus | Sun | Slow-running streams, springs, with grassy margins; irrigation ditches, rice fields, seepage areas | Remains in houses and cow sheds after feeding | Always important; especially so in India, Burma, S. China up to 5,500 ft. |
| | India, Burma, Malaya, Thailand, Indo-China, Dutch Indies, Philippine Islands | A. philippinensis | Sun to partial shade | Pools, drains, ditches, tanks, swamps, borrow pits, rice fields; grass-covered stagnant waters | Found in houses, stables, cattle sheds | Important in Bengal; probably *not* vector in Philippine Islands |
| | See Persian Gulf, etc. for: | A. stephensi | | | | |
| | India, Burma, Thailand, Malaya, Sumatra, Java, Borneo, Lesser Sunda Islands, S. Celebes | A. sundaicus | Sun | Brackish or salt water in lagoons, swamps and behind coastal embankments | Prefers human blood (?); found in large numbers in cow sheds, houses; strong fliers | Important in Bengal, Malaya, Indo-China, East Indies |
| | See Persian Gulf, etc. for: | A. superpictus | | | | |
| | India, Burma | A. varuna | Sun or shade | Stagnant water of pools, ditches, wells; slow streams, irrigation ditches | Feeds readily on man; found in houses, cow sheds | Proved vector in some localities |
| | India, Ceylon, Burma, Thailand, Cochin-China, Malaya, Sumatra, Java, Borneo, Celebes | A. aconitus | Sun to partial shade | Irrigation ditches, swamps, ponds, rice fields, pools in creek beds, storm drains; reservoirs with grassy margins | Feeds readily on man, animals; found in houses, cow sheds (1200 to 2500 ft.); strong fliers | Important in French Indo-China |

| Distribution | Species | Sun/shade | Breeding water | Habits | Importance |
|---|---|---|---|---|---|
| See Afghanistan, etc. for: N.E. India, Burma, Indo-China, China, Korea, Japan, Formosa, Okinawa | A. culicifacies / A. hyrcanus sinensis | ......... | Stagnant water in rice fields, pools, ponds, swamps; rarely stream or lake margins | Not recorded as domestic | Vector in S. Japan, Korea, Okinawa and in China |
| Malaya, Sumatra, Borneo, Java, Celebes | A. hyrcanus williamsoni | Sun | Same as for A. hyrcanus sinensis | Same as for A. hyrcanus sinensis | Important vector in Java and Celebes |
| India, China, Tonkin Prov., Burma, Formosa | A. jeyporiensis candidiensis | Same as for A. hyrcanus sinensis | Running water in ditches | Not recorded as domestic | Vector in Tonkin Prov. |
| India, Ceylon, Burma, S. China, Thailand, Malaya, Indo-China, East Indies, Formosa, Philippines | A. maculatus maculatus | Sun to slight shade | Stream and river beds, seepages; also pools, rice fields, lake margins, ditches | Enters houses temporarily; bites humans | Important in Malaya and East Indies |
| See Afghanistan, etc. for: | A. minimus | Sun to very slight shade | | ......... | ......... |
| See Afghanistan, etc. for: | A. sundaicus | ......... | | | |
| E. India, Tonkin Prov., Malaya, Cochin-China, Sumatra, Java, Borneo, Celebes | A. umbrosus | Shade (can tolerate sunlight) | Stagnant jungle pools and morasses; brackish water in mangrove swamps | Fierce biter, found in dense forests, jungles, also in houses; strong fliers | Important in some areas |
| Philippine Islands: Philippine Islands | A. manganus | Partial shade | Clear water among bamboo roots; in slow-flowing ditches or streams with sandy or rocky beds, close to mountain areas | Bites man; not found above 2000 ft. | Probably a vector |
| Philippine Islands | A. minimus flavirostris | Sun and shade | Clear water of shaded streams (bamboo roots); rivers, irrigation ditches, pools, wells | Enters houses to attack man; leaves after feeding, rests, under overhanging banks | The important vector in the Philippines |
| Indonesia: See Burma, etc. for: India, Ceylon, Burma, Thailand, Indo-China, China, Malaya, Sumatra, Borneo, Java, Lesser Sundas, Celebes, New Guinea, Philippines | A. aconitus / A. barbirostris barbirostris | Sun and shade | Clear water of shaded streams, rivers, vegetated ponds, pools, flowing ditches, canals; borrow pits, rice fields, salt water swamps; wells | Flies by day (in shade); enters houses rarely; prefers blood of domestic animals | Of little importance (found infected in Malaya, East Indies) |
| India, Ceylon, Burma, Thailand, Indo-China, China, Malaya, Sumatra, Java, Celebes, Borneo, Philippine Islands | A. hyrcanus nigerrimus | Sun, largely | Rice fields especially; stagnant vegetated canals, borrow pits, lakes, impounded areas; slow streams | A wild species, invades houses rarely; feeds on man or animals | Of some importance in Malaya and East Indies |
| India, Burma, Malaya, Sumatra, Java, Lesser Sundas, Moluccas, Borneo, Philippine Islands | A. kochi | Sun or shade | Small muddy pools (rainy season); unplanted rice fields; streams, irrigation ditches, artificial containers | Moderately domestic; bites man, prefers animals; found in houses, stables | Not considered important |

*Table 25   Principal Vectors of Human Malaria (Continued)*

| REGION | AREA | SPECIES | TYPE OF BREEDING PLACE — LIGHT REQUIREMENTS | TYPE OF BREEDING PLACE — WATER, VEGETATION, ETC. | ADULT BEHAVIOR | EFFICIENCY AS VECTOR |
|---|---|---|---|---|---|---|
| Oriental (cont'd) | India, Ceylon, Burma, Indo-China, Malaya, Sumatra, Java, Borneo, Philippines | A. leucosphyrus leucosphyrus | Heavy shade required | Rock pools; stagnant pools in beds of mountain streams | A wild species; found in dense jungles | Found infected in East Indies |
|  | See Burma, etc. for: | A. maculatus, A. minimus | .......... | .......... | .......... | .......... |
|  | See Afghanistan, etc. for: India, Malaya, East Indies, New Guinea | A. subpictus subpictus | Sun or shade | Fresh, brackish, or contaminated pools, borrow pits, wallows; roof-gutters, containers | Feeds on man, other animals, but prefers cattle; numerous in cow sheds, houses, barracks | Believed important in Celebes |
|  | See Afghanistan, etc. for: See Burma, etc. for: | A. sundaicus, A. umbrosus | .......... | .......... | .......... | .......... |
| Australian | Australia, New Guinea, Pacific Islands; Australia, Tasmania | A. annulipes annulipes | Sun to slight shade | Shallow, grassy pools; edges of marshes, slow creeks, surface wells, rock pools (tolerates brackish water) | Enters houses; readily bites man (occurs up to 5000 ft.) | Evidence epidemiological only |
|  | New Guinea, Queensland, Northern Australia | A. bancroftii | Some shade | Shallow, slow-running overgrown water | Bites during evening hours; prefers man but rarely enters houses | Vector in New Guinea (?) |
|  | New Guinea, New Britain, Solomons, New Hebrides, Admiralties, N. Australia | A. farauti (= punctulatus moluccensis of authors) | Sun or slight shade | Fresh or brackish water, natural or artificial, clear or polluted | Bites freely both at night and in day time shade; exclusively anthropophilic | Dominant carrier in this area |
|  | New Guinea, Bismarck Archipelago and Solomon Islands | A. punctulatus punctulatus | Sun | Small rain pools, stream margins; rarely in larger bodies of water | Frequents houses; bites throughout night; strong flier | Important in New Guinea, probably also in Solomons |

of temperature, humidity and rainfall affecting both the breeding of anopheline vectors and the development of the exogenous phase of the parasites in them. Thus the optimum temperature for the exogenous phase of *P. vivax* is 25° C. (77° F.), of *P. falciparum* 30° C. (86° F.), and of *P. malariae* 22° C. (72° F.).

It is obvious that average climatic conditions in the temperate zone permit development and transmission of *P. vivax* and *P. malariae* but are less favorable to *P. falciparum.* These factors undoubtedly are important in the seasonal incidence of the types of malaria in cooler parts of the endemic areas. In such regions *P. vivax* infections are the earliest to appear in the spring while *P. falciparum* and *P. malariae* do not reach their peak until late summer and early autumn.

In the true tropics rainfall is the determining factor controlling anopheline breeding. In areas where there are wet and dry seasons each year there are commonly two peaks of incidence. The first follows shortly after the beginning of the rains. The second, and frequently the more important, appears at the end of the rainy season when ample anopheline breeding areas are present and when the destructive action of heavy rainfall upon the larvae is diminished.

In mountainous tropical countries both *P. vivax* and *P. falciparum* are prevalent in the hot, moist lowlands. At higher altitudes as the average temperatures more nearly approach those of temperate zones *P. falciparum* gradually disappears. *Plasmodium vivax*, however, may be heavily endemic in certain regions at altitudes even in excess of 8000 feet.

Evaluation of the malaria problem in any area entails study of all the known factors which contribute to the endemicity and the transmission of the disease.

*Malaria reconnaissance* provides a rapid, superficial and statistically inexact estimate of the situation. The data provided by such an investigation are insufficient for the preparation of a detailed control program.

A *malaria survey*, on the other hand, is an intensive, detailed, often time-consuming study of all relevant local factors. It should be carried on throughout a year to secure accurate information adequate for planning a control program.

EVALUATION OF INFECTION OF THE HUMAN RESERVOIR. Evaluation of the degree of infection of the human reservoir is based upon the following findings:

1. SPLEEN RATE. This is the per cent incidence of splenomegaly in children of the indigenous population two to nine years of age inclusive. The age group may be varied in certain regions, but in each case the inclusive ages must be so stated. It is also important to specify the position of the child when splenic palpation was performed (standing or recumbent) since only slightly enlarged spleens vary in their palpability depending upon the method of examination. The size of the spleen should be noted in each case according to standard measurements proposed by various authors.

2. ADULT SPLEEN RATE. When the number of children is insufficient adults may be included in the figures. The incidence of splenomegaly in the adult population is lower, however, and consequently the qualifying term "adult" must be included to avoid misinterpretation of the data.

3. PARASITE RATE. This is the per cent incidence of blood films showing malarial parasites in children of the indigenous population two to nine years of age inclusive.

4. TRANSMISSION INDEX. This is the per cent incidence of blood films showing malarial parasites in infants of the indigenous population under one year of age. It provides important information concerning variations in the seasonal transmission rate of malaria in the particular area.

Certain arbitrary terms have been accepted to express the *intensity of infection* in a given area. These are:

1. Low endemicity—spleen rate under 10 per cent.
2. Moderate endemicity—spleen rate 10 to 25 per cent.
3. High endemicity—spleen rate 25 to 50 per cent.
4. Hyperendemicity—spleen rate 50 per cent or over.

These levels of endemicity are accompanied by characteristic differences in the general health of the populations concerned. In areas of low and moderate endemicity human infections are comparatively scarce and immunity is practically nonexistent. The incidence and severity of clinical malaria are more or less uniform throughout all age groups. Severe and fatal cases occur at all ages. The incidence and the severity of the disease are approximately the same among both the indigenous population and newcomers.

In hyperendemic areas, on the other hand, *P. falciparum* is the predominant parasite. Children up to two years of age have a high incidence of acute disease and show recurring attacks of severe malaria accompanied by high parasitemia and a heavy mortality rate. Nearly all severe and fatal cases occur in childhood. Sickness is universal and intense during the early years of life, declining in the older age groups as tolerance to the plasmodia is established. In such areas adult native survivors of the universal childhood infection are relatively healthy while nonimmune newcomers rapidly succumb unless adequately protected or treated.

Epidemic malaria cannot occur among the population indigenous to a hyperendemic region. This is obvious since the surviving population has acquired satisfactory immunity to the local strains of plasmodia. Epidemics do occur, however, in areas of low endemicity when transmission suddenly becomes intense. Furthermore, epidemic malaria is a constant threat to incoming nonimmune population groups irrespective of the existing level of endemicity among the indigenous population with whom they come in contact. It can be avoided only by the continuous application of effective methods of control.

THE INSECT VECTOR. The definitive host of the plasmodia is the anopheline mosquito. There are over 200 known species of anophelines of which only some fifty have been incriminated as vectors of malaria.

Determination of the particular species which are or may be efficient vectors and estimation of their relative abundance in an area are essential functions of the malarial survey. The marked variation in the capacity among different species to transmit the disease depends upon certain fundamental biologic differences. Certain individuals within each species are physiologically unsuitable hosts and the plasmodia cannot complete their development in them. Some anophelines are domestic in behavior, breeding and remaining in the vicinity of human habitations. Others are forest dwellers, breeding in and rarely leaving the jungle. Many anophelines feed almost exclusively on animal rather than human blood while others feed with equal frequency on blood from man or animals. Certain ones remain in or close to dwellings after obtaining a blood meal, while others immediately leave the human environment. Similarly there are great variations in flight range. Some anophelines are weak fliers and travel only short distances while the normal flight range of others may be several miles.

Malaria tends to be a "place" disease with highest incidence close to important mosquito-breeding areas. Therefore the location and description of such areas are likewise essential functions of the survey. In general anopheline larvae require clear water with an adequate content of algae for optimal growth. The typical habitats of different species vary greatly. Some species seek only sunlit water; others flourish in shade. Certain ones cannot utilize water containing even small amounts of salt, while others thrive in brackish water containing 40 to 60 per cent sea water. Some species utilize streams or seepage areas, others only swamps and marshes. Such variations in specific habitats form the basis for so-called naturalistic control methods which are designed to alter the natural characteristics of a breeding area, rendering it unsuitable for larval development.

The final evaluation of the importance of a particular anopheline species as a vector of malaria is based upon certain specific procedures.

1. EPIDEMIOLOGIC INDEX. This expression represents the attempt to establish a significant correlation between the prevalence of a particular species of anopheline and the transmission of the disease. It is seldom a practicable procedure and rarely affords dependable evidence.

2. EXPERIMENTAL INDEX OF INFECTION. Laboratory-raised female anophelines of a given species are fed upon a human gametocyte carrier. They are subsequently dissected and the percentage showing oocysts on the stomach wall and sporozoites in the salivary glands is noted. This procedure may give accurate information of the biologic suitability of the particular anopheline to serve as a definitive host for the *Plasmodium*. It does not provide information as to the importance of the species as a *natural* vector. A number of species, of no

practical importance in the transmission of malaria, may nevertheless yield a high index of experimental infection.

3. NATURAL INDEX OF INFECTION. Large numbers of captured
anopheline mosquitoes are dissected and the per cent incidence of
oocyst formation on the stomach wall and of sporozoite infection in
the salivary glands is noted. The incidence of salivary gland infection
provides the more important information, for in certain species
oocysts do not often undergo complete development and hence the
insect is of no importance as a vector. A salivary gland index as low
as 0.1 per cent or even lower nevertheless indicates an important
transmitter when the species is very abundant. Much higher rates
may be encountered exceptionally. In the course of epidemic malaria
in northeastern Brazil the salivary gland infection rate of *Anopheles
gambiae* reached 30.2 per cent.

4. THE PRECIPITIN TEST. The precipitin test applied to the gut
contents of engorged mosquitoes provides a useful means of distinguishing between androphilic and zoophilic species (p. 847).

**Pathology** Malaria is accompanied by the destruction of enormous
numbers of red blood cells, both parasitized and nonparasitized, and
a consequent increase in the bilirubin content of the blood. The
hemolysis may be so intense in *P. falciparum* infections as to cause
hemoglobinuria and blackwater fever. Severe grades of anemia may
be produced and reticulocyte crisis may follow upon effective therapy.
In chronic cases, however, the anemia may be refractory. At least
three factors appear to contribute to this—continued destruction of
erythrocytes, failure of the liver to reconvert liberated iron and, in
*P. vivax* infections, the selective parasitization of reticulocytes.

In chronic malaria there is characteristically a moderate leukopenia with an absolute increase in the number of monocytes.

Malarial pigment is taken up by circulating polymorphonuclear
leukocytes and monocytes and is deposited in the reticulo-endothelial
cells of the viscera. One of the striking features of the gross pathology
in patients who have died after prolonged infection is a slaty or
blackish pigmentation of the organs, especially the spleen, liver and
brain.

The spleen varies in size, color and consistency depending upon
the duration and severity of the infection. Usually it is more or less
enlarged and dark in color. It may reach a weight of 1000 gm. (four
times normal) or even larger. In acute malaria it is congested and
soft; spontaneous or traumatic rupture may occur. In chronic cases
there is fibrous overgrowth of the connective tissue of the capsule
and the trabeculae (Fig. 141). There is compensatory hyperplasia of
the reticulo-endothelium and the splenic phagocytes are filled with
pigment. In fatal cases there may be hemorrhagic areas in the pulp,
thrombi in the arterioles and capillaries, and areas of infarction.
Torsion of the pedicle may occur.

The liver is usually somewhat enlarged and dark in color. On
microscopic examination the endothelial and Kupffer cells are seen to

be packed with black pigment. The cells of the parenchyma may contain considerable amounts of hemosiderin and show cloudy swelling and vacuolization. Occasionally necrotic foci are seen in the portal areas and in the central zones of the liver lobules (Fig. 142).

The brain is frequently leaden colored due to the malaria pigment

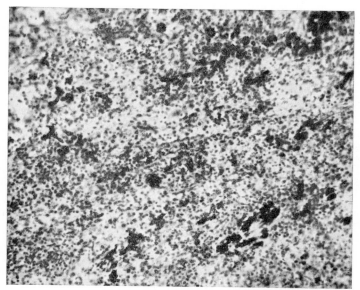

Fig. 141. Agglutinated pigment granules in spleen in chronic malaria.

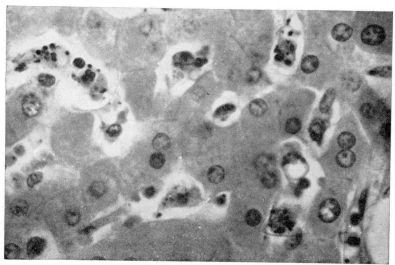

Fig. 142. Malaria pigment in Kupffer cells of liver.

and there may be extensive capillary plugging by masses of parasitized red cells. In fatal cases of cerebral malaria granulomatous lesions are frequently seen in the white matter (Figs. 143, 144).

Toxic acute focal or interstitial myocarditis with capillary obstruction in the myocardium may also be present in fatal cases. In the presence of prominent gastro-intestinal symptoms, lesions in the stomach and intestines are not uncommon. These consist of punctate hemorrhages, capillary obstruction by parasitized erythrocytes, necrosis of epithelium and occasionally hemorrhage into the lumen.

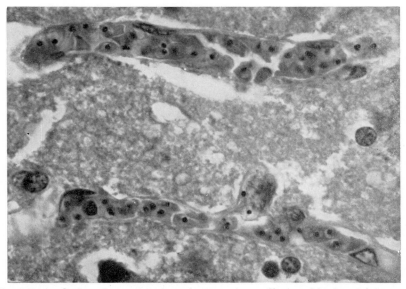

Fig. 143. Agglutinated parasitized erythrocytes in capillaries of brain—*falciparum* malaria.

The bone marrow may reveal large numbers of parasitized cells and considerable amounts of malarial pigment.

Acute malaria may be associated with profound disturbances of body chemistry. There is reduction of the total plasma proteins with reversal of the albumin-globulin ratio but usually not above unity. Water balance is frequently disturbed and the viscosity of the blood altered. In certain instances there is sufficient interference with renal function to produce varying degrees of nitrogen retention and uremia.

**Clinical Characteristics** The clinical phenomena accompanying infection by *P. falciparum* differ greatly in their evolution, and in the hazard to the infected individual, from those accompanying infection by *P. vivax, P. malariae* or *P. ovale.*

*Falciparum* malaria, often called malignant tertian, is always dangerous and may be fatal. The other types, although capable of producing severe illness, are commonly free from dangerous complications and grave menace to life. The term *benign tertian* is therefore often applied to infections by *P. vivax*. This difference, in part at least, is due to special characteristics of *P. falciparum*. Its capacity to invade both mature erythrocytes and reticulocytes is probably directly related to the intense and rapidly increasing parasitemia which accompanies this infection. Furthermore the infected red blood cells tend to agglutinate and to adhere to capillary endothelium, forming

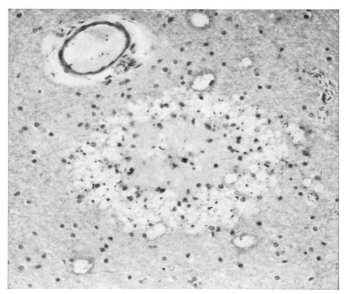

Fig. 144. Early phase of malarial granuloma in brain: necrosis and edema.

emboli and thrombi which produce areas of local anoxemia and ischemia in the viscera.

The intrinsic incubation period for both benign and malignant tertian malaria is usually eleven to thirteen days but its duration is four to five weeks in quartan malaria. Prodromes consisting of malaise, muscle pains, headache, anorexia and slight fever may exist for a few days before the onset of the acute phenomena. In many instances, however, the initial attack comes on abruptly without prodromes.

VIVAX AND QUARTAN MALARIA. The classic clinical picture of malaria with its alternation of "good" and "bad" days is much more the exception than the rule. Even in *P. vivax* infections the initial clinical attack seldom exhibits tertian fever at the outset; on the contrary there are usually two groups of parasites out of phase with one another and these, maturing on alternate days, produce daily, or quotidian, rather than tertian fever. Later one group drops out and the release of a new generation of parasites occurs every forty-eight hours. Only then does the fever become tertian.

The typical paroxysms of benign tertian and quartan malaria are identical except for the difference in periodicity. The onset is abrupt and frequently initiated by a rigor which may vary from a slight subjective chilliness to a frank chill accompanied by a sensation of extreme cold although the temperature meanwhile rises rapidly to 104° to 106° F. The pulse is rapid and of small volume. Polyuria, nausea and vomiting are common. After twenty to sixty minutes the hot stage begins, accompanied at first by relief from the sense of intense cold, but shortly followed, however, by an increasing and severe headache and a sensation of intense heat. At this stage the face is flushed and the pulse full. Epigastric discomfort, nausea and vomiting are more prominent. There is frequently mild delirium and although the temperature does not remain long at the fastigium, the sweating stage, ushered in by the appearance of moisture on the previously dry skin, increases to a profuse diaphoresis of the entire body. With this change the temperature falls rapidly and the pulse returns to normal. This is frequently followed by sleep after which the individual awakes somewhat exhausted but otherwise feeling well. The sweating stage lasts two to three hours and the entire paroxysm eight to twelve hours.

During the paroxysm there is a moderate leukocytosis while in the afebrile period leukopenia with an increase in the number of large mononuclears is usual.

In quartan malaria the attacks occur every seventy-two hours. The rise of temperature is less abrupt, the fall more rapid and the total duration of the paroxysm is usually four to five hours.

Falciparum Malaria. The onset of malignant tertian malaria is frequently insidious, the individual complaining of gradually increasing headache, of gastro-intestinal symptoms, or of a clinical complex suggestive of influenza and frequently misdiagnosed unless examination of the blood is carried out. In other instances it is abrupt and dramatic. Characteristically there are: a sensation of chilliness rather than a frank chill; a prolonged and intensified hot stage; and lack of the marked terminal sweating, with its accompanying drop in temperature, characteristically observed in *P. vivax* infections. The fever curve frequently shows prolongation of the fastigium, often with primary fall and secondary rise, before returning to or toward normal. This double peaked elevation is characteristic when it is observed. Frequently, however, the fever is continuous or remittent instead of intermittent. During the periods of remission there is little or no return of the sense of well-being. Commonly the tertian periodicity of the infection is indicated by exacerbation of a continuous fever. Defervescence in *falciparum* malaria frequently occurs by lysis rather than by crisis. In those instances in which the fever curve is intermittent the paroxysm often lasts twenty to thirty-six hours. These variations in the fever curve are to be explained by the phenomena of anticipation and retardation of the events of schizogony as a result of which the new generation of parasites is released over a prolonged period.

Prostration is more marked and the tendency to delirium greater than in benign tertian and quartan infections. Nausea and vomiting are prominent in most instances and the spleen is generally palpable and tender. It is frequently difficult to demonstrate the parasites in the peripheral blood on the day of the paroxysm and it may be necessary to make repeated smears at intervals of several hours in order to find them.

PERNICIOUS TYPES. *Falciparum* malaria is notorious for its tendency to produce, suddenly and without warning, severe and dangerous types of disease to which the term, *pernicious* or *malignant* malaria have been applied. These may be rapidly fatal if not promptly recognized and adequately treated. Several clinical types are known.

BILIOUS REMITTENT FEVER. Bilious remittent fever is the most common and the least dangerous of the pernicious forms of *falciparum* malaria. The onset is characterized by marked nausea and profuse continuous vomiting. Jaundice customarily appears about the second day, earlier than in yellow fever and later than in blackwater fever. The urine frequently contains bile pigment and yields a yellow foam test. Epigastric distress and liver tenderness are marked and hemorrhage from the stomach may occur, producing coffee-ground vomitus. The temperature tends to be high and the fever curve is usually remittent rather than continuous. Dehydration and disturbance of the alkali reserve and of mineral balance may develop rapidly.

CEREBRAL MALARIA. The onset of cerebral malaria may be sudden or gradual and the clinical picture may be varied. The patient may complain of progressively increasing headache with little or no fever and gradually lapse into coma; or a clinical picture in which there appears little cause for immediate concern may be superseded without warning by a progressive and uncontrollable rise of temperature to levels in excess of 108° F. These clinical phenomena may occur within a few hours and lead to a rapidly fatal termination. In other instances the onset may be sudden and characterized by mania or other acute psychotic manifestations. The initial stages of cerebral malaria have not infrequently been mistaken for acute alcoholism. The results of such a diagnostic error are usually disastrous.

The extensive interference with the vascular supply to the central nervous system in cerebral malaria may produce any combination of symptoms and signs indicative of severe and extensive involvement of the brain. In children convulsions are a frequent presenting symptom.

There are no constant or significant changes in the spinal fluid. The spinal fluid pressure, however, may be considerably elevated above normal. In such instances repeated lumbar drainage is an important therapeutic procedure.

ALGID MALARIA. The algid forms of *falciparum* malaria accompany extensive vascular involvement in the gastro-intestinal tract and other abdominal viscera. Profound prostration, with a tendency to fatal syncope, and marked coldness of the skin accompanied by high internal temperatures usually occur. Severe grades of hemolytic anemia may develop rapidly. Acute diarrhea unaccompanied by fever and often ending fatally has long been recognized as an algid form of pernicious malaria.

Other recognized types of algid malaria are the gastric, which is characterized by persistent vomiting, and the dysenteric, in which there is a bloody diarrhea due to extensive capillary thrombosis in the intestinal walls. The blood in the stools frequently contains immense numbers of parasites.

The general mortality for the pernicious forms of *falciparum* malaria varies between 25 and 50 per cent.

**Diagnosis**    The diagnosis of malaria is frequently difficult. It may be confused with many diseases, both cosmopolitan and tropical. This situation is inevitable in view of the pathology, which consists mainly of mechanical interference with the vascular supply in many organs of the body. Among the tropical diseases it may be confused with kala-azar, amebic liver abscess, relapsing fever and yellow fever. Among the cosmopolitan diseases it may frequently simulate typhoid fever, tuberculosis, brucellosis, influenza, pyelitis and other septic conditions including malignant endocarditis as well as acute or chronic organic disease of the central nervous system. Malaria is commonly associated with positive Wassermann and Kahn reactions.

Definitive diagnosis depends upon demonstration of the parasites. For this purpose the thick blood film is far superior to the thin film technique since in light infections it may be impossible to find plasmodia in the thin film. The thick film will yield three to four times as many positive findings and will reveal the plasmodia in 91 to 95 per cent of active clinical cases (Diagnostic Methods, pp. 810–811). It may be necessary to examine stained thin blood films for positive identification of the particular species present.

Other characteristics of the stained thin blood films may be suggestive. Leukocytes containing ingested malarial pigment may be seen. There is often a leukopenia with a relative increase of monocytes. In chronic cases a sustained submaximal reticulocyte crisis beginning four to seven days after the institution of specific therapy is suggestive.

Periodicity of the febrile curve and splenomegaly should arouse suspicion of malaria. In chronic cases, however, there may be little if any significant splenic enlargement.

In instances when it is impossible to prove the infection by the thick blood film, subcutaneous injection of 0.5 to 1 ml. 1–1000 Adrenalin may be followed by the appearance of plasmodia in the peripheral blood. Four or five smears should be made thereafter at intervals of fifteen minutes. Sternal puncture and examination of the stained marrow smear may likewise be useful. Splenic puncture is hazardous and should not be undertaken.

In view of the marked differences in severity and prognosis between *falciparum* malaria and the other forms of the disease, accurate identification of the species of *Plasmodium* is essential. The following table presents the significant differential characteristics which may be seen in the stained thin blood film:

*Table 26    Differential Characteristics of the Plasmodia of Man in Stained Thin Films*

| CHARACTERISTICS | P. falciparum | P. vivax | P. ovale | P. malariae |
|---|---|---|---|---|
| Infected erythrocyte enlarged.............. | — | + | ± | — |
| Infected erythrocyte not enlarged.......... | + | — | ± | + |
| Infected erythrocyte oval, crenated margin*.. | — | — | + | — |
| Infected erythrocyte decolorized........... | — | + | + | — |
| Infected erythrocyte, Schüffner's dots*...... | — | + | + | — |
| Infected erythrocyte, Maurer's dots*........ | + | — | — | — |
| Multiple infections in erythrocytes*........ | + | Rare | — | — |
| Parasite, all forms in peripheral blood....... | — | + | + | + |
| Parasite, large coarse rings................ | — | + | + | + |
| Parasite, double chromatin dots*.......... | + | Rare | — | — |
| Parasite, accolé forms*................... | + | Rare | — | — |
| Parasite, band forms*.................... | — | — | + | + |
| Parasite, crescentic gametocytes........... | + | — | — | — |
| Number of merozoites.................... | 8–24 | 12–24 | 8–12 | 6–12 |

* Not invariable but suggestive when seen.

Because of the importance of the thick film in the differential diagnosis of human malaria the characteristics of the three principal species are summarized in Table 27.

**Prognosis**    The prognosis for recovery from the primary attack of malaria due to *P. vivax*, *P. malariae* or *P. ovale* is excellent. *Falciparum* malaria carries a good prognosis if adequately treated; untreated its mortality is sometimes 25 per cent. Radical cure of malaria due to *P. falciparum* and *P. vivax*, in the great majority of cases, is possible with proper use of the new antimalarial drugs. The prognosis with respect to relapses of infections by *P. malariae* has not yet been evaluated.

**Treatment**    The recommended drugs fall into three classes: for the treatment of acute clinical malaria—*chloroquine, Amodiaquin* and *quinine;* for the prevention of relapses of vivax malaria—*primaquine;* for suppressive treatment—*chloroquine, Amodiaquin, chlorguanide, pyrimethamine,* and *quinacrine.*

*Chloroquine.* Synonyms: Aralen, Nivaquine. The drug is available in tablets for oral administration, each 0.5 gm. equivalent to 0.3 gm. of base, and in ampules 3 ml. and 1 ml., each containing 50 mg.

*Table 27   Differential Diagnosis of Malarial Parasites in Stained Thick Blood Films**

| STAGE OF PARASITE | *Plasmodium falciparum* | *Plasmodium vivax* | *Plasmodium malariae* | COMMENTS |
|---|---|---|---|---|
| Small trophozoite (early ring) | Small size rings, with small chromatin dot and delicate, scanty cytoplasm. Frequently rings have double chromatin dots. Tendency toward large number of rings. Many ring forms with no older stages—practically certain to be *falciparum* infection. Diagnosis on small number of rings may often be assisted by finding distinguishing gametocyte, though this stage is not necessarily present. | Larger, heavier, ring form than in *falciparum*, often with variety of cytoplasmic pattern and irregularities in shape. Usually older stages of the parasite can be found also. | Ring is likely to be heavy, with large dot of chromatin and small amount of cytoplasm, which is often "filled in," without a vacuole. Pigment forms early and may appear as haze in cytoplasm of this stage. Rings practically always associated with older forms. The ring phase is brief, so this stage is not found as often as older stages. | Ring forms often not complete circle—may be "swallow" forms, "exclamation mark," "comma" forms, or "interrupted rings." When rings only are present and number is small, it is practically impossible to differentiate species. |
| Growing trophozoite | Heavy large ring forms—resemble young rings of *vivax*. Sometimes show pigment grains or haze rather clearly in cytoplasm. | Stage usually ameboid in appearance, with large variety of shapes. Cytoplasm frequently fragmented and arranged irregularly in cluster of varying sized pieces or streamers, about or close to a large chromatin mass. Small yellowish brown pigment granules scattered through parts of the cytoplasm. This is the most characteristic stage of *vivax*. Frequently other younger or older stages accompany this one. | Small, usually rounded compact forms, "like marbles in a ring." Profuse, heavy, dark, large-grained pigment. Forms frequently so solid that chromatin seems buried in the mass. This stage and the one that follows are the commonest forms of this parasite seen. | In heavily stained films and in films which have been kept for several days before staining, the "ghost" of the enlarged host cell and persistence of Schüffner's stippling or a pinkness remaining from the stippling, may assist in diagnosis of *vivax*. |
| Large trophozoite | Ring vacuole lost or almost lost. Parasite quite small and compact, cytoplasm often quite pale, irregularly circular or oval. One large chromatin dot. Pigment in blurred mass or small, very dark clump or clumps. Stage is usually found only when the infection is intense and usually accompanied by numbers of ring-form trophozoites. | Frequently quite solid and dark staining. More or less irregular in outline, possibly with one or more vacuoles. Fine brown pigment scattered throughout the cytoplasm. May be confused with macrogametocyte. | Compact, dark, larger than "growing" stages. Sometimes in thinner portion of the smear spreads to normal size. Profuse, fairly coarse, dark brown pigment—often masking the chromatin. May be confused with "rounded up" *falciparum* gametocyte or with gametocyte of *malariae*. | On rare occasions Maurer's dots have been observed in thick films of *falciparum*. The infrequently found stages of *falciparum* are, of course, more readily found in thick films. Band forms have tendency to become rounded in thick films of *malariae*—except perhaps in very thin edge of smear. |
| Schizont (presegmenting) | Stage not often seen and is usually accompanied by large numbers of growing trophozoites when present. Parasite is very small. Contains 2 or more divisions of chromatin and very little cytoplasm (often pale) in which there is located one or more small, dense blocks of very dark pigment. | Irregular or compact clusters of chromatin divisions, often dark reddish-purple in color. Cytoplasm in irregular broken masses and wisps, containing light brown pigment granules which are clumping in spots. Usually accompanied by other stages. May be confused with same stage of *malariae*. | Much like *vivax* of the same stage except that parasites are often smaller with darker, larger pigment granules. Often so compact that internal structure is difficult to define. Usually accompanied by other stages. May be confused with presegmenting schizonts of *vivax*. | Schizonts are much like thin film forms of same stages—more compact, smaller in thicker portions of smear. This is most difficult stage (except infrequent ring forms) on which to diagnose species. |

| | | | |
|---|---|---|---|
| Mature schizont | Seldom seen except in severe cases. Always associated with many small trophozoites. Usually contains around 20 or more tiny merozoites clustered around a small, very dark, pigment mass. | Usually contains around 16 merozoites which are individually larger than those of *falciparum*. Usually relatively larger than other species. Nearly always associated with other stages. Not so often found as other stages. | Most distinctive stage of *malariae* in thick film. Often found in large numbers—usually with trophozoites or presegmenting forms or both. About 8 merozoites each with large chromatin dot and small amount of cytoplasm—may be compact or clearly separated. Frequently the chromatin and pigment only are seen, the chromatin dots being bare and well separated. The dark heavy pigment is more often concentrated, though sometimes dispersed. · Usually smaller than same stage in thin film. |
| Young gametocyte | Sometimes long, slender and pointed, with pigment scattered to the ends. Usually associated with many trophozoites. | When found is a small, compact, usually rounded parasite, with one chromatin mass which is often in the center of cytoplasm and frequently has unstained area around chromatin mass. Sex is almost impossible to determine. | Same as *vivax* except that parasite is even less frequently found and resembles compact trophozoite so closely that differentiation is absolutely impossible. |
| Mature gametocyte | Differentiation of sex is difficult or impossible. As "crescent" or "sausage" shapes, may be quite diagnostic of species. In thicker portion of smear may take on oval or rounded, somewhat eroded appearance, which may be confused with *malariae* trophozoite or gametocyte. Oftimes may be distinguished by difference in amount and appearance of pigment or by pink or red "flag", protruding from the edge of the parasite. May be accompanied by ring form trophozoites or appear alone and infrequently. Often appears in "showers." | Macrogametocyte is larger, as a rule, than in other species; pigment is light, delicate, well dispersed through nonvacuolated cytoplasm. Except in thin edge of film cannot be differentiated from some mature trophozoites of same species. Microgametocyte often distinguishable as large blob of chromatin (varying from pink to purplish red) surrounded by halo of pale or colorless cytoplasm in which pigment granules are more or less evenly dispersed. Other stages of the parasite can usually be found. | As a rule, few in number, somewhat smaller than *vivax*, otherwise have the same distinguishing features except that pigment is coarser and darker. May resemble rounded *falciparum* gametocytes. |

* Courtesy of Aimee Wilcox, Laboratory of Tropical Diseases, Microbiological Institute, National Institutes of Health, in "Manual for The Microscopical Diagnosis of Malaria in Man." 2nd ed., 1950; and the American Public Health Association, Standard Methods Committee on Diagnostic Procedures and Reagents: "Diagnostic Procedures and Reagents." 2nd ed., New York, 1945.

equivalent to 40 mg. of base for intramuscular and intravenous use.

The drug is a 4-aminoquinoline, a white crystalline powder with bitter taste, freely soluble in water.

Absorption is relatively complete and rapid when taken by mouth. It is stored in the tissues, excreted slowly and does not discolor the skin. Chloroquine is usually well tolerated in the dosages used clinically. No serious toxic effects have been observed. In certain individuals it may cause mild transient headache, visual disturbances, pruritus, trivial gastro-intestinal complaints, psychic stimulation and rarely a lichen planus–like eruption. When given intravenously undiluted, there is a fall of systolic blood pressure with little or no change in the diastolic pressure. When well diluted and given slowly no significant change occurs. Excretion is accelerated by acidification of the urine.

Chloroquine is highly active against the erythrocytic forms of the plasmodia and is approximately three times as effective as quinacrine against *P. vivax* and *P. falciparum*. It acts more slowly against *P. malariae* but is more effective than either quinine or quinacrine.

It is the drug of choice for the treatment of acute malaria. In the majority of cases fever is controlled within twenty-four hours and thick blood films usually become negative in from forty-eight to seventy-two hours. It will terminate infection by *P. falciparum* and, when given in conjunction with primaquine, it will prevent relapses of *vivax* malaria in the great majority of cases.

*Amodiaquin.* Synonyms: Camoquin, Cam-aqi. The drug is prepared as the hydrochloride and is distributed in tablets each containing 0.2 gm. of Amodiaquin base.

It is a 4-aminoquinoline, a yellow crystalline powder having a bitter taste. It forms a 5 per cent solution in water at room temperature, and it is rapidly absorbed from the gastro-intestinal tract. No toxic effects have been reported, although long continued administration in amounts considerably above the recommended therapeutic dosage may be accompanied by loss of energy, insomnia, epigastric discomfort and anorexia.

Amodiaquin acts rapidly against the asexual forms of the plasmodia, commonly causing their disappearance from the peripheral blood in from twenty-four to forty-eight hours with accompanying cessation of fever. It is much less active against the gametocytes of *P. vivax* and *P. malariae* and has little or no action against the gametocytes of *P. falciparum*.

Good results have been reported in the treatment of acute malaria using a single dose of 0.6 to 1.0 gm. for adults. The recommended dosage for children is 10 mg. per kilogram of body weight.

Amodiaquin has likewise proved to be an efficient suppressive agent. For this purpose a single dose of 0.6 gm. taken once every two weeks has proved sufficient under most conditions.

*Quinine.* This is a general protoplasmic poison. It is rapidly absorbed from the gastrointestinal tract; 60 to 70 per cent is oxidized in the body and the remainder rapidly excreted in the urine. Indications of poisoning appear when the blood level rises to about 10 mg. per 100 ml.

In therapeutic doses it has little effect on the circulatory system. In excessive dosage it produces an initial rise in pulse rate and blood pressure followed by a depression of both. When given intravenously in too large a dosage or too quickly, rapid progressive fall of blood pressure occurs with the appearance of circulatory collapse due to cardiac depression and vasodilatation.

Cinchonism is the expression of toxic action of quinine upon the central nervous system. It is characterized by mental depression, giddiness, headache, sense of fullness in the head, tinnitus, deafness, amblyopia and occasional blindness. There may be mental confusion and somnolence as well. True idiosyncrasy to quinine results in the symptoms of cinchonism after small doses which are well within the normal therapeutic range.

*Primaquine Diphosphate.* This is an 8-aminoquinoline chemically related to pamaquine. It is an orange crystalline solid with bitter taste, slightly soluble in water, and is supplied in tablets, 26.5 mg. of the salt being equivalent to 15 mg. of the base.

Like paraquine, the drug has a dangerous toxic potential. In overdosage or in susceptible individuals it produces severe hemolytic reactions. The colored race is particularly susceptible. Anemia, methemoglobinemia and leukopenia should be watched for during therapy by repeated blood and urine examinations. Primaquine should be discontinued immediately if signs suggestive of hemolytic anemia occur such as darkening of the urine, or significant fall of hemoglobin or of the erythrocyte count. Quinacrine appears to increase the toxicity. The two drugs should never be used together and primaquine should not be given to a patient who has received quinacrine until the latter drug has been excreted.

Primaquine is active against the presumed exo-erythrocytic stage of *P. vivax.* It is relatively ineffective against the erythrocytic forms of the plasmodia. Its use is restricted to the prevention of relapses of *vivax* malaria.

*Chlorguanide Hydrochloride.* Synonyms: proguanyl, Guanatol, Paludrine. Chlorguanide hydrochloride is a colorless, bitter pyrimidine compound which is rapidly absorbed from the gastro-intestinal tract and is excreted in the feces and urine. There are no significant toxic effects at therapeutic dosage levels.

Chlorguanide is a slowly acting schizonticide which inhibits chromatin division. It is not gametocidal but it inhibits the development of female gametocytes in the mosquito, thus interrupting the exogenous cycle of the plasmodia. Resistant strains of plasmodia are produced when the drug is used at suboptimal levels.

It is an effective therapeutic agent but slower in action than chloroquine, quinine or quinacrine. The effectiveness, however, varies between different geographic areas. In general, the fever is controlled and trophozoites disappear from the peripheral blood in the course of forty-eight to seventy-two hours. In many instances, but not in all, a single course of therapy terminates infection by *P. falciparum.*

It is not the drug of choice for the treatment of acute clinical malaria, especially since the serious complications are brought under control only slowly.

*Pyrimethamine.* Synonyms: Daraprim, Malocide. Pyrimethamine is a diaminopyrimidine chemically related to chlorguanide. It is a tasteless, odorless, freely soluble white powder. The drug is concentrated in the liver, spleen, brain and bone marrow. It is entirely free from toxic or unpleasant side effects at recommended dosage levels. When administered to experimental animals in amounts far exceeding the therapeutic levels it produces megaloblastic changes in the marrow, inhibition of leukopoiesis, reduction of erythrocyte and leukocyte counts, atrophy of lymphatic tissue and degenerative changes in the intestinal epithelium.

It is a slowly acting schizonticide. It inhibits the development of female gametocytes of *P. falciparum* in the mosquito. When used in suboptimal dosage resistant strains of plasmodia are produced.

Pyrimethamine is not a preferred drug for the treatment of acute malaria. Although a single dose of 0.25 to 0.5 mg. per kilogram of body weight causes disappearance of parasites from the blood, the speed of action in controlling fever and parasitemia is less than that of chloroquine. Furthermore, in certain areas it has not proved effective against the local strains of *P. falciparum.*

It is a potent malaria suppressive for nonimmunes and has been shown to bring malaria transmission to a virtual standstill when given in single doses of 25 mg. weekly. The fact that it is tasteless and may be given in syrup makes it particularly useful for children (12.5 mg. weekly) and for mass suppression.

*Quinacrine Hydrochloride.* Synonyms: Atabrine, mepacrine. Quinacrine is a yellow acridine dye with bitter taste, soluble in water. The dihydrochloride, Atabrine, is absorbed rapidly, deposited in the tissues especially the liver and gallbladder, and causes a yellow discoloration of the skin. Excretion is slow. The drug is present in the breast milk of nursing mothers.

Quinacrine is usually well tolerated although in certain individuals it acts as a gastro-intestinal irritant causing epigastric pain, nausea, vomiting and diarrhea. These symptoms are usually transient phenomena which may be controlled by giving the drug with food or sweetened fluids. With rare exceptions quinacrine may be taken over long periods of time without ill effect. Rarely dermatitis occurs. This may take the form of atypical lichen planus, eczematoid or exfoliative lesions. There may be leukoplakia or pigmentation of the mucous membrane of the mouth. Quinacrine should not be administered in conjunction with pamaquine or primaquine because of the danger of acute hemolytic crises.

The drug is active against the erythrocytic forms of the plasmodia. Although a single course of therapy will commonly terminate infections by *P. falciparum* it is not as effective as chloroquine. It does not affect the relapse rate of *vivax* or *malariae* malaria and when taken as a suppressive will completely prevent *falciparum* malaria.

It is an efficient suppressive agent when taken in dosage of 0.1 gm. daily. Clinical attacks begin to appear about two weeks after discontinuing the medication.

*Pamaquine.* Synonyms: Plasmochin, Plasmoquine. Pamaquine is an 8-aminoquinoline which is rapidly absorbed when taken by mouth and excreted in the urine. It regularly causes some degree of methemoglobinemia and may precipitate serious hemolytic crises especially if given in conjunction with quinacrine or primaquine. It is more toxic for Negroes than whites.

It has been used in the past to destroy the gametocytes of *P. falciparum* and to limit the relapses of *vivax* malaria. It has been displaced by the newer antimalarial drugs. It is not recommended, especially in view of the narrow margin of safety between the therapeutic and toxic dosage.

DEFINITIVE TREATMENT OF CLINICAL MALARIA. GENERAL. *Falciparum* malaria in the nonimmune individual is a highly dangerous infection which requires immediate and effective therapy. The grave complications presented by the pernicious forms of the disease may develop with great rapidity and are commonly accompanied by high mortality rates. Acute *falciparum* malaria and the paroxysms of *vivax* malaria are frequently accompanied by profuse nausea and vomiting. Particularly, in the former, it may be necessary to initiate treatment by parenteral therapy. This, however, should be superseded as early as is practicable by oral medication.

1. Oral treatment by chloroquine: 2.5 gm. (1.5 gm. of base) in three days:
    Initial dose 1.0 gm.;
    0.5 gm. six to eight hours later;
    0.5 gm. on each of two consecutive days.
    Infants up to one year: 0.25 gm.;
    0.25 gm. six hours later.
    Children two to five years: 0.5 gm.;
    0.25 gm. eight hours later.
    Children six to ten years: 0.5 gm.:
    0.25 gm. two doses at intervals of eight hours.
    Children eleven to fifteen years: 0.75 gm.;
    0.25 gm. eight hours later;
    0.25 gm. twenty-four hours later.
2. Treatment by quinine: 15 gm. in seven days:
    Quinine sulfate 1.0 gm. three times daily after meals for two consecutive days. Followed by 0.6 gm. three times daily after meals for five days.

Dosage for children should be reduced in proportion to the age.

3. Parenteral therapy: The drug of choice is chloroquine dihydrochloride (Aralen). This may be given intramuscularly in individual doses up to 3 ml., 50 mg. of the salt equivalent to 40 mg. of chloroquine base, or it may be administered intravenously in slow infusion in physiologic saline solution. The latter route is preferable. As much as 400 mg. of the base may be given to an adult in a single infusion of 500 ml. of saline solution.

Intravenous quinine: The parenteral administration of quinine should not be used if chloroquine dihydrochloride is available because of the risk of toxic reaction. Quinine dihydrochloride: 0.6 gm. in 300 to 400 ml. of sterile physiologic saline solution may be given slowly intravenously. During the injection indications of toxic effect—rising pulse rate and falling blood pressure—should be watched for and treatment discontinued immediately if they appear. This treatment may be repeated every six to eight hours if necessary until the patient is able to take medication by mouth.

Parenteral treatment should be resorted to in the presence of the serious complications of malaria, or in a severly ill patient when vomiting makes oral therapy impracticable. It should be seriously considered for the treatment of any *falciparum* infection in which 5 per cent or more of the red blood cells are parasitized.

PREVENTION OF RELAPSES OF VIVAX MALARIA. Relapses of *vivax* malaria may be prevented in the great majority of cases by the standard course of treatment of the acute attack using chloroquine and concurrent administration of primaquine diphosphate 26.5 mg. daily for 14 consecutive days. Patients receiving this treatment should be under observation and watched for evidence of hemolytic anemia, an imperative indication for discontinuing medication. Particular caution is required in the case of colored patients.

The dosage of primaquine has not been determined for children and its use should be restricted to adults at the present time.

SUPPRESSIVE TREATMENT. Although prevention of infection is not possible, clinical attacks of *vivax* and *malariae* malaria can be held in abeyance for prolonged periods of time by the administration of various antimalarial drugs. However, following cessation of medication, clinical attack due to infection by *P. vivax* and *P. malariae* begin to occur after ten days or two weeks. In the case of infections by *P. falciparum* certain of the available drugs will eradicate the infection without the development of clinical malaria. The following routines for suppressive treatment are recommended:

1. Chloroquine 0.5 gm. weekly, to be taken on the same day each week.
2. Chlorguanide 0.3 gm. weekly, to be taken on the same day each week.
3. Amodiaquin, adult dose 0.6 gm., dose for children 10 mg. per kilogram of body weight, to be taken in a single dose every fourteen days.
4. Pyrimethamine (Daraprim), adult dose 25 mg., for children 12.5 mg., weekly, to be taken on the same day each week. This drug has the advantage of being tasteless and can be given dissolved in syrup.
5. Quinacrine 0.1 gm. daily. Suppressive treatment should be begun two weeks before the probable first exposure.

To be effective, suppressive treatment must be taken regularly. Break-through of clinical activity will occur when administration is irregular or insufficient in amount. It may likewise occur in the presence of excessive fatigue, acute infections, trauma and hemorrhage or exposure to high altitudes since these conditions tend to activate latent malaria.

## Blackwater Fever

Blackwater fever is one of the most dangerous complications of malaria. It is characterized by prostrating chills, profuse vomiting, early jaundice, the passage of dark red to black urine, and a rapidly developing anemia. It is essentially an acute intravascular hemolysis with hemoglobinemia, hemoglobinuria and renal insufficiency.

**Etiology** The great majority of cases of blackwater fever occur in the course of demonstrable infection by *P. falciparum*. Although *P. vivax* alone has been reported occasionally, double infection in these instances has not been ruled out. Irregular or inadequate suppressive or therapeutic dosage with antimalarial drugs are factors of extreme importance in many cases. There is a high coefficient of correlation between the last dose of quinine and the appearance within fifteen hours of hemoglobinuria. Many cases have been reported after administration of quinacrine and of pamaquine. However, the disease may occur in persons who have never taken any of these medications.

The mechanism of the sudden intravascular hemolysis is not understood. It is possible that immunity reactions may play a part since blackwater fever is apt to occur in individuals who have lost immunity, or premunition, to a particular strain of *P. falciparum* if they acquire an additional infection by the same strain. However, it is unlikely that the hemolysis depends upon an antigen-antibody reaction. Hemolytic strains of plasmodia have not been found. There is some experimental evidence in support of the hypothesis that the process may represent an imbalance between a lysin present in normal tissue and inhibitory substances in the plasma together with some abnormality of the erythrocytes.

**Epidemiology**   Blackwater fever occurs predominantly in hyperendemic areas of *falciparum* malaria, particularly during the rainy season when transmission is high. It is not necessarily associated with long residence, and observations during and since World War II indicate that dark-skinned races have little if any more natural immunity than the white race.

Among white British forces in Africa the majority of cases occurred between eight and eighteen months after arrival. In native African troops the rates for blackwater fever per 10,000 of strength increased progressively from 0.86 in 1941 to 32.40 in 1945. There was no suppressive treatment but other control measures presumably reduced malaria transmission. The increased prevalence of the condition was attributed to loss of premunition due to decreased frequency of, but not freedom from, bites of infected mosquitoes. The disease has likewise been encountered more frequently among African children. This is associated with more widespread but irregular use of suppressive treatment.

**Pathology**   Sudden destruction of red blood cells occurs and large amounts of hemoglobin are released. Although the osmotic fragility of the erythrocytes is not altered, there is abnormal fragility to lysolecithin, and the red blood cells have a reduced survival time when transfused into a normal individual. Erythrocytes from a normal donor when transfused into a case of acute blackwater fever are lysed as rapidly as the patient's own cells.

The mechanism for the disposal of blood pigment is overloaded. Hemoglobin, methemalbumin and hemobilirubin accumulate in the plasma. When the renal threshold is reached hemoglobinuria appears and methemoglobin and bile pigments are present in the urine.

Renal insufficiency, anuria and azotemia, in the past, have been incorrectly attributed to precipitation of hemoglobin and its products in an acid medium causing obstruction of renal tubules. Renal anoxia and ischemia are probably of great importance in reducing glomerular filtration and tubular re-absorption. Dehydration increases the hazard of renal failure.

The pathologic changes in the viscera are predominantly those of chronic malaria. In addition, the liver may show either cloudy swelling or necrosis of parenchymal cells, particularly in the regions of the central veins.

Discoloration and granular degeneration of the epithelium lining the renal tubules occur. Granular eosinophilic material may be observed within the straight and collecting tubules (Fig. 145).

**Symptomatology**   Blackwater fever presents three cardinal symptoms—hemoglobinuria, fever and jaundice. The onset is usually sudden with very severe chill, marked prostration, pain over the region of the kidneys and a rapid rise of temperature to 104° or 105° F. The fever may be continuous or remittent and rather profuse sweating is apt to accompany drops of temperature. Severe nausea and vomiting accompanied by epigastric distress usually appear early and may be continuous and serious. Jaundice appears within a few hours after the onset and may become intense if the hemolysis is extensive or long continued. Not infrequently the onset of symptoms is accompanied by the desire to void and the urine specimen presents the appearance characteristic of the disease. The pulse is usually rapid, feeble and of low tension. Pallor proportionate to the

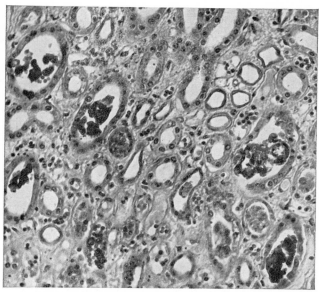

Fig. 145. Kidney in blackwater fever showing hemoglobin casts in distal convoluted tubules and degeneration and regeneration of tubular epithelium.

degree of anemia rapidly becomes apparent and the red blood count may fall by as much as two million within a period of twenty-four hours.

The clinical course may terminate after one such abbreviated episode or there may be recurring hemolytic crises, or the process may be continuous, extending over several days in the course of which the fever, hemolysis and hemoglobinuria continue.

**Prognosis**   The general mortality rate is 25 to 50 per cent. In approximately half of the fatal cases death results from renal failure. Marked and persistent vomiting and hiccough are unfavorable signs as are, likewise, a rising curve of the blood urea and a falling urinary output. One attack of blackwater fever seems to predispose to subsequent attacks.

**Diagnosis**   The occurrence of hemoglobinuria, fever and jaundice in an individual known to have had malaria is strong presumptive evidence of blackwater fever. Other causes of hematuria, however, must be considered. Hemolysis due to pamaquine may be identified by the presence of methemoglobin in the erythrocytes.

It is frequently impossible to demonstrate plasmodia in the blood during an attack. Parasites are found in only 50 to 70 per cent of cases and when present they may be difficult to find after the first twenty-four hours. Failure to demonstrate plasmodia, therefore, is insufficient evidence to exclude this condition.

In addition to the characteristic color of the urine, microscopic examination reveals the presence of much amorphous sediment, occasional red blood cells and casts of various types. Albumin is present in considerable amounts.

**Treatment** Absolute rest is essential. A cardinal rule should be never to move the patient after the onset of the disease. A lower mortality rate will be obtained by the institution of limited therapy than by transportation of the patient to a hospital where all necessary facilities may be available.

FLUIDS. Dehydration increases the hazard of the disease and must be watched for especially in the presence of severe vomiting. Administration of excessive amounts of fluid in the presence of oliguria or anuria may precipitate pulmonary edema. It is desirable to maintain a daily urine output of 1200 to 1500 ml., which may require a fluid intake of 2000 to 5000 ml. Parenteral administration is frequently necessary because of vomiting. For this purpose intravenous physiologic saline with or without plasma should be used.

The bladder should be emptied completely every four hours, by catheterization if necessary, and accurate record kept of the volume of urine excreted. Samples of each voiding acidified with acetic acid should be retained in individual test tubes as a guide to the degree and persistence of hemolysis.

TRANSFUSION. Transfusion of whole blood has proved beneficial especially in cases in which there is a rapidly developing severe anemia. A procedure said to have equal or even greater value in view of the fact that red blood cells rather than plasma have been lost is the repeated administration of washed, packed erythrocytes resuspended in normal saline solution.

ANTIMALARIA THERAPY. When malaria parasites are present in the peripheral blood immediate intensive treatment with a rapidly acting plasmocidal drug is essential. The drug of choice is chloroquine dihydrochloride (Aralen). This is distributed in 3 ml. and 1 ml. ampules each containing 50 mg. of chloroquine dihydrochloride, equivalent to 40 mg. of chloroquine base. This may be administered intramuscularly or intravenously. The latter route is preferable. As much as 400 mg. of the base may be given to an adult in a single infusion of 500 ml. of physiologic saline solution. When injected slowly there is no appreciable fall in blood pressure or other toxic effect.

Quinine and quinacrine are contraindicated.

Administration of alkali in the presence of acid urine has been advocated in the past. This was based upon the erroneous concept that the oliguria and anuria were the result of the precipitation of acid hematin in the renal tubules, producing obstruction. It is now recognized that the mechanism of renal insufficiency is quite different and that administration of alkalis is of no value and may be dangerous.

Diuretics do not increase the urine output in blackwater fever and should not be used.

**Prophylaxis** In the prevention of blackwater fever, malaria prophylaxis and adequate treatment of clinical malaria, especially when due to *P. falciparum*, are essential. Recognition of the so-called *pre-blackwater state* is important. This is characterized by toxemia, slight jaundice, enlargement and tenderness of the liver and abnormally dark colored urine. In the presence of this condition hospitalization and careful antimalarial therapy are essential.

## Malaria Control

The prevention and control of malaria are accomplished by the application of five general methods which necessarily overlap in practice.

1. Protection of the individual against the bite of the anopheline mosquito.

2. Destruction of anopheline mosquitoes.

3. Control of anopheline breeding areas.

4. Suppressive drug treatment for individuals who will probably be exposed.

5. Adequate treatment of clinical cases and gametocyte carriers.

The suppressive drug treatment and the treatment of clinical malaria have been discussed previously (pp. 311–319).

**Measures for Individual Protection** The measures which are appropriate for protection of the individual against the bite of the anopheline mosquito vary depending upon the environment of the individual.

LOCALE. The situation of permanent villages and buildings as well as temporary camps is important. They should be at least one-half mile and preferably one mile distant from actual or potential breeding areas. Whenever possible they should be placed to windward of such areas.

Native villages should be avoided particularly at night since indigenous populations constitute the source of infection for newcomers.

SCREENING. All buildings should be carefully and completely screened using good quality plastic or electrogalvanized 18-mesh wire. In tropical areas close to the sea non-corrosive wire such as bronze or aluminum is preferred.

BED NETS. Good quality bed nets should be used even in screened buildings in areas where malaria is highly endemic. They must be used religiously in temporary camps and tents. The lower edge of the net must be folded carefully under the bedding so that mosquitoes cannot enter. They should not be allowed to hang free to the floor or the ground and should be inspected each evening to be sure that no mosquitoes are present inside them.

The flight time of many species of anophelines begins very shortly after sundown. Whenever possible individuals should remain within properly screened buildings or under their bed nets from sundown to sunrise.

KILLING ADULT MOSQUITOES. Control of adults is accomplished by the use of (1) quick-killing contact insecticide sprays or (2) by the application of residual type insecticides. The first may be applied by individuals as needed to rooms, bed nets, etc. Such a space type spray provides a rapid knockdown of adults through the use of such contact insecticides as pyrethrins, pyrenones, rotenone, cubé, etc. These may be applied by means of "aerosol bombs," pressure-operated paint gun sprayers or even hand-operated sprayers of the Flit-gun type, the last type being least satisfactory.

The residual type insecticide may be applied to screening on buildings, tents, other shelter used for sleeping quarters or even bed nets. Such sprays should be "coarse" but should not drip. Screens should be painted with the insecticide.

Both space and residual sprays containing the following insecticides are listed in descending order of effectiveness: lindane, DDT, BHC, chlordane and toxophene. (For a more detailed consideration see p. 748.)

REPELLENTS. When it is necessary to be outside at night one of the efficient repellents must be used. The following preparations are available:

1. Refined indalone. The effectiveness of this preparation does not exceed two hours in the presence of sweating.

2. Insect Repellent No. 612. This is effective for two to four hours except under conditions of marked sweating, when it should be used more frequently.

3. Dimethyl phthalate. This preparation has a longer period of effective action and is a better repellent against certain species of anophelines.

4. The following mixture of these three preparations is useful and possesses repellent action against a wide variety of annoying pest insects as well as mosquitoes. It has been termed 6–2–2 mixture.

| | |
|---|---|
| Dimethyl phthalate | 6 parts |
| Indalone | 2 parts |
| No. 612 | 2 parts |

5. The Armed Forces of the United States have two new repellents, M-2020 and M-2043, which are superior to those listed above for repelling mosquitoes, biting flies, gnats, fleas or chiggers.

A few drops should be taken into the palm of one hand, the hands then rubbed together and the repellent carefully rubbed over all exposed skin areas. Care should be taken to avoid the mouth, the eyes and the eyebrows since these preparations are irritating to mucous membranes.

PROTECTIVE CLOTHING. Individuals who must be outside screened buildings at night should wear long trousers, preferably with leggings or mosquito boots, and shirts with long sleeves. The shirt must be completely buttoned and the sleeves rolled down and buttoned. In heavily malarious regions head nets and gloves should likewise be worn whenever practicable. Clothing impregnated with any of the standard repellents is of some use against mosquitoes.

**Destruction of Anopheline Mosquitoes.**    The destruction of anopheline mosquitoes is accomplished by the use of various measures including insecticides lethal to the adult mosquito and larvicides which destroy the aquatic larval forms in the breeding areas.

LARVICIDES. The larvicides useful for the destruction of the aquatic forms of the anopheline mosquito comprise volatile oils, such as Diesel oil No. 2 or kerosene, Paris green and DDT.

The reader is referred to the section on mosquito control (p. 738) for more detailed consideration of these measures.

# 33  Toxoplasmosis

**Synonyms**   None.

**Definition**   Toxoplasmosis is a disease of man and animals produced by the organism, *Toxoplasma gondii* (Nicolle and Manceaux). The infection is usually inapparent and unrecognized in adults. In children it may take the form of various syndromes in which involvement of the central nervous system or viscera predominates.

**Distribution**   Infection is widespread in animals (dogs, guinea pigs, hares and pigeons) throughout the world. Human infections have been reported from every continent including Europe, the Middle East, Ceylon, North, Central and South America, Australia and Hawaii.

**Etiology**   Toxoplasmosis of man is caused by *Toxoplasma gondii* which was originally described from a North African rodent, the gondi. All strains recovered from man and animals that have been tested are morphologically and immunologically identical. The organism is an obligate intracellular parasite presenting typical morphology and staining characteristics in exudate or impression films of fresh tissue. It is pathogenic for small laboratory animals and shows immunologic relationship with established strains. Parasites fulfilling these criteria have been found in man, dogs, swine, guinea pigs and pigeons. *Toxoplasma* recovered from the gondi, wild rats and wild mice must still be tested immunologically.

*Toxoplasma gondii* may be found free in the body fluids of its host, or it may occur as an intracellular parasite of the mononuclear leukocytes, endothelial, parenchymal and other tissue cells. In the free stage *T. gondii* is typically curved or crescent shaped and measures 4 to 6 microns in length and 2 to 3 microns in breadth in fresh exudate or on films. One extremity is more rounded than the other. In fresh preparations it appears as a hyaline body and when recovered from the peritoneal exudate of experimentally infected animals it is found singly or in pairs. When stained by Wright's or Giemsa's method the cytoplasm stains blue and the nucleus stands out as a red to purple irregular mass occupying only one-fifth to one-fourth of the cell. Typically the nucleus is eccentric and is situated nearer the round end of the parasite (Fig. 146 *a*).

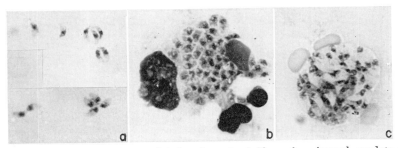

Fig. 146. Toxoplasm as seen (*a*) free in stained films of peritoneal exudate or tissue, (*b*) intracellularly, and (*c*) as pseudocyst in film of brain. Wright's stain (800 ×) reduced from a photomicrograph with a magnification of 1,000 diameters. (Courtesy of Dr. A. B. Sabin in J.A.M.A., vol. 116.)

In the intracellular stages *T. gondii* may appear singly or in clusters within the parenchymal and reticulo-endothelial cells of many organs. When so situated the parasites appear to lose their crescent shape (Fig. 146 *b*) and may be readily confused with the leishmanias, especially when found in endothelial and mononuclear cells. Clusters of pseudocysts have also been described (Fig. 146 *c*).

**Epidemiology** Toxoplasmosis may be congenital or acquired. In mice the disease has been transmitted experimentally in utero as well as through the milk of lactating females. Although the actual method of transmission to man is unknown *Toxoplasma* organisms have been transmitted in experimental animals orally and by inoculation (intracutaneous and subcutaneous, intravenous, intraperitoneal, intracerebral and intranasal). This suggests the possibility of transmission by the droplet method, or by contact with excreta or infected tissues. Various arthropods have been suspected but no vectors have been incriminated.

Large scale dye- and skin-test surveys have been conducted in various parts of the world. The results suggest that inapparent infection with *Toxoplasma* is widespread since the incidence of positive tests increases with age until, in some areas, after the age of twenty, 50 per cent or more are positive.

**Pathology** The pathology of congenital toxoplasmosis differs from that of the usual infections in adults. In the former the acute involvement may be present in every organ. Parenchymal cells as well as those of the reticulo-endothelial system are generally affected and lesions occur in the brain, spleen, kidneys, adrenals and lymph nodes. Serous fluids accumulate in the body cavities. Lesions of the central nervous system frequently require diligent search of sections of the brain and spinal cord.

In the usual postnatally acquired infections of adults, which are typically inapparent, lesions are detected only accidentally. In the rare acute cases, however, they may be widespread throughout the body.

**Clinical Characteristics** The most commonly recognized clinical picture of human toxoplasmosis is the result of congenital infection in infants and young children. It usually appears as a form of encephalitis accompanied by such features as chorioretinitis, hydrocephalus or microcephaly, microphthalmos, intracerebral calcification and mental retardation. Convulsions are not infrequent.

Immunologic studies of human sera indicate that inapparent or unrecognized infections are not uncommon among the adult population. Active toxoplasmosis among adults, however, is rare, and frequently fatal. It is usually accompanied by prolonged remittent fever, often with such features as pneumonitis suggestive of primary atypical pneumonia, encephalitis and myocarditis. There may be disseminated myositis accompanied by generalized aching and pain, and there may be generalized lymphadenopathy with firm, discrete, painless lymph nodes. Often there is a maculopapular erythematous rash which typically does not appear on the hands, feet or scalp.

**Diagnosis** *Toxoplasma gondii* may be demonstrated by a variety of laboratory procedures (see p. 845) in blood, bone marrow, cerebrospinal fluid or exudates from the serous cavities of patients. Usually *Toxoplasma* can be recovered from suspect patients following intracerebral and intraperitoneal inoculation of laboratory mice. Other diagnostic aids include complement fixation, or the methylene blue dye technique (see p. 845). The organisms can also be recovered at necropsy. A presumptive diagnosis is generally made by serologic means and confirmed by the inoculation of exudate or blood into laboratory mice.

**Treatment** Treatment is unsatisfactory and consequently the prognosis is poor. Sulfadiazine has been shown to arrest the disease in early infections in experimental animals. It is the drug of choice for the treatment of human infections. The antibiotics have not proved useful.

# 34   The Trypanosomidae

**Introduction**   The genera *Leishmania* and *Trypanosoma* are the only members of the family TRYPANOSOMIDAE which are pathogenic for man or animals. There are six important diseases of man caused by these flagellates. Three are produced by species of the genus *Leishmania* while the remainder are caused by members of the genus *Trypanosoma* (Table 28).

*Table 28   Diseases of Man Caused by the* TRYPANOSOMIDAE

| DISEASE | ETIOLOGIC AGENT |
|---|---|
| Kala-azar | *Leishmania donovani* |
| Oriental sore | *L. tropica* |
| Mucocutaneous leishmaniasis | *L. brasiliensis* |
| Trypanosomiasis, West Africa | *Trypanosoma gambiense* |
| Trypanosomiasis, East Africa | *T. rhodesiense* |
| Chagas' disease | *T. cruzi* |

All species listed in the above table have both vertebrate and invertebrate hosts. Their life cycles are carried on partly in certain insects and partly in man or other mammals, the parasites living alternately in the blood or other tissues of the vertebrate and in the gut of the insect. The leishmanial parasites all occur as intracellular organisms, principally in cells of the reticulo-endothelial system. The

*Table 29   Stages in Life Cycles of the* TRYPANOSOMIDAE *of Man*

| SPECIES OF PARASITE | STAGE IN MAN | STAGE IN INSECT | STATION |
|---|---|---|---|
| *Leishmania donovani* | *Leishmanial | Leptomonad | A† |
| *L. tropica* | *Leishmanial | Leptomonad | A |
| *L. brasiliensis* | *Leishmanial | Leptomonad | A |
| *Trypanosoma gambiense* | *Trypanosomal | Crithidial, trypanosomal | A |
| *T. rhodesiense* | *Trypanosomal | Crithidial, trypanosomal | A |
| *T. cruzi* | *Leishmanial, crithidial, trypanosomal | Crithidial, trypanosomal | P‡ |

* = the multiplicative stage in man
† A = anterior station
‡ P = posterior station

trypanosomes, on the other hand, are extracellular parasites occurring in the blood, lymph or cerebrospinal fluid. *Trypanosoma cruzi* is the only member of the family producing both trypanosomal forms in the blood and leishmanial stages in the tissue cells of man (Table 29).

**Developmental Stages**   In the course of the life cycle in the invertebrate and the vertebrate hosts multiplication occurs and certain

**328**

members of the family pass through developmental stages in which they resemble other genera within the family (Fig. 147).

In the *leishmanial stage* the parasite is an intracellular organism which occurs only in the mammal. It is a nonflagellated round or ovoid body measuring 1.5 to 5 microns in greatest diameter and con-

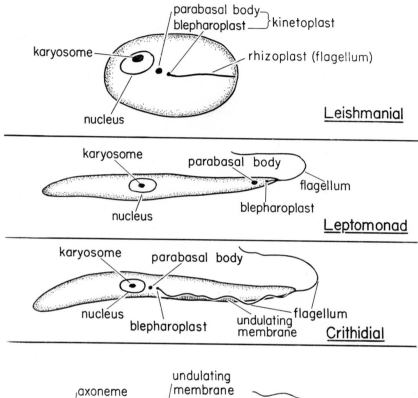

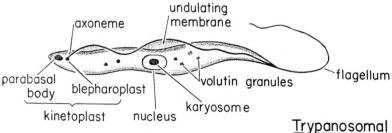

Fig. 147. Leishmanial, leptomonad, crithidial, trypanosomal forms of the Try-
PANOSOMIDAE.

taining a spherical vesicular nucleus and a rod-shaped parabasal body. In close proximity to this latter structure is a dotlike blepharoplast which, together with the parabasal body, constitutes the kineto-plast. Occasionally a fibril, the rhizoplast, may be seen extending from the blepharoplast to the periphery of the parasite (Fig. 147).

The *leptomonad stage* occurs in the life cycle of members of the genus *Leishmania* in the insect host and in culture. It has not been found in man. The leptomonad form is slender and elongate with a more or less centrally placed vesicular nucleus. A single anterior flagellum arises from a well developed kinetoplast near the anterior extremity of the body. In some specimens the component parts of the kinetoplast are visible—the parabasal body and the blepharoplast from which the flagellum originates. There is no undulating membrane.

The *crithidial stage* occurs in the course of the life cycle of members of the genus *Trypanosoma*. It is found primarily in the insect vector and is the predominant multiplicative stage of the parasite. *Trypanosoma cruzi*, unlike the other members of the genus, manifests both leishmanial and crithidial stages in the human host. Trypanosomes in culture revert to the forms characteristic of the invertebrate phase of their cycle. The typically slender crithidial form resembles the leptomonad in general contour. The vesicular nucleus is centrally placed. The kinetoplast, with its prominent parabasal body and less conspicuous blepharoplast, is situated near and anterior to the nucleus. The single flagellum originating from the blepharoplast emerges and continues as the free border of a short undulating membrane which extends to the anterior extremity of the parasite. At this point the flagellum becomes free.

The *trypanosomal stage* occurs only among members of the genus *Trypanosoma*. It is represented by a metacyclic phase and a mature phase. The metacyclic form is the young infective trypanosome which develops only in the insect vector. It represents the culmination of the reproductive crithidial stage, which is not infective to the mammal. When the metacyclic trypanosome is found in the salivary glands of the insect it is said to have an anterior station. When it is developed in the hind gut and is passed in the feces the term posterior station is used. The metacyclic trypanosome has a relatively short stumpy body with a centrally placed, ovoid or spherical nucleus. The kinetoplast is situated posterior to the nucleus. The single flagellum originating from the blepharoplast emerges from the cytoplasm to form the free border of an undulating membrane which extends along the greater portion of the body of the parasite. The flagellum, becoming free at the anterior extremity, is relatively short. The mature trypanosome is longer and more slender. The nucleus is usually centrally placed. The kinetoplast, consisting of an oval or rod-shaped parabasal body and the usually indistinguishable blepharoplast, is situated near the posterior extremity. The flagellum emerges after a short course through the cytoplasm, is continued as the border of a long undulating membrane and becomes free anteriorly. Volutin granules are scattered through the cytoplasm. Two forms of mature trypanosomes may be encountered. In the monomorphic type all individuals are morphologically similar, each possessing a central nucleus, a posteriorly placed kinetoplast, a long undulating membrane and a long anterior flagellum. Those of the polymorphic type, on the other hand, exhibit morphologic differences particularly with respect to variation in size, position of the nucleus and length of the flagellum.

*Multiplication* of the parasites in these genera occurs by longitudinal fission. Division of the blepharoplast, the parabasal body and the nucleus precedes division of the cytoplasm. The flagellum when present does not divide but as division of the blepharoplast occurs a new flagellum rapidly develops while the old flagellum persists. With fission of the cytoplasm two flagellated organisms are produced.

The diagnosis of leishmanial and trypanosomal infections in man is based upon demonstration of the parasites in stained smears of blood, spinal fluid, material aspirated from cutaneous lesions, lymph nodes, spleen, or bone marrow, or in fixed and stained tissue sections. The species of *Leishmania* and the trypanosome, *T. cruzi*, may be isolated in culture (pp. 836–837). African trypanosomes have been grown on various media although cultivation is often difficult or unsuccessful. Xenodiagnosis also may be useful in the identification of *T. cruzi* infections; an uninfected reduviid bug is allowed to feed upon the infected individual and subsequently the crithidial forms of the trypanosome may be demonstrated in its gut.

When stained with the Romanowsky or common tissue stains the cytoplasm of these parasites appears blue, the nucleus pink and the parabasal body a deep red.

Dogs, cats, monkeys, mice, rats, guinea pigs, Chinese and European hamsters, the gerbil and certain species of squirrels have all been shown to be susceptible in varying degree to infection by species of *Leishmania*. The hamster is the best experimental animal.

# 35   Leishmaniasis

The term leishmaniasis includes a variety of conditions which may conveniently be subdivided into the visceral and the superficial infections. These diseases are produced by protozoal parasites belonging to the genus *Leishmania*. Although the different organisms are morphologically identical they are classified as different species within the genus (Table 30).

The leishmania localize in the reticulo-endothelial cells of the viscera or the skin. Thus in kala-azar the pathologic changes occur predominantly in the spleen, liver and bone marrow. In post–kala-azar dermal leishmaniasis the localization of the parasites is more widely distributed throughout the skin of the body. In oriental sore, on the other hand, only the exposed skin areas are affected. The Central and South American form of leishmaniasis likewise involves exposed skin areas and there is invasion of the mucous membranes of the nose, mouth and pharynx as well.

Oriental sore occurs as a natural disease of dogs. Human and canine infections are frequently found to be endemic in the same area and the lesions in the dog do not differ from those in man. Several other mammalian species are susceptible. Animals which have recovered from oriental sore have a solid immunity against reinfection by *L. tropica*. They are not immune, however, to *L. donovani*, the etiologic agent of kala-azar. On the other hand, infection by *L. donovani* confers immunity both to this parasite and to *L. tropica*. Such evidence suggests that these parasites, although

*Table 30    Human Leishmaniasis*

| TYPE | COMMON NAME | ETIOLOGIC AGENT |
|------|-------------|-----------------|
| Visceral | Kala-azar (Indian and Oriental) | *Leishmania donovani* |
|  | Kala-azar (Mediterranean) | *L. donovani* |
| Dermal | Post–kala-azar dermal leishmaniasis | *L. donovani* |
| Cutaneous | Oriental sore | *L. tropica* |
| Naso-oral | Mucocutaneous leishmaniasis | *L. brasiliensis* |

related, are not identical. This is further supported by the distinctly different geographic distribution of oriental sore and kala-azar (Fig. 148).

The various leishmaniases have essentially the same epidemiology. Several species of biting flies belonging to the genus *Phlebotomus* are chiefly responsible for the transmission of the parasites (Table 31). These flies are small and hairy. They are weak fliers, remaining near the ground and in close proximity to the breeding area. Their larvae develop in cracks in masonry and walls, and in rubbish and stone piles.

Man, the dog, wild rodents and possibly other mammals serve as endemic reservoirs for species of *Leishmania* in various parts of the world.

*Phlebotomus* flies acquire the protozoan by direct ingestion from the infected skin or from parasites present in the ingested blood of the reservoir host. Leishmanial organisms, after entrance into the insect's gut, develop into leptomonad flagellates, undergo multiplication and ultimately come to occupy an anterior station in the insect's pharynx. It is believed that when the flies subsequently feed on man these leptomonad forms gain access to the human body, localizing in the cells of the reticulo-endothelial system where they undergo extensive multiplication as leishmanial forms.

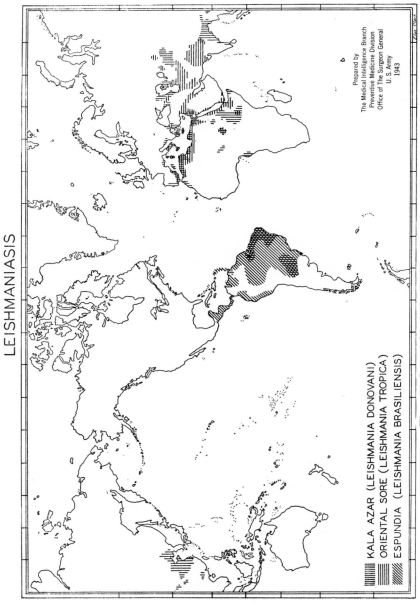

LEISHMANIASIS

Prepared by
The Medical Intelligence Branch
Preventive Medicine Division
Office of The Surgeon General
U. S. Army
1943

KALA AZAR (LEISHMANIA DONOVANI)
ORIENTAL SORE (LEISHMANIA TROPICA)
ESPUNDIA (LEISHMANIA BRASILIENSIS)

Fig. 148. Geographical distribution of leishmaniasis.

## *Table 31*   *Known and Probable Vectors of Leishmaniasis*

| *Leishmania donovani:* Kala-azar | |
|---|---|
| Asia: India, China, Pakistan | * *Phlebotomus argentipes*<br>* *P. chinensis*<br>* *P. sergenti* var. *mongolensis* |
| Middle East: Palestine, Turkey | *P. perfiliewi*<br>* *P. papatasi* |
| Mediterranean: Greece, Sicily, Italy, Spain, Cyprus, Portugal | * *P. perniciosus*<br>*P. major*<br>* *P. papatasi*<br>* *P. tobbi*<br>* *P. chinensis*<br>* *P. perfiliewi* |
| North Africa: Sudan, Ethiopia, Algiers | *P. sergenti*<br>*P. orientalis*<br>* *P. perniciosus*<br>* *P. longicuspis* |
| South America: Brazil, Venezuela, Argentina, Paraguay, Bolivia | *P. intermedius* (= *lutzi*)<br>* *P. longipalpis* |
| *Leishmania tropica:* Cutaneous Leishmaniasis | |
| Asia: Middle Asia (USSR): Turkmenistan (only rodents), Iran | * *P. papatasi*<br>* *P. caucasicus* |
| Mediterranean: Palestine, Turkey, Italy, Syria | *P. caucasicus*<br>* *P. perfiliewi* |
| Africa: Algeria, Tunisia, Libya, Egypt, Central Africa | * *P. sergenti*<br>† *Stomoxys calcitrans* |
| *Leishmania braziliensis:* Mucocutaneous Leishmaniasis | |
| Central and South America: Brazil, Peru, Venezuela | * *P. intermedius* (= *lutzi*)<br>‡ *P. migonei*<br>*P. evansi*<br>‡ *P. whitmani*<br>*P. gomezi*<br>‡ *P. pessoai*<br>*P. paraensis*<br>*P. squamiventris*<br>‡ *P. fischeri* (experimental)<br>*P. verrucarum*<br>*P. peruensis* |

* Vectorship generally accepted by most authors; in regard to all others there is a difference of opinion. In many cases evidence is epidemiologic only.

† Mechanical experimental transmission.

‡ Only to monkeys—experimentally.

# 36  Kala-Azar

**Synonyms**  Dumdum fever, tropical splenomegaly, black sickness, splenic anemia of infants, ponos.

**Definition**  Kala-azar is a disease produced by a protozoal organism, *Leishmania donovani*. It is characterized by irregular fever of long duration, chronicity, enlargement of the spleen and often of the liver, emaciation, anemia and leukopenia.

**Distribution**  Kala-azar is widely distributed in certain portions of the world but has rather strict geographic limitations within these areas.

ASIA. It is endemic in the eastern portion of India in Assam, Bengal, Bihar, Madras and Sikkim where extensive epidemics with high mortality rates have occurred in the past. In China it occurs from Peking in the north, south to Canton, and in southern Manchuria and central Asia.

EUROPE. It is present in southern Russia, Transcaucasia, Turkestan and the Mediterranean littoral including southern Italy, France, Spain and the Mediterranean islands.

AFRICA. It is present in Morocco, Algeria, Tunis, Tripolitania, Cyrenaica, Egypt, Sudan, Kenya, French Equatorial Africa and Nigeria.

WESTERN HEMISPHERE. Visceral leishmaniasis or kala-azar occurs in Paraguay, Argentina and Brazil.

INFANTILE KALA-AZAR. Infantile kala-azar is limited in its geographic distribution to the Mediterranean basin, Portugal, Spain, southern France, Turkey, Yugoslavia and Hungary.

**Etiology**  Kala-azar of India and the Orient and the disease in children in the Mediterranean area were formerly considered to be caused by two different parasites, *L. donovani* and *L. infantum*, but *L. donovani* is now accepted as the etiologic agent of both diseases. This is a round or ovoid organism measuring 2 to 5 microns in diameter containing a relatively large and peripherally placed vesicular nucleus. A rod-shaped or oval parabasal body and a dotlike blepharoplast in close proximity to it together form the kinetoplast. Occasionally a short fibril, the rhizoplast, may be seen arising from the blepharoplast and extending to the periphery.

When stained with a Romanowsky stain the cytoplasm appears faintly blue, and the nucleus and kinetoplast red or reddish purple.

The leishmania, or Leishman-Donovan bodies, are found within cells of the reticulo-endothelial system and in large wandering phagocytic cells of the mammalian host.

**Epidemiology**  In both India and China kala-azar is a rural disease, occurring principally in low alluvial plains. It rarely occurs at altitudes in excess of 2000 feet. There are three factors essential for transmission—a reservoir of infection, a suitable vector, and a susceptible population. Susceptibility of the population appears to be highly important. Recovery from infection is accompanied by relatively complete immunity of long duration. Under endemic conditions the disease affects chiefly children. It appears to become epidemic only when the general resistance of the population is lowered. Adults then are affected with increasing frequency. Kala-azar occurs in both sexes at all ages. It is a disease primarily of the

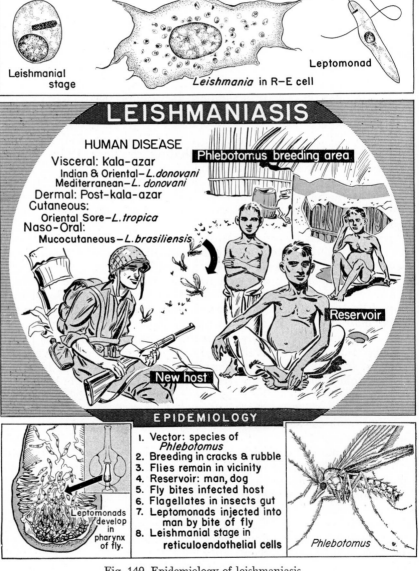

Fig. 149. Epidemiology of leishmaniasis.

poorer classes. Epidemics have been restricted principally to India (Fig. 149).

In most areas where the leishmanial diseases are endemic it is probable that infected man, particularly in the case of post–kala-azar dermal leishmaniasis, constitutes the most important reservoir. In the Mediterranean region, however, infected dogs are believed to be reservoirs for the infantile form of the disease. In China, also, cutaneous leishmaniasis of dogs is not uncommon, and naturally infected dogs have been found in Brazil. These animals, however, are not found infected in India and presumably play no part in the epidemiology of Indian kala-azar. *Phlebotomus sergenti* var. *mongolensis* and *P. chinensis* in China, and certain of the Brazilian and Paraguayan species have been shown to acquire infection from these animals.

The *sandfly vectors* (various species of *Phlebotomus*) are weak fliers and are most numerous in the immediate proximity of the breeding places. They remain, for the most part, close to the ground and consequently are much less numerous above the first floor in houses. They breed in cracks in the walls and masonry and in collections of rubbish and rubble. The average life of the sandfly is estimated to be fourteen to sixteen days. *Phlebotomus argentipes* is considered the most important vector in India and *P. chinensis* in China.

Leishmanial bodies present in the peripheral blood in the course of the active disease are ingested by the vector. Leptomonad forms may be observed in the gut of the insect by the third day after the infective blood meal. They move forward to occupy an anterior station in the pharynx and mouth parts by the fourth or fifth day. From the seventh to the ninth day the flagellates often invade the proboscis and the flies are then infective. The organisms are presumed to enter the new host during subsequent biting. Successful transmission by the sandfly to hamsters and to man has been accomplished.

Leishmanial bodies have been demonstrated in the urine and feces of infected humans. They have also been found in material obtained by swabbing the nasal mucosa and the tonsil, and have been demonstrated in the saliva of infected individuals. This implies the possibility of direct man-to-man transmission by droplet infection. It seems probable, however, that this method of spread, if it occurs, is of minor importance because of the sharp geographic limitations, the failure of the disease to extend outside these regions, and its absence at altitudes above 2000 feet within the endemic areas.

Animals have been shown to acquire leishmaniasis by the eating of infected carcasses. It is possible that this may be a factor in maintaining the animal reservoir.

**Pathology**   The chief lesion of kala-azar is essentially a marked hyperplasia of the cells of the reticulo-endothelial system, particularly of the spleen and liver. The leishmania multiply within these cells which ultimately rupture, releasing the parasites which are then taken up by other reticulo-endothelial cells. They are ingested to a lesser extent by leukocytes and monocytes, which not infrequently may be found containing leishmania in films of the peripheral blood.

The spleen may be greatly enlarged owing principally to the enormous increase of reticulo-endothelial cells, many of which are parasitized. There is replacement of splenic pulp by these parasitized cells and often pressure atrophy of the malpighian bodies. There may be some fibrosis in advanced chronic cases (Fig. 150).

The liver is usually, but not always, enlarged in kala-azar. There is marked proliferation of the Kupffer cells which contain large numbers of leishmanial bodies. Pressure atrophy of the liver cords occurs,

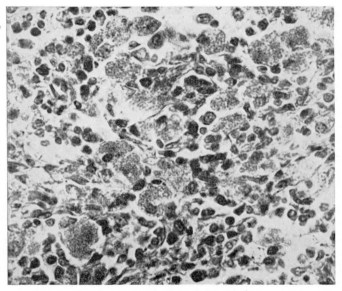

Fig. 150. Kala-azar spleen: parasitized reticulo-endothelial cells in splenic pulp.

and cloudy swelling and fatty degeneration may both be observed. In advanced chronic cases there may be some fibrosis of the parenchyma (Fig. 151).

The villi of the small intestine, especially the duodenum and jejunum, may be crowded with parasitized reticulo-endothelial cells and ulceration of the overlying mucosa occasionally occurs. Less often similar lesions are reported in the colon, and, rarely, cells containing parasites may be observed in the mucous membrane of the stomach.

In the bone marrow there is a progressive replacement of the hematopoietic tissue and the fatty marrow by masses of heavily parasitized reticulo-endothelial cells.

There are no characteristic lesions of other organs. Scattered infected phagocytic cells may be observed. The lymph nodes are often enlarged owing to obstruction of the lymph sinuses by parasitized reticulo-endothelial cells (Fig. 152).

*Post–kala-azar dermal leishmaniasis* usually does not appear until some two years after the acute stage of the disease in India. In the Sudan it commonly appears as the visceral disease subsides. The early lesions are depigmented areas which may be one-half inch in diam-

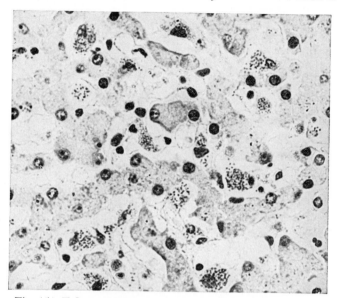

Fig. 151. Kala-azar: *L. donovani* in Kupffer cells of the liver.

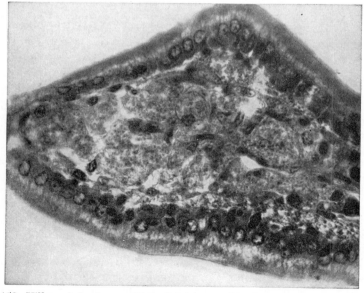

Fig. 152. Villus of duodenum distended by parasitized reticulo-endothelial cells. Experimental infection in hamster.

eter, occurring particularly on the face, neck, extensor surface of the forearms and the inner aspect of the thighs. There is little change in the epidermis but the pigment in the basal layer is diminished. The subpapillary layer is edematous, the vessels are dilated and there is infiltration by macrophage cells. Parasites are scanty.

A second type of skin lesion, nodular in character, likewise occurs in post–kala-azar dermal leishmaniasis. In this type there is a thinning of the epidermis over a nodular granulomatous mass of reticulo-endothelial cells, some of which contain leishmanial bodies.

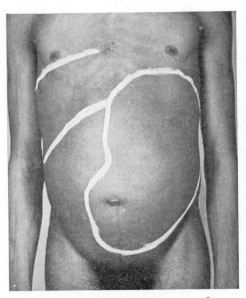

Fig. 153. Chronic kala-azar: extreme splenomegaly.

Less commonly xanthomatous lesions of the skin are observed. In these there is a marked increase of connective tissue. Parasites are rare.

**Clinical Characteristics**    The duration of the incubation period is not known exactly. It is usually considered to be two to four months; rarely it may be only ten to fourteen days.

The onset may be sudden or gradual. In some instances it is acute, accompanied by chills, high fever and vomiting. In others it resembles typhoid and is characterized by general malaise and rising fever which reaches 103° to 104° F. in about a week. In still others it is insidious, slow and unaccompanied by any significant febrile reaction.

During the acute stage the fever is frequently intermittent, with two daily remissions, and each drop in temperature is often accompanied by profuse sweating. Characteristically the patient's temperature rises in the early afternoon, subsides toward evening and rises again usually before midnight. This type of daily double-remitting fever is pathognomonic. It may be observed in only 5 to 10 per cent of the early cases. The initial fever may last two to six weeks. Thereafter, if the disease becomes chronic, it is characterized by recurring febrile waves resembling those observed in brucellosis.

The first noticeable enlargement of the spleen may occur as late as five months after the onset of the acute phase although it is usually at or below the costal margin by the end of the first month. In the early stages of the disease it has a doughy consistency. Each wave of fever is accompanied by further enlargement followed by some reduction in size during the apyrexial periods. In chronic cases the spleen is often hard and greatly enlarged, extending to the umbilicus or even to the anterior superior spine of the ilium (Fig. 153). Soft enlargement of the liver is usually evident after the first month.

Diarrhea, and at times even dysentery, are not uncommon during the acute stage. As the disease progresses there is marked emaciation, most noticeable in the limbs and the chest wall. Drenching night sweats are common. Despite these symptoms and the height of the fever curve, toxemia is inconspicuous. The appetite usually remains good and the tongue clean.

As the disease advances a characteristic grayish color of the skin develops from which the synonym, "black disease," is derived. This pigmentation is most noticeable on the hands, the nails, the forehead and the central line of the abdomen.

The replacement of hematopoietic marrow by parasitized reticuloendothelial cells is probably responsible for the characteristic changes in the blood picture. There is a leukopenia with a relative increase of lymphocytes and monocytes. Although anemia is usual, the red blood cells seldom fall below two and one-half million and more commonly range between three and four million per cubic millimeter. The erythrocytes are frequently macrocytic and hyperchromic.

Progressive alteration of the plasma proteins occurs early in the disease. The serum euglobulin is three to thirteen times normal and may constitute 30 to 63 per cent of the total serum globulins. There is an absolute decrease in the serum albumin. In the late stages of the disease these changes in the plasma proteins commonly lead to ascites and edema.

Purpura, gingivitis, stomatitis and trophic changes of the hair are common. It is probable that they are to be attributed, at least in part, to nutritional deficiencies. Pneumonia, cancrum oris or intercurrent disease are frequent terminal phenomena.

**Diagnosis**   In endemic areas the diagnosis of kala-azar may be made with reasonable assurance on clinical grounds by about the fourth month, when the characteristic features, splenomegaly, hepatomegaly, and leukopenia usually below 4000 per cubic millimeter, are ordinarily well established. The serum tests provide additional but not conclusive evidence. In early cases the characteristic fever curve may be the only significant clinical finding.

1. DEFINITIVE DIAGNOSIS. This depends upon the demonstration of *L. donovani* in the blood or other tissues and may be accomplished by microscopic examination of stained smears, by cultures, or by inoculation into hamsters.

BLOOD SMEARS. Parasites are always present in the peripheral blood of untreated cases. Careful examination of the leukocytes and monocytes in stained blood films will reveal *Leishmania* in many of the cases.

BLOOD CULTURE. Inoculation of the sedimented cells from citrated blood into N.N.N. medium and subsequent cultivation at 20° to 24° C.

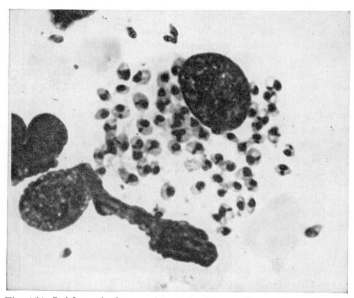

Fig. 154. *Leishmania donovani* in stained smear from spleen puncture.

may yield a positive culture of leptomonad forms in one to four weeks. With proper technique positive cultures should be obtained in all cases.

SPLEEN PUNCTURE. In 95 per cent of the cases Leishmania will be found in large numbers in stained smears of the splenic aspirate. Inoculations of N.N.N. medium will yield positive cultures in all cases (Fig. 154).

STERNAL PUNCTURE. Leishmania may be demonstrated in stained smears of sternal marrow in approximately 90 per cent of the cases. The parasites, however, are usually much less numerous than in smears of spleen pulp. Culture will frequently yield positive results.

2. SEROLOGIC DIAGNOSIS. The serum tests for kala-azar are based upon the increase of the euglobulin fraction. When positive they provide suggestive but not conclusive evidence. The techniques are described on page 846.

ALDEHYDE (NAPIER) TEST. The reaction does not become strong until the third to the fifth month of the disease and it persists for about four months after the conclusion of successful treatment.

ANTIMONY (CHOPRA) TEST. This reaction becomes positive earlier in the course of the disease than does the aldehyde test. It usually gives a doubtful reaction by the end of the first month or even before and becomes strongly positive at the end of the second or third month. False positives are obtained in some cases of splenomegaly from other causes.

COMPLEMENT FIXATION TEST. A very promising complement fixation test using an antigen prepared from human tubercle bacilli has been developed. Positive reaction is obtained in approximately 90 per cent of cases as early as the third week of the disease. A negative reaction is obtained in all conditions entering into the differential diagnosis with the exception of about 10 per cent of cases of clinically obvious chronic pulmonary tuberculosis.

DIFFERENTIAL DIAGNOSIS. The clinical picture of kala-azar frequently may resemble that produced by other diseases which occur in the endemic areas. The early acute stage may be confused with malaria, especially since it may appear to respond to quinine, and in the early weeks it may also resemble atypical typhoid fever. In the chronic stage it may be confused with tuberculosis, brucellosis and amebic abscess of the liver. Infantile kala-azar has been confused with Banti's disease. The onset of kala-azar in children is frequently insidious. The clinical course is associated with splenomegaly, anemia and general lymphadenitis. The lesions of post–kala-azar dermal leishmaniasis may suggest leprosy.

**Treatment** Malnutrition is frequently serious. It complicates the problem of specific treatment, contributes to the incidence of complications and significantly affects the prognosis. Severe cases of the disease, therefore, should be hospitalized whenever it is possible.

A high protein high vitamin diet is essential. Oral hygiene is of great importance because of the frequency of the highly fatal complication, cancrum oris. Likewise respiratory infections must be guarded against because of the susceptibility of kala-azar patients to pneumonia. The presence or absence of pulmonary tuberculosis must be determined prior to the institution of specific therapy since all of the antimonial drugs are contraindicated in the presence of this infection.

SPECIFIC TREATMENT. The susceptibility of kala-azar to specific drug treatment appears to vary considerably between different geographic areas. The disease in India seems to be most easily cured. The Chinese and Mediterranean forms occupy intermediate positions and visceral leishmaniasis of the Sudan is notoriously resistant. Prior to the introduction of the currently used drugs the mortality was 95 per cent; it is now 2 to 5 per cent.

Two groups of compounds are recommended: pentavalent organic antimonials, and certain aromatic diamidines. One or more of these will meet the requirements of almost all cases.

PENTAVALENT ORGANIC ANTIMONIALS. 1. *Sodium antimony gluconate.* Synonyms: pentostam, Bayer 561, Solustibosan. This drug has been widely used and found to be effective in resistant forms of the disease. Toxic effects are rare. It should be given daily for eight to twelve days intravenously in 5 per cent solution for adults, and intramuscularly in 25 per cent solution for children. The individual injection must be a *freshly prepared* solution in sterile distilled water.

Dosage. For adults: initial dose 0.2 gm., subsequent doses 0.3 gm. The adult dose may be used for children weighing 30 kilograms or more.

A preparation of sodium antimony gluconate issued under the name of Pentostam is distributed in a form suitable for immediate injection. It may be administered intravenously or intramuscularly. The recommended adult dosage is one intravenous injection of 6 ml. daily for six days.

2. *Neostibosan.* Synonym: Bayer 693. Neostibosan is a phenyl-stibonic acid derivative. The methods of administration and dosage are the same as for sodium antimony gluconate.

3. *Urea stibamine.* The drug is a mixture of compounds of phenyl-stibonic acid. It has been widely used in India where it has proven effective. It has greater toxicity than Neostibosan and should be administered by the intravenous route only since it is too irritating to give by intramuscular injection. It should be given on alternate days or every third day in 5 to 10 ml. of sterile distilled water. It must not be heated.

Dosage. The initial recommended dose for an adult is 0.05 gm., the second 0.1 gm., the third 0.15 gm., and the fourth and subsequent doses 0.2 gm.

The mode of action of antimony on the leishmania is not known. The parasites may continue to be present and viable on culture during at least part of the course of treatment, and even for a short period after completion of therapy.

The antimonyl tartrates no longer have a place in the treatment of kala-azar.

AROMATIC DIAMIDINES. The aromatic diamidines are the most powerful known drugs for the treatment of kala-azar. Particularly when given intravenously, reactions of some degree occur in a considerable proportion of cases. These include headache, flushing, faintness, epigastric pain and vomiting, collapse and unconsciousness. There is associated fall in blood pressure and, at times, lowering of the blood sugar. These reactions can be largely prevented or controlled by intramuscular injection of 0.25 ml. 1/1000 Adrenalin or an antihistaminic immediately prior to administration of the drug.

1. *Pentamidine isethionate.* Synonym: M&B 800, Lomidine. This may be given intravenously or intramuscularly. The latter route is preferred since it is rarely associated with any of the symptoms refer-

able to the depressor action of the drug. It should be given daily or on alternate days to a total of twelve to fifteen injections. Only freshly prepared solutions in sterile distilled water should be used.

Dosage. For intramuscular injection, 4 mg. ker kilogram of body weight, in 3 ml. of sterile distilled water. For intravenous injection, 2 to 4 mg. per kilogram of body weight, dissolved in 5 to 10 ml. of sterile distilled water.

2. *Stilbamidine isethionate*. Stilbamidine is the most effective drug for the treatment of kala-azar but it should *not* be used for routine treatment. Solutions of the drug are unstable when exposed to light and, unless freshly prepared, cause immediate toxic reactions. It is frequently followed by a late and troublesome complication, "diamidino stilbene neuropathy" of the trigeminal nerve.

Use of this preparation should be restricted to such special cases as antimony-resistant, antimony-sensitive cases, and cases complicated by pulmonary tuberculosis. It is the drug of choice for the treatment of the latter group since there is no adverse effect upon the tuberculous infection.

Stilbamidine must be administered intravenously and slowly in a *freshly prepared* 1 per cent solution in sterile distilled water. It should be given daily. A minimum of ten injections totalling 0.75 gm. of drug per 45 kilograms of body weight is required. Weak, emaciated persons and children are relatively tolerant of the drug.

Dosage. No total individual dose should exceed 2 mg. per kilogram of body weight. The initial dose for an adult irrespective of weight should be 0.025 gm. The subsequent doses should be increased by increments of 0.01 to 0.02 gm. to a total individual dose of 2 mg. per kilogram of body weight.

Treatment of Complications. Appropriate use of penicillin and the sulfonamide drugs has greatly reduced the mortality from cancrum oris and pneumonia.

Favorable response to treatment consists of definite subjective improvement within the first four or five days except in the case of therapy by stilbamidine, together with rise of the white blood count to at least 6000 per cubic millimeter, appreciable reduction in the size of the spleen and improvement in the erythrocyte count becoming evident about a week after completion of the course of therapy.

Post–kala-azar dermal leishmaniasis usually responds better to pentavalent antimony compounds than to the aromatic diamidines. The dosage recommended for the visceral infections should be used but the injections should be spaced two or more days apart.

Relapses in kala-azar are not uncommon if insufficient treatment has been given. The relapse is usually accompanied by fever and progressive enlargement of the spleen.

**Prognosis** The serious prognosis which attends untreated or incompletely treated cases necessitates long continued observation of the patient in the post-treatment period. The *criteria of cure* may be stated as complete cessation of fever for a period of several months, gain in weight, disappearance of splenomegaly, restoration of normal white blood cell and differential counts, and disappearance of the anemia.

Certain cases fail to respond to medical treatment despite repeated courses and adequate dosage of the various recommended drugs. In such instances it is justifiable to consider splenectomy before undertaking further treatment.

**Prophylaxis**   There are no specific prophylactic measures for kala-azar. The basic problem centers around the control of the species of *Phlebotomus* which act as vectors. Insect repellents furnish temporary protection for the individual. However, residual DDT and other insecticides have given remarkable results, even when directed primarily against mosquitoes. Since *Phlebotomus* is a weak flier, some communities can be protected by residual spraying of potential resting and breeding places for 200 yards beyond the outskirts.

# 37   Cutaneous Leishmaniasis

**Synonyms**   Oriental sore; Aleppo, Bagdad, or Delhi boil; bouton d'Orient, bouton de Biskra, chiclero ulcer, forest yaws.

**Distribution**   Oriental sore is prevalent in many tropical and subtropical regions in both the Eastern and Western Hemispheres. Its distribution, however, does not coincide with that of visceral leishmaniasis (kala-azar).

ASIA. Prevalent in parts of China. In Asia Minor, especially prevalent in Syria, Palestine, Armenia, Mesopotamia, Arabia, Persia, Iran, the Caucasus, southeast Russia, Turkestan, Pakistan.

EUROPE. In the Mediterranean littoral, in the Mediterranean islands, southern Italy, Spain, the South of France and Greece.

AFRICA. Morocco, Tunis, Algiers, the Sudan, Abyssinia, French Congo, Lake Chad area, Nigeria and on the west coast south as far as Angola.

WESTERN HEMISPHERE. Reported from every country in Central and South America except Chile.

**Etiology**   The etiologic agent of oriental sore or cutaneous leishmaniasis is *Leishmania tropica*. It is morphologically identical with *L. donovani*.

**Epidemiology**   Experimental and epidemiologic evidence indicates that sandflies are natural vectors of the disease, particularly *Phlebotomus papatasii* and *P. sergenti* in the Near East, and *P. macedonicum* in Italy. Successful inoculation of man by the bite of *P. papatasii* has been accomplished. In Central and South America *P. intermedius* is generally regarded as a vector and several other species may be concerned. Although infection by *L. tropica* occurs by direct inoculation, the parasites do not penetrate the unbroken skin.

Cutaneous leishmaniasis may occur in almost epidemic form. Children are more commonly affected than adults. There is no distinctive sex incidence. A fairly solid immunity follows infection in man. This has long been the basis for deliberate inoculation of children in endemic areas, the inhabitants knowing that the induced attack confers protection against naturally acquired infection. Sites are chosen where the resultant scar will be least disfiguring.

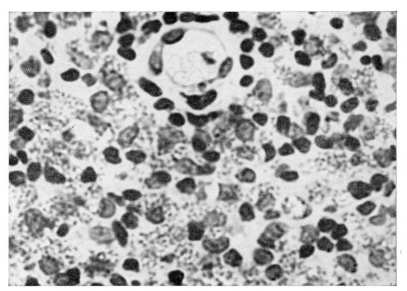

Fig. 155. Section through the indurated edge of oriental sore, showing cellular infiltration including heavily parasitized reticulo-endothelial cells.

**Pathology**   Following inoculation of the skin either through the bite of an infected sandfly or by some other means, a nodule develops produced by infiltration of the corium with plasma cells, lymphocytes and large endothelial macrophages. There are often thinning and atrophy of the overlying epidermis. Perivascular infiltration then becomes prominent and polymorphonuclear leukocytes more numerous. Focal accumulations of endothelial phagocytes filled with leishmania are seen (Fig. 155).

With further progression an ulcer develops having a granulation tissue base and surrounding zone of inflammation. Infiltration extends into the subcutaneous connective tissue in which reticulo-endothelial cells, plasma cells and lymphocytes are prominent. Occasional giant cells are present.

The leishmania are often difficult to demonstrate in the fully developed ulcer and may be found only at the margin of the lesion or in scrapings from its floor. There is no general dissemination of the parasites. Ultimately the leishmania disappear, granulation tissue becomes more abundant and healing occurs, leaving a depressed fibrous scar (Fig. 156).

**Clinical Characteristics** The incubation period of oriental sore may vary from a few weeks to several months. The lesions may be multiple. They appear first as slowly growing papules on an exposed skin area. As ulceration develops they become covered with a crust which exudes a sticky secretion. On removal of the crusts, moist, freely bleeding ulcers are revealed. These ulcers are usually not deep

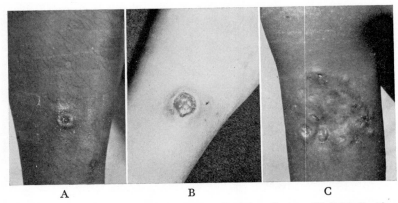

A          B          C

Fig. 156. The extremities are favorite sites for oriental sores (Delhi boil, Aleppo boil). Beginning as a small papule, the lesion becomes a plaque, called "Biskra button" (*A*); later, the ulceration extends showing rolled indurated edges (*B*). Complete healing with scarring usually occurs but satellite lesions may be formed (*C*) with central scarred areas and secondary ulcerated nodules. (Courtesy Ash and Spitz, Pathology of Tropical Diseases.)

and ordinarily vary from 1 cm. to 3 cm. in diameter. Secondary infection is usual and, when severe, greater tissue destruction may result. After effective treatment or after a number of months if no treatment is given, healing occurs by granulation and a lasting immunity is produced.

**Diagnosis** The development of one or more cutaneous ulcers on exposed skin areas of the body in a region where oriental sore is known to be endemic and where sandflies are present should arouse suspicion of this condition. Definitive diagnosis depends upon the demonstration of *L. tropica* obtained from the lesion. Examination of the exudate will seldom be successful. Smears made from curettings of the base or the sides of the ulcer should be used or a fine hypodermic needle introduced through normal skin may be inserted into the indurated margin of the lesion and material aspirated for preparation of a stained smear. Material aspirated thus, under sterile conditions, from the margin of the lesion may be inoculated into N.N.N. medium and leptomonad forms recovered after incubation at 22° C. (p. 836).

The other diagnostic procedures of value in kala-azar are not appropriate for oriental sore. Leishmania are not found in the blood, the aldehyde and antimony tests are negative, and anemia is not a feature of this infection.

The *differential diagnosis* of cutaneous leishmaniasis must include blastomycosis, yaws, tertiary syphilis and lupus.

**Treatment** The optimal method of treatment varies with the type and number of lesions. In early cases in which there are only one or a limited number of nonulcerating papules, infiltration with quinacrine (Atabrine) or with berberine sulfate usually results in cure in from two weeks to two months. In more advanced cases parenteral administration of Neostibosan with or without surgical treatment is required.

1. *Quinacrine.* The indurated edge and base of the lesion should be infiltrated with 2 ml. of a 10 to 20 per cent solution of quinacrine using a fine needle. Two to three treatments at intervals of a week to ten days may be required. Results are frequently excellent and the procedure is relatively free from pain.

2. *Berberine Sulfate.* Similar infiltration of the lesion should be done using 2 ml. of a 1 per cent solution of berberine sulfate. Not more than two or at most three lesions should be treated at one sitting. From three to six weekly treatments are usually required. These are commonly painful.

3. When the lesions are numerous, *sodium antimony gluconate* in the dosage recommended for kala-azar should be used parenterally. However, the injections should be given on alternate days; a total of ten or twelve may be required.

4. All cases of ulceration with secondary bacterial infection require combined treatment. Standard surgical procedures for the control of infection and the promotion of healing, including use of the sulfonamides and appropriate antibiotics, should be utilized in addition to specific therapy. When the ulcers are numerous or extensive, sodium antimony gluconate should be given as indicated above.

# 38 Naso-oral or Mucocutaneous Leishmaniasis

**Synonyms** American leishmaniasis, uta, bubas, espundia.

**Distribution** This infection is widely distributed throughout Central and South America with the exception of Chile. Although a clinically similar condition has been observed in India and Africa its identity is uncertain.

**Etiology** The etiologic agent is *Leishmania brasiliensis*. It is identical morphologically and culturally with *L. donovani* and *L. tropica*.

**Epidemiology** Naso-oral or mucocutaneous leishmaniasis occurs predominantly in forest workers. Men are more frequently affected than women. This difference in sex incidence, however, is probably occupational in character. It is believed, on epidemiologic grounds, that various species of sandflies, *Phlebotomus,* are the vectors and that transmission from infected man or animals is accomplished by the bite of these insects. The disease has occurred in epidemic form in Paraguay.

It is questionable whether this form of leishmaniasis should be separated from oriental sore on any grounds other than clinical.

**Pathology**   American leishmaniasis is distinguished from oriental sore primarily by the fact that in 10 to 20 per cent of cases of "oriental sore" in South America the mucous membranes are involved, leading to extensive ulceration and necrosis of the nose, mouth and pharynx. During the period of active infection there is frequently profound cachexia and healing is often accompanied by great deformity of the affected structures. The mucosae may be invaded by direct extension from an adjacent cutaneous lesion; or the nasopharyngeal process may be secondary to a distant primary focus, the latter in some cases having healed prior to the onset of the secondary development.

The development of the lesion is similar to that of oriental sore. It appears first as a small papule, later becoming crusted and exuding sticky exudate. Removal of the crust reveals a freely bleeding ulcer. This extends slowly into adjacent tissues, increasing both in size and depth as secondary infection is established. The cartilage and bony support of the nose are often destroyed and the hard and soft palate and walls of the pharynx are sometimes similarly affected. Death occurs from sepsis or malnutrition.

Leishmania may be recovered from nodules and the indurated margins of ulcers. There is no general dissemination, although rarely they may be found in the regional lymph nodes adjacent to an active lesion.

**Clinical Characteristics**   The disease begins as a small papule appearing on an exposed skin surface, often on the margins of the ears. Ulcer formation follows and the process at this stage does not differ from oriental sore. Later ulcers develop about the margins of the nose and mouth and may extend causing widespread destruction of tissue in the naso-oral region.

**Diagnosis**   In advanced cases with extensive secondary infection it may be impossible to demonstrate leishmania. Material for staining or culture should be obtained by curettage of the indurated margin of the lesion or by aspiration from this area.

The *differential diagnosis* of this condition involves consideration of yaws, leprosy, tertiary syphilis, blastomycosis, lupus, and nasal myiasis.

**Treatment**   The prognosis is much more serious than is that of oriental sore because of the destructive mucocutaneous lesions. In order to prevent these serious complications intensive treatment should be instituted at the earliest possible moment.

The early cutaneous lesions should be intensively treated by infiltration with a 10 to 20 per cent solution of quinacrine or a 1 per cent solution of *berberine sulfate* as recommended for the treatment of oriental sore. Because of the risk of secondary development of nasopharyngeal lesions, the local treatment should be supplemented by parenteral administration of *sodium antimony gluconate.* Treatment should be continued until apparent cure is obtained, and the patient should be held under observation for an additional period of time.

The extensive lesions encountered in the later stages of the disease require intensive antimony treatment. This should be initiated with neostibosan. Subsequently if required, *sodium antimony tartrate,* which has been considered very useful in this form of leishmaniasis, may be used. It should be administered intravenously on alternate days. A 2 per cent freshly prepared solution should invariably be used, the initial injection being 2 ml. (equals 0.04 gm.) and each dose thereafter increased by 1 ml. to a total individual dose of 5 ml. The latter should then be maintained until completion of the course. A total of 40 or more injections should be given.

Secondary bacterial infection must be treated by the appropriate antibiotics and sulfonamides.

# 39   African Trypanosomiasis

**Synonyms**   Sleeping sickness; maladie du sommeil (French); Schlafkrankheit (German).

**Definition**   African trypanosomiasis is an acute and chronic protozoal disease produced by a hemoflagellate of the genus *Trypanosoma,* family TRYPANOSOMIDAE. It is transmitted by various species of tsetse flies, all of which fall in the genus *Glossina.* The acute disease is distinguished by fever, adenitis, rash and transitory edemas. The chronic form appears when the central nervous system is invaded and is characterized clinically by meningo-encephalitis and meningomyelitis with wasting and mental and physical apathy which may progress into coma and death.

**Distribution**   The disease is limited to the tsetse fly areas of Africa. It is endemic throughout most of the tropical area of the continent. Roughly the boundaries extend from Senegal, east to Bahr el Ghazal province of the southern Sudan; then south through the lake country of East Africa into Portuguese East Africa; and then west to Angola (Fig. 157).

**Etiology**   *Trypanosoma gambiense, T. rhodesiense* and *T. brucei* have been regarded in the past as separate species. They are morpho-

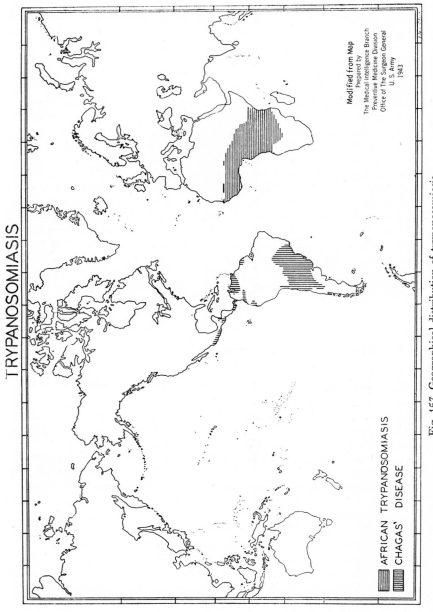

Fig. 157. Geographical distribution of trypanosomiasis.

logically identical and no significant or dependable distinctions among them have been found.

*Trypanosoma rhodesiense* is said to be more virulent for man than *T. gambiense*. It has been suggested that the former is identical

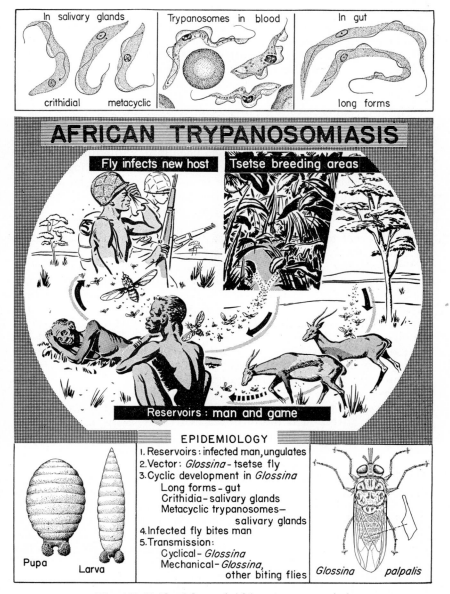

Fig. 158. Epidemiology of African trypanosomiasis.

with *T. brucei,* the parasite causing nagana, a disease of cattle, horses and game.

These trypanosomes are slender flagellates tapering to a fine point anteriorly and having a relatively blunt posterior extremity. They vary from about 8 to 30 microns in length. There is a large centrally placed nucleus. The kinetoplast is situated near the posterior end of the trypanosome. It consists of the parabasal body and a dotlike blepharoplast which is the origin of an axial filament or axoneme which extends forward as the free edge of an undulating membrane and becomes free anteriorly to form the single flagellum. The free edge of the undulating membrane is longer than its base, producing numerous folds. Motion is usually in the direction of the flagellar end.

These trypanosomes are polymorphic, some having a free flagellum and some lacking it. When the parasites are present in the blood in considerable numbers both long, narrow and short, stumpy forms may be seen. The former have a long flagellum, while the latter have none or at most a very short one. At times the nucleus may be situated posteriorly, occasionally close to the kinetoplast. The posterior position of the nucleus was formerly regarded as the distinguishing morphologic characteristic of *T. rhodesiense.* This view is no longer accepted.

At different stages of the disease trypanosomes may be found in the blood, the lymph and the tissues of the central nervous system.

**Epidemiology**  RESERVOIR. Man is the principal reservoir for *T. gambiense* and *T. rhodesiense.* It is believed that certain domestic animals, notably the pig, may likewise serve in this capacity, particularly for *T. gambiense.* The morphologic identity of the two human trypanosomes and *T. brucei,* which is widely prevalent in various antelopes and other ungulates, has given rise to the belief that the human strains may be variants of *T. brucei* and that the wild game is the ultimate and important reservoir of infection. This continues to be a controversial question (Fig. 158).

VECTOR. These trypanosomes undergo cyclical development in various species of *Glossina,* which are the only insect hosts. Endemicity of the infection is therefore limited to tsetse fly infested areas. The genus *Glossina* contains some twenty species of which only a limited number has so far been proven to be of importance in the epidemiology of trypanosomiasis (Table 32).

When these trypanosomes are ingested by the fly they multiply in the mid-gut and hind-gut. Depending upon conditions of temperature and humidity, long slender forms appear from the eighth to the eighteenth day. These move anteriorly to the proventriculus and thence to the salivary glands and ducts where crithidial forms are produced. The infective metacyclic trypanosomes, which are similar to the short stumpy trypanosomes observed in the patient's blood in the presence of a heavy infection, are derived from these. They pass down the salivary ducts, entering the bite wound through the channel in the hypopharynx. The fly becomes infective in eighteen to thirty-four days after the infecting meal.

In the presence of epidemic outbreaks of the disease it is possible that mechanical transmission of the trypanosomes from man to man occurs both by the tsetse flies and possibly the biting fly, *Stomoxys*, as the result of interrupted feedings in the course of which the proboscis has become contaminated with trypanosomes.

**Incidence**   There is no significant variation in incidence as regards age, sex and occupation except insofar as these factors may contribute to exposure to the flies. While there is no true racial immunity, it is

*Table 32   Principal Vectors of African Trypanosomiasis*

| SPECIES OF *Trypanosoma* | SPECIES OF *Glossina* |
| --- | --- |
| *T. gambiense* | *G. palpalis\*; G. tachinoides\*; G. pallidipes; G. brevipalpis; G. fusca* |
| *T. rhodesiense* | *G. morsitans\*; G. swynnertoni; G. brevipalpis* |
| *T. brucei* | *G. morsitans\** |

\* Much more important than other species listed.

*G. palpalis*—always in vicinity of water; pupates close to water in dry shaded places; closely associated with man; feeds on crocodiles, animals, man.

*G. tachinoides*—pupates in dry sandy soil near water; never closely associated with man; feeds largely on game.

*G. morsitans*—open country; pupates in dry friable earth: feeds on animals and man.

generally considered that the disease tends to be more acute in the white race than in the colored. There is no definite acquired immunity.

**Pathology**   The essential pathologic changes of trypanosomiasis are found in the lymph nodes and in the central nervous system. In the early stages there is proliferation of lymphoid tissue. In the chronic stages a productive endarteritis occurs with endothelial proliferation, involving especially the small vessels and accompanied by perivascular infiltration with plasma cells and lymphocytes, giving many of the lesions a histologic appearance similar to those of syphilis. Chronic inflammation of the lymphatic system results in enlargement of the lymph nodes which in the early stages frequently contain trypanosomes. At this stage there is usually some enlargement of the spleen.

Central nervous system involvement results essentially in a meningoencephalitis and meningomyelitis. These are accompanied by perivascular plasma and round cell infiltration which is most marked in the pia-arachnoid of the brain and cord, particularly about the vessels of the pons and medulla. The brain and cord are congested; hemorrhages may be present and trypanosomes are frequently scattered through the brain substance. At times small granulomatous lesions are encountered, especially in the cortex (Fig. 159).

Prior to involvement of the nervous system the cerebrospinal fluid reveals no abnormalities. When lesions are established, however, the fluid is usually under increased pressure and the cell count may reach 1000 per cubic millimeter. There is a positive globulin reaction and the centrifuged fluid frequently reveals trypanosomes.

**Clinical Characteristics** The clinical manifestations of trypanosomiasis may vary greatly in their intensity and duration. The bite of the infected tsetse fly is often followed by a local inflammatory reaction of the skin which may last forty-eight to seventy-two hours. The incubation period of the disease may show great variation, in

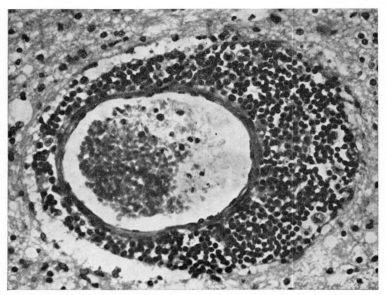

Fig. 159. African sleeping sickness: section of brain showing perivascular infiltration (cuffing) and edema.

occasional instances lasting apparently two to five years before the appearance of clinical symptoms. Its usual duration, however, is ten days to three weeks.

The disease may be divided into *two clinical stages*. The first, that of invasion by the trypanosomes, is characterized by fever and lymphadenopathy. The second stage is marked by the onset of central nervous system involvement and is characterized by the symptoms and signs of a meningo-encephalitis and meningomyelitis with cachexia and ultimately, in the most severe cases, coma and death.

In the *stage of invasion* trypanosomes are present in the peripheral blood but may be more readily demonstrated in fluid aspirated from enlarged lymph nodes (Fig. 160). The irregularly remitting fever may be high. Characteristically the temperature is normal or close to normal in the morning, rising to 103° or 104° F. at night. The pulse and respiration are correspondingly elevated. Early in the disease headache, neuralgic pains, insomnia and loss of ability to concentrate are common. In white individuals there is frequently an irregular circinate rash, most commonly observed on the trunk and thighs. This usually appears as irregular oval, pinkish, erythematous areas, having a clear center. Pruritus is common and often severe. Painful local edemas of the hands, the feet, about the eyes and in the vicinity of various joints are frequent and characteristically transitory. All these symptoms and signs, including the febrile reaction, may be irregular and inconstant, disappearing and reappearing after varying intervals.

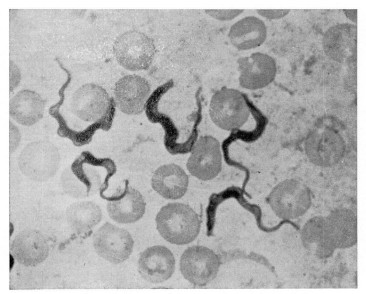

Fig. 160. *Trypanosoma gambiense* in stained blood film.

As the infection becomes established the superficial lymph nodes become enlarged. This is most evident in the posterior cervical chain where the swelling constitutes one of the most important diagnostic criteria, Winterbottom's sign. This is such a constant accompaniment of African trypanosomiasis that examination for enlargement of the posterior cervical nodes is a useful procedure for survey purposes (Fig. 161). The individual nodes are discrete, varying from 1.0 to 1.5 cm. in diameter. At first they are soft and elastic, later becoming hard as the result of fibrotic changes. The enlargement usually persists from the second to the sixth month of the disease. With the involvement of the lymphatic system there may be some enlargement of the spleen and liver which, with the fever, may be suggestive of a malarial infection.

During this first stage of the disease deep hyperesthesias, especially over the ulna, Kerandel's sign, are frequent.

Involvement of the central nervous system may occur early in the disease. In consequence lumbar puncture and careful spinal fluid examination are essential.

The total leukocyte count is usually normal. There is characteristically a relative mononucleosis with increased numbers of both large and small mononuclear cells which may constitute 50 to 70 per cent of the total white blood cells.

The *second stage*, that of involvement of the central nervous system, may occur early in the clinical course of the infection or may not develop until months or even years later. The onset of this stage

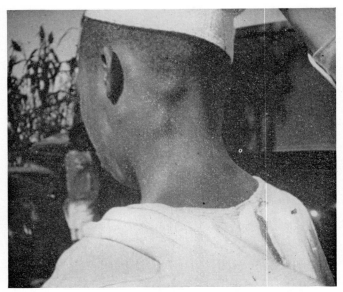

Fig. 161. Enlargement of posterior cervical lymph nodes—Winterbottom's sign. (Courtesy of Dr. James R. Busvine, London School of Hygiene and Tropical Medicine.)

is usually insidious. It may be ushered in by tremor of the tongue and fingers, headache, delusions, hysteria, mania and other signs of meningo-encephalitis and meningomyelitis. The common presenting symptom is a gradually increasing languor and lassitude. This is followed shortly by the appearance of tremor of the tongue and fingers. With further progression the facial expression is altered; the patient appears apathetic, morose and lethargic; somnolence is common. Speech is slow and mumbling, the gait becomes shuffling, and fine fibrillary tremors of the tongue and of the muscles of the forearms are prominent.

With still further progression the typical *sleeping sickness stage* is reached. The somnolent state is almost continuous and it becomes increasingly difficult to arouse the patient. Ultimately this progresses to true coma. Concurrently there is progressive development of marasmus with wasting, increasing muscular weakness, increasing tremor and dribbling of saliva. Late in the disease epileptiform convulsions may occur. Death ensues as the result of sleeping sickness itself, malnutrition, or intercurrent infection (Fig. 162).

**Diagnosis** The diagnosis of trypanosomiasis depends upon the demonstration of the trypanosomes in the peripheral blood, in fluid aspirated from enlarged lymph nodes or in the spinal fluid. In the majority of instances trypanosomes are rare or impossible to find in the peripheral blood.

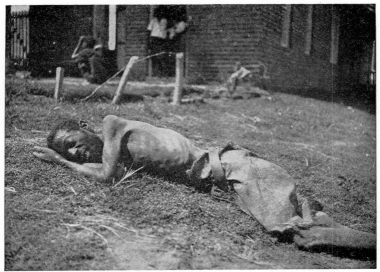

Fig. 162. Comatose stage of sleeping sickness. (Courtesy of E. R. Kellersberger in Strong: Stitt's Diagnosis, Prevention and Treatment of Tropical Diseases. The Blakiston Co.)

Examination of a stained smear of fluid aspirated from an enlarged elastic lymph node is the most dependable diagnostic procedure in the early stages of the disease. It is not of value in the later stages when the nodes have become hard and sclerotic. A fine hypodermic needle should be introduced into the substance of a lymph node and the aspirate used to prepare thick and thin films. These should be stained with Wright's, Giemsa's or Leishman's stains.

Examination of the blood should include the study of both thick and thin smears. In fresh unstained cover-slip preparations the motility of the trypanosomes may reveal their presence even when few are present. The most certain method, however, entails the use of centrifuged citrated blood. The technique is described on page 810.

The cerebrospinal fluid should be examined in all cases. In the stage of early involvement of the central nervous system there may be only a slight increase in the cell count and a positive globulin reaction. Even in this stage trypanosomes may be demonstrable after centrifuging the fluid. As the involvement becomes more extensive the cell count rises, the pressure is increased and the fluid may have a ground glass appearance or may even be turbid. The cells are predominantly mononuclears.

Examination of the blood of rats, guinea pigs or monkeys after inoculation with lymph node aspirates, blood or spinal fluid from the patient may reveal trypanosomes when other methods fail.

**Treatment**   GENERAL MEASURES. Lumbar puncture should be performed immediately, periodically through the course of treatment, and at least twice at intervals of six months after completion of treatment to ensure early recognition of central nervous system invasion. It is important to emphasize that the earlier efficient therapy is initiated, the greater are the possibilities of cure.

The drug treatment of trypanosomiasis presents three aspects: the early case; the intermediate and advanced case in which invasion of the central nervous system has occurred; and chemoprophylaxis.

EARLY CASES. Two drugs are recommended for treatment in the stage prior to invasion of the central nervous system.

*Naphuride.* Synonyms: Naphuride sodium, suramin, Bayer 205, Antrypol, Moranyl, Fourneau 309, Germanin. The drug is a complex organic chemical which contains no heavy metal. It combines with the plasma proteins and remains in the circulating blood for long periods of time. It is excreted through the kidneys and frequently acts as a renal irritant causing albuminuria with yellowish granular casts. More rarely, administration of the drug may be followed by nephritis and uremia. Urinalyses should be performed the day after each treatment and therapy must be discontinued if evidence of renal irritation appears.

Suramin is effective in the early stages of trypanosomiasis and is considered to be particularly useful in cases of infection by *T. rhodesiense*. It is ineffective against infection of the central nervous system. The drug may be given intramuscularly or intravenously; the latter is the preferred route of administration. It must not be given intrathecally because of its irritating effects.

Dosage. Suramin is administered intravenously at four day intervals dissolved in 10 ml. of distilled water. The initial dose should not exceed 0.3 gm. to 0.5 gm. because of possible idiosyncrasy. Subsequent doses should be 1.0 gm. and should be continued until a total of 10.0 gm. has been administered. The dosage for children is reduced in accordance with age and weight.

*Pentamidine.* Synonyms: M&B 800, Lomidine. The drug is an aromatic diamidine available in two forms:

Pentamidine: the isethionate, 1.74 mg. equivalent to 1 mg. of the base.

Lomidine: the methanesulfonate, 1.56 mg. equivalent to 1 mg. of the base.

Although it may be administered by mouth, the recommended

routes are by intramuscular or intravenous injection. When given too rapidly by vein it may cause sudden fall of blood pressure. This pressor effect may be prevented by slow administration with the patient in the recumbent position or by intramuscular injection of 0.25 ml. of 1/1000 Adrenalin or by an antihistaminic given just before the injection of pentamidine. In some instances blood sugar levels are depressed.

Intramuscular injection is usually employed since this method of administration is seldom accompanied by any of the symptoms referable to the depressor action of the drug. It is dangerous when given intrathecally, and oral dosage is often associated with vomiting and diarrhea.

Pentamidine is extremely effective in early cases of infection by *T. gambiense*. It cannot be relied upon when increased cell count and the protein content of the spinal fluid indicate invasion of the central nervous system. In such cases cryptic infection of the nervous system may continue without the appearance of trypanosomes in the blood or lymphatics.

Dosage. Solutions of pentamidine must be freshly prepared using sterile distilled water. For intramuscular injection the average dose is 4 mg. per kilogram of body weight dissolved in not more than 3 ml. of sterile distilled water; for intravenous administration the dose is 2 to 4 mg. per kilogram of body weight dissolved in 5 to 10 ml. of sterile distilled water.

The drug may be given daily or on alternate days to a total of 8 to 10 injections. When administered concurrently with suramin the depressor effects of pentamidine seem to be reduced.

Later Cases. The onset of the later stages of the disease is marked by the development of central nervous system symptoms and signs and abnormalities of the cerebrospinal fluid. There are two drugs which are useful for the treatment of advanced cases, tryparsamide and Mel B. Tryparsamide is still the mainstay in therapy of central nervous system infections. Unfortunately, there is an increasing number of resistant strains of trypanosomes, especially in the Belgian Congo.

*Tryparsamide.* Synonyms: Fourneau 270, Orsanine, tryponarsyl. Tryparsamide contains approximately 25 per cent of pentavalent arsenic which is reduced in the body to the active trivalent form. It is freely soluble in water. The margin of safety between the therapeutic and the toxic dose is small. In a susceptible person even a small dose may cause circulatory collapse and a full dose, death. The common toxic effect, however, is optic atrophy. This may lead to permanent blindness. The development of actual optic atrophy is commonly preceded by definite ocular symptoms, including photophobia, lacrimation, ocular pain or dimness of vision. On the appearance of any of these symptoms the dose should be reduced or the interval between doses lengthened and further administration of the drug should be controlled by repeated measurements of the visual fields.

Patients receiving this drug should be under close observation and, prior to treatment, careful examination of the eyes should be performed, including measurement of the visual fields and ophthalmoscopic examination of the fundi.

Tryparsamide penetrates through the "blood-brain barrier" and kills trypanosomes in the nervous tissue. Because of its relative ineffectiveness against the parasites in the blood and lymph, pentamidine or suramin are usually given in the intervals between the weekly injections of tryparsamide. Incomplete treatment is an important factor in the development of tryparsamide-resistant strains.

Dosage. It is preferable to administer the drug intravenously dissolved in 10 ml. of sterile distilled water, although it may be given intramuscularly. Salt solution *must not* be used. Individual doses should be 0.04 to 0.05 gm. per kilogram of body weight. Children up to twelve years of age seem to tolerate this drug and may be given up to 0.08 gm. per kilogram of body weight. The initial adult dose should be 1.0 to 1.5 gm. and subsequent doses 2.0 to 3.0 gm., depending upon the weight of the patient. Fifteen weekly injections should be given.

*Mel B.* The drug is a compound of Melarsen oxide and dimercaprol containing trivalent arsenic. It is administered in the form of a 5 per cent solution in propylene glycol. At times it causes serious toxic side effects and fatalities have not been infrequent. Because of this Mel B should be given only under close supervision in hospital and not in field dispensaries.

It has given good results in advanced cases and in infections which are refractory to other forms of treatment. It is usually effective against tryparsamide-resistant strains but will itself produce drug resistance when insufficient dosage is used. Mel B is not regarded as superior to tryparsamide and should be reserved for treatment of tryparsamide-resistant cases.

Dosage. The recommended dosage is 3.6 mg. per kilogram of body weight given intravenously on each of four consecutive days. After a rest period of one week the course is repeated.

There are no dependable criteria of cure. Relapses are frequent, especially in the advanced cases, and additional treatment is then required. Further therapy, however, should not be undertaken until a period of from one to three months has elapsed after the end of the previous treatment course. The spinal fluid affords a guide to the efficacy of treatment. Disappearance of trypanosomes and decrease of the cell count and globulin are favorable signs.

It is necessary to keep the patient under periodic observation for at least two years. Examination of the spinal fluid at intervals of two to three months is essential regardless of the patient's state of health.

Toxic reactions due to arsenic should be treated with British antilewisite (BAL). The recommended dosage is four intramuscular injections of 1.5 ml. BAL daily for six to ten days. If relapse occurs, treatment should be resumed immediately.

**Prophylaxis** The recognition, isolation and effective therapy of infected persons constitutes one of the most important measures in the prophylaxis of trypanosomiasis. Individuals entering disease-free areas from regions in which the disease is endemic should invariably be examined and subjected to medical control and treatment if infected. This is particularly true of native populations which may be imported for labor purposes.

The second important control measure is directed against the vector. In fly-infested areas individuals should wear suitable clothing, including long sleeves and long trousers. The flies are attracted by moving objects and will frequently follow individuals or automobiles for considerable distances. They bite easily through thin clothing. Motor vehicles passing into a controlled area should be carefully examined for the presence of the tsetse. Insofar as possible heavily infested areas should be avoided. It has been necessary, on occasion in the past, to evacuate population groups of considerable size from regions where satisfactory control of *Glossina* was not practicable.

Two drugs have proved to be effective chemoprophylactic agents: *Naphuride* and *pentamidine*. Suramin in dosage of 1.0 gm. every two to three months exercises a definite protective action. However, pentamidine has been shown to confer a high degree of protection over a longer period of time.

Mass chemoprophylaxis using pentamidine has been greatly extended and has given highly encouraging results. In areas where injection has been repeated four to five times at intervals of six months the new infection rate has been reduced by 90 to 95 per cent. It appears that mass treatment may prove to be a most important factor in the control of trypanosomiasis. Pentamidine does not cause abortion.

Dosage. Naphuride 1.0 gm. every two to three months. Pentamidine 3 mg. per kilogram of body weight every six months.

# 40 Chagas' Disease

**Synonyms** South American trypanosomiasis; schizotrypanosomiasis; opilaçao; enfermedad de Chagas.

**Definition** This is a relatively uncommon acute and chronic disease produced by infection with *Trypanosoma cruzi* especially affecting children. It is characterized pathologically by the presence of trypanosomes in the blood and leishmanias in the tissues. The acute stage is manifested by fever, facial and general edema, adenitis and anemia. The symptoms in the chronic stage depend upon the localization of the parasite, especially in the heart muscle, the central nervous system and the liver.

**Distribution**    The disease is limited to rural areas of Mexico and of Central and South America. Cases have been reported from Mexico, Guatemala, San Salvador, Costa Rica, Panama, Colombia, Venezuela, the Guianas, Brazil, Argentina, Uruguay, Paraguay, Bolivia, Ecuador, Chile and Peru. *Trypanosoma cruzi* has been found in wild rodents in California, Arizona, New Mexico and Texas and in armadillos and opossums in Texas, but as yet an autochthonous human infection has not been reported within the United States.

**Etiology**    *Trypanosoma cruzi* is a pleomorphic trypanosome having two phases in its life cycle. One occurs in man and other mammals, and one in the transmitting insects. In the infected mammal

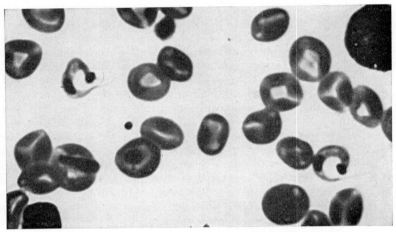

Fig. 163. *Trypanosoma cruzi* in stained blood film.

typical trypanosomes are present in the blood, while leishmanias and transformation stages occur in the endothelial and tissue cells.

The trypanosome is approximately 20 microns in length, often spindle-shaped and presents both long and short forms. The nucleus is centrally placed and the characteristically large oval kinetoplast is situated posteriorly. An axoneme arises from the dotlike blepharoplast and is extended along the free margin of a narrow undulating membrane, presenting few folds, becoming a free flagellum anteriorly. Characteristically this trypanosome presents a sharp wedge-shaped posterior extremity. In stained films the parasites usually appear C- or U-shaped. Dividing forms do not occur in the blood (Fig. 163).

The trypanosomes invade tissue cells, losing the flagellum and undulating membrane. Division occurs by binary fission, producing groups of leishmanias giving the appearance of intracellular cysts. These eventually fill and destroy the infected cell.

The leishmanias are round or oval bodies 3 to 5 microns in diameter, presenting both a nucleus and a kinetoplast. As the invaded cells are destroyed parasites are liberated, apparently as leishmanial, crithidial or trypanosomal forms. Only the trypanosomes, however, are demonstrable in the peripheral blood. *Trypanosoma cruzi* may be grown on artificial culture media. (See pp. 836–837.)

**Epidemiology** The reservoirs of *T. cruzi* are man and other mammals, especially the armadillo and opossum. Dogs, cats, bats, the domestic pig, the house rat and various other mammals including at least two species of monkeys have been found naturally infected.

The infection is transmitted from man to man and from a reservoir animal to man by the reduviid (cone-nose) bugs, also known as "assassin" or "kissing" bugs. The latter designation is based on the fact that they are vicious biters and attack the face especially.

The reduviid becomes infective eight to ten days after ingestion of *T. cruzi* and may remain infective for as long as two years. The reduviids particularly concerned in the transmission of Chagas' disease are *Panstrongylus megistus* and *P. infestans*. Other species of the genus are also vectors. The infection may likewise be transmitted by allied genera such as *Rhodnius, Eratyrus* and *Eutriatoma*.

The reduviid bugs frequently inhabit the burrows of armadillos and likewise adapt themselves to living in poorly-constructed types of rural houses. They are also commonly found in outbuildings such as stables and pigsties. During the day they remain in cracks and holes or in thatch, coming out at night to feed. They tend to remain in the same house as long as it is inhabited (Fig. 164).

After ingestion by the bug the trypanosomes multiply in the mid-gut by longitudinal fission with the development of noninfective crithidia which have a centrally placed nucleus and a kinetoplast at the anterior end. Subsequently, intermediate forms with a kinetoplast variously situated and metacyclic trypanosomes with the kinetoplast at the posterior extremity are formed. The latter have a well developed undulating membrane and flagellum. The metacyclic trypanosomes are found in the hind-gut of the reduviid and are passed in its feces. When the insect feeds, the feces containing metacyclic trypanosomes contaminate the bite wound, or an abrasion of the skin, or the organisms may penetrate directly through the mucous membranes of the conjunctiva or mouth.

There is no racial or sex distribution of the infection in man. The disease, however, is one predominantly of children under two years of age although adults are occasionally infected.

**Pathology** The basic lesion of Chagas' disease is a degeneration of various types of tissue cells after their invasion by the leishmanias. This is accompanied by replacement fibrosis. In acute cases the parasites may be found in almost every organ. The most marked lesions, however, occur in the heart muscle, brain and liver. In the individual cell rapid multiplication of the parasites produces a cystlike structure, ultimately leading to destruction of the cell and release of the contained organisms.

Cardiac muscle fibers are commonly and often intensely infected, the fibers containing enormous numbers of leishmanias. Muscle fibers often appear separated and exhibit both fragmentation and hyaline degeneration with large nests of parasites between them. Perivascular collections of lymphocytes and plasma cells are not uncommon in the myocardium. The epicardium and endocardium like-

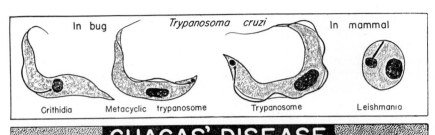

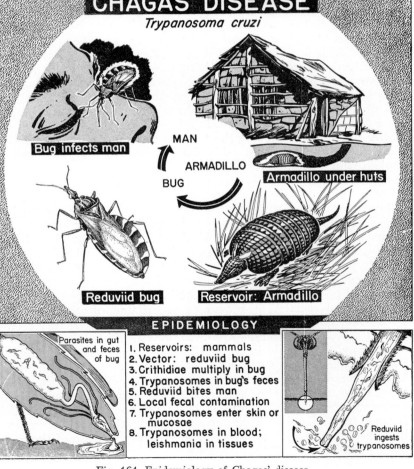

Fig. 164. Epidemiology of Chagas' disease.

wise may be invaded. Skeletal muscle is also frequently parasitized, the fibers containing large numbers of leishmanias (Fig. 165).

In severe cases of the acute form of the disease the brain and meninges may be congested and edematous and there may be scattered small inflammatory foci in the brain substance in which occa-

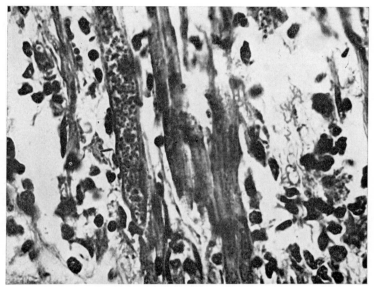

Fig. 165. Cardiac muscle showing extensive invasion by leishmanial forms, and degeneration of muscle fibers.

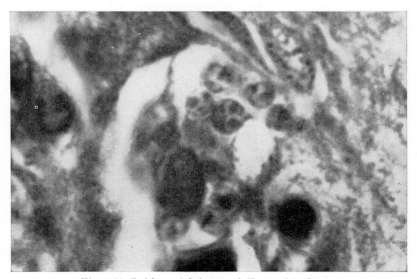

Fig. 166. Leishmanial forms of *T. cruzi* in brain.

sional leishmanias are present. The parasites, however, do not attack the nerve cells (Figs. 166, 167).

The liver is frequently enlarged, exhibiting cloudy swelling and fatty degeneration. Parasites, however, are rarely present and then only in the Kupffer cells. The spleen is often enlarged and may con-

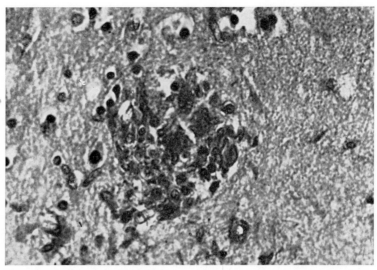

Fig. 167. Nodules in brain: necrosis, cellular proliferation and infiltration.

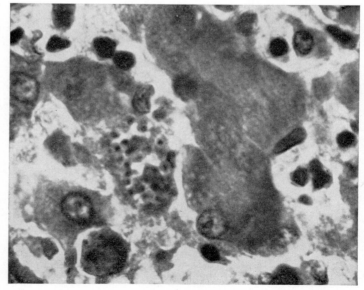

Fig. 168. Leishmanial forms of *T. cruzi* in Kupffer cells of the liver.

tain leishmanias. There is enlargement of peripheral lymph nodes with congestion and hyperplasia. Parasites, however, are rarely present in them (Fig. 168).

**Clinical Characteristics**  The clinical features of Chagas' disease vary markedly. In general the younger the individual the greater is the severity. The acute form of the disease predominates in the younger age groups, whereas the chronic form is usual among adults.

Early accounts of Chagas' disease, particularly of the chronic form, refer to a high incidence of thyroid enlargement and the not infrequent occurrence of myxedema in adults and cretinism in children. These features are not encountered in all areas where Chagas' disease has been observed and it is believed, therefore, that the association is an accidental one, with the trypanosome infection occurring in individuals already the subjects of endemic goiter.

*Acute Chagas' disease* occurs usually in children under one year of age. High continuous fever, which may reach 104° F., follows an incubation period of seven to fourteen days. The infection is often associated with unilateral conjunctivitis and edema of the face (Romaña's sign). This syndrome is very suggestive and may indicate the eye as the site of inoculation. In severe cases an elastic non-pitting edema may extend from the face to involve the body. The liver and spleen are enlarged and there is likewise enlargement of the superficial lymph nodes, especially the inguinal and axillary groups. During the febrile stage trypanosomes may be demonstrated in the blood stream, usually disappearing when the temperature falls to normal. As the blood becomes negative and the fever ceases the edema commonly disappears. The acute stage of the disease is usually of short duration, not infrequently with fatal outcome in very young children. The parasitization of the myocardium producing cardiac failure is a frequent cause of death.

The *chronic form* of the disease may follow in young children who survive the acute stage and is the type of disease commonly observed in older children and adults. In the latter individuals the infection frequently produces no important symptoms. It is probable that many of the phenomena attributed in the past to chronic Chagas' disease are the result of endemic goiter rather than chronic infection by *T. cruzi*. Notable among these are the enlargement of the thyroid, alopecia, mental dullness, circulatory disturbances, and certain of the nervous disorders. Invasion of the thyroid gland, however, may be a factor in causing thyroid dysfunction, and similar involvement of the suprarenal glands may produce a syndrome having much in common with Addison's disease. The liver, spleen, and peripheral lymph nodes may be enlarged, and there may be irregular fever and anemia. *Trypanosoma cruzi* is not commonly found in the blood during the chronic stage of the disease.

**Diagnosis**  The diagnosis of Chagas' disease depends upon the demonstration of the trypanosomal stage of *T. cruzi* in the blood or the leishmanial stage in other tissues. Trypanosomes when present in the blood may be demonstrated by the following procedures (see pp. 811–836):

1. Examination of fresh blood films.

2. Examination of stained thick and thin blood films.

3. Examination of stained films after centrifuging 5 to 10 ml. of citrated blood.

4. Animal inoculation using 5 to 10 ml. of the patient's blood. Most laboratory animals are easily infected and the white rat is a suitable test animal.

5. Culture of blood on N.N.N. medium or culture in blood broth.

6. Xenodiagnosis: clean, uninfected laboratory-bred reduviid bugs are allowed to feed on the suspected patient. Two weeks later the contents of the hind-gut are examined for the presence of crithidia and particularly metacyclic trypanosomes. In conducting this test it is essential to use clean insects properly protected, since they can become infected by coprophagy.

These procedures directed to the recovery of trypanosomes from the blood stream are usually unsuccessful except during the acute febrile stage of the disease in children and during the febrile periods of chronic disease in adults.

When blood examinations are negative, biopsy of skeletal muscle may demonstrate the leishmanial forms within the muscle fibers.

*Trypanosoma cruzi* may be found in the enlarged lymph nodes. It is rarely present in the spinal fluid except in instances when there is a meningo-encephalitis.

**Treatment**    The treatment of Chagas' disease is unsatisfactory. None of the drugs effective against the African trypanosomes affects *T. cruzi*. Bayer 7602 and Eagle's 70A are the only available drugs. While they appear to be useful in controlling acute symptoms in young children they do not free the blood of trypanosomes. There is no preparation which is effective against the leishmania forms in the tissues. In consequence, treatment is largely symptomatic.

**Prophylaxis**    Native houses and adobe and thatched huts in the endemic area should not be used for sleeping quarters, since they constitute the normal harborage of the insect vector. Some protection of individuals resident in such structures may be afforded by proper use of bed nets, since the vectors are nocturnal feeders.

Reports concerning the value of residual spraying with DDT are conflicting. However, Gammexane is highly effective in controlling the reduviid bug population when used as a residual spray inside of buildings and huts. It is claimed that entire reduviid bug populations have been eliminated by the use of this chemical.

While complement fixation tests are not dependable for clinical diagnosis they do provide an important tool for use in screening prospective blood donors. Numerous instances of infection by *T. cruzi* have followed transfusion. In endemic areas the complement fixation test should be used routinely and persons having a positive reaction should not be used as donors.

# 41  Introduction

Parasitic worms infect man in almost all regions of the world but they are especially abundant in number both of species and of individuals in the tropics. This is the result of important climatic and sociologic factors. Many of these parasites require special conditions of temperature and humidity for survival and multiplication. Many others require particular vertebrate or invertebrate hosts such as fish, snails, crustacea or insects for the completion of their life cycles. These hosts in turn gain ready access to man in tropical regions owing to the lack of preventive measures by the indigenous populations. Insect vectors such as various mosquitoes, midges and biting flies are particularly important among these intermediate hosts.

The distribution of those helminth parasites whose eggs are passed in human dejecta is affected not only by the climatic conditions of rainfall, temperature and humidity but likewise by the sanitary practices of the human population. The almost universal custom in many regions of the world of using human excreta (nightsoil) for fertilizer results frequently in widespread pollution of soil, water supplies and certain foods by which infection is transmitted to others.

Moreover racial food habits often determine the incidence of certain of these parasites in man. The practice of eating raw or partially

**371**

cooked fresh-water fish and shellfish, meat and certain aquatic plants in which, or on which, encysted larvae of parasitic worms occur permits completion of the biologic cycle and infection of man. Root vegetables pickled in weak concentrations of vinegar or brine are an important potential source of infection, since eggs of *Ascaris* and *Trichuris* have been shown to remain viable in such foods for considerable periods of time.

The parasitic helminths of man fall into two main groups, the roundworms or Nemathelminthes and the flatworms or Platyhelminthes. The former are characterized by their unsegmented, undifferentiated external appearance (except the spiny-headed worms), slender shape and the smooth or occasionally striated cuticula. The Nemathelminthes consist of three groups only one of which, the threadworms, roundworms (*sensu strictu*) or Nematoda, contains important human parasites.

The flatworms or Platyhelminthes are flattened dorsoventrally and sometimes exhibit pseudosegmentation. The flatworms parasitizing man include the leaflike flukes or Trematoda and the ribbonlike, pseudosegmented tapeworms or Cestoda.

One other group, the spiny-headed worms or Acanthocephala, should be mentioned briefly. These are often placed in the same phylum as roundworms or Nemathelminthes. The sexes are separate and both males and females have a retractile proboscis armed with spines, and a cylindrical body which lacks a digestive tract but contains other organ systems.

Only two species of *Acanthocephala* parasitize man, and infections by these are rare. Therefore they will not be considered further in this book.

The parasitic way of life has brought about numerous modifications in structure, function and even life cycles. Some of these changes are characteristic of groups while others may be peculiar to given genera or species. For example, the integument or cuticula of helminths, secreted by the underlying cells, forms a hardened, tough and elastic, or delicate covering which is resistant to digestion during the life of the parasite. Often it is specialized to form hooks or cutting plates such as occur in the buccal cavity of hookworms, the stylets of the microfilariae, or other spines, spicules or hooks. Both the trematodes and tapeworms may possess circular suckers, or acetabula, that serve as holdfast or locomotor organs. However, in some species of tapeworm, such as *Diphyllobothrium latum*, the holdfast device is a poorly developed, although very efficient, pair of sucking grooves. Many helminths possess glands which open near the mouth and are believed to secrete an enzyme-like substance which causes tissue destruction. Some parasites use this tissue directly as food, while for others the destruction merely makes it possible for them to penetrate to a definitive location within the host.

Many organs of locomotion, nutrition and reproduction have undergone marked changes in parasitic organisms. Parasites are usually transported from place to place by the host and in many instances may be transmitted passively from one host to another. This has been associated with a reduction in the development of locomotor devices. Organs of nutrition have become modified or even lost as in the case of the tapeworms. On the other hand, the reproductive organs have undergone considerable development and are often larger and more complicated than those found in free-living relatives. Frequently the production of tremendous quantities of eggs is associated with the slender chance that an egg or larva will succeed in reaching, and establishing itself on or within, another host. These structural or physiologic differences may be characteristics of the large groups, or perhaps only of genera or species.

Helminths almost without exception do not multiply in man as adults, thus differing signally from other disease-producing organisms. The pathologic changes which they induce in the host are the effects of a variety of mechanisms. Thus the hookworm is a voracious feeder upon blood which it obtains through lacerations of the intestinal mucosa produced by its cutting plates or teeth. Certain of the tapeworms merely rob the host of food while others, utilizing man as an intermediate host for their larval forms, produce single or multiple expanding tumors in many anatomic locations. Other parasites entering the skin cause more or less severe dermatitis, probably the result of toxic secretions or excretions of the larvae after penetration. Certain helminths produce pathologic changes in the subcutaneous tissues, the eye, the lungs and other viscera in the course of the migrations of the larvae or adult worms. Certain of the filarial worms which localize in the vessels of the lymphatic system cause acute and chronic inflammation which is followed by extensive lymphatic obstruction. The spined eggs of the schistosomes, deposited in the smaller venous channels of the bowel and vesical walls, produce vascular damage and ulceration into the viscus. Further, the mechanical irritation from the eggs or chemical irritation from products of the contained embryo appears to induce epithelial hyperplasia and metaplasia which may be followed occasionally by carcinoma.

Thus the pathologic changes accompanying helminthic infections may be both varied and severe, and the resulting clinical phenomena those of serious and acute or chronic disease. The diseases caused by parasitic worms constitute a most important segment of tropical medicine. The physician practicing in the tropics must be familiar with this group of conditions, their epidemiology, pathology and clinical manifestations, and the life cycles of the parasites if he is to practice either therapeutic or preventive medicine successfully.

# 42   Intestinal Nematodes

## Morphology of the Nematodes in General

*Introduction*   All parasitic nematodes possess certain common characteristics. These will be briefly considered. Other pertinent data dealing with the morphology and biology of the specific subdivisions will be taken up in subsequent chapters. *Strongyloides stercoralis* is believed by many workers to be the only heterogenetic nematode infecting man, i.e., it has both free-living and parasitic generations. All the others are parasitic during part or all of each life cycle.

All nematodes are characterized by their elongate, cylindrical, unsegmented bodies and glistening cuticula. The sexes are separate, the males being smaller than the females and usually curved ventrally. Nematodes possess a simple, tubular alimentary canal which includes an anterior mouth and a posterior anus.

Intestinal species range in size from a fraction of a millimeter to a maximum of 49 cm. (*Ascaris*) while some of the nematodes inhabiting blood or other tissues may approximate a meter (*Dracunculus medinensis*).

*Nematode Structure*   Externally nematodes are covered with a non-nucleated, shiny *cuticula* secreted by underlying subcuticular cells. This integument may be smooth, striated or covered with bosses (elevations), or occasionally spines. Some regions contain specialized *sensory papillae* (phasmids and amphids).

Beneath the subcuticula lies a *dermo-muscular layer* composed of a syncytium of cells and muscle fibers which constitute the lining of the pseudocoelom or body cavity. The *excretory system* as well as six longitudinal nerve trunks lie in this syncytium. In addition there is a *nerve ring* surrounding the esophagus and also sensory devices, previously mentioned, such as *phasmids* and *amphids* (papillae) which are caudal receptor organs. Amphids are located also in the cephalic or cervical regions.

The *digestive system* of the nematodes is simple, being composed of a straight tube running from the anteriorly placed mouth to a ventral, posteriorly situated anus. The *buccal* or *pharyngeal cavity* is lined with cuticula and may vary in length; it is surrounded by lips or papillae and is sometimes provided with teeth or cutting plates. Behind the buccal cavity is the typically muscular *esophagus* which, lined with cuticula, varies in structure and shape, and functions as a sucking organ. The esophagus is surrounded by well-developed valves at its juncture with the *intestine* or "mid gut" which is lined with a single layer of cells capable of absorbing food material. Posteriorly the intestine passes into a rectum, followed by the anus which in males opens into a ventral cloaca. Rectal glands are present in both sexes, except those males (like those of the hookworm) which have

**374**

a posterior cloaca modified to form a holdfast device called a *copulatory bursa*. In such cases the rectal glands are modified to serve as cement glands.

The *reproductive system* of the male consists of a single tubule which begins as a testis and passes successively into a vas deferens, seminal vesicle, and ejaculatory duct which opens into the cloaca. Special copulatory devices, such as spicules, a *gubernaculum*, or a posterior extremity modified to form a bursa or holdfast disk, may also occur.

The female reproductive system consists of a delicate threadlike, tubular ovary which passes successively into an oviduct, seminal receptacle, uterus, ovijector, vagina and externally opening vulva. This system may be single as in the trichina- and whipworms, double as in hookworms and pinworms, or multiple as in others.

**Nematode Eggs** The eggs contain the fertilized cell and yolk granules which are surrounded by a vitelline membrane in a chitinous shell (Fig. 169). Sometimes this in turn has an outer protein covering as in *Ascaris* eggs. Unsegmented, partially developed, or embryonated eggs may be discharged or the larvae may be already hatched. Unsegmented eggs are typical of *Ascaris* and whipworm, while the eggs of hookworms usually show signs of development. Pinworm eggs are embryonated when passed while in the case of some microfilariae (*W. bancrofti*) the original shell is stretched to form the sheath which characterizes them. Larvae or nonsheathed microfilariae are liberated respectively by such parasites as *Trichinella spiralis* and *Onchocerca volvulus*.

## The Generalized Cycle of the Intestinal Nematodes

The life cycles of the intestinal nematodes fall into one of several categories on the basis of developmental sequences: (1) the direct type, such as pinworm and whipworm; (2) the modified direct type, such as *Ascaris;* (3) the skin-penetrating or hookworm type, such as is seen in hookworm and *Strongyloides*.

**The Direct Type** No intermediate host is required; the adult worms develop directly from eggs reaching the alimentary canal of man. Whipworm, *Trichuris trichiura*, and pinworm, *Enterobius vermicularis*, are examples of this type. Whipworm eggs passed in the stool require a period for the development of infective larvae within the shell, after which time they become infective for man. Pinworm eggs are embryonated when deposited and become infective for man in a few hours after deposition (Fig. 170).

**The Modified Direct Type** *Ascaris* eggs are unsegmented when passed in the feces and require a period for embryonation before becoming infective for man. Ingested embryonated eggs hatch in the intestine of man, the larvae penetrating the intestinal wall to reach the circulatory system. Surviving larvae leave the capillary beds of the lung and migrate up the respiratory tract to the esophagus and

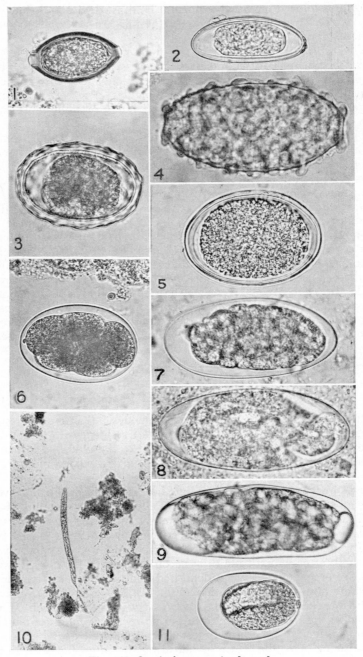

Fig. 169. *See facing page for legend.*

thence down through the stomach to the intestine where they mature (Fig. 171).

**The Skin Penetrating Type**  Members of this group pass partially developed eggs or rhabditiform larvae in the stool. The former eventually hatch into noninfective rhabditiform larvae. Such larvae continue to grow, molt several times, and become transformed into infective or filariform larvae, capable of penetrating the exposed skin surface of man. Developing eggs are found in the stools of persons

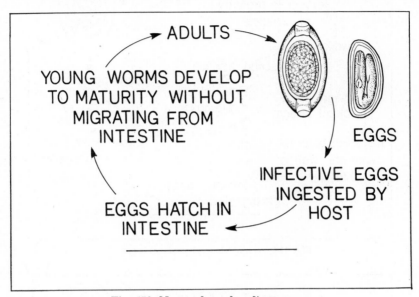

Fig. 170. Nematode cycle—direct type.

infected with hookworms, but larvae are characteristically present in the feces of those infected with *Strongyloides stercoralis*.

In both hookworm disease and strongyloidiasis, the filariform larvae which penetrate the skin of man reach the circulatory system and eventually the capillary beds of the lungs. There they leave the capillaries, pass to the alveoli and migrate up the respiratory tract and down the esophagus to the intestine where maturation takes place (Fig. 172).

Fig. 169. Some common nematode eggs: (*1*) whipworm, *Trichuris trichiura*; (*2*) pinworm, *Enterobius vermicularis*; (*3*) large roundworm, *Ascaris lumbricoides*, fertilized egg; (*4*) *Ascaris*, unfertilized egg; (*5*) *Ascaris*, decorticated egg; (*6*) hookworm egg; (*7*) immature egg of *Trichostrongylus orientalis*; (*8*) embryonated egg of *T. orientalis*; (*9*) egg of *Heterodera marioni*, a plant nematode, which sometimes is found in stools; (*10*) rhabditiform larva of *Strongyloides stercoralis*, the stage usually found in the stool; (*11*) egg of *S. stercoralis*, rarely seen in the stool. All figures 500 × except (*10*) 75 ×. (Nos. 5 and 6 courtesy of the Photographic Laboratory, AMSGS; photos by Milt Cheskis. Nos. 7, 8 and 9 courtesy of Dr. T. B. Magath, Mayo Clinic. All others courtesy of Dr. R. L. Roudabush, Ward's Natural Science Establishment, Rochester, N.Y.; photos by T. Romaniak.)

*Strongyloides stercoralis* differs from hookworm in several important respects. Under some conditions the rhabditiform larvae may become established as free-living organisms which survive and reproduce in the soil. In other cases dwarf filariform larvae are produced

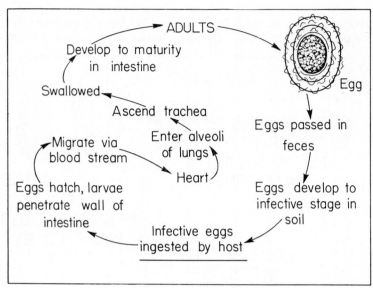

Fig. 171. Nematode cycle—*Ascaris* type.

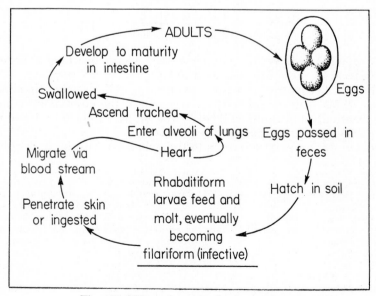

Fig. 172. Nematode cycle—hookworm type.

in the intestine; these directly penetrate the lower or small bowel or the perianal skin, resulting in an additional and sometimes fatal infection of the host.

## Trichuriasis

**Synonyms**   Trichocephaliasis, whipworm infection.

**Definition**   Trichuriasis is an infection of the human intestinal tract caused by the nematode, *Trichuris trichiura.*

**Distribution**   Whipworm is a cosmopolitan parasite, being most abundant in the warm, moist regions of the world. In various areas studied it has been found in 1 to over 96 per cent of the population.

**Etiology**   MORPHOLOGY. Adult whipworms, *Trichuris trichiura* (Linnaeus 1771) Stiles 1901 (= *Trichocephalus trichiurus* [Linnaeus 1771] Blanchard 1895), are usually attached to the cecal mucosa. The parasites have a characteristic whiplike shape, the "handle" of the whip comprising the posterior two-fifths of the worm. The female parasites range between 35 and 50 mm. while the males are slightly smaller, measuring 30 to 45 mm. in length. Anteriorly the mouth opens into a delicate esophagus characterized by a narrow lumen surrounded by a single row of cells which extends through most of the narrow anterior three-fifths of the body. The male reproductive organs open into a posterior cloaca. The caudal region of the male is often coiled. There is a retractile penial sheath with a bulbous spined tip through which protrudes the single copulatory spicule. The female reproductive system also consists of a single set of reproductive organs the external pore of which opens at the anterior extremity of the thickened body proper.

The barrel-shaped eggs when passed in the stool are undeveloped, ranging between 50 and 54 microns by about 22 microns, and are provided with a characteristic knob or mucoid plug at either end. The eggs have a double shell, the outer portion of which is usually bile-stained. A normal female produces over 1000 eggs per day, the average probably being between 3000 and 7000.

DEVELOPMENT. The unsegmented eggs require a minimum of ten days under optimal conditions of moisture and temperature for development in soil. Under less favorable circumstances embryonation may require several months.

After ingestion the infective eggs hatch in the upper duodenum and the larvae become attached to the villi of the intestines where they remain and grow for about a month. At maturity the adult parasites leave their primary site of attachment and pass down the intestine to their final habitat in the cecum and proximal colon. In heavy infections they may also localize in the terminal ileum, appendix and much of the remaining colon.

**Epidemiology**   The distribution of whipworm is co-extensive with that of *Ascaris*. The former, however, predominates in areas of heavy rainfall, high humidity, dense shade and moist soil. *Ascaris*, on the other hand, is more prevalent in regions of lesser rainfall and shade. The eggs of *Trichuris trichiura* do not withstand exposure to direct sunlight and are destroyed by drying. They are unlikely to develop to the infective stage on cinders, ashes or hardened clay.

Infection results from the ingestion of embryonated eggs present in contaminated soil. This may occur through the medium of food or water or directly from the hands of the individual. Children particularly may be heavily infected and constitute important reservoirs.

**Pathology** The anterior portions of the parasites are attached to, or interlaced through, the mucosa of the cecum and appendix or less frequently the lower ileum and colon. Ordinarily there is no marked tissue reaction although liquefaction of the cells in immediate proximity to the parasites may occur. Secondary bacterial infection may cause inflammatory lesions.

Severe infections may be accompanied by a moderate eosinophilia and by anemia with hemoglobin values as low as 25 per cent.

**Clinical Characteristics** Whipworm infection is asymptomatic in most persons in temperate climates. Children tend to acquire heavier infections and some of them experience nausea, irritability, sleeplessness and abdominal pain. In very young infants bloody diarrhea has been reported occasionally. Heavy chronic infections extending into the rectum may cause *prolapsus recti*. The prognosis is good in most cases although complete eradication of the parasites is difficult.

**Diagnosis** Diagnosis depends upon the recovery from the feces of the characteristic double shelled, bile-stained eggs with mucoid plugs. These may be detected in direct smears, flotations, or by the MGL or AMS III centrifugation sedimentation techniques (see p. 822).

**Treatment** Treatment is unsatisfactory. The drug of choice is leche de higuerón. Since this preparation is obtainable only in Central America and parts of South America it is frequently not available. Several drugs have been recommended. Hexylresorcinol Crystoids by mouth combined with retention enemeta of 1:1000 solution of hexylresorcinol, or a mixture of tetrachloroethylene, and oil of chenopodium (2.7 ml. and 0.3 ml., respectively) are reasonably effective. Although emetine hydrochloride in enteric coated pills has given good results, severe toxic reactions, including sloughing of the colonic mucosa, may occur. It is doubtful if this preparation should be used.

The complete removal of whipworms is more likely to occur if the large bowel is emptied with a high cleaning, tepid, salt solution enema the previous night following the prepurgation treatment. This is believed by some to make it possible for the anthelmintic to come into direct contact with the worms (see pp. 545, 553, 556 for details of treatment).

**Prophylaxis** Prophylaxis depends upon sanitary disposal of human feces, washing of the hands before eating and avoidance of raw vegetables in areas where human excreta are used for fertilizer. The maintenance of a safe water supply is also of importance.

## Enterobiasis

**Synonyms**   Oxyuriasis, pinworm or seatworm infection.

**Definition**   Enterobiasis is an infection of the human intestinal tract by the pinworm, *Enterobius vermicularis*.

**Distribution**   Enterobiasis is a cosmopolitan infection. Surveys in various parts of the world indicate that *E. vermicularis* is probably the most common and widely distributed human helminth, its incidence varying from 1 to 100 per cent in the group studied.

**Etiology**   MORPHOLOGY. *Enterobius vermicularis* (Linnaeus 1758) Leach 1853 (= *Oxyuris vermicularis* [Linnaeus 1758] Lamarck 1816) is a spindle-shaped parasite of man. It is usually attached to the mucosa of the lower ileum, cecum or ascending colon. The female measures 8 to 13 mm. in length and the male 2 to 5 mm. The anterior

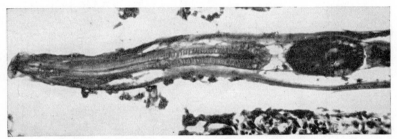

Fig. 173. *Enterobius vermicularis:* section of adult showing characteristic esophagus and esophageal bulb.

extremity lacks a true buccal capsule but is characterized by three labia and laterally a pair of cephalic, winglike alae. The muscular esophagus terminates in a distinct bulb (Fig. 173). The male possesses a strong, ventrally curved tail with caudal alae and a single, large copulatory spicule. The posterior tip of the female is distinctly attenuated, constituting the posterior third of the worm. The paired reproductive system is "T" shaped, the vulva opening at the base of the "T" near the juncture of anterior and middle thirds of the body.

Females lay embryonated eggs which are flattened on one side and measure 50 to 60 microns in length and 20 to 30 microns in breadth. The shell consists of three parts, a thick outer albuminous layer, an inner thinner hyaline one and the embryonic membrane. An average female produces about 11,000 eggs during the course of her life.

DEVELOPMENT. Pinworm eggs are infective shortly after being deposited. After ingestion the eggs hatch in the upper intestine, liberating the larvae which migrate to the region of the ileum, moulting twice en route. It is not uncommon for migrating larvae to attach themselves temporarily to the folds and crypts of the jejunum and upper ileum. Copulation of worms takes place in the lower small intestine, the female then migrating into the cecum or lower bowel. As their eggs develop, the worms' hold on the intestinal wall is relaxed and the parasites pass through the anus where upon contact with the air they shower their sticky eggs over the perianal skin. Development from egg to egg requires a minimum period of about fifteen days. Usually infections build up from repeated reinfections and may not be noticed for approximately two months after they are acquired.

**Epidemiology**  Pinworm eggs are relatively resistant and withstand desiccation in a humid environment for about ten days. Infection occurs by ingestion of the eggs which reach the mouth on soiled hands or in contaminated food or drink. Since the eggs are resistant,

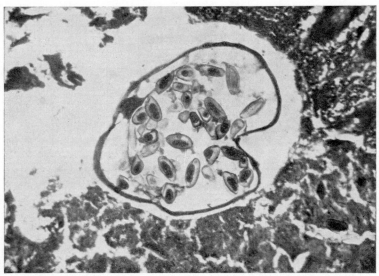

Fig. 174. *Enterobius vermicularis* in lumen of appendix, cross section of female containing eggs.

dust-borne infections may occur in households, eggs adhering to the fingers of persons handling contaminated clothing and bedding.

The intense pruritus ani which is frequently present is an important factor in autoinfection and maintenance of the primary reservoir.

Pinworm infection is commonly a group problem affecting families and others living under crowded conditions. When one individual in a household is infected, it is usual to find several others also harboring *E. vermicularis*.

**Pathology**  *Enterobius vermicularis* produces no significant intestinal pathologic changes. A mild catarrhal inflammation may occur in the immediate vicinity of the sites of attachment of the young worms; appendiceal colic is rarely attributable to their presence in the appendix (Fig. 174).

The most important effect is the cutaneous irritation in the perianal region produced by the migrating gravid females and the presence of eggs. The intense pruritus and constant scratching may lead to dermatitis, eczema, and severe secondary bacterial infections of the skin.

A moderate eosinophilia may occur.

**Clinical Characteristics**   While pinworm infection may be asymptomatic the most common symptom is an intense pruritus ani. This provokes scratching of the affected parts which may result in eczema and pyogenic infections of the anal and perianal regions. Anorexia, restlessness and insomnia are usual in cases of severe involvement. Rectal colic may also occur.

**Diagnosis**   Eggs are commonly present in scrapings from the perianal skin and are more rarely encountered from under the fingernails or in the feces. The most satisfactory method of diagnosing pinworm infections is by the use of a perianal swab. The modified Graham swab utilizes Scotch tape held sticky side out over the closed end of a test tube or over a tongue depressor, which is then applied to the perianal region. The tape is placed sticky side down on a clean glass slide (to which a drop of toluene has been added), and examined. This method is believed to be more practical than either the NIH swab or the wet pestle method. For details of the technique, see p. 829.

**Treatment**   Oxytetracycline (Terramycin) is the drug of choice. Demonstration of the effectiveness of this drug against *E. vermicularis* has greatly simplified the problem of treatment. In the past the lack of a fully effective drug and the ease with which the infection may be transmitted within the household have necessitated complicated regimes of hygienic measures together with the oral and rectal administration of anthelmintic drugs to members of the entire family group. Such difficult and time-consuming measures have been largely superseded.

The effectiveness of Terramycin approaches 100 per cent. If this antibiotic is not available, hexylresorcinol or phenothiazine may be used. For detailed outline of treatment see pages 545, 554, 556.

Cutaneous perianal lesions should be treated with antiseptic and palliative ointments such as yellow oxide of mercury or Benadryl cream.

**Prophylaxis**   Prevention centers around personal hygiene and cleanliness of living quarters. It is important to avoid overcrowding and to bear in mind that enterobiasis is definitely a familial or group disease.

## Ascariasis

**Synonym**   Large roundworm infection.

**Definition**   Ascariasis is an infection by *Ascaris lumbricoides*, one of the most common helminthic parasites of man. The adults commonly remain in the small intestine. Passage of the larvae through the lungs is accompanied by pneumonitis of varying intensity.

**Distribution** Ascariasis has a worldwide distribution and is particularly common in unsanitated or poorly sanitated regions. The incidence in some areas of Europe and the Orient is reported to be as high as 90 and 94 per cent respectively. Highly endemic regions exist in the United States, especially in southeastern parts of the Appalachian range, where 30 to 40 per cent of the population has been found to be infected.

**Etiology** MORPHOLOGY. Adult *A. lumbricoides* Linnaeus 1758 are white or pale yellow in color. They are the largest intestinal nematodes and their macroscopic appearance is characteristic. The females usually range between 20 and 35 cm. in length while the males vary between 15 and 30 cm. The cuticula is finely striated. The anterior extremity is characterized by three lips, one dorsal and two ventrolateral in position. Each lip carries a pair of small papillae on its lateral border.

The male possesses a single set of reproductive organs composed of a long, single, tortuously coiled tubule which is sometimes faintly visible through the cuticula. The copulatory spicules are simple and unequal. The vulva of the female is situated midventrally where the anterior and middle thirds of the body meet. The paired female reproductive system is coiled in the posterior two-thirds of the body and, like that of the male, sometimes may be seen through the cuticula.

The female produces between 25,000,000 and 27,000,000 eggs during her life, laying them at the rate of about 200,000 per day. Eggs are deposited in an undeveloped stage and may be fertilized or unfertilized. These measure 45 to 75 microns and 88 to 94 microns respectively in length. The eggs may be covered with an outer roughened (mammillated) albuminous coat. If this is lacking the egg is said to be decorticated.

DEVELOPMENT. The adults live in the small intestine where they may persist for six months or longer. Eggs reach the external environment with the feces. Under conditions of sufficient moisture and oxygenation, and at an optimum temperature of 25° C., they develop and become infective in about three weeks. Before eggs become infective for man the contained embryo must have undergone one molt within the egg. These eggs hatch in the intestine, liberating minute larvae which promptly penetrate blood or lymph vessels in the intestinal wall. Some larvae thus reach the portal circulation and are carried to the liver. Others pass through the thoracic duct, but by either route must finally reach the lungs where they are filtered out of the blood stream and in a few days many perforate the alveoli. After increasing in size and molting twice the larvae migrate up the respiratory passages to the epiglottis and then down the esophagus. In this way the parasites again reach the small intestine where maturation and copulation occur. During the migration the larvae increase from about 0.2 to 1.5 mm. in length and undergo a total of four

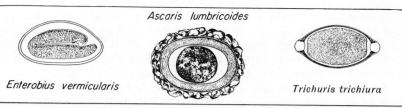

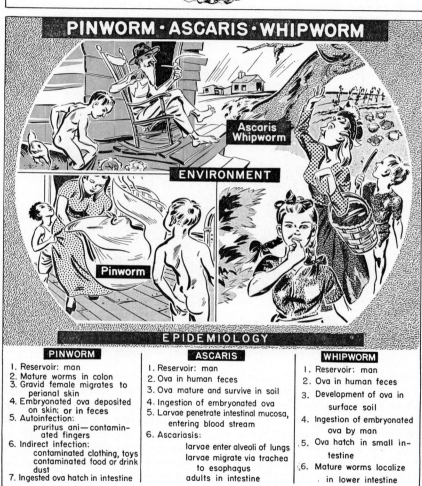

Fig. 175. Epidemiology of pinworm, whipworm and ascaris infections.

molts. A new generation of eggs appears in the feces within approximately two months after the ingestion of embryonated eggs.

**Epidemiology**    Man may acquire *A. lumbricoides* by the ingestion of embryonated eggs in contaminated food or, rarely, in drink. More frequently eggs containing embryos reach the mouth directly from the soil via dirty hands. For this reason it is not uncommon to find children more often infected than adults (Fig. 175).

Ascariasis is primarily a dooryard and household infection. It is well known that *Ascaris* eggs are highly resistant to desiccation and to thermal changes under 70° C.; they therefore remain infective for a considerable period of time. Adequate sanitary practices will pre-

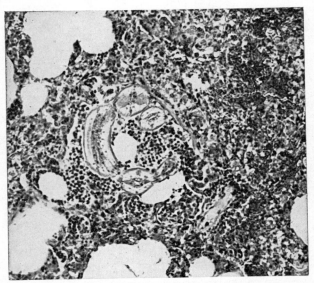

Fig. 176. Larva of *A. lumbricoides* surrounded by hemorrhage and purulent exudate in lung. Experimental infection in guinea pig.

vent the spread of this parasite only if they are applied by the entire population. Since children are less likely to use sanitary facilities than are adults they constitute the important reservoir of infection.

**Pathology**    Reactions to Larvae. Minute hemorrhages occur at the penetration sites of the parasites through the intestinal wall or into the alveoli of the lungs. As the larvae are considerably larger than the diameter of the capillaries some trauma and petechial hemorrhage take place. In experimental animals exudation of erythrocytes and white blood corpuscles, including many eosinophils, and desquamation of the pulmonary alveolar epithelium occur (Fig. 176).

Large numbers of infective eggs, or repeated ingestion of eggs produce marked pathologic changes in the lungs characterized by a lobular pneumonitis. This is most commonly seen in children since they are usually more heavily infected than are adults.

Larvae which pass through the lungs to reach the general circulation may cause lesions in other areas, notably the brain, spinal cord, and the kidneys.

REACTIONS TO ADULTS. The adult worms cause no specific pathologic response in the small intestine. If, however, they are present in sufficient numbers they occasionally form a bolus which produces obstruction necessitating surgical intervention. This happens particularly following the injudicious administration of anthelmintics, e. g., therapeusis directed at a co-existing hookworm infection. *Ascaris* infrequently causes appendicitis and rarely perforates the gut

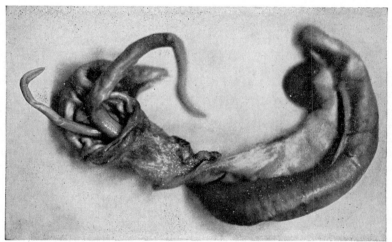

Fig. 177. Ascariasis: adults in appendix. (Strong: Stitt's Diagnosis, Prevention and Treatment of Tropical Diseases. The Blakiston Co.)

wall or invades the bile duct. A moderate eosinophilia is often noted in individuals infected by this worm (Fig. 177).

**Clinical Characteristics** REACTION TO LARVAE. Children are particularly susceptible to ascariasis. If numbers of infective eggs are ingested there may be an elevation of temperature to 103° or 105° F. within a period of five days corresponding to the period of migration of the larvae. This may be associated with frequent spasms of coughing, bronchial râles, evidence of lobular consolidation and hemoptysis. The physical signs often simulate an atypical pneumonia. A fatal pneumonia may supervene, especially when secondary bacterial infection occurs (see Fig. 176).

REACTION TO ADULTS. If only a few parasites are present it is unlikely that symptoms will occur. In heavier infections abdominal pain or discomfort, passing ascarids prior to treatment, vomiting, abdominal or epigastric tenderness, fever, constipation, distention of the abdomen, cough, nausea, headache and diarrhea may be noted. Less frequently convulsions, malaise, anorexia, palpable abdominal mass and dyspnea may be encountered. Evidence of other digestive disturbances or systemic toxemia sometimes occurs.

**Diagnosis** Diagnosis depends upon the demonstration of characteristic eggs in the stool or the recovery of an adult worm. Recognition of both mammillated and decorticated eggs is important (see Fig. 169, p. 376). Eggs presenting several different appearances may be encountered in the stool as follows:

(1) FERTILIZED EGGS. These range from 45 to 75 microns by 35 to 50 microns in diameter. Ordinarily they are covered by a coarsely mammillated albuminoid bile-stained outer shell beneath which is a thick, transparent, hyaline inner shell.

(2) UNFERTILIZED EGGS. These measure 88 to 94 microns by 39 to 44 microns; these are longer, narrower and have a slightly thinner outer and inner shell than typical fertilized *Ascaris* eggs.

(3) DECORTICATED EGGS. Occasionally the roughened mammillated outer shell is absent and only the thick hyaline inner shell remains; these are known as decorticated eggs. They may be fertile or infertile.

Ascariasis can usually be detected by direct smears; however, concentration techniques such as the MGL or AMS III insure a diagnosis (see p. 822).

DIFFERENTIAL DIAGNOSIS. In heavily endemic areas the clinical picture of an acute diffuse bronchitis or bronchopneumonia is not unusual in children. In cases due to pulmonary ascariasis there may be bloody sputum in which the larvae are demonstrable by microscopic examination.

**Treatment** Crystoids anthelmintic (Caprokol) for adults and diethylcarbamazine (Hetrazan) syrup for children, are the drugs of choice in the treatment of uncomplicated ascariasis. Although these drugs are highly effective against adult worms in the intestine, more than one course of treatment may be necessary.

Mixed infections by *A. lumbricoides* and hookworm should be treated as for ascariasis. If large numbers of hookworms still remain, tetrachloroethylene may be administered a week following the last administration of Caprokol. Some recommend tetrachloroethylene and oil of chenopodium for mixed infections by hookworm and *A. lumbricoides*. For details of treatment see pages 545, 548.

The therapy of ascaris pneumonia is symptomatic and supportive.

**Prophylaxis** Effective prophylaxis against ascariasis consists especially of sanitary disposal of human excreta and prevention of fecal contamination of top soil. Children are the most important reservoirs of infection. The protection of food and water supplies, and the institution of proper habits of personal cleanliness are important secondary measures.

# Hookworm Disease

**Synonyms** For *Ancylostoma duodenale* infections: uncinariasis, ancylostomiasis, Old World hookworm infection. For *Necator ameri-*

*canus* infections: necatoriasis, New World hookworm infection, American hookworm infection.

**Definition**  Hookworm disease is an infection of the small intestine by *Ancylostoma duodenale* or *Necator americanus*. Tissue destruction and blood loss attributable to the parasites occur in proportion to the abundance of these invaders. Malnutrition and avitaminosis aggravate the detrimental effects of infection.

**Distribution**  Hookworm disease is widespread and is one of the most important helminthic diseases of man. It occurs in nearly all subtropical and tropical countries. The ranges of the two species of hookworm infecting man overlap and both are present in many regions of the world. The current distribution of these parasites is not an indication of their original endemicity.

*Ancylostoma duodenale*, the Old World hookworm, is prevalent in southern Europe, northern Africa, northern India, China, and Japan; it is also present in southern India, Indonesia, Burma, Malayan archipelago, the Philippines, South and Central Pacific islands, Portuguese West Africa, Australia and Paraguay. *Necator americanus* is the predominant human hookworm in southern Asia, Indonesia, the Philippines, Polynesia, Melanesia, Micronesia, Central and South Africa, the southern United States, Central and South America and the West Indies. Consult map (Fig. 178) for other details.

**Etiology**  MORPHOLOGY. *Ancylostoma duodenale* (Dubini 1843) Creplin 1845 and *Necator americanus* (Stiles 1902) Stiles 1903, cause ancylostomiasis and necatoriasis, respectively. While morphologic differences exist between them, only *A. duodenale* will be described here. Other important diagnostic differential features are presented in Table 33.

The adults have a pinkish or creamy white, tough cuticula and are provided with a pair of prominent laterally situated cervical papillae situated behind the esophageal nerve ring. The oval buccal capsule contains, on the ventral (or apparently upper) side, two pairs of fused teeth of which the outer is the larger and the inner is provided with a small inconspicuous accessory median process (Figs. 179, 180, 181, 182).

The males measure 8 to 11 mm. in length while the females range between 10 and 13 mm. The posterior tip of the male is expanded to form a typical copulatory bursa supported by fleshy rays with a pattern that is characteristic of the species. The alimentary canal and genital ducts open into this bursa. A pair of long copulatory spicules are regulated by an accessory copulatory device or *gubernaculum*.

The females have a subterminal, ventrally located anus on the conical posterior extremity. The reproductive system is double, the tubules of the ovary being coiled intricately over the alimentary canal and confined to the posterior two-thirds of the body. The vulva is located ventrally at the beginning of the posterior third of the body. During copulation the copulatory bursa of the male surrounds the vulva, thus permitting the spermatozoa access to the reproductive

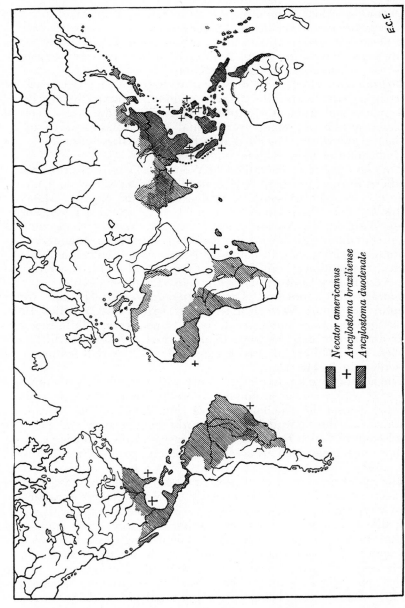

Fig. 178. Geographical distribution of hookworms. (Craig and Faust: Clinical Parasitology, Lea & Febiger.)

*Necator americanus*
*Ancylostoma braziliense*
*Ancylostoma duodenale*

system of the female. After mating the male becomes detached. Fertilization takes place in the upper portion of the uterus or in the seminal receptacle.

*Differential diagnosis* of the various species of hookworms depends upon their length, the number and arrangement of the teeth or cut-

Fig. 179.  Fig. 180.

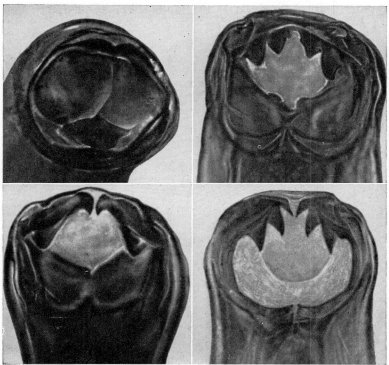

Fig. 181.  Fig. 182.

Fig. 179. Mouthparts of *Necator americanus*. Note two pairs of chitinized cutting plates characteristic of this species. (Courtesy J. M. Edney through A. O. Foster.)

Fig. 180. Mouthparts of *Ancylostoma duodenale*. Note two large pairs of teeth, each of the medial pair bearing a small accessory process. (Courtesy J. M. Edney through A. O. Foster.)

Fig. 181. Mouthparts of *Ancylostoma braziliense*. Note two pairs of teeth, a large outer pair and a small inner pair without accessory processes. (Courtesy J. M. Edney through A. O. Foster.)

Fig. 182. Mouthparts of *Ancylostoma caninum*. Note three well developed pairs of teeth. (Courtesy J. M. Edney through A. O. Foster.)

ting plates, the length of the esophagus, the detailed morphology of the bursa of the male, the position of the vulva in the female and the size of the eggs. Table 33 summarizes these points in tabular form for the two common hookworms of man and two closely related species.

DEVELOPMENT. Since the life cycles of these two species are essentially identical they will be considered together. Adult hookworms live attached to the intestinal mucosa. Females liberate eggs into the lumen which are eliminated with the feces in two- to eight-celled stages of cleavage. Eggs vary between 56 and 76 microns in length by 35 to 40 microns in breadth. Those of *Necator* usually are somewhat longer than the eggs of *Ancylostoma*. Eggs which remain in undiluted feces develop slowly. Under optimum conditions of dilution,

*Table 33   Differential Characteristics of Common Hookworms*[1]

| | NECATOR AMERICANUS | ANCYLOSTOMA DUODENALE | ANCYLOSTOMA BRAZILIENSE | ANCYLOSTOMA CANINUM |
|---|---|---|---|---|
| Shape | Head curved opposite to curvature of body, giving a hooked appearance to anterior end | Head continues in same direction as curvature of body | Similar to *A. duodenale* | Similar to *A. duodenale* |
| Length Female | 9 to 11 mm. × 0.35 mm. | 10 to 13 mm. × 0.60 mm. | 9 to 10.5 mm. × 0.38 mm. | 14 mm. × 0.6 mm. |
| Male | 5 to 9 mm. × 0.30 mm. | 8 to 11 mm. × 0.45 mm. | 7.8 to 8.5 mm. × 0.35 mm. | 10 mm. × 0.4 mm. |
| Buccal capsule | One pair of ventral semilunar cutting plates | Two pairs of curved ventral teeth of nearly the same size, rudimentary inner pair | Two pairs of ventral teeth, inner smaller | Three pairs of ventral teeth, inner smallest |
| Length of esophagus | 0.5 to 0.8 mm. in length. Opening small, oval, long axis dorsoventral | 1.3 mm. in length. Opening oval, long axis transverse | Opening very small, long axis dorsoventral | Opening large, oval, long axis dorsoventral |
| Bursa of male | Long, wide and rounded, dorsal ray small, bipartite | Broader than long, dorsal ray tripartite | Small, almost as broad as long, with short stubby rays | Large and flaring, with long slender rays |
| Caudal spine in female | Absent | Present | Present | Present |
| Vulva | Anterior third to middle of body | Posterior to middle of body | Posterior to middle of body | Posterior to middle of body |
| Size of eggs (microns) | 64 to 76 × 35 to 40 | 56 to 60 × 35 to 40 | 55 to 60 × 35 to 40 | 60 to 75 × 38 to 45 |

[1] From Belding, 1952, "Textbook of Clinical Parasitology," p. 285. 2nd ed. D. Appleton-Century Co., Inc., N. Y.

moisture and temperature, however, they hatch within twenty-four to forty-eight hours, each liberating a rhabditiform larva which measures approximately 250 to 300 microns in length. Its anterior extremity is bluntly rounded and is characterized by a long narrow buccal cavity. Hookworm larvae in this stage of development may be confused with the rhabditiform larvae of *Strongyloides* (see Table 34, p. 399). The rhabditiform larvae of hookworm may migrate several inches beneath the soil where they feed on bacteria, molt, gradually double in size and finally undergo a metamorphosis to become infective, or filariform, larvae. During this period of growth a second molt, or ecdysis, occurs, the parasites frequently remaining within their sheaths.

The worms then enter a period during which no food is consumed, but active vertical migration may continue. When these infective larvae come into contact with unprotected human skin they penetrate the superficial layers, enter the blood stream and are transported to the lungs. There they leave the vascular system, emerge into the alveoli and migrate up the bronchi and trachea and down the esophagus to reach the small intestine where maturity is attained.

**Epidemiology**  Both *A. duodenale* and *N. americanus* occur in the small intestine of man. Eggs deposited in stools under proper conditions of moisture, shade and temperature hatch and develop to the infective stage. These infective filariform larvae ordinarily enter the skin. As penetration is difficult, mud caked on the foot or between the toes gives the larvae a purchase for the actual penetration. It is also possible for infective larvae to be swallowed directly with food and drink. In such cases development usually takes place directly in the intestine without any period of migration.

In the tropics, coffee and banana groves as well as sugar cane and sweet potato fields are ideal for the growth and development of the larvae. Conditions most favorable to embryonic development include a loose moist soil, loam or humus, through which the filariform larvae are able to crawl vertically. They cannot, however, climb up rocks or the sides of concrete-lined latrines. Temperatures ranging between 80° and 90° F. are optimal. Because eggs and larvae are readily killed by freezing and desiccation, hookworm disease is endemic only in those tropical and subtropical areas where the rainfall averages fifty or more inches a year (Fig. 183).

In many parts of the world special habits or customs of the people are factors in maintaining hookworm infections. In some regions, for example, there are usually certain defecation areas which adults use. These spots often provide the proper environment for the development of infective hookworm larvae. Adults revisit these sites daily, thus exposing themselves to infection and reinfection. In such families young children often defecate beside the house or in the area in which they play. Chickens ingesting the feces facilitate the distribution of eggs as these are not destroyed in passing through their digestive tracts. In many regions such a combination of factors results in a high incidence of hookworm infection.

In other parts of the world, such as China, dissemination is furthered by the utilization of untreated nightsoil as fertilizer. Infection results as the fields are worked.

There is a fundamental distinction between hookworm infection and hookworm disease; the two terms are not synonymous and the medical implications are quite different. It is difficult to obtain adequate data on the incidence and distribution of hookworm disease. The method for routine stool examination merely demonstrates the presence of the parasite; it provides no exact evidence of the magnitude of the hookworm burden. Other methods involving egg count techniques give data on the *intensity* of the infection, thus furnishing a basis for estimating the worm burden of an individual. Persons harboring hookworms may be divided into two groups:

(1) The hookworm "carrier"—a person with few worms and no clinical evidence of hookworm disease.

(2) The clinical case—a patient carrying many worms who presents clinical evidence of hookworm disease. Clinical cases are severe
only when large numbers of the parasites are present.

It is frequently stated that the highest incidence of hookworm
infection occurs in the teen-age group. While this may be true in the
United States and certain other areas, it does not conform to the

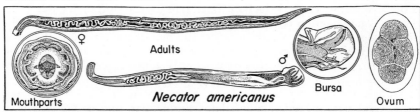

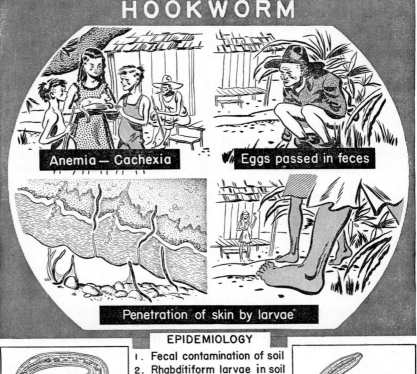

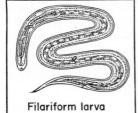

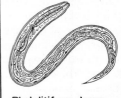

EPIDEMIOLOGY

1. Fecal contamination of soil
2. Rhabditiform larvae in soil
3. Filariform larvae on soil
4. Penetration of exposed skin
5. Migration of larvae
6. Localization, small intestine
7. Feeding on blood of host
8. Ova passed in stool

Fig. 183. Epidemiology of hookworm disease.

findings in Okinawa, Southern Korea and Japan, where the incidence increases until old age is reached and the individuals cease working in fields contaminated by nightsoil. In many areas males may be more heavily infected than females, but in Okinawa, Southern Korea and Japan, this is not true; the incidence is approximately the same but the *worm burden* is higher in women.

It appears probable that some human immunity to hookworm develops; otherwise large numbers of people would die from the disease. The incidence is lower and heavy infections are more rarely encountered in Negroes than in whites. Knowledge of the development of immunity is based upon experimental studies made with the dog hookworm. It has been found that small repeated infections give almost complete immunity. When such immunity develops, the worms in the gut are eliminated; anemia, however, may prevent the development of such immunity. Further experiments demonstrate that pre-existing malnutrition and avitaminosis determine the appearance of hookworm disease after doses of worms that ordinarily would produce only a subclinical infection. If immunity has been established it can be lost if the diet becomes deficient; it can likewise be restored after an adequate diet has been resumed. This immunity to the invasion of the larvae seems to be a response to their secretions and excretions, the mechanism of which is the formation of precipitates which are deposited around the larvae. Their motion is then slowed and they soon disintegrate and are phagocytized.

There is also evidence of a gradual and spontaneous reduction in the numbers of hookworms in cases where there is no re-infection. It has been estimated that in *N. americanus* and *A. duodenale* infections there is a 90 per cent reduction of the worm burden within one or two years and a total elimination by the end of five or seven years.

**Pathology**  The penetration of the skin by the filariform larvae of *Necator americanus* often causes a *local dermatitis*, "ground- or dew itch," with edema, erythema and a vesicular or papular eruption which usually subsides spontaneously in about two weeks unless secondary bacterial infection occurs. *Ancylostoma duodenale*, however, seems much less prone to produce a cutaneous reaction.

As the migrating larvae leave the capillaries of the lungs and penetrate into the alveoli minute *hemorrhagic lesions* are produced. In heavy infections these may be numerous and may be accompanied by round cell infiltration. In general, however, the pulmonary reaction is much less severe than that accompanying ascariasis or strongyloidiasis.

The adults of both human species inhabit the upper half of the small intestine where they become attached and suck blood (Fig. 184). Of these *N. americanus* is believed to be the more benign. Injury to the host results from the mechanical and lytic destruction of tissue at the point of attachment. A secondary hemorrhagic anemia is the chief pathologic condition. It has been estimated that a single hookworm may remove as much as 0.38 to 0.84 ml. of blood a day.

When this figure is multiplied by thousands of worms and repeated day after day for long periods of time, the resulting anemia is readily understood. Hookworms digest only part of the blood they ingest. Previous points of attachment bleed for some time after the worm moves on to a new site, due to the anticoagulant secreted by the worm.

**Clinical Characteristics**   The clinical picture of hookworm disease is variable and dependent primarily upon the severity of the infection and the dietary of the individual. Common symptoms are weak-

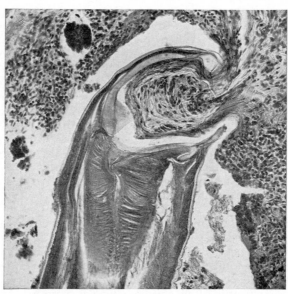

Fig. 184. Longitudinal section through hookworm attached to intestinal mucosa.

ness, fatigue, dyspnea on exertion, cardiac palpitation, pallor, epigastric tenderness, digestive symptoms, and mental and physical retardation. Children harboring this parasite in large numbers are frequently pot-bellied. Depravity of appetite with a craving for earth (geophagy), wood, charcoal or other abnormal substances is not unusual. Advanced cases with severe anemia may present extensive edema and even anasarca.

In many areas where the infection is heavily endemic, malnutrition is widespread in the population. Furthermore the clinical picture may be complicated by concurrent malaria and other parasitic infections of the intestinal tract. Hookworm disease therefore seldom appears as a clear-cut entity. The most serious effects occur in children (Fig. 185).

The *anemia* of hookworm disease may be severe, with hemoglobin values under 15 per cent and erythrocyte counts below 1,000,000 per cubic millimeter. The cells are usually microcytic and hypochromic.

However, when the disease is complicated by malnutrition the anemia may be macrocytic or normocytic in type.

There may be a moderate leukocytosis; more commonly the white blood count is within normal limits or a slight neutropenia with a moderate macrocytosis may exist. Eosinophilia usually ranging between 15 and 35 per cent is characteristic. It is less marked, however, in advanced cases.

The pentration of the skin by infective hookworm larvae produces an intense *pruritus* sometimes called "ground itch" or "dew

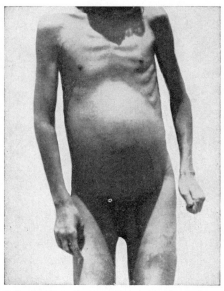

Fig. 185. Clinical hookworm disease showing emaciation and protuberant abdomen. (Maj. D. S. Glusker, M.C., A.U.S., for the Office of the Coordinator of Inter-American Affairs.)

itch" which frequently occurs between the toes where secondary infections due to contamination easily develop. Edema of the ankles and feet is common and an urticarial rash is sometimes seen.

Estimates of the worm load should not govern too strictly the decision as to whether or not specific therapy should be undertaken. Infection alone without symptoms or significant signs is not necessarily an indication for treatment. When, however, definite clinical effects can be attributed to the parasites, therapy should not be withheld irrespective of the numbers which may be present.

**Diagnosis**  Diagnosis depends upon finding typical eggs in the stool (Fig. 169, p. 376). Differentiation between the eggs of *N. americanus* and *A. duodenale* is not necessary or possible. It is important, however, that the rhabditiform larvae of hookworm, *Strongyloides, Trichostrongylus,* and the free-living *Rhabditis* be dis-

tinguished from one another (Fig. 186). In the diagnostic laboratory
it is usually a question of differentiating between the larvae of hookworm and *Strongyloides,* since those of *Trichostrongylus* and
*Rhabditis* are rarely encountered. Rhabditiform larvae of hookworm

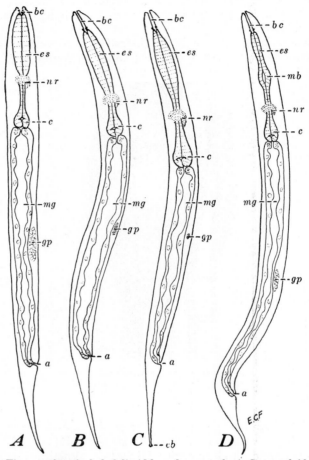

Fig. 186. Figures of typical rhabditoid larval stages of: *A, Strongyloides; B,* hookworm; *C, Trichostrongylus;* and *D, Rhabditis.* ca. 400 ✕. Explanation of labels: *a,*
anus; *bc,* buccal chamber; *c,* cardiac bulb of esophagus; *cb,* beadlike swelling of
caudal tip, etc. (Courtesy of E. C. Faust in Craig and Faust's Clinical Parasitology,
3d ed., 1951, Lea & Febiger.)

will occasionally be found in constipated stools or in stool samples
which are held too long before examination. The presence of embryonated eggs together with rhabditiform larvae in the stool is
highly suggestive of hookworm infection. If only rhabditiform larvae
are present strongyloidiasis should be suspected. It should be borne
in mind that mixed infections are common, especially in the tropics.
Rhabditiform larvae of hookworm and *S. stercoralis* may be differentiated by the following characteristics (see Table 34).

Stools should be examined by some concentration method such as the MGL, AMS III or zinc sulfate technique (p. 822). If it is desired to determine the worm burden the Beaver or Stoll technique should be utilized (p. 824).

DIFFERENTIAL DIAGNOSIS. Hookworm disease may be confused with wet beriberi, malarial cachexia and chronic nephritis. Both beriberi and malaria may coexist with hookworm disease and complicate the diagnostic and the therapeutic problems.

**Treatment** In hookworm infections uncomplicated by ascariasis the drug of choice is tetrachloroethylene. This will remove up to 97 per cent of the worms and those remaining will do the patient no harm provided an adequate diet is maintained.

*Table 34    Rhabditiform Larvae*

| CHARACTER | STRONGYLOIDES | HOOKWORM |
|---|---|---|
| Size, average | 225 × 16 microns | 275 × 17 microns |
| Posterior tip | Blunter | Sharper |
| Buccal chamber | Shorter—not longer than width at tip of head | Longer—longer than width at tip of head |
| Genital primordia | Larger | Smaller |

If both hookworm and *A. lumbricoides* are present, treat first with Crystoids anthelmintic (Caprokol) as for ascariasis (p. 545) and if numbers of hookworms are still present tetrachloroethylene may be administered in one week. Tetrachloroethylene in conjunction with oil of chenopodium has been recommended also by some workers (p. 553).

Such specific treatment may need to be supplemented or preceded by the institution of a balanced diet to restore normal nutrition, and by the administration of iron or liver extract to overcome the anemia. Generally, however, removal of the worms, together with an adequate dietary, is sufficient.

**Prophylaxis** The prophylaxis of hookworm infection is based upon sanitary disposal of human excreta and the prevention of soil pollution. In heavily endemic areas it is usually necessary to carry out mass treatment of the population to eliminate the reservoir of infection; to construct adequate latrine facilities; and, perhaps of even greater importance, to instruct the population concerning the epidemiology of the infection and the necessity for the prevention of soil pollution.

## Trichostrongyliasis

**Synonym** *Trichostrongylus* infection.

**Definition** Trichostrongyliasis is an infection caused by one of several species of *Trichostrongylus*. Adult worms lie with their heads embedded in the epithelium of the duodenum and jejunum.

**Distribution** Although several species normally parasitizing lower animals have been reported in isolated instances from man in various parts of the world it is only *Trichostrongylus orientalis* which has been found as a common intestinal parasite in certain areas of Armenia, Japan, Korea, Formosa and China. In some areas of Japan *Trichostrongylus* sp. is the most common helminth encountered. Eggs are present in over 80 per cent of the stools examined. Recently trichostrongyliasis has been reported from Chile.

**Etiology**  MORPHOLOGY. Adult *Trichostrongylus* sp. are small roundworms, the males measuring 4 to 6 mm. in length and the females 5 to 8 mm. The head is unarmed; a distinct buccal capsule is absent but a definite notch occurs where the excretory pore opens. Males are characterized by a copulatory bursa with characteristic rays and spicules which is diagnostic for each species. In the female the paired reproductive system opens through a common vulva. The eggs of these species are elongate, oval, possess a transparent hyaline shell and resemble those of hookworms except that they are much larger (85 to 115 microns). When found in the feces they are usually in the morula stage (Fig. 169).

DEVELOPMENT. Under favorable conditions of humidity and temperature the eggs hatch within 24 to 36 hours. However, they are remarkably resistant to long periods of cold or drought. The larvae undergo two ecdyses and reach the infective stage in 60 hours or more. Infection normally occurs when infective larvae are ingested *per os*, although adult parasites have been recovered following penetration of the skin. They mature in the small intestine within 25 to 30 days without undergoing a migration through the lungs.

**Epidemiology**  Man is believed to acquire the infection through contaminated food or drink. The universal use of nightsoil in the Orient and the resistance of eggs and infective larvae to desiccation often create conditions in farming communities which are ideal for the spread of *Trichostrongylus*.

**Pathology and Clinical Characteristics**  Little is known concerning the pathology of trichostrongyliasis. In severe infections a mild anemia, dry skin and general emaciation have been reported. In Japan significant clinical phenomena were not observed even in individuals with heavy egg burdens.

**Diagnosis**  Diagnosis depends upon the detection of characteristic eggs or the recovery of adult worms from the stool (Fig. 169, p. 376). For recommended techniques see p. 822.

**Treatment**  No satisfactory drug is known.

**Prophylaxis**  Effective prophylaxis against trichostrongyliasis comprises the sanitary disposal of human excreta and the prevention of fecal contamination of the topsoil by infected animals or man.

## Creeping Eruption

**Synonyms**  "Larva Migrans," ancylostomiasis braziliensis.

**Definition**  Creeping eruption results from the presence of the larvae of the dog and cat hookworm, *Ancylostoma braziliense,* in the epidermis of man.

**Distribution** Ancylostomiasis braziliensis is endemic in the southeastern part of the United States while sporadic cases have been reported as far north as Massachusetts. It is present to a lesser degree along the coastal regions of Texas, Mexico and Central America. Colombia, Venezuela, the Guianas and Brazil are regarded as centers of infection. In Africa, ancylostomiasis braziliensis exists in a band across the tropical portion of the continent with another endemic center on the beaches of Port Elizabeth, Union of South Africa. It is also reported in Ceylon, Malaya, Burma, Siam, Java, Formosa, Hongkong and the Philippines. Adult worms have been reported in scattered instances from the intestine of man in the Philippines, East Indies, Ceylon, India, Siam, parts of Africa and Brazil.

**Etiology** MORPHOLOGY. The dog and cat hookworm, *A. braziliense* de Fairo 1910, is the smallest of the "human" hookworms. The male measures 7.8 to 8.5 mm. and the females 9 to 10.5 mm. in length. The general morphology of this species is essentially similar to that of *A. duodenale. Ancylostoma braziliense* has two pairs of teeth, a small, curved, inner pair and a larger, outer pair, making the buccal capsule diagnostic of the species. The bursa of the male is smaller than that of other hookworms, and is likewise diagnostic: it is almost as broad as it is long and is supported by short stubby rays. The eggs cannot be readily distinguished from those of *A. duodenale.*

DEVELOPMENT. The females produce about 4000 eggs a day. The extra-human developmental cycle parallels that of the other hookworms. The filariform larvae, however, usually remain localized in the skin of man and do not undergo further development.

**Epidemiology** Wild and domestic members of the dog and cat families constitute the normal and reservoir hosts of *A. braziliense.* The eggs are passed in the stools and contaminate the soil where, under adequate conditions of temperature and humidity, infective filariform larvae develop (Fig. 187). These, coming in contact with the skin of man, readily penetrate and produce "creeping eruption." Sandy areas of the southeastern states constitute the chief endemic foci in this country. Beaches, children's sand piles and the area beneath cottages where dogs and cats defecate are often hotbeds of infective larvae. Less extensive lesions of creeping eruption have been reported for the European dog hookworm, *Uncinaria stenocephala,* and experimentally by the dog hookworm, *Ancylostoma caninum.*

**Pathology** The larvae after penetrating the epidermis produce serpiginous tunnels in the stratum germinativum of the skin, progressing at a rate of several millimeters or a few centimeters each day. The course of the tunnels is marked by erythema, induration, and at times overlying vesiculation. Histologic examination reveals local eosinophilic and round cell infiltration. The larvae may remain active in the skin for several months. They rarely enter the blood stream.

The pathologic changes resulting from intestinal infections with the adult worms are not well known. However, *A. braziliense* has penetrated the submucosa, the invasion resulting in peritonitis and death.

**Clinical Characteristics**   A reddish papule, accompanied by pruritus, occurs at the site of invasion within a few hours after the larvae

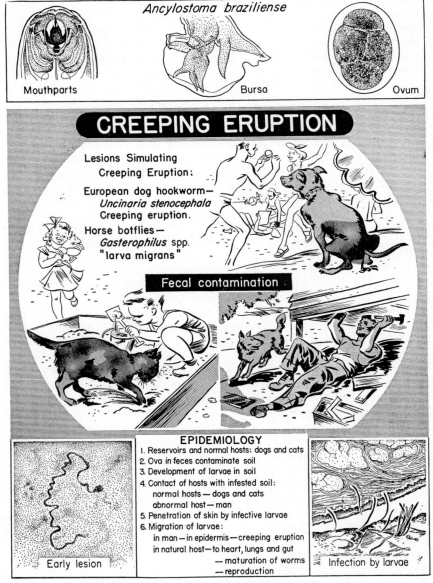

Fig. 187. Epidemiology of creeping eruption.

have penetrated the skin. Within two or three days the parasites begin to migrate, producing an erythematous, serpiginous, linear and elevated tunnel. This migration is accompanied by an intense pruritus. The unoccupied portion of the tunnel soon dries and becomes crusted. Scratching of these lesions frequently leads to secondary infection. The infected person may suffer intolerably, the local symptoms producing insomnia, anorexia and even loss of weight. The clinical picture resulting from the presence of adults in the intestine of man is not well known (Fig. 188).

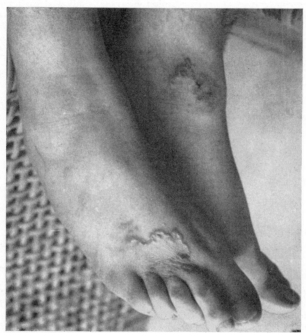

Fig. 188. Creeping eruption caused by the larvae of *Ancylostoma braziliense*. (Courtesy of Dr. K. F. D. Sweetman, Australia.)

**Diagnosis**   *Ancylostoma braziliense* infection may be diagnosed most readily on the basis of the characteristic serpiginous lesions and a history of exposure in a typical "creeping eruption environment."

A *differential diagnosis* between "creeping eruption" and other types of dermatitis caused by metazoan parasites is sometimes difficult. Considerable confusion is possible but a careful analysis and reference to the accompanying table should prove helpful (Table 35).

**Treatment**   Permanent relief is secured only by killing the parasite. This is accomplished by freezing the area just ahead of the tunnel with ethyl chloride or carbon dioxide snow. Considerable difficulty is frequently experienced in reaching the parasite and destroying it. Recently both Hetrazan and Fuadin have given promising results; the former appears to be the drug of choice. In severe infections elevation of the part and the application of wet dressings of a saturated solution of magnesium sulfate will give partial and temporary relief.

### Table 35    Differential Diagnostic Chart of Cutaneous Lesions Produced by Some Metazoan Parasites

| PARASITE | CHARACTER OF THE LESIONS |
|---|---|
| *Necator americanus* "American" hookworm | Penetration of larvae is followed by itching, burning, erythema and edema. Later a papule appears, followed frequently by a vesicle. If secondary infection does not occur, the dermatitis disappears spontaneously in two weeks. This is known commonly as "ground itch," or "dew itch." |
| *Ancylostoma duodenale* "Old World" hookworm | May cause "ground itch" as above, but not invariably, some cases being asymptomatic. |
| *Ancylostoma braziliense* Dog and cat hookworm | The commonest type of "creeping eruption." Lesions serpiginous, extending sinuously through the stratum germinativum from several mm. to several cm. daily. Erythema, or even purpura, make the "burrows" superficially visible, in addition to elevation of the skin over the tunnels. The chief symptom is intense itching. The worms live for weeks or months. Secondary infection may complicate the disease. |
| *Ancylostoma caninum* The dog hookworm | Penetration is followed by itchy papules with little or no linear extension by "burrowing." Symptoms disappear in two weeks. |
| *Uncinaria stenocephala* European dog hookworm | This nematode, the European dog hookworm, produces a condition practically identical with the "creeping eruption" of *Ancylostoma braziliense* but is of shorter duration. |
| *Strongyloides stercoralis* The strongylid threadworm | Infections may produce a violent pruritus at the site of entry within an hour, characterized by an erythematous macule. |
| *Gnathostoma spinigerum* Gnathostomes | This nematode forms boils, abscesses, or deep burrows. Infiltration by WBC, especially eosinophils, is seen histologically. |
| *Dermatobia hominis* The tropical warble fly | Deeply penetrating, with an open "breathing hole" in skin. No migration. Elevated red itchy painful boil or "bot" or "warble." Duration about six weeks (see p. 781). |
| *Gasterophilus* sp. Horse bot fly | Penetrates to stratum germinativum, then burrows parallel to skin surface, migrating slowly for several months. Looks more like true "creeping eruption" of *A. braziliense* than any other similar lesion and is called "larva migrans" (see p. 779). |
| *Hypoderma* sp. Cattle warble fly | Deeply penetrating to subcutaneous tissue. Slow migration occurs during the course of a month. Quite painful. Little itching (see p. 785). More serious than *Gasterophilus*. |
| *Schistosoma*, species for which man is an abnormal or unfavorable host Blood flukes | Known as schistosome dermatitis or swimmers' itch. Urticarial wheals immediately after penetration of cercariae. Several hours later itching and edema, followed by papules and pustules. Symptoms begin to subside after three days (see p. 484). |

**Prophylaxis** Avoid contact with sandy soil which dogs and cats may leave polluted with feces. Sand boxes and the like should be protected from dogs and especially cats which may select these as defecation sites.

## Gnathostomiasis

**Synonyms** *Gnathostoma spinigerum* infection, "larva migrans" or "creeping eruption."

**Definition** Gnathostomiasis is an infection by immature *Gnathostoma spinigerum,* an uncommon helminthic parasite of man. The worm may localize in the internal organs but occurs more typically in the peripheral tissues in nodules or in subcutaneous tunnels in which the worms migrate (hence "larva migrans" or "creeping eruption"). Adult parasites are usually found in wild or domestic cats and more rarely in dogs, hogs or mink.

**Distribution** Gnathostomiasis is known from Palestine, India, Java, Malaya, Thailand, China and Japan. In certain areas of Thailand it is highly endemic.

**Etiology** Morphology. The adult nematode, *Gnathostoma spinigerum* Owen 1836, is stout, reddish in color and possesses a globose cephalic bulb or head which is separated from the body proper by a slight constriction and is armed by 4 to 8 transverse rows of recurved spines. The anterior half of the body is spinose also. Males and females range respectively from 11 to 25 mm. and 25 to 54 mm. in length. The mature female produces ovoid, unsegmented eggs with a greenish tinged, irregularly pitted shell, marked by a transparent plug at one end; the eggs measure 63 to 70 microns in length by 37 to 41 microns in breadth.

Development. The adult worms lie coiled in tumors along the alimentary canal of cats, dogs and other reservoir hosts. Eggs reach the lumen of the intestine from these lesions, and are passed in the feces where they become embryonated; they hatch upon reaching water, releasing a cylindrical, ensheathed rhabditiform larva which, if ingested by a copepod (*Cyclops*), continues to develop. When the infective copepod is eaten by a fish, frog or snake a third stage larva is produced which becomes encapsulated in the flesh of the host. Upon ingestion by the definitive host, the parasite usually becomes localized in the stomach wall where it matures after about seven months.

**Epidemiology** Although the epidemiology has been inadequately studied, it appears probable that man becomes infected through the ingestion of improperly cooked fish, frogs and possibly snakes containing encapsulated larvae. It appears doubtful that man becomes infected by swallowing infected copepods in water.

**Pathology** Man appears to be an abnormal host. Only immature worms have been encountered and these were usually situated superficially. In some cases abscesses or cutaneous nodules were produced while in others deep or subcutaneous tunnels were formed through which the larvae migrated. Ocular involvement occurs rarely, as does visceral encapsulation.

**Clinical Characteristics**    The worms are usually encountered between the stratum germinativum and the corium of the skin, producing local inflammatory symptoms, edema, eosinophilia, and leukocytosis. Other symptoms depend upon the location of the parasite.

**Diagnosis**    Residence in an endemic area is suggestive, but definitive diagnosis depends upon the recovery and identification of the parasite. In the nonmigrating type the infection must be differentiated from abscesses of bacterial origin, while in the migrating form it must be distinguished from cases of cutaneous myiasis (p. 404) or the migrations of larval hookworms, especially *Ancylostoma braziliense* (p. 392).

**Treatment**    Hetrazan is believed to be the most effective drug. See p. 400 for details of treatment.

**Prophylaxis**    Both man and other hosts acquire the infection through the ingestion of infected fish, frogs or snakes. Adequate cooking, especially of fish, is recommended, although immersion in vinegar for at least 5½ hours has also been found to be effective. On the basis of the evidence at hand the possibility of acquiring the infection by ingesting infested copepods (*Cyclops*) in water cannot be entirely disregarded.

## Strongyloidiasis

**Synonyms**    Strongyloidosis, *Strongyloides stercoralis* infection, the strongylid threadworm.

**Definition**    Strongyloidiasis is an infection by the nematode, *S. stercoralis*, which usually is embedded in the mucosa and submucosa of the small intestine of man.

**Distribution**    Strongyloidiasis occurs primarily in the tropics and subtropics although it has been reported sporadically from temperate regions. It is nearly as widespread as hookworm infections, but accurate data on its distribution are lacking. The chief known endemic centers are located in tropical Africa, Central and South America, and southern Asia (especially Burma, Siam and Malaya). Autochthonous cases have been reported from the United States and Canada. Over 13 per cent of the population were infected on Okinawa, but it is uncommon in South Korea, Japan, China, and French Indo-China.

**Etiology**    MORPHOLOGY. The adult parasite, *S. stercoralis* (Bavay 1876) Stiles and Hassall 1902, is small, the female measuring about 2.2 mm. in length. The cuticula is delicately striated and in the parasitic females the esophagus occupies one-third to two-fifths of the body length. The paired ovaries, oviducts and uteri open through a short vaginal opening near the beginning of the posterior third of the body.

The mature female lies buried in the mucosa and submucosa of the human intestine where it liberates thin-shelled, ovoid eggs, resembling those of hookworm and measuring 50 to 58 microns by 30 to 34 microns. These are usually embryonated and soon hatch to produce the typical rhabditiform larvae encountered in the stools of individuals with strongyloidiasis. These larvae measure 200 to 250 microns in length and closely resemble the rhabditiform larvae of hookworm but differ from them chiefly in having a shorter buccal capsule and a more robust posterior extremity (Table 34, p. 399). The little-known rhabditiform male measures about 0.7 mm. It possesses two spicules and a gubernaculum, but no caudal alae. The tail is pointed and ventrally curved.

DEVELOPMENT. The larvae of *S. stercoralis* which are passed in the stool are believed to develop in either of two ways: (1) as free-living adults or (2) as infective filariform larvae. A free-living generation of rhabditiform adults including both males and females may develop under suitable conditions of moisture and temperature and it is believed by some workers that this cycle may continue until unfavorable conditions stimulate the production of filariform larvae. The latter are infective for man. Under other circumstances the rhabditiform larvae passed in the stool may become transformed within 24 hours directly into infective larvae capable of penetrating the skin of man.

The infective filariform larvae of *Strongyloides* resemble hookworm larvae at the corresponding stage of development but differ in that they are smaller and possess a much longer esophagus and a minute but distinct tridigitate tail which is diagnostic of *Strongyloides*.

The filariform larvae which pentrate the skin eventually reach the lymphatics or capillaries and are carried to the right side of the heart and the pulmonary capillaries. Here the larvae leave the capillary beds and penetrate into the alveoli of the lungs. Most of these parasites migrate up the respiratory passages, reach the esophagus and pass down into the stomach and intestines. Mating is reported to occur in the duodenum or jejunum. After fertilization the females burrow into the mucosa and submucosa to oviposit, thus completing the life cycle.

It is probable that not all parasites leave the respiratory tract of man. Some precocious individuals may migrate into the pulmonary tissues and develop there. In such cases rhabditiform and, rarely, filariform larvae may be demonstrated in the sputum.

In certain cases the cycle is completed entirely within one host. The rhabditiform larvae that would ordinarily be passed in the stool rapidly metamorphose into dwarf filariform larvae. These directly penetrate either the lower bowel or the perianal skin, producing hyperinfection.

**Epidemiology**  While much remains to be learned concerning the epidemiology of strongyloidiasis, it is known that man usually acquires the infection by skin contact with the infective filariform larvae. Penetration is effected in the same manner as in hookworm infection. While contamination of the skin is the usual avenue of invasion, it appears probable that contaminated food or drink may occasionally be a factor in transmission.

Little is known of the adaptability of the free-living generation to unfavorable environmental conditions. It is believed, however, that these organisms cannot survive in water or withstand desiccation.

**Pathology**   Penetration of the skin is followed by petechial hemorrhage and edema but without inflammatory reaction unless bacterial infection occurs. Larvae which reach the blood stream are carried to the lungs where they migrate into the alveoli, causing hemorrhage

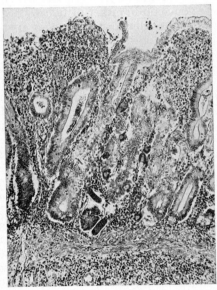

Fig. 189. Strongyloidiasis showing adult worm in a section through the mucosa.

and cellular infiltration. Certain of the larvae may fail to complete the normal migration, undergo precocious development in the lung and mature in the bronchial or tracheal epithelium, producing pulmonary strongyloidiasis. In this condition larvae may be present in the sputum accompanying a lobular pneumonitis. *Strongyloides* larvae have also been recovered from pleural and pericardial effusions.

Normally the immature females develop rapidly after reaching the the duodenum and upper jejunum where they invade the mucosa and the submucosa (Fig. 189). Less frequently they may be found in the mucosa of the pyloric region of the stomach, ileum or colon. The females soon produce eggs which occur singly or in nests near the bases of the villi and in the interglandular stroma. Upon hatching, the young larvae gradually work into the lumen of the intestine. In heavy infections where the mucosa may be honeycombed by both the adult worms and the hatched larvae there may be extensive ulceration and sloughing which may result in the rare appearance of eggs in the stool.

In hyperinfections filariform larvae may be encountered in the connective tissue spaces and lymphatics of the mesentery and in the mesenteric lymph nodes. Occasionally they may be observed in the portal areas of the liver and in the subserosal lymphatics and connective tissue of the gallbladder wall. *Strongyloides* larvae have been recovered also from pleural and pericardial effusions. In some cases there is an eosinophilia of 50 per cent and a polymorphonuclear leukocytosis in excess of 20,000.

**Clinical Characteristics**   There is no characteristic clinical picture. Variability of location of the parasite in the host is marked. There may be a long latent period between infection and the development of symptoms.

A pruritic erythema resembling the "ground itch" of hookworm infection may appear within an hour at the site of entry. The subsequent migration of the larvae through the lungs may be accompanied by signs and symptoms of bronchitis or pneumonitis which may be quite severe.

The symptomatology of intestinal strongyloidiasis is varied. The parasite frequently produces severe gastro-intestinal disturbances. Diarrhea almost invariably occurs at some time during the course of the infection. It is usually intermittent, often alternating with mild constipation. Occult blood may be present in the stools while in severe cases they may be grossly bloody. Abdominal pain, near the midepigastrium commonly to the right of the midline, is often the chief complaint, accompanied by general abdominal tenderness. Dyspepsia characterized by vague distress, heartburn and flatulence are common. There may be nausea and vomiting attributable to reflex nervous stimulation or direct irritation of the gastric mucosa. Jaundice and other evidence of biliary tract involvement may be strongly suggestive of cholecystitis. Recurring attacks of urticaria occur in certain individuals. Fever is variable and probably related to the degree of secondary bacterial infection.

In the presence of hyperinfection there may be severe involvement of the lungs with lobular pneumonitis accompanied by dyspnea, cough and hemoptysis. Extensive invasion of the gastro-intestinal tract with ulceration and sloughing of the mucosa may produce grave symptoms with progressive emaciation and cachexia resulting in death.

Except in cases of hyperinfection the prognosis is favorable although eradication of the parasite is difficult.

**Diagnosis**   Eosinophilia is the most characteristic feature of the blood picture; polymorphonuclear leukocytosis may be marked or absent.

The finding of motile rhabditiform larvae in a stool is highly suggestive of strongyloidiasis. Confirmation consists in carefully checking the morphology of the larvae to distinguish them from those of hookworm. As the length and diameter of rhabditiform larvae of these two species are comparable when in the same stage of development, the most satisfactory criteria are the length of the buccal capsule and the attenuation of the tail (Table 34 and Fig. 186). The rhabditiform larvae of hookworm have an attenuated posterior tip and a buccal capsule that is longer than the diameter of the head of the worm, while the rhabditiform larvae of *Strongyloides* possess a bluntly pointed posterior tip and a short buccal capsule. The MGL (Formalin-ether) or AMS III techniques usually reveal larvae if they are in the feces (see p. 822 for details of the method).

In a high percentage of the cases of strongyloidiasis the larvae will not be found in the stool. If an infection with this parasite is suspected, aspirated duodenal fluid and sputum specimens should be examined for the presence of these larvae (Fig. 186).

**Treatment** Gentian violet medicinal has been recommended but it is uniformly unsatisfactory. It is administered either in enteric coated tablets or, in refractory cases, in solution by vein or duodenal intubation. Hospitalization is necessary only when intravenous injections of the drug are indicated (see p. 547 for other details).

**Prophylaxis** The prophylaxis of strongyloidiasis does not differ from that of hookworm disease. In both, the essential feature is prevention of soil pollution by human feces.


# 43 Tissue-Inhabiting Nematodes: The Filarioidea

### Biology of the Filarioidea

**Introduction** Nematodes inhabiting the tissues of man include the filarial worms, the guinea worm, and the trichina worm. These belong to the superfamilies FILARIOIDEA, DRACUNCULOIDEA and TRICHUROIDEA respectively. Parasites in only the first subdivision will be considered here. Members of the FILARIOIDEA infecting man may be characterized as follows: (1) The threadlike adults inhabit the tissues or body cavities of a vertebrate where the females produce eggs which are partially or completely embryonated. (2) At the time of oviposition, or just prior thereto, the embryos uncoil and are known as microfilariae. (3) The eggshell may persist, accommodating itself to the elongated larva, thus producing a "sheathed" microfilaria. If the shell ruptures a naked or "unsheathed" microfilaria results. (4) All microfilariae must pass a developmental stage in a blood-sucking insect vector (Fig. 190).

Some of the tissue-inhabiting nematodes produce diseases in man. Thus Bancroft's filariasis is an infection by *Wuchereria bancrofti* or filariasis malayi by *W. malayi*, onchocerciasis by *Onchocerca vol-vulus* and loiasis by *Loa loa*. Two other FILARIOIDEA, *Acantho-cheilonema perstans* and *Mansonella ozzardi*, which are found in man do little if any damage and produce few if any symptoms. In addition to these well recognized parasites a number of rarer forms

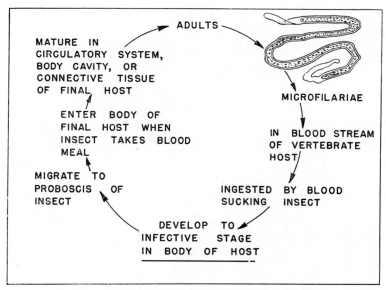

Fig. 190. Nematode cycle—filarial worm type.

have also been reported in man. Since records of these are based either upon a single infection or on an inadequate description of a single worm, these parasites will not be considered.

## Morphology of the Filarioidea

**Adults** The adult parasites vary between 19 mm. and 60 cm. in length, the females often being twice as long as the males. Most are creamy white, filiform worms whose cuticle may be smooth, trans-versely striated, or covered with annular rings or knoblike bosses. There are species-specific papillae about the head, mouth and usually the tail. In some species the males possess caudal alae and all have spicules which vary in size and shape. Further details will be found in the discussion of the appropriate species.

**Microfilariae** Adult females produce prelarvae known as micro-filariae which range from 177 to 300 microns in length. Some of these embryonic forms retain their shells as "sheaths" while others break out and hence are "unsheathed." Sheaths appear as delicate close-fitting membranes that may be detected only where they project beyond the head or tail of the microfilariae.

Internally each parasite is seen to consist of columns of nuclei which are believed to represent the anlagen of various systems and structures. The best means of differentiating among various species of microfilariae lies in the position of organ precursors of parts of the digestive, excretory and reproductive systems and in the position of the caudal nuclei. These stain deeply with hematoxylin and occupy

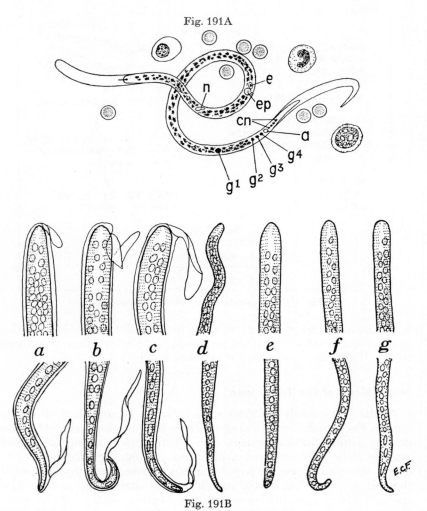

Fig. 191A

Fig. 191B

Fig. 191*A*. Diagram of an unsheathed microfilaria of *Wuchereria bancrofti* from peripheral blood showing characteristic features: *a*, anal pore; *cn*, caudal nuclei; *e*, excretory cell; *ep*, excretory pore; *g1–4*, genital cells; *n*, nerve ring. (Original.)

Fig. 191*B*. Differential characteristics of head and tail ends of the microfilariae of *a*, *Wuchereria bancrofti*; *b*, *W. malayi*; *c*, *Loa loa*; *d*, *Onchocerca volvulus*; *e*, *Acanthocheilonema perstans*; *f*, *A. streptocerca*; and *g*, *Mansonella ozzardi*. Greatly enlarged, drawn to scale. (Craig & Faust: Clinical Parasitology, 5th ed., Lea & Febiger.)

characteristic positions. Certain anatomic landmarks differ in their distances from the anterior tip of the worm. Such structures include the nerve ring, excretory pore, excretory cell in relation to the excretory pore, anal pore, and the four genital cells, $G_{1-4}$ (Figs. 191$A$ and $B$).

A determination of the type of periodicity displayed by the microfilariae is of value in making tentative species identifications, although periodicity can be reversed if the individual works at night

*Name:* Jam Basha.     *Race:* Indian male, *aet.* 26.     *Physical State:* Normal.

*Residence in Fiji:* Three years.

April, 1910.

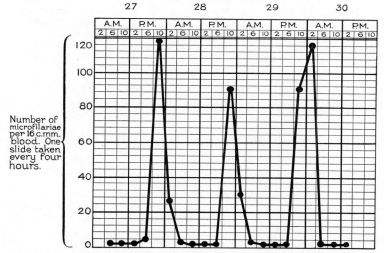

Fig. 192. Periodicity of *Wuchereria bancrofti* in peripheral blood. (After Manson Bahr in Strong: Stitt's Diagnosis, Prevention and Treatment of Tropical Diseases. The Blakiston Company.)

and sleeps during the day. For example, the microfilariae of the periodic form of *W. bancrofti* occur in greatest numbers in the peripheral blood between 8 p. m. and 2 a. m. while the microfilariae of the diurnal or nonperiodic strain appear in infected individuals both day and night (Fig. 192). However, in the case of loiasis the microfilariae are diurnal.

**Developmental Stages**    All members of the Filarioidea require an insect intermediate host. As this vector feeds on man, microfilariae are ingested. The parasites soon leave the vector's alimentary canal, undergo a period of development in the thoracic muscles and finally migrate into the mouthparts where they are infective for man. When the insect next feeds on man the parasites leave the vector, penetrate the skin surface and migrate to the internal site specific for the development of the given species of worm. After maturing and mating, the adult females produce new microfilariae (Figs. 191$A$ and $B$). The better known vectors are summarized in Table 36.

**Differentiation of Microfilariae**   Microfilariae in onchocerciasis may occur in the fluid aspirate of nodules or in thin sections of skin. Microfilariae of other species of the Filarioidea are found in films of the peripheral blood, some being diurnal, others noc-

*Table 36   Vectors of Human* Filarioidea

| PARASITE | HOSTS |
|---|---|
| *Wuchereria bancrofti* and *Wuchereria malayi* | Many species of mosquitoes belonging to the genera *Culex, Aedes, Mansonia, Anopheles* |
| *Onchocerca volvulus* | Black flies: *Simulium damnosum, Simulium neavei, Eusimulium avidum, Eusimulium ochraceum, Eusimulium mooseri,* and probably others. |
| *Loa loa* | Tabanid flies: *Chrysops dimidiata, Chrysops silacea* |
| *Mansonella ozzardi* | Midge: *Culicoides furens* |
| *Acanthocheilonema perstans* | Midge: *Culicoides austeni, Culicoides grahami* |

turnal, while still others display no periodicity. These larvae or prelarvae may be differentiated by the key presented in Table 37.

*Table 37   A Key to the Common Microfilariae Infecting Man*

```
 1  (10)  Microfilariae in peripheral blood...............................  2
 2   (7)  Microfilariae sheathed.........................................  3
 3   (4)  Nuclei do not extend to tip of tail; cephalic space equal to
          diameter of head; nocturnal periodicity (or non-
          periodic ?)..................................Wuchereria bancrofti
 4   (3)  Nuclei extend to tip of tail in broken or unbroken chain; diurnal or noc-
          turnal periodicity...........................................  5
 5   (6)  Nuclei extend in solid row to tip of tail; diurnal periodicity.........Loa loa
 6   (5)  Nuclei extend in broken row to tip of tail, resembling W. ban-
          crofti except for two small terminal nuclei; cephalic space
          twice diameter of head; nocturnal periodicity...........Wuchereria malayi
 7   (2)  Microfilariae unsheathed.......................................  8
 8   (9)  Nuclei extending to tip of tail, often appearing as a
          double row...............................Acanthocheilonema perstans
 9   (8)  Nuclei not extending to tip of tail.....................Mansonella ozzardi
10   (1)  Microfilariae in skin and subcutaneous tissues; nuclei not to
          tip of tail.....................................Onchocerca volvulus
```

A more detailed summary of the microfilariae infecting man occurs in Table 38.

## Filariasis Bancrofti

**Synonyms**   Bancroft's filariasis. *Wuchereria bancrofti* infection.
**Definition**   Filariasis bancrofti is due to the presence of adult *W. bancrofti* in the lymphatic system or connective tissues of man. The infection may be accompanied by important pathologic conditions related to the lymphatic system which include inflammatory lesions, dilatation and rupture of lymphatics, hypertrophy, hyperplasia and fibrosis. Offspring of the parent worms, known as microfilariae, are

characteristically present in the circulating blood; their presence while alive does not contribute to the pathologic changes listed above. Many species of *Anopheles*, *Culex*, *Mansonia* and *Aedes* are vectors.

*Table 38   The Differentiation of the Microfilariae of the*
FILARIOIDEA *of Man**

| SHEATHED MICROFILARIAE FROM PERIPHERAL BLOOD | | | |
|---|---|---|---|
| Characteristics | *Wuchereria bancrofti* | *Wuchereria malayi* | *Loa loa* |
| Periodicity | Usually nocturnal | Nocturnal | Diurnal |
| Appearance | Graceful sweeping curves | Stiff, secondary kinks | Stiff, secondary kinks |
| Tail | Tapers to a delicate point, terminal nuclei absent | Slight bulb at tip, 2 terminal nuclei | Gradual tapering, caudal nuclei continuous row into tail |
| Length | 244–296 $\mu$ (thick films) | 177–230 $\mu$ (thick films) | 250–300 $\mu$ (thick films) |
| Excretory cell | Small, near excretory pore | Large, far behind excretory pore | Large, far behind excretory pore |
| G cells | Small, similar in size; $G_2$–$G_4$ far behind $G_1$; $G_1$–70.14% ‡ | Larger; $G_1$ relatively near and larger than $G_2$–$G_4$; $G_1$–68.33% ‡ | Similar to those of *W. malayi*; $G_1$–68.6% ‡ |
| Anal pore | 82.48% ‡ | 82.28% ‡ | 81.9% ‡ |
| Intermediate host | Best—*Culex quinquefasciatus* (= *Culex fatigans*), *A. gambiae* | Best—*Mansonia* spp.† *Anopheles* spp. | *Chrysops* spp. |
| Cephalic space | As long as broad | Twice as long as broad | ? |
| Stylets | 1 | 2 | ? |
| Body nuclei | Well defined | Blurred, intermingled | Larger and stain less deeply |

| UNSHEATHED MICROFILARIAE FROM PERIPHERAL BLOOD | |
|---|---|
| Characteristics | *Mansonella ozzardi* | *Acanthocheilonema perstans* |
| Stylet | 1 | 0 |
| Tail | 5 terminal nuclei not reaching tip of tail | Nuclei extend to tip of tail, often in 2 rows |

| MICROFILARIA OF SKIN AND SUBCUTANEOUS TISSUES | |
|---|---|
| Characteristics | *Onchocerca volvulus* |
| Sheath | Absent |
| Stylet | None |
| Tail | Curved |
| Nuclei | 5–7 near tip |

* Modified from Faust's adaptation from Feng, 1933.
† Subgenus *Mansonioides*.
‡ Distance from anterior end.

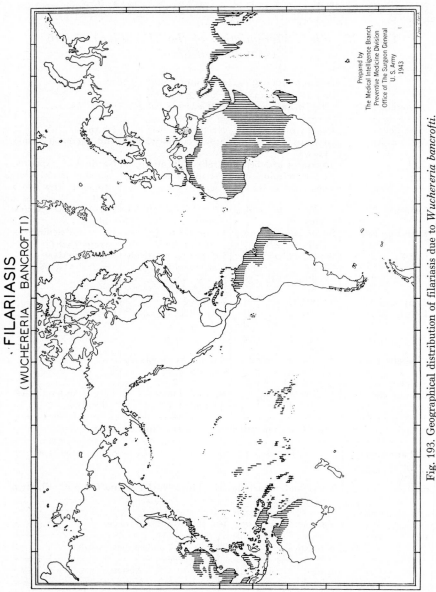

Fig. 193. Geographical distribution of filariasis due to *Wuchereria bancrofti.*

Some workers regard periodic filariasis bancrofti as different from the diurnal or nonperiodic form. Variations in the clinical development of these two entities, their mutual geographic isolation and their different types of periodicity suggest the possibility that two species, or perhaps varieties, of etiologic agent exist. The name, *W. pacifica*, has been proposed for the diurnal or nonperiodic form.

**Distribution**  The periodic or classic form of filariasis bancrofti is widespread throughout the tropics and subtropics except in the Southwest Pacific (Fig. 193). In the western hemisphere it was formerly established as far north as Charleston, S. C., but has become extinct. The disease occurs throughout the West Indies, Colombia, Venezuela, Panama and the coastal portions of the Guianas and Brazil.

In Europe it appears to be limited to Spain (Barcelona), Hungary, Jugoslavia and Turkey, while along the North African Coast it occurs spottily from lower Egypt to Morocco. Other areas include a wide belt across the central portion of Africa, as well as Madagascar, the neighboring islands and the east coastal region.

The disease is endemic in the Orient. In many localities its distribution overlaps that of *W. malayi*, which was not described until 1927. The periodic form has also been reported from coastal Arabia to India and is found with the Malayan form in India, Southeast Asia, southern China, Philippines and southern Japan. Although both are generally present, filariasis malayi predominates in Sumatra, Borneo, Celebes and Ceram in Indonesia but not in New Guinea or tropical Australia.

The diurnal or nonperiodic type of filariasis bancrofti appears restricted to the islands of the South Pacific area.

**Etiology**  MORPHOLOGY. Adult *W. bancrofti* (Cobbold 1877) Seurat 1921 localize in the lymphatic vessels and the lymph nodes. The males and females are often closely intertwined. The mature worms are threadlike, cylindrical and creamy white with a smooth cuticula and bluntly tapering extremities. The slightly swollen cephalic region bears two rings of small papillae. The unarmed mouth opens directly into a cylindrical esophagus which is divided into an anterior muscular and a posterior glandular portion. The male worm measures as much as 40 mm. in length. On the ventrally curved tail may be found a maximum of eight preanal and four postanal pairs of papillae supporting narrow inconspicuous alae, while farther caudad are two pairs of larger, and one pair of smaller papillae. Copulatory spicules which vary in size and shape, and a crescent-shaped gubernaculum, characterize the male.

The females are longer, ranging between 80 and 100 mm. in length. The vulva opens about 0.8 or 0.9 mm. from the anterior tip. The vagina extends to a long, bilateral, coiled uterus which has its origin about 1 mm. from the posterior tip.

Developing microfilarial embryos are coiled in a membrane or shell averaging about 38 by 25 microns in size; later this structure elongates to form the microfilarial sheath.

Fully developed, sheathed microfilariae measure 244 to 296 microns in length by 7.5 to 10 microns in breadth. The tip of the head is described as bearing a stylet and the cephalic space between the column of nuclei and the anterior tip is approximately equal to the diameter of the head. Adequate staining of smears is necessary to determine that the nerve ring is 20 per cent of the body length from the anterior tip, the excretory pore 29.6, the excretory cell 30.6, the $G_1$ cell 70.14 and the anal pore 82.4 per cent (see Fig. 191$A$). The last 5 per cent of the body length, i. e., the tail, is devoid of nuclei, a point of importance in distinguishing between the microfilariae of

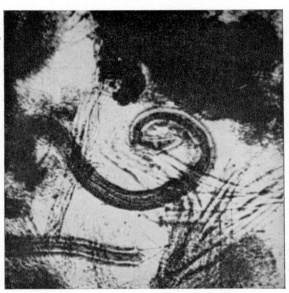

Fig. 194. Developing larva of *W. bancrofti* in thoracic muscle of *C. quinquefasciatus.* (S.E.S.P. Brazil, for the Office of the Coordinator of Inter-American Affairs.)

this species and *W. malayi* (see Table 38). Microfilariae of periodic and nonperiodic *W. bancrofti* are indistinguishable.

DEVELOPMENT. Adult *W. bancrofti* normally inhabit the lymphatics, where they liberate microfilariae. The latter either remain in the lymph or reach the peripheral circulation where they are ingested by the mosquito vector as it feeds. They complete their intermediate development in the gut and tissues of the insect host (Fig. 194).

Within an hour after ingestion, the larvae exsheath and those that are not passed in the mosquito's feces penetrate the stomach wall and migrate within twenty-four hours to the thoracic muscles. Here the parasites undergo a series of complex morphologic changes including two molts. During this period the developing larvae pass from a sausage-shaped stage to mature, infective filariform (third stage) larvae measuring between 1.4 and 2 mm. in length. Under optimum conditions ten to eleven days are required for this transformation to occur. The larvae then migrate to the mouthparts of the mosquito from which point they reach the new host when it next feeds. Since the larvae usually leave the mosquito by breaking through Dutton's membrane, it is believed they actively penetrate the skin, entering either the puncture site, or possibly even forming their own portal of entry. The filiform larvae which succeed in establishing entrance eventually reach the lymphatic system and are thought to mature within about a year. The details of the migrations and development of these worms within man are not fully known.

**Epidemiology** Complete development of the larval forms of *W. bancrofti* has been shown to occur in over thirty species of mosquitoes included in the genera *Anopheles, Culex, Aedes,* and *Mansonia.* However, these mosquitoes are not all necessarily concerned with the transmission of the infection in nature. The most important known vectors are *C. quinquefasciatus* (*C. fatigans*), *C. pipiens, Aedes scutellaris* and *Anopheles gambiae.* In the South Pacific and Australian regions *C. quinquefasciatus* and *Anopheles punctulatus* are regarded as the most important transmitters. *Anopheles farauti* is an important vector in the Solomons and New Hebrides (Table 39).

The importance of a particular mosquito will depend to a large extent upon its biology, especially its feeding on human rather than animal blood and its breeding in areas in close proximity to man. The conditions necessary for maintaining filariasis at a high level of endemicity comprise an adequate human reservoir, a sufficient number of cases having numerous microfilariae in the peripheral blood, and ample breeding of suitable mosquitoes within range of the infected population. Since some vectors are daytime feeders and others purely nocturnal, the infection may be transmitted by day as well as by night in certain areas (Fig. 195).

The roles of occasional or continuous infection in the development of the syndromes of the disease are not known. It is said that demonstrable infection is rare in young children and infants and that the incidence is highest after the twentieth year. It is also said that the incidence of clinical disease varies between the sexes in different parts of the world. This may be an expression of differences in occupation of the infected individuals and of variations in the behavior and habitats of the important vectors in different regions. It is probable that persons experiencing asymptomatic infections and the early clinical stages of the disease constitute the important human reservoir. In the early or advanced stages, particularly in the presence of elephantiasis, microfilariae may not be present in the peripheral blood.

As previously indicated, periodicity is the alternate increase and decrease in the number of microfilariae present in the peripheral blood. The epidemiologic importance of the phenomenon of periodicity is that it will determine which species of mosquito become

*Table 39 Some Known and Probable Vectors of* Wuchereria bancrofti *by Countries*

| | | |
|---|---|---|
| Africa: | Belgian Congo | *Aedes aegypti* |
| | | *Anopheles funestus* |
| | | *Anopheles gambiae* |
| | Central Africa | *Mansonia uniformis* |
| | Egypt | *Culex quinquefasciatus* ( = *C. fatigans*) |
| | | *Culex pipiens* |
| | Nigeria | *Aedes ochraceus* |
| | Sierra Leone | *Anopheles squamosus squamosus* |
| | | *Anopheles funestus* |
| | | *Anopheles rhodesiensis* |
| | Tanganyika | *Culex quinquefasciatus* ( = *C. fatigans*) |
| | Tunis | *Anopheles algeriensis* |
| | West Africa | *Aedes aegypti* |
| | | *Anopheles funestus* |
| | | *Anopheles gambiae* |
| | Zanzibar | *Culex quinquefasciatus* ( = *C. fatigans*) |
| | | *Anopheles funestus* |
| | | *Anopheles gambiae* |
| Asia: | China | *Culex vagans* |
| | Central China | *Culex pipiens* |
| | (Shanghai area) | *Culex pipiens pallens* |
| | | *Anopheles hyrcanus sinensis* |
| | South China | *Culex quinquefasciatus* ( = *C. fatigans*) |
| | India | *Culex quinquefasciatus* ( = *C. fatigans*) |
| | | *Culex vagans* |
| | | *Culex vishnui* |
| | | *Mansonia annulifera* |
| | | *Anopheles annularis* ( = *A. fuliginosus*) |
| | | *Anopheles barbirostris barbirostris* |
| | | *Anopheles pallidus* |
| | | *Anopheles philippinensis* |
| | | *Psorophora confinnis* (Ceylon) |
| | | *Anopheles stephensi* subsp. |
| | | *Anopheles subpictus subpictus* ( = *rossi*) |
| | | *Anopheles sundaicus* |
| | | *Anopheles vagus vagus* |
| | | *Anopheles varuna* |
| | | *Anopheles ramsayi* ( = *A. pseudojamesi*) |
| | Travancore | *Anopheles hyrcanus nigerrimus* |
| | Japan | *Culex pipiens* |
| | | *Culex pipeins pallens* |
| | | *Culex sinensis* |
| | | *Aedes togoi* |
| | | *Anopheles hyrcanus sinensis* |
| | Philippines | *Culex quinquefasciatus* ( = *C. fatigans*) |
| | Formosa | *Culex quinquefasciatus* ( = *C. fatigans*) |
| | Okinawa | *Culex quinquefasciatus* ( = *C. fatigans*) |
| | | *Culex tritaeniorhynchus* (?) |
| | | *Anopheles hyrcanus sinensis* |
| Australia: | New South Wales | *Aedes aegypti* |
| | Queensland | *Anopheles amictus* |
| | General | *Culex quinquefasciatus* ( = *C. fatigans*) |
| | | *Aedes vigilax* |
| Central Pacific Islands | | *Aedes tongae* |
| Indonesia | | *Culex fuscocephalus* |
| | | *Culex whitmorei* |

## *Table 39   Continued*

| | |
|---|---|
| Central Pacific Islands | *Culex annulirostris* |
| Indonesia | *Culex alis* |
| | *Culex bitaeniorhynchus* |
| | *Culex sitiens* |
| | *Culex tritaeniorhynchus* |
| | *Aedes vigilax* |
| | *Mansonia annulata* |
| | *Mansonia indiana* |
| | *Mansonia longipalpis* |
| | *Mansonia uniformis* |
| | *Anopheles aconitus* |
| | *Anopheles bancroftii* |
| (also Kabaema Is.) | *Anopheles leucosphyrus hackeri* |
| Solomon Islands | *Anopheles farauti* and related species |
| Certain Indonesian Islands | *Culex quinquefasciatus* ( = *C. fatigans*) |
| | *Culex vishnui* |
| | *Anopheles hyrcanus nigerrimus* |
| South Pacific Islands | *Aedes scutellaris* |
| | *Aedes tongae* |
| | *Anopheles koliensis* |
| Celebes | *Culex quinquefasciatus* ( = *C. fatigans*) |
| (East Indies and other Pacific Islands) | *Anopheles aconitus* |
| | *Anopheles bancroftii* |
| | *Anopheles maculatus* |
| | *Anopheles punctulatus moluccensis* |
| | *Anopheles punctulatus punctulatus* |
| New Guinea | *Mansonia indiana* |
| | *Anopheles farauti* |
| | *Anopheles punctulatus* |
| Samoa | |
| Fiji | *Aedes pseudoscutellaris* |
| Other Pacific Islands | |
| Malaya | *Mansonia uniformis* |
| | *Anopheles hyrcanus nigerrimus* |
| New Hebrides | *Culex quinquefasciatus* ( = *C. fatigans*) |
| | *Anopheles farauti* |
| North America: West Indies | *Culex quinquefasciatus* ( = *C. fatigans*) |
| | *Culex habilitator* |
| | *Aedes aegypti* |
| | *Aedes taeniorhynchus* |
| | *Anopheles albimanus* |
| Trinidad | *Culex quinquefasciatus* ( = *C. fatigans*) |
| South America: Brazil | *Culex quinquefasciatus* ( = *C. fatigans*) |
| | *Mansonia pseudotitillans* |
| | *Mansonia juxtamansonia* |
| | *Anopheles aquasalis* |
| | *Anopheles darlingi* |
| | *Anopheles albitarsis* |
| Dutch Guiana and | *Culex quinquefasciatus* ( = *C. fatigans*) |
| British Guiana | *Aedes aegypti* |
| Dutch Guiana | *Aedes aegypti* |

infected. Microfilariae with nocturnal periodicity are therefore transmitted almost exclusively by night-biters, while nonperiodic microfilariae are carried by any suitable species regardless of its time of feeding.

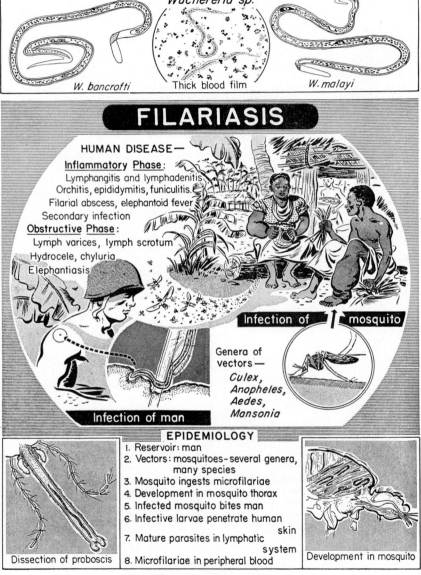

Fig. 195. Epidemiology of filariasis.

There is no natural immunity to filariasis.

**Pathology** The essential pathologic changes in filariasis consist of inflammatory reactions and subsequent progressive obstruction of lymphatic channels by scar tissue. These changes occur especially in the vicinity of adult worms which are commonly found in the lymphatic vessels, especially those of the abdominal cavity. However, worms may be present in the lymphatics in any part of the body. Common sites are the elephantoid tissues of the external genitalia and the mammary gland; the lymph nodes of the extremities; and the

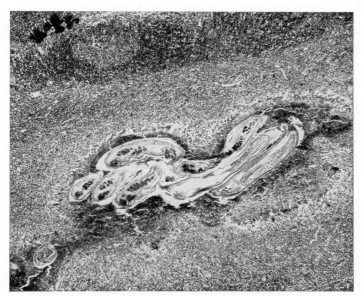

Fig. 196. Filariasis: acute inflammatory reaction about female worm in a lymph node.

retroperitoneal tissues particularly about the kidneys. There is no evidence to indicate that circulating microfilariae participate in the production of lesions (Fig. 196).

Biopsy studies performed on United States troops in the Southwest Pacific infected by the nonperiodic *W. bancrofti* during World War II have thrown some light on the genesis and the progression of the pathologic changes. The acute stages of filariasis of the lymphatic system may occur as early as three months after exposure. Essentially the same lesions were found whether or not adult worms, living or dead, were present. Furthermore, there was no indication that either microfilariae or bacteria participate in the early pathology.

The lesions in the lymph nodes were characterized by granulomatous inflammation, proliferation of the macrophage (reticulo-endothelial) system and eosinophilia of adjacent tissues. The dilated sinuses showed a wide zone of macrophages with variable numbers of eosinophils, lymphocytes and foreign body giant cells at the periphery. Necrosis was slight in amount and there was no increase of collagenous connective tissue.

The lymphatic vessels showed a variety of lesions including hyperplasia of the lining endothelium and of reticular cells in the walls; acute lymphangitis with or without thrombosis of the vessel; and finally fibrous obliteration. It would appear that the latter constitutes the basis for the development of lymph blockage and elephantiasis by successive thrombosis, organization of the thrombus and fibrosis with obliteration of the lymph channel.

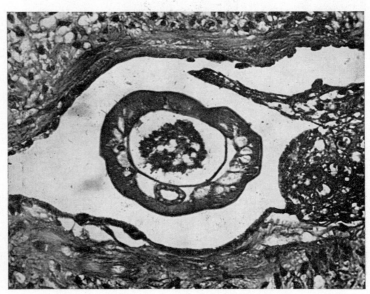

Fig. 197. Filariasis: adult worm in lymphatic vessel of the epididymis.

In the past the exact role of the adult worm has been controversial. Some authorities have held that the parasite itself does not cause a significant host reaction and that the tissue changes result from concomitant bacterial infection. Others have maintained that the living or dead worm itself causes inflammation or fibrosis, the result of toxic secretions of the parasite, from mechanical irritation and from disintegration products after the death of the worm.

Lymphatic obstruction (Fig. 197) is almost invariably followed by acute lymphangitis, which may be accompanied by leukocytosis and eosinophilia.

The inflammatory reaction is followed by the deposition of scar tissue about the involved lymphatics and lymph nodes. Degenerated worms ultimately may become calcified. Streptococcal and staphylococcal infections undoubtedly play a part in the production of some of the lesions. Particularly in old chronic cases, bacterial lymphangitis is not uncommon and abscess formation may occur (Fig. 198).

Following repeated inflammatory episodes, chronic obstruction to the lymphatic circulation occurs and there is progressive fibrosis. The distal lymph channels are distended or thrombosed, and the tissues become edematous and infiltrated with connective tissue. When the thoracic duct is involved, distended lymphatics in the urinary tract may rupture causing chyluria. When the extremities and superficial structures are involved the lymphatic obstruction and fibrosis lead to great thickening of the skin and subcutaneous tissues and the development of elephantiasis.

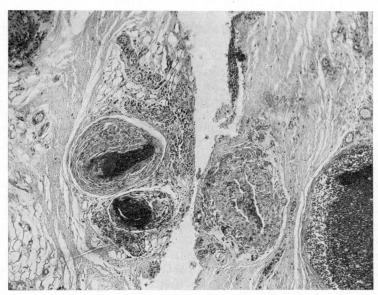

Fig. 198. Filariasis: fibrotic reaction about partially calcified worms in the capsule of a lymph node.

**Clinical Characteristics**  The clinical phases of filariasis may be classified as inflammatory or obstructive. The effects of inflammation may include lymphangitis, lymphadenitis, orchitis, epididymitis, funiculitis, filarial abscess, elephantoid fever, and secondary bacterial infections especially by streptococci and staphylococci. The obstructive phase is accompanied by a variety of clinical syndromes. Lymphatic dilatation without rupture produces lymph varices, lymph scrotum, and hydrocele. Rupture of the distended lymphatics is responsible for chyluria, chylous ascites, chylous diarrhea, lymphorrhea and lymphuria. The advanced stages of the obstructive phase are characterized by elephantiasis which commonly affects the leg, the scrotum, the arm, and the mammae.

Clinical filariasis normally has a prolonged incubation period which is seldom of less than eight to twelve months' duration and may be much longer. However, it is now well established that clinical phenomena may appear within three months of exposure. The early stages of the infection are usually accompanied by inflammatory phenomena and fever which frequently suggest other conditions.

The initial symptoms are largely local and unaccompanied by significant constitutional reaction. They usually consist of pain, swelling or redness of an arm or leg; or pain and swelling in the scrotal region. Stiffness of an involved extremity is common. Local lymphangitis with enlargement of the regional lymph nodes, particularly the epitrochlear, the axillary, the femoral or the inguinal nodes, depending upon the site of infection, frequently accompanies the early symptoms. Fever is usually mild when present. Characteristically, the acute local symptoms are transitory, rarely persisting more than a week or ten days. Enlargement of lymph nodes, however, tends to persist. Repeated recurrences of these phenomena are usual in the early stages of the disease.

THE INFLAMMATORY PHASE. *Acute lymphangitis* is a common early manifestation, usually involving the lower extremities, accompanied by fever ranging from 101° to 104° F., often with chills, and by more or less severe toxemia. The onset is frequently preceded by a "focal spot" of sharply circumscribed pain and tenderness often in the region of one of the malleoli and followed by ascending lymphangitis originating in this area. In other instances the lymphangitis begins centrally and follows a centrifugal course. The affected part is swollen, often tender and painful, and the involved lymphatics are frequently palpable. The skin may be diffusely reddened or red streaks may be seen over the inflamed lymphatic vessels. When the abdominal lymphatics are involved the clinical picture may suggest malaria or an acute abdomen. Involvement of the testes and spermatic cord is common. Spontaneous resolution occurs after several days and the skin of the affected part may return to normal or there may be residual induration. Recurring attacks are usual.

*Inguinal lymphadenitis* commonly accompanies or may precede filarial lymphangitis. The nodes are usually enlarged, painful and tender during the attack.

*Filarial orchitis* is a frequent acute manifestation. The onset is usually sudden, with pain in the testicle, fever, and occasionally rigors. The testicle rapidly enlarges in size and is extremely tender; this condition is commonly accompanied by hydrocele. Recurrences are frequent.

*Funiculitis*, a lymphangitis of the spermatic cord, and *epididymitis* are likewise common complications of filariasis (Fig. 199).

*Filarial abscesses* are often deeply seated in intermuscular fascial planes but frequently occur about infected lymph nodes, particularly those of the inguinal, axillary, and epitrochlear regions. Dead filarial worms may be present in the abscess cavity. The pathologic process apparently is the combined result of the presence of the parasite and secondary bacterial infection.

*Elephantoid fever* is a recurrent acute febrile condition which may be associated with elephantiasis or lymphangitis. Inflammatory phenomena may be absent; in these instances it is probable that there is an acute lymphangitis of the visceral lymphatics. The onset is usually sudden, with fever ranging from 102° to 104° F., rigors and sweating. An attack may last from a few hours to several days. Recurrences are common and often frequent.

THE OBSTRUCTIVE PHASE. This phase of filariasis is characterized by interference with the lymphatic circulation, edema, and accumulations of serous fluid. These manifestations frequently appear in the course of the various phenomena of the inflammatory phase which

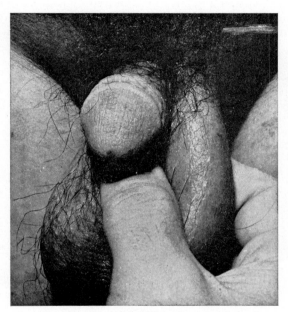

Fig. 199. Filariasis: thickened spermatic cord.

commonly leave evidence of progressive lymphatic obstruction in their wake. The two phases of the disease therefore often exist concurrently, each contributing to the progressive pathologic changes.

*Lymph varices,* or "varicose glands," commonly affect the inguinal or femoral lymph nodes of one or both sides, and less often the axillary nodes. These are soft lobulated swellings which usually develop slowly as the result of obstruction and dilatation of the lymphatic vessels. They are not attached to the overlying skin. The dilated lymphatics are palpable and tense, having a soft elastic consistency. The condition is usually painless and insidious. Aspirated fluid may contain microfilariae. Incision may be followed by a persistent lymph sinus (Fig. 200).

*Lymph scrotum* in many instances is associated with inguinal lymph varices and with chyluria. The onset often occurs with fever, swelling of the scrotum, varicose lymphatics and occasionally vesicles in the skin which may rupture and drain for considerable periods of time. Microfilariae may be present in this fluid. Elephantiasis of the part may follow.

*Hydrocele* is a frequent accompaniment of filariasis because of the common localization of adult worms in the epididymis. It may develop acutely in the course of filarial orchitis or epididymitis or more slowly and with relatively little local symptomatology. Microfilariae are often demonstrable in the serous fluid.

*Chyluria* is the result of obstruction and dilatation of the thoracic duct or its chyle-carrying tributaries followed by rupture of distended lymphatics into the urinary tract and the appearance of chyle in the urine. The urine frequently has the appearance of milk. Blood is

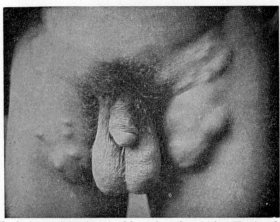

Fig. 200. Filariasis: varicose inguinal lymph nodes. (After Taniguchi—Kumamoto in Strong: Stitt's Diagnosis, Prevention and Treatment of Tropical Diseases. The Blakiston Company.)

often present in varying amounts, giving a pinkish coloration. On standing, the urine separates into an upper fatty layer, a semitransparent gelatinous layer of coagulated lymph, and a pinkish sediment containing lymphocytes, red blood cells and frequently microfilariae.

The onset is usually abrupt, often preceded by pain in the back, or aching in the lower abdomen and thighs. Fever may or may not be present. The attack commonly lasts only a few days. Recurrences are usual with intermissions of varying duration.

*Elephantiasis* occurs particularly in the legs and scrotum, less frequently in the arms, mammae or vulva, as a late complication of filariasis. Commonly it develops gradually in the course of repeated attacks of acute filarial lymphangitis. The skin and subcutaneous tissues are greatly thickened and fibrotic and the regional lymph nodes draining the affected area are usually enlarged. In the majority of cases of elephantiasis, microfilariae are not demonstrable in the blood (Figs. 201, 202).

**Diagnosis**  In the early stages of filariasis, microfilariae may not be demonstrable in the peripheral blood and the diagnosis must be based on clinical data alone. A history of exposure in an area of known endemicity, of an incubation period of at least three months' duration prior to the appearance of symptoms, and of recurrent inflammatory phenomena is highly suggestive.

Certain objective signs should be carefully sought. Commonest of these is enlargement of the regional lymph nodes draining the affected area with or without swelling of an extremity or of the scrotal contents. The spermatic cord is frequently thickened, in-

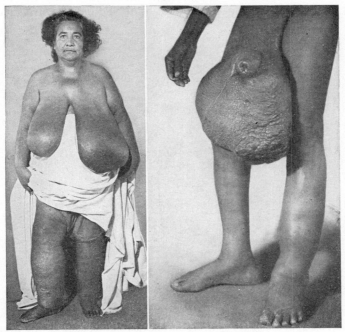

Fig. 201.          Fig. 202.

Fig. 201. Filariasis: elephantiasis of legs and breasts. Cook Islands.
Fig. 202. Filariasis: elephantiasis of scrotum, lymphedema of leg. (Alan Fisher for the Office of the Coordinator of Inter-American Affairs.)

durated and nodular. Hydrocele of moderate degree is common even in the early stages of the disease and there may be enlargement of the testicle as well.

There is at present no laboratory test which provides dependable diagnostic criteria in the absence of demonstration of the microfilariae. Complement fixation tests using antigen prepared from related worms (*Dirofilaria immitis*) have not proved to be reliable. However, skin tests using antigen from adult *D. immitis* or from microfilariae of *W. bancrofti* have given few false reactions even during the preclinical stage of the disease.

Although adult worms may be present in affected lymph nodes, biopsy is emphatically contraindicated since it further augments lymphatic obstruction. Between acute inflammatory attacks subjection of the individual to heavy physical exertion often initiates an acute recurrence accompanied by characteristic clinical phenomena. The acute episodes are commonly accompanied by leukocytosis and eosinophilia.

In the intermediate stages of the disease microfilariae may be demonstrated in the peripheral blood. They are commonly absent in the early phases and in the stage of advanced elephantiasis. A thick film of fresh blood is useful in light infections since the actively motile microfilariae are easily found. Stained thick smears should be

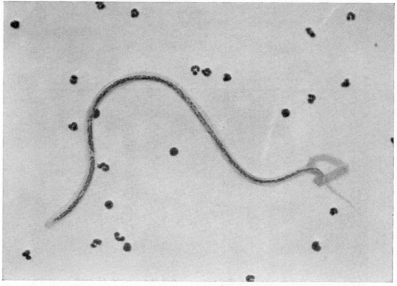

Fig. 203. Microfilaria of *W. bancrofti* in thick blood film stained with hematoxylin to show sheath and characteristic tail. (Courtesy National Institutes of Health, U.S.P.H.S.)

used in preference to thin films. Smears of the sediment from laked centrifuged blood should be used when other methods fail. When infection by nocturnally periodic forms is suspected blood for examination should be taken at night, preferably after nine o'clock. Day-time specimens are preferable for the diurnally periodic form (Fig. 203).

Microfilariae may sometimes be demonstrated in fluid aspirated from a hydrocele or enlarged lymph nodes.

**Treatment and Prophylaxis** See p. 434.

## Filariasis Malayi

**Synonyms** Brug's filariasis, *Wuchereria malayi* infection.
**Definition** Filariasis malayi is due to the presence of adult *W.*

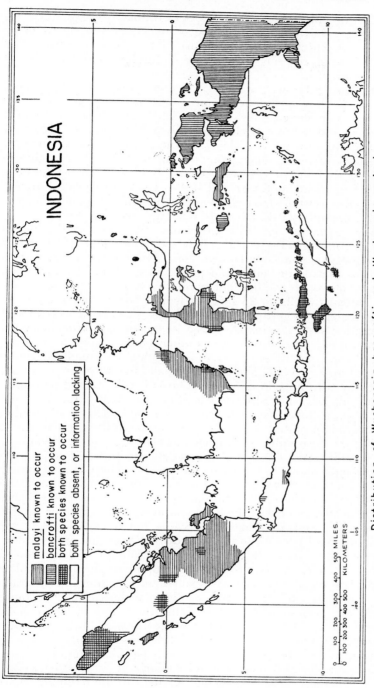

Distribution of Wuchereria bancrofti and Wuchereria malayi. (Courtesy Preventive Medicine Division, Bureau of Medicine and Surgery, U. S. Navy.)

Fig. 204. Distribution of filariasis in Indonesia. (Courtesy Preventive Medicine Division, Bureau of Medicine and Surgery, U. S. Navy.)

*malayi* in the lymphatics, lymph nodes or connective tissues of man. Characteristic sheathed microfilariae occur in the peripheral blood only at night. Species of *Mansonia* are of particular importance as vectors. In other respects this disease is fundamentally similar to filariasis bancrofti.

**Distribution**  Filariasis malayi is found in India, Indo-China, China, Korea, Japan, Indonesia and Malaya. The following areas are known as endemic centers for Brug's filariasis: Malaya; India—Travancore; Indo-China—Delta of the Red River; China—Huchow and Changsha; Indonesia—Celebes, Borneo, Ceram, Java, Sumatra. It has also been found among the Tonkinese in the New Hebrides and among Koreans in Hawaii (Oahu). It appears to be the only filarial worm found in Korea and it also has been reported among Japanese on a coastal island off Honshu. In some areas the distribution of *W. malayi* and *W. bancrofti* overlaps (see Fig. 204).

**Etiology**  MORPHOLOGY. Filariasis malayi is caused by the filarial parasite *W. malayi* (Brug 1927) Rao and Maplestone 1940, which bears a close resemblance to *W. bancrofti*. The adults are white, delicate worms that occur coiled and paired in the dilated lymphatics. Two rows of small papillae surround the mouth. The males are smaller, measuring 22 to 23 mm. in length and their posterior extremities undergo about three complete loops. The cloaca is 0.1 to 0.14 mm. from the posterior tip. There is a large pair of papillae near the cloaca and one posteriad, while two other smaller pairs are nearby. The copulatory spicules are unequal in length and a small naviculate gubernaculum is present. The known females measure about 55 mm. in length by 0.16 mm. in diameter. The vulva is situated 0.92 mm. from the anterior end while the anal pore is 0.94 mm. from the posterior tip. Although the measurements made by Dutch and Indian scientists are in essential accord, the description of the papillae differ, indicating the desirability of further morphological observations.

The sheathed microfilariae of *W. malayi* measure 177 to 230 microns in length and 5 to 6 microns in breadth. There is an anterior cephalic space about twice as long as the diameter of the head, the latter bearing double stylets. Staining reveals that an excretory pore is situated 30.09 per cent of the body length from the anterior tip, the large excretory cell 37.07 per cent, while the $G_1$ cell is 68.33 per cent and the anal pore 82.28 per cent distant from the anterior end. The body tapers from the anal pore, the column of large nuclei terminating some distance before the acuminate tip of the tail is reached. The distal extremity is swollen to accommodate a single distinct nucleus, while a second smaller one lies a short distance anteriad. The position of these nuclei and the length of the cephalic space constitute the two characteristic features of this essentially nocturnal microfilaria (see Table 38, p. 415).

DEVELOPMENT. The developmental cycle parallels that of *W. bancrofti* in all essential details. The microfilaria of this species undergoes two molts and completes its development in the mosquito in six days under optimum conditions.

**Epidemiology** Although the epidemiology is very similar to that of filariasis bancrofti, certain differences exist in the identity of the vectors, their ecology and the periodicity of the microfilariae. The generally accepted mosquito vectors belong to the genera *Mansonia* (subgenus *Mansonioides*) and *Anopheles*. The known and other suspected vectors are summarized by countries in Table 40.

The *Mansonia* group constitutes a difficult larval control problem because these organisms secure their oxygen by attaching themselves to such green aquatic plants as *Pistia* spp. or water lettuce, *Eichhornia*

*Table 40    Known and Suspected Vectors of* Wuchereria malayi *by Countries*

| | |
|---|---|
| China | *Anopheles hyrcanus sinensis* |
| India | *Mansonia annulifera* |
| Indo-China | *Mansonia indica* |
| Indonesia | *Mansonia annulata* |
| | *Mansonia annulifera* |
| | *Mansonia indiana* |
| | *Mansonia longipalpis* |
| | *Mansonia uniformis* |
| | *Anopheles barbirostris barbirostris* |
| Japan | *Anopheles hyrcanus sinensis* |
| Malaya | *Mansonia annulata* |
| | *Mansonia annulipes* |
| | *Mansonia longipalpis* |
| | *Mansonia uniformis* |
| | *Mansonia indiana* |
| | *Anopheles letifer* |
| | *Anopheles barbirostris* |
| | *Anopheles hyrcanus sinensis* |
| Philippines | *Mansonia annulata* |
| South Korea | *Anopheles hyrcanus sinensis* |

*crassipes* or *Lemna* sp. In Travancore, India, filariasis malayi was reduced by removing the water plant, *P. striatioles*, on which live the larvae of the principal vector, *Mansonoides annulifera*. Ordinary larviciding measures, such as the use of oil, Paris green, or DDT are ineffective.

The microfilariae are essentially nocturnally periodic. Although they are present in the peripheral blood nearly twenty hours a day, there is a peak which is reached about 4 A. M., thus differing from the condition noted in nocturnally periodic filariasis bancrofti.

**Pathology and Clinical Characteristics** The pathologic changes and the clinical syndromes associated with infections by *W. malayi* range from asymptomatic adenitis to periodic attacks of fever and lymphangitis, and to elephantiasis, typically involving the feet and legs. Lymph scrotum, chyluria and chylous hydrocele have not been observed and elephantiasis of the genitalia is rare. Treatment as outlined for filariasis in general is indicated.

**Diagnosis** The diagnosis rests upon a clinical picture suggestive of filariasis and its confirmation by the demonstration of characteristic microfilariae of *W. malayi* (see p. 415). The morphology of the sheathed microfilaria differs from that described for *W. bancrofti* chiefly in the cephalic space, which is twice as long as broad, and the posterior extremity of the worm, which has a slight bulb at the tip with two minute terminal nuclei; the remainder of the tapering posterior extremity is devoid of nuclei (Fig. 205). Skin tests may be of value if microfilariae cannot be demonstrated.

**Treatment of Filariasis Bancrofti and Malayi**   There is no known drug which is a specific therapeutic agent for infections by *W. bancrofti* or *W. malayi*. A number of preparations of antimony or arsenic

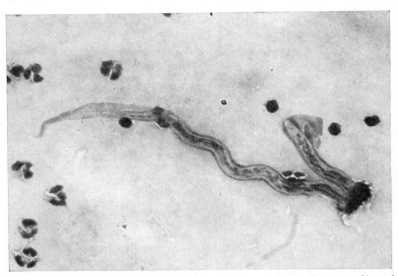

Fig. 205. Sheathed microfilaria of *W. malayi* in thick blood film (hematoxylin stain). Note position of characteristic terminal caudal nuclei and cephalic space.

have been found to reduce, at least temporarily, the number of microfilariae in the circulating blood. No drug is known to cause the death of the adult worm or to alter the clinical course of the disease, nor is it certain that killing of adult worms may not cause exacerbation due to absorption of the degenerating parasites.

Recently it has been shown that both diethylcarbamazine (Hetrazan, Banocide) and suramin will eliminate the microfilariae from the circulating blood of a significant proportion of infected persons and will greatly reduce the numbers of microfilariae in the remainder. However, it does not reduce the frequency or the severity of clinical filariasis, nor does it affect favorably the late complications. Hetrazan is the drug of choice.

Although Hetrazan is generally well tolerated, reactions occur in more than 50 per cent of treated individuals. These tend to be more severe in older persons than in children. The early reactions frequently appear during the first day of treatment. Fever is the most common manifestation. It may be accompanied by a variety of other symptoms including anorexia, headache, pain in the abdomen, femoral area or the joints, pruritus and nausea.

A delayed reaction occurs a week or two later in over one-half of the clinical cases of filariasis and in approximately one-third of the asymptomatic carriers. This appears to be, in part at least, allergic in nature. The clinical phenomena include pruritus, inflammatory reactions of lymph nodes and of the scrotal contents, and skin eruptions varying from urticaria and vesicular rashes to bulla formation. The inflammatory reaction may be followed by abscess formation.

Concurrent administration of an antihistaminic drug may lessen the incidence and severity of the allergic reactions. The treatment of asymptomatic cases to prevent clinical filariasis is of doubtful value. For details of dosage see pages 548, 551.

Since the acute inflammatory phenomena may be associated with secondary streptococcal or staphylococcal infections, administration of one of the absorbable sulfonamides or one of the antibiotics may be desirable. For involvement of the extremities or scrotum, elevation of the part with or without continuous wet dressings should be used.

Chyluria should be treated by complete bed rest with elevation of the foot of the bed. Cystoscopic treatment and bladder irrigations may be required in severe cases when more conservative measures fail.

Surgical procedures are completely contraindicated except for definitive treatment of elephantiasis, especially of the scrotum. Palliative operations directed to improve lymph circulation in elephantiasis of the extremities are seldom successful. Such conditions are best managed by a period of continuous elevation of the affected part followed by constant wearing of an elastic stocking or elastic bandage. In cases of early elephantiasis of the lower extremities, elevation and pressure bandages are particularly successful in reducing the swelling. Care must be taken not to bandage too tightly and the limb must be exercised lest venous stasis result. In mild cases the leg may assume its original size and the skin a natural texture, remaining normal for a prolonged period without further treatment.

Painful lymph scrotum may be relieved by the use of a suspensory and by keeping the affected parts clean and protected.

**Prophylaxis of Filariasis Bancrofti and Malayi** The essential features of prophylaxis against filariasis are mosquito control and individual protection against possibly infected mosquitoes (pp. 738–752). The various species which may serve as vectors and their different behaviors as regards breeding areas and times of flight are complicating factors. The largest numbers of infected insects will be found in and near villages of the indigenous population in the endemic areas. Since certain of the vectors are daytime transmitters and others nocturnal, mosquito-infested communities in endemic regions should be avoided at all times.

Specific control measures applicable to a particular area will depend upon locally important mosquito vectors (pp. 420–421). In regions where a suitable species of *Mansonia* (*Mansonioides*) is prevalent the problem is difficult. The breeding of this group cannot be readily controlled since the larvae secure their oxygen by attaching to the stems of floating aquatic plants such as *Pistia* or water lettuce. Consequently, the use of oil or surface application of Paris green or DDT is ineffective. Removal of the aquatic vegetation or the introduction of minnows are the only satisfactory measures; the former has been quite successfully carried out experimentally.

Mass treatment of infected population groups using Hetrazan in dosage of 2.0 mg. per kilogram of body weight may prove to be a useful and practical measure in some regions to reduce the prevalence of the infection. It significantly reduces the number of persons having microfilariae in the circulating blood and the number of infective mosquitoes, and thus diminishes the cycle of transmission.

## Onchocerciasis

**Synonyms**  Onchocercosis, "blinding filarial disease."

**Definition**  Onchocerciasis is due to the presence of the filarial parasite, *Onchocerca volvulus*, in the skin and in subcutaneous and other tissues of man where it may produce fibrous nodules. Blindness is a serious complication of this infection. The disease is transmitted by species of buffalo gnats or black flies of the family SIMULIIDAE.

**Distribution**  In the Western Hemisphere onchocerciasis is largely confined to Mexico and Central America although cases have been reported from Venezuela and Dutch Guiana. It is widespread in tropical Africa. In the Americas it occurs principally in persons inhabiting the western slope of the Sierras at altitudes of 600 to 2000 meters. Guatemala and the southern states of Mexico constitute the chief endemic centers. In Africa, onchocerciasis is found from Sierra Leone and Liberia southward through the Gold Coast, Dahomey, Nigeria, and the Cameroons to the Congo; then east to the southern Sudan, Uganda, Nyasaland, Kenya, Tanganyika and Kavirondo (Fig. 206).

**Etiology**  MORPHOLOGY. The adult parasite, *Onchocerca volvulus* (Leuckart 1893) Railliet and Henry 1910 (= *Onchocerca caecutiens* Brumpt 1919), occurs in tumors in the subcutaneous connective tissue. The living parasites are white or cream colored and transparent, with a cuticula showing distinct striations. Both extremities are blunt. Anteriorly about the mouth are two concentric circles of four papillae each. In addition there is a pair of large, oval, lateral papillae situated between these two circles. Posteriorly the tightly coiled males show copulatory spicules and a number of perianal and caudal papillae which, although diagnostic, nevertheless show considerable variation in position. The males measure 19 to 42 mm. in length and the females 33 to 50 cm. The vulva of the female opens posterior to the esophagus. Microfilariae of two sizes, 285 to 368 by 6 to 9 microns and 150 by 287 by 5 to 7 microns are produced.

DEVELOPMENT. The microfilariae of *O. volvulus* probably ex-

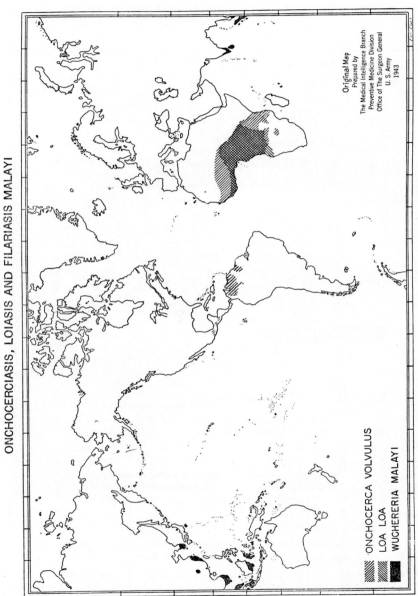

Fig. 206. Geographical distribution of onchocerciasis, loiasis, and filariasis malayi.

sheath soon after leaving the female worm. Both extremities and the excretory pore region of these larvae lack nuclei. The absence of nuclei from the tip of the tail is of diagnostic value. These microfilariae do not occur in the peripheral blood but are found typically

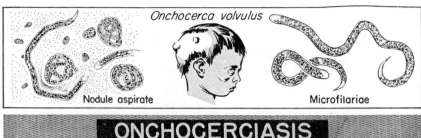

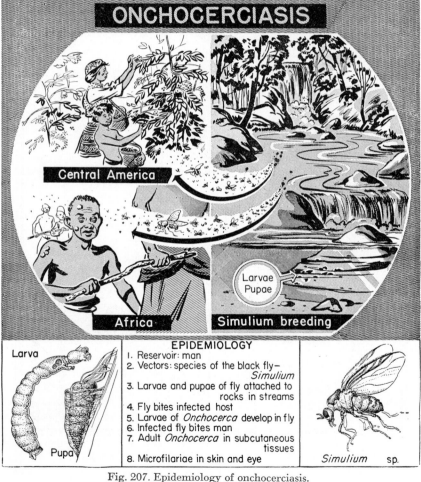

Fig. 207. Epidemiology of onchocerciasis.

in the subcutaneous nodules near the parent worms, in the dermis, and in the tissues of the eye.

The vectors of onchocerciasis are species of black flies of the family SIMULIIDAE. These become infected as they suck blood and tissue juices from the skin of an infected host. Ingested microfilariae leave the food reservoir of the fly and penetrate the thoracic muscles where development of the larvae takes place. A period of at least six days, during which time two molts occur, is required for development. The

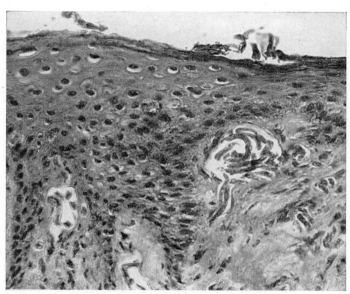

Fig. 208. Onchocerciasis—microfilariae in skin. (Courtesy of Dr. M. Martínez Baez, Mexico, D. F.)

infective larva then travels to the labium of the fly, at which time the insect becomes infective.

**Epidemiology** Man is the reservoir for the filarial worm, *O. volvulus*. In Africa *S. damnosum* and *S. neavei* are the chief vectors of onchocerciasis while in Guatemala, Venezuela and Mexico, *Eusimulium avidum* (= *S. metallicum*), *E. ochraceum* and *E. mooseri* (= *S. callidum*) transmit the disease; *S. exiguum*, *S. veracruzanum* and *S. hematopotum* have been infected experimentally and should be added to the potential vectors in Guatemala. Most of the species of the SIMULIIDAE transmitting onchocerciasis breed in the riffles of rapidly flowing streams where the larvae and pupae may be found attached to submerged stones, logs, or even vegetation. A few species prefer the more slowly flowing water of roadside ditches (Fig. 207).

Buffalo gnats, turkey gnats, or black flies, as these simuliids are called, are small "hump-backed" flies measuring 1 to 5 mm. in length. Ordinarily they are outdoor day biters but in Guatemala they will bite indoors even at night in the presence of artificial light. African species apparently do not enter houses. The bite is painless and the fly is not easily disturbed when it has started feeding.

Transmission of the disease occurs only through the female fly which feeds on an infected person.

**Pathology**   In some cases the adult worms provoke no tissue response in the human host. More commonly, however, they cause a local inflammatory reaction followed by fibrous encapsulation and the production of subcutaneous nodules. These tumors are distributed

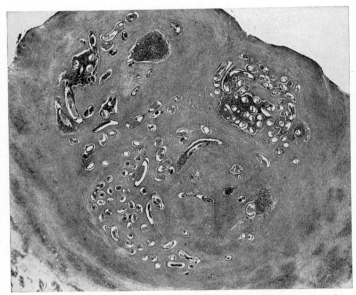

Fig. 209. Section through onchocercal nodule showing small abscesses and numerous adult worms. Large worms are females, small ones males.

over regions of the body where there is convergence of the superficial lymphatics. In Guatemala they occur predominantly on the head and thorax while in Africa they are most numerous on the pelvis and thorax. Histologically they show a relatively low grade of inflammation, a leukocytic infiltration in which eosinophils are conspicuous, and a heavy deposition of collagen fibrils. As a rule the nodules are solid, though infrequently where the adult parasites die and degenerate, or where secondary bacterial infections have occurred, abscesses have resulted. Usually microfilariae are very abundant within the nodules and in the skin. They are not found in the circulating blood (Figs. 208, 209).

The incidence and the severity of the ocular pathologic changes in onchocerciasis bear no relation to the anatomic situation of the nodules, the duration of the infection or the age of the individual. Accumulating evidence indicates that the underlying mechanism is related to the development of sensitivity to antigenic substances of the parasite or its products of metabolism or disintegration.

The essential pathologic process is a low grade chronic iritis and iridocyclitis with occasional acute exacerbations which lead to synechia, distorted, contracted, eccentric pupils, pigment deposits and corneal opacities. Superficial punctate keratitis is so common as to be almost pathognomonic. Dead microfilariae have been identified in these minute opacities and the latter have been observed to increases in number following treatment which kills the microfilariae. Blindness results from pupillary occlusion, corneal opacity or both.

**Clinical Characteristics** The subcutaneous nodules are the most characteristic lesions of onchocerciasis. However, they are frequently not demonstrable. In the Central American form of the disease they are most numerous over the head and thorax; in Africa they are predominantly on the trunk.

In the typical case, following the bite of an infected fly, there is an incubation period of several months before nodules appear. There is little if any systemic reaction. The nodules grow slowly, attaining full size in three or four years when they may reach a diameter of 2 to 3 cm. There may be few on one individual and over a hundred on another. Ordinarily they cause little inconvenience although in the vicinity of joints they are often painful. Inflammatory reactions may occur in and about certain nodules, occasionally followed by abscess formation. These may be due to secondary bacterial infection or to an allergic reaction. Pruritus may be troublesome. A facial complication observed in Guatemala, "erysipelas de la costa," formerly considered to be bacterial in origin, is almost certainly allergic in nature since it is reproduced exactly in hypersensitive patients following treatment with Hetrazan.

The ocular pathology is the most serious feature of onchocerciasis. The incidence of eye lesions has been reported as high as 30 per cent in certain groups in Central America and up to 85 per cent in Africa. In Guatemala blindness occurs in about 6 per cent of the cases having ocular lesions. These complications usually do not appear until some years after the initial infection. The early symptoms include conjunctivitis, lacrimation and photophobia. Serious involvement is indicated by circumcorneal congestion, iritis and punctuate keratitis of the cornea.

**Diagnosis** Blood smears do not demonstrate the microfilariae of *O. volvulus*. An eosinophilia averaging about 35 per cent is frequently present.

Diagnosis depends upon demonstration of the microfilariae in the skin or nodules (Fig. 210). Ordinarily they are not found in greatest numbers over, or adjacent to, subcutaneous nodules. In the Central American disease they are most consistently found in the skin of the scapular region, and in the African form in the scapular, or pelvic girdle and thigh regions.

Skin biopsy, taking a thin section of superficial skin with a razor blade, is the simplest and probably the easiest method. The excised skin should be mounted in saline under a cover glass (Fig. 210). A second useful method is by scarification, making several closely approximated superficial incisions into the skin and preparing a smear of expressed blood and lymph for staining with hematoxylin. Aspiration of a subcutaneous nodule and examination of the fluid will frequently reveal large numbers of microfilariae.

When the eye is involved, examination of the cornea under oblique illumination will frequently reveal minute superficial opacities, the superficial punctate keratitis which is almost pathognomonic of onchocerciasis.

The prognosis is good unless ocular complications have appeared.

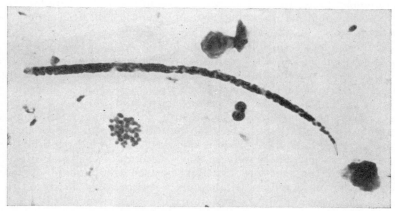

Fig. 210. Unsheathed microfilaria of *O. volvulus* in aspirate from skin. Caudal nuclei do not reach tip of tail.

**Treatment**   Whenever possible all tumors should be excised, particularly in view of the danger of later ocular complications. This is frequently impracticable, however, when large numbers of the nodules are present. Such treatment is not always followed by disappearance of the microfilariae, probably because other adult worms remain in the host's tissues.

Drug treatment of onchocerciasis must be undertaken with caution in the presence of ocular involvement since severe reactions may occur in sensitive patients, producing further damage to the eye.

Suramin (Naphuride, Bayer 205, Antrypol, Germanin) is the drug of choice. Reported reactions include fever, headache, muscle and joint pains, abdominal pain and nausea. These should be treated symptomatically. Hyperesthesia of the soles of the feet may be troublesome in some individuals. Pruritus and subjective ocular reactions, apparently allergic in nature, may be controlled by antihistamine preparations. Treatment should be discontinued if severe symptoms or peripheral edema occur.

Suramin causes the death of adult worms and slow disappearance of microfilariae. Whenever possible large subcutaneous nodules should be excised, since abscess formation may follow death of the adult worms.

Diethylcarbamazine (Hetrazan) is of less value in the treatment of onchocerciasis. Although it rapidly kills the microfilariae, severe allergic reactions are not uncommon in sensitized patients, and in the presence of ocular pathology severe damage to the eye may result. Hetrazan has little or no effect upon the adult worms.

For details of dosage see pp. 548, 551.

**Prophylaxis**  Satisfactory control measures directed against the breeding places of the vector are difficult and often impractical. In Africa, aerial spraying of DDT and the introduction of DDT into larger streams and rivers has proved effective. In Central America, however, the vectors breed in much smaller, more rapidly flowing streams which renders effective control difficult if not impossible. There is no satisfactory personal prophylaxis other than avoidance of endemic areas and the doubtful value of repellents.

## Loiasis

**Synonyms**  Calabar or fugitive swelling disease, eye-worm disease of Africa.

**Definition**  Loiasis is due to the presence of the parasitic filarial worm, *Loa loa*, in man where it frequently causes calabar or fugitive swellings. Tabanid flies, *Chrysops* spp., are the intermediate hosts and vectors.

**Distribution**  Loiasis is a disease of tropical Africa where it is endemic along the Congo River watershed. It is also prevalent on the coastal plains and delta regions of Sierra Leone as well as in Angola and the Cameroons.

**Etiology**  MORPHOLOGY. The loa or eye-worm, *L. loa* (Cobbold 1864) Castellani and Chalmers 1913, produces loiasis or fugitive swellings as the adult migrates about the subcutaneous tissues of man.

The male averages 30 to 34 mm. while the female ranges between 50 and 70 mm. in length. In both sexes the body is filiform, semi-transparent and is bluntly tapered at both extremities. The head is characterized by two lateral and four small, semi-median papillae lying in the same transverse plane a little below the mouth. The latter passes directly into a slender, muscular esophagus. The cuticula of these parasites is covered with small bosses, except for a portion of either extremity of the male which lacks these knoblike protuberances.

The posterior end of the male is ventrally curved and possesses narrow lateral alae and eight pairs of perianal papillae (five anterior and three posterior) which are diagnostic. The copulatory spicules are unequal in length and shape and the cloacal orifice is surrounded by a powerful sphincter.

The broadly rounded posterior tip of the female carries a pair of terminal papillae. The vulva which opens about 2.5 mm. from the anterior tip passes into a posteriorly extending vagina which, within 9 mm. of its external aperture, bifurcates to form twin uteri and other paired structures of the reproductive system. The uterus contains developing embryos in various embryonic stages. When these are mature, sheathed microfilariae are liberated which measure 250 to 300 microns in length and 6 to 8.5 microns in breadth. These are similar in size to corresponding stages of *W. bancrofti*. The percentage distances of the worm's length from the anterior end to various anatomic landmarks are as follows: the widely separated excretory cell and pore, 31.6 and 36.6 per cent respectively; the $G_1$ cell, 68.6 per cent; and the anal pore, 81.9 per cent. The nuclei extend caudally to the tip of the gradually tapering tail. In many respects the microfilariae of *L. loa* resemble those of *W. malayi* but may be distinguished by the arrangement of the caudal nuclei and the shorter cephalic space.

DEVELOPMENT. The female liberates sheathed microfilariae which enter the blood stream and are diurnal in their periodicity. The intermediate hosts for these worms consist of certain tabanid or "deer" flies belonging to the genus *Chrysops*. The parasites undergo development in the thoracic muscles and fat body of the fly. About ten days after infection the mature larvae, about 2 mm. in length, migrate to the proboscis and remain infective for about a week. After reaching man by the bite of the fly the parasites disappear into the subcutaneous tissues and mature slowly.

***Epidemiology*** Infection is acquired through the bite of infected tabanid flies of the species *Chrysops dimidiata, C. silacea, C. longicornis, C. distinctipennis,* and possibly *C. centurionis*. These flies are diurnal biters, feeding primarily between dawn and 10 A.M. and again between 4 P.M. and dusk. Only the females bite. It has been noted that they prefer darker colors and hence are found more frequently in wooded areas and are believed to have a biting preference for the Negro. However, whites remaining in endemic areas for three to five years almost invariably become infected. Such infections develop slowly and are known to persist for at least fifteen years.

The incidence of loiasis in man varies with the prevalence of the native reservoir and dipterous intermediate hosts. Loiasis has been reported from 15 per cent of the population along the Welle River in Rio Muni, Central Africa, while other investigators have found infection rates of 90 per cent or more among the indigenous populations of the Belgian Congo.

***Pathology*** Loiasis is a chronic disease frequently characterized by inflammatory processes and fugitive swellings of the subcutaneous tissues. The adult worms migrate through the subcutaneous tissues at a maximum rate of about a centimeter per minute and have been removed from such locations as the back, axilla, groin, breast, penis, scalp, eyelids, the anterior chamber of the eye and the bulbar conjunctiva. Adult *L. loa* are rarely encapsulated but usually migrate more or less continuously. A marked eosinophilia, sometimes as high as 50 to 70 per cent, may be present. The microfilariae are diurnal and are found in greatest numbers in the peripheral blood during the middle of the day.

**Clinical Characteristics** The most outstanding clinical feature of the disease is the occurrence of the transient tumors known as fugitive or calabar swellings. These are about the size of a small hen's egg. They appear suddenly, are frequently preceded by pain, and in most cases persist for only two or three days. As a rule no serious inconvenience is suffered, although prickling sensations as well as pruritus may occur.

A number of theories has been advanced in an attempt to explain the occurrence of calabar swellings. It has been suggested that the

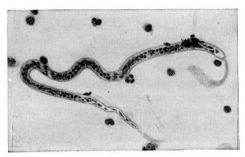

Fig. 211. Sheathed microfilaria of *Loa loa* in thick blood film. Caudal nuclei extend to tip of tail. (From slide of Liverpool School of Tropical Medicine, loaned by Puerto Rico School of Tropical Medicine. From Bercovitz, Z. T., Clinical Tropical Medicine, Paul B. Hoeber, Inc. 1944).

swellings may be due to: (1) the wanderings of the worm; (2) the liberation of large numbers of microfilariae by the female; (3) toxins secreted by the parasite; and (4) an allergic response on the part of the host. A typical calabar swelling has been produced experimentally in a patient with loiasis by injecting antigen from the dog heartworm, *Dirofilaria immitis*, thus supporting the concept of the allergic nature of such responses.

External heat tends to bring the worm close to the surface of the body.

**Diagnosis** Diagnostic findings in cases of loiasis include one or more of the following: (1) calabar swellings; (2) worm crossing the eye; (3) edematous outline of the worm under the skin; (4) microfilariae in films of the peripheral blood, or in fluid aspirate of the calabar swellings. A marked eosinophilia is usually present.

Microfilariae may be demonstrated in the usual thick smear or by concentration methods (see pp. 816–817) (Fig. 211).

Differentiation between the microfilariae of *L. loa* and the other sheathed species, *Wuchereria bancrofti* and *W. malayi*, is necessary.

A detailed comparison is given on p. 412. Diurnal periodicity, a tapering tail and the position of the caudal nuclei characterize the present form (Table 38).

**Treatment** Loiasis responds well to treatment with diethylcarbamazine (Hetrazan) and both microfilariae and adult worms are killed. However, the first course of therapy is accompanied by allergic reactions in approximately 70 per cent of patients. These occur particularly in the first three or four days and, in highly sensitized patients, may appear shortly after the first dose of the drug. The most common reactions are the appearance of calabar swellings, creeping sensations under the skin, pruritus and fugitive papular erythematous eruptions. Other symptoms include headache, nausea and arthralgia; more rarely there may be fever, vomiting and diarrhea. These reactions may be controlled by antihistaminic drugs and do not necessitate termination of treatment.

The microfilariae are phagocytized in the liver and rapidly disappear from the circulating blood. The adult worms tend to appear under the skin where they are destroyed and small nodules are formed. The initial course of Hetrazan therapy is commonly accompanied by a marked rise of the eosinophil count.

Mild symptoms of loiasis may reappear in the course of the second week following treatment; these are due, in part at least, to the allergic mechanism. A second course of Hetrazan should be given two or three weeks after completion of the first, and it is probably desirable to give one or two additional courses to ensure eradication of the infection.

See p. 548 for details of dosage.

Surgical removal of the migrating adult worms as formerly practiced is not recommended.

**Prophylaxis** Protection from bites of *Chrysops* in endemic areas will prevent the disease. Oiling of the surface of the pools over which the flies skim will aid in their elimination as the spiracles or tracheal tubes become occluded by the oil, thus causing suffocation. Repellents such as indalone or 6-2-2 are reported to be effective against these flies.

Elimination of carriers by mass treatment of local population groups with Hetrazan will interrupt transmission of the disease.

## Filariasis Ozzardi

**Synonyms** Mansonelliasis ozzardi, Ozzard's filariasis.

**Definition** Filariasis ozzardi is due to the presence of *Mansonella ozzardi* in man. The adults inhabit the body cavities while the nonperiodic microfilariae are found in the blood stream. The intermediate host and vector is a midge of the genus *Culicoides*.

**Distribution** *Mansonella ozzardi* is confined exclusively to the Western Hemisphere, being native to parts of South America, particularly the Guianas, Colombia, Venezuela and northern Argentina.

It is also present in Panama, Puerto Rico and Yucatan, as well as St. Vincent and Dominica in the West Indies.

**Etiology** MORPHOLOGY. *Mansonella ozzardi* (Manson 1897) Faust 1929 is a nematode, the adults of which are found in the mesenteries, body cavities and visceral fat of man. A complete male has not been described. The female ranges between 65 and 81 mm. in length and possesses an unarmed head, a smooth cuticula and a pair of fleshy lappets or flaps at the caudal extremity. The unsheathed microfilariae measure 185 to 200 microns in length and about 5 microns in breadth. Both the cephalic and caudal extremities lack nuclei, the nucleus-free region comprising the anterior 2.2 to 2.5 per cent and the posterior 1.8 to 2.0 per cent of the worm. Other measurements from the

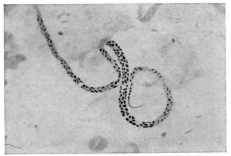

Fig. 212. Unsheathed microfilaria of *M. ozzardi* in thick blood films. (Courtesy of F. W. O'Connor, from Bercovitz, Z. T., Clinical Tropical Medicine, Paul B. Hoeber, Inc. 1944.)

anterior tip are as follows: the nerve ring, 21.9 to 22.2 per cent; excretory pore and excretory cell, 30.9 to 31.5 and 35 per cent respectively; the $G_1$ cell, 67.9 to 69.3 per cent, and the $G_4$ cell just in front of the anal pore at 79.4 per cent. The outstanding diagnostic characteristics are the lack of a sheath and the absence of nuclei in the posterior tip of the tail (see Table 38, on p. 415).

DEVELOPMENT. The unsheathed microfilariae are nonperiodic. The larvae require five to seven days for development in the vector, *Culicoides furens.*

It appears probable that the *Microfilaria tucumans* of Argentina is identical with the microfilaria of *M. ozzardi.*

**Epidemiology** Even though the epidemiology of Ozzard's filariasis has not been adequately studied, it has been demonstrated that transmission occurs through the bite of an infected *Culicoides furens; C. paraensis* may prove to be another vector.

The prevalence of this infection is not definitely known for most areas. In endemic areas of the Argentine about 30 per cent of the population are believed to be infected.

**Pathology and Clinical Characteristics** The adult worms apparently produce few if any pathologic changes or symptoms. An occasional hydrocele or enlarged lymph node has, however, been attributed to *M. ozzardi* infections.

**Diagnosis**   This is based upon the recovery and the identification of the unsheathed microfilariae from the peripheral blood. The pointed tail and absence of nuclei extending to the posterior tip are important diagnostic characters (see Table 38, p. 415 for additional details) (Fig. 212).

**Treatment**   None recommended.

**Prophylaxis**   No effective control measures are known, other than the use of repellents against midges. These insects are so small that screening will not exclude them.

## Acanthocheilonemiasis

**Synonyms**   Dipetalonemiasis, *Acanthocheilonema perstans* infection.

**Definition**   Acanthocheilonemiasis is due to the presence of *Acanthocheilonema perstans* in man. The adults inhabit the peritoneal cavity, the pleural cavity, pericardium, mesenteries or retroperitoneal tissues, while the nonperiodic microfilariae are found in the blood stream. The vectors are various species of *Culicoides*.

**Distribution**   *Acanthocheilonema perstans* is common in the tropical regions of South America, Africa and New Guinea. In the Western Hemisphere it has been reported from British and Dutch Guiana, Venezuela, the lower Amazon Valley, northern Argentina, Trinidad and Panama. In Africa it has been found in Sierra Leone, the Gold and Ivory Coasts, Nigeria, Rhodesia, Uganda, the Cameroons and the Congo River Basin. Cases have also been found in Tunis and Algiers. These parasites are often found in persons infected with *Wuchereria bancrofti*.

**Etiology**   Morphology. Adult *Acanthocheilonema perstans* (Manson 1891) Railliet, Henry and Langeron 1912 (= *Dipetalonema perstans* [Manson 1891] Yorke and Maplestone 1926) inhabit the body cavities of man, being found most commonly in the peritoneal and pleural cavities. The parasites are elongated, cylindrical, creamy white Filarioidea with a smooth cuticle. The anterior tip is unarmed and bluntly rounded, although a shield possessing two large lateral papillae and two pairs of submedian papillae are present. The caudal extremity is somewhat curved ventrally in both males and females and is bifurcated so as to form a pair of triangular nonmuscular flaps. The female measures 70 to 80 mm. in length while the male averages about 45 mm. The latter possesses four pairs of preanal papillae and one postanal pair with unequal rodlike copulatory spicules.

Development. The female produces unsheathed microfilariae measuring about 200 by 4.5 microns. These enter the blood stream and are nonperiodic. The intermediate hosts of this parasite include several species of *Culicoides*. Development occurs in the midge which then transmits the infection when it next feeds, allowing the infective stage to reach the skin of man.

**Epidemiology**   In Africa *C. austeni* and perhaps *C. grahami* serve as the vectors for this disease. The vectors in other areas are unknown.

The incidence of parasitism in man varies markedly. The infection rates in northern Argentina range between 39.1 and 50.6 per cent. In some areas of Africa, such as Uganda, the parasite has been found in about 90 per cent of the population, and in the heavily

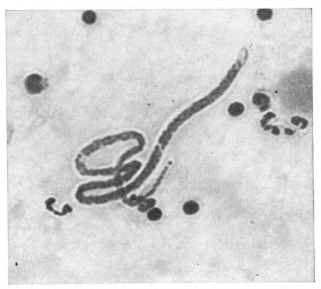

Fig. 213. Unsheathed microfilaria of *A. perstans* in thick blood film (hematoxylin stained). Note caudal nuclei extending to tip of tail and other morphological characteristics. (What appears to be a sheath is merely a halo.)

wooded portion of the Cameroons the infection rate is more than 92 per cent. As noted above, the parasite is endemic in the Congo River Basin and often appears concomitantly with *W. bancrofti* in Africa and with *M. ozzardi* in South America.

**Pathology and Clinical Characteristics**   Little is known concerning the pathology and symptomatology of this disease.

**Diagnosis**   The detection and identification of the unsheathed microfilariae of *A. perstans* in the peripheral blood are diagnostic. These may be differentiated from the microfilariae of *M. ozzardi* by the position of the caudal nuclei which, in the case of *A. perstans*, extend into the posterior tip of the blunt tail, and stop short thereof in the case of *M. ozzardi* (Fig. 213).

**Treatment**   None recommended.

**Prophylaxis**   At present it does not seem feasible to control the breeding of *Culicoides*. Ordinary screening does not exclude these midges. Avoidance of endemic areas or the use of repellents are the only available prophylactic measures.

# 44 Tissue-Inhabiting Nematodes: The Dracunculoidea

The DRACUNCULOIDEA are tissue-inhabiting nematodes of which but a single representative, *Dracunculus medinensis,* infects man. The adults may be distinguished from members of the FILARIOIDEA on the basis of their great size, while the characteristic larvae, which are rather large, measure 500 microns or more in length. Copepods (minute crustacea) serve as intermediate hosts.

## Dracunculiasis

**Synonyms** Dracontiasis, dracunculosis, medina, serpent, dragon or guinea worm infection.

**Definition** Dracunculiasis is due to the presence of the guinea worm, *Dracunculus medinensis,* in the deep connective and subcutaneous tissues of man. Superficial lesions are formed through which the larvae are discharged.

**Distribution** The medina or guinea worm produces a disease which has been recognized in man for many centuries. It is highly endemic in a number of regions in tropical Africa and over large areas of India. Dracunculiasis occurs also in Arabia (especially along the Red Sea), Iran, Afghanistan and Russian Turkestan. The endemic centers in Africa lie between the equator and the Tropic of Cancer where they are scattered from Mauritania to Gabun, especially in Mauritania, Senegal, Upper Volta, Ivory and Gold Coasts, Northern territories, Togo, Dahomey, Nigeria and the Cameroons. Endemic centers extend east to Lake Chad and to the southern parts of the Anglo-Egyptian Sudan and into Uganda. It is also found in the Nile Valley and in Iraq.

The western half of India constitutes the next important endemic center; there is little infection east of Delhi and the central provinces. Dracontiasis also occurs in limited areas of New Guinea, some of the islands of the West Indies and in the Guianas.

Guinea worms morphologically similar to those infecting man have been reported from monkeys, baboons, dogs, leopards, polecats, cattle and horses from the Old World and possibly an identical species from foxes, mink and raccoons in North America. However, many authorities are inclined to consider infections of the latter hosts as due to *D. insignis.*

**Etiology**    Morphology. *Dracunculus medinensis* (Linnaeus 1758) Gallandant 1773, is an elongate, cylindrical, threadlike worm that is known commonly as the dragon, medina, serpent, or guinea worm. Males of the species are rare, only one complete specimen measuring 40 mm. in length having been recovered from man. Experimental infections in dogs and monkeys have yielded a few additional specimens which are smaller, varying between 12 and 29 mm. in length. The female has a smooth cuticula and is much larger than the male, averaging about one meter in length.

Development. As the female becomes gravid she migrates to the subcutaneous tissues, usually in the lower extremities. As she ap-

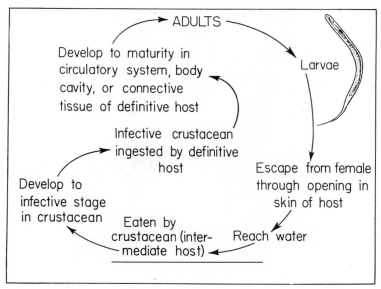

Fig. 214. Nematode cycle—guinea worm type.

proaches the skin a small papular induration is produced in the dermis which develops into a blister within twenty-four to thirty-six hours. Shortly thereafter this blister bursts and if the affected part comes in contact with water a loop of the uterus of the parasite prolapses through its body wall, ruptures, and liberates large numbers of larvae. These larvae measure 500 to 750 microns in length and have a maximum diameter of 15 to 25 microns. Their anterior extremity is bluntly rounded while their caudal extremity is long and attenuated. In order that the life cycle of these parasites be completed the larvae must be ingested by one of several species of copepods (Fig. 214). Here they undergo a developmental period averaging ten to twelve days, after which time the copepods become infective. Following ingestion of the intermediate host by man the parasites probably mate and the female migrates through the tissues. After eight months to a year the fertilized female approaches the skin to liberate her young, thus completing the cycle.

**Epidemiology**   Human infection results from swallowing water containing infected copepods. These become infected following ingestion of the larvae liberated from the gravid females.

The character of the drinking water is of great epidemiologic importance in the spread of this disease, since infected persons must have access to it. The parasite is usually absent from those individuals who obtain their drinking water from small streams or rivers where

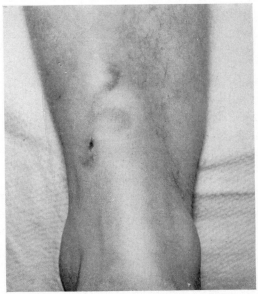

Fig. 215. Dracontiasis. Track of part of the worm which became visible in the skin following the appearance of the vesicle. Note that the blister is now crusted and that there is discoloration of the surrounding skin.

the proper species of copepod does not thrive. The parasite is more often established in small open wells, step-wells, temporary cisterns and the like which are of easy access to infected persons. In some parts of India religious ablutions include rinsing the mouth and this custom may facilitate infection.

Lesions in man occur most frequently on the appendages. In endemic areas step-wells facilitate the dissemination of larvae and the infection of copepods, since persons with lesions on the foot, ankle or leg wade into these sources of water.

Although many species of copepods have been found to serve as intermediate hosts, it is probable that further study would reveal an even larger number of vectors.

**Pathology**   After an incubation period of eight to twelve months the female parasite approaches the skin and in 85 to 90 per cent of the cases migrates to some portion of the lower extremities. Here a reddish papular lesion appears; it has a domelike vesicular center, the margin of which gradually becomes indurated. The entire lesion measures between 2 mm. and 7 cm. in diameter. The size depends upon the amount of exudate underneath the blister and the time elapsing before the blister ruptures (Fig. 215). Usually not more than twenty-four to forty-eight hours elapse between the first symptoms and the bursting of the lesion. In many instances patients do not present themselves for treatment until after the blister has ruptured, with the result that secondary infection occurs in nearly half

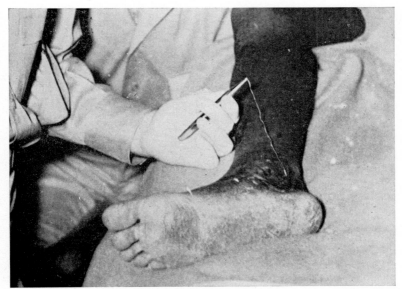

Fig. 216. *Dracunculus medinesis* partially extracted. (Courtesy of Dr. J. M. Hulsey, Jr., through Dr. Hardy A. Kemp, Baylor University.)

the cases. An eosinophilia up to 15 per cent has been recorded in some infected individuals (Fig. 216).

**Clinical Characteristics**   The infection is asymptomatic during the entire incubation period of approximately eight to twelve months. A few hours before the appearance of the worm beneath the skin there are pronounced symptomatic prodromes. These consist essentially of erythema, generalized urticaria, severe pruritus, giddiness, asthma-like symptoms, severe dyspnea, and sometimes vomiting and diarrhea. It is believed that these are reactions associated with toxic secretions of the parasite. As the anterior extremity of the worm reaches the skin, intense itching or burning sensations are frequently experienced.

**Diagnosis**   Diagnosis cannot be made until the cutaneous lesion has developed or until the adult worm presents itself immediately below the surface of the skin. Although intradermal tests may be performed they are seldom needed as a diagnostic aid. Partially or completely calcified worms may be detected by x-ray. The larvae are found only in the washings of the ulcers through which the gravid females discharge their young (Fig. 217).

**Treatment** It is advisable to immobilize or elevate the affected part, since continued use of the limb may aggravate secondary infections.

Satisfactory results are reported in the treatment of dracunculiasis when olive oil emulsions of phenothiazine are injected. This kills

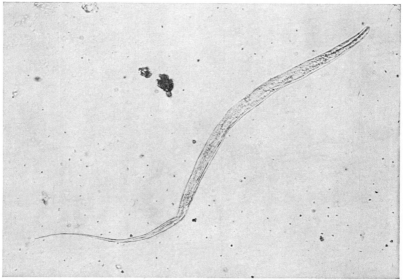

Fig. 217. Larva of *D. medinensis* as discharged from cutaneous lesion; note long tapering tail.

the worms and is believed to lead to the rapid dissolution and absorption of the parasite. Other drugs have been suggested by a number of workers, but phenothiazine emulsion is the drug of choice (see p. 550).

The time-honored custom of "forcing" parturition by the use of wet pads and then rolling the worm on a stick is not recommended. However, this method will doubtless continue to be used in some remote areas.

**Prophylaxis** As infection comes from swallowing water containing infected copepods, control centers around the destruction of the copepods or the covering of wells so that the water may not be contaminated by infected persons. This may be accomplished as follows: (1) Eliminate the so-called step wells. (2) Treat the water with quicklime in dilution of 1:1000. When used in a strength of one ml. per liter (80 per cent CaO) this water is potable in two days and remains free of copepods for two weeks. (3) Copper sulfate in combination with Perchloron is also effective. (4) Biological methods of control may be introduced. Almost any small plankton-feeding minnow will keep down the copepods. In Indian step wells *Barbus puckelli* has been found to be a voracious feeder on copepods and their larvae.

# 45   Tissue-Inhabiting Nematodes: The Trichuroidea

The TRICHUROIDEA contains two common parasites of man: *Trichinella spiralis*, whose larvae inhabit the muscles of man and other

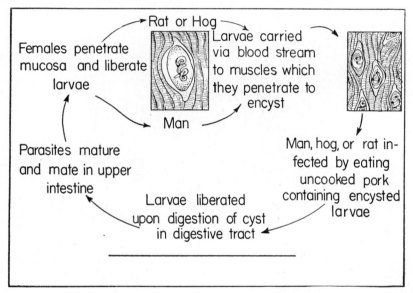

Fig. 218. Nematode cycle—*Trichinella spiralis*.

mammals, and *Trichuris trichiura*, which occurs as an adult in the alimentary canal of man. Only the former, which is a tissue-inhabiting species, is considered here. Members of the *T. spiralis* group may be distinguished from the FILARIOIDEA by their location as adults in the alimentary canal and the liberation of morphologically characteristic larvae which circulate only for a brief period in the blood stream and then penetrate into, and encyst within, the muscles (Fig. 218). Both adult and larval *T. spiralis* possess a thin esophagus surrounded by glandular cells arranged in columnar fashion.

## Trichinosis

*Synonyms*    Trichiniasis, trichinelliasis.

**Definition**    Trichinosis is a disease caused by the parasite, *Trichinella spiralis*. It runs an acute and rapid course and is characterized by fever, gastro-intestinal symptoms, myalgia and eosinophilia. The mortality may be high.

**Distribution**    Trichinosis is widespread through the temperate regions of the world wherever pork or pork products are eaten. It is endemic in the United States, Central and South America (Mexico, Guatemala, Venezuela, Brazil, Uruguay), Hawaii, Alaska, Africa

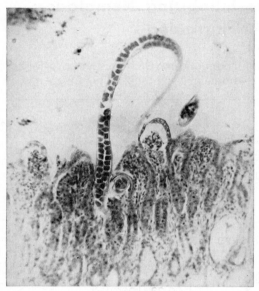

Fig. 219. Adult female *T. spiralis* penetrating mucosa between villi of experimentally infected mouse. (From Dr. Irving Rappaport, in Nauss' Medical Parasitology and Zoology, Paul B. Hoeber, Inc.)

(Uganda, Kenya, Tanganyika, Nigeria), and Europe, while sporadic outbreaks have been reported from subtropical and tropical areas of Africa and South America.

**Etiology**    MORPHOLOGY. The trichina worm, *T. spiralis* (Owen, 1835) Railliet 1895, is a white roundworm just visible to the naked eye. The adult male ranges from 1.4 to 1.6 mm. in length by 40 to 60 microns in diameter, while the female is 3 to 4 mm. in length and about one and one-half times as broad as the male. Both sexes are somewhat attenuate anteriorly and are characterized by a long slender esophagus extending one-third to one-half the body length surrounded by a single layer of esophageal cells. Posteriorly the eversible cloaca of the male is guarded by two papillae. The vulva of the female lies in the anterior third of the worm and through this the small infective larvae, measuring only 100 microns in length by 6 microns in cross-section, are discharged.

DEVELOPMENT. The worms gain entrance to the digestive tract as larvae encysted in muscle tissue. By the time they reach the small intestine they are freed from their cysts, penetrate the duodenal epithelium and mature within a few days. Within five to seven days the females are fertilized, invade the intestinal mucosa (Fig. 219) and produce larvae. It is believed that an adult female discharges between 1000 and 1500 larvae during the three to sixteen week period she parasitizes man. If many females are present, large numbers of larvae are soon circulating in the blood. The larvae leave the blood stream between the eighth and twenty-third day. They may invade various tissues or cavities of the body, which they may subsequently leave to re-enter the blood stream; those finally reaching striated muscles will encyst. Musculature low in glycogen is the site of greatest invasion by the larvae of *T. spiralis*, which usually begins eight to nine days following the infecting meal. After reaching this final destination the larvae require a minimum period of at least sixteen days to complete their development and to become infective. Larvae which are filtered out and remain in other organs fail to develop to the infective stage and are destroyed. The encapsulated larvae continue to grow until they reach a size of 0.8 to 1 mm. In man these cysts usually become calcified within six months, although some are believed to remain viable for thirty years. Under normal conditions the cycle is completed when viable cysts are ingested by a new host. While both adults and encysted larvae develop in the same animal, two hosts are nevertheless necessary to continue the cycle.

**Epidemiology**    The most important reservoir of human infection is the hog, although many other flesh-eating mammals occasionally serve as reservoirs. In the United States hogs become infected chiefly from feeding on garbage containing uncooked pork scraps, and thus complete a hog-to-hog cycle. Both hogs and rats having access to the offal remaining after the slaughter of an infected hog may thereby acquire the infection. Other hogs may thus be infected at once, or they may later feed upon infected rats, thus completing a rat-to-hog cycle. Rats, because of their cannibalistic habits, show a high incidence of natural infection (Fig. 220).

Outbreaks of human trichinosis follow group consumption of fresh, insufficiently-cooked pork products containing striated muscle. A sampling of a large proportion of the population reveals that nearly 18 per cent of the people in the United States are infected. A small number of worms does not produce clinical signs and consequently such infections are discovered only by postmortem studies in which the diaphragm is examined.

Occasional outbreaks have also been traced to such unusual sources as jerked infected bear meat.

**Pathology**    Trichinosis causes localized inflammation and necrosis in muscle tissue. The penetration of striated muscle fibers by the larvae of *T. spiralis* causes the destruction both of the fibers in which the larvae lie and of the adjacent ones. The parasites grow rapidly and even after encystment distention of the cysts occurs, causing further damage to adjacent tissues. In severe infections the

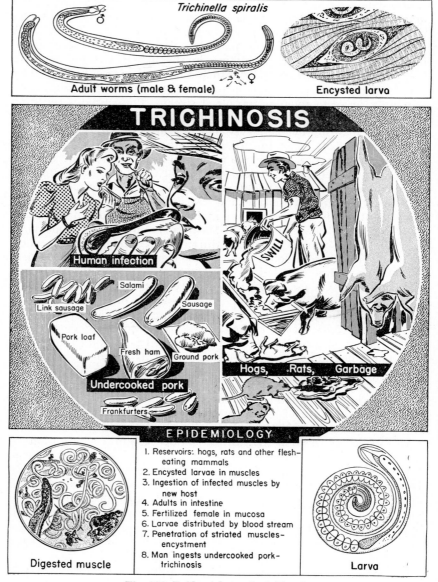

Fig. 220. Epidemiology of trichinosis.

myocardium may be extensively damaged and present cellular infiltration and necrosis and fragmentation of the muscle fibers. Encystment, however, does not occur in cardiac muscle. It is believed that the destruction and absorption of host tissue and of many of the larvae causes the generalized toxemia. A high eosinophilia, sometimes reaching 70 per cent, is typical of this disease. In fatal cases death, usually intervening four to eight weeks after the infection, is due to toxemia, secondary pneumonia and myocardial failure (Figs. 221, 222).

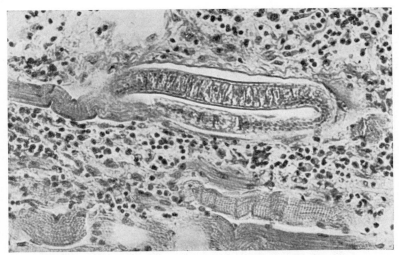

Fig. 221. Early stage of encystment of larva of *T. spiralis* in man, showing degeneration of muscle fiber and surrounding myositis.

**Clinical Characteristics** The clinical picture may be divided roughly into the stages of intestinal invasion, muscle penetration, and tissue repair (encystment). Twenty-four hours following the ingestion of viable larvae, signs of gastro-intestinal disturbance in the form of nausea, vomiting, diarrhea and abdominal pain may become evident. In about a week the females begin to larviposit and the stage of muscle penetration commences. This period is characterized by periorbital edema which usually occurs between the twelfth and fourteenth day, and irregular but persistent fever lasting one or two weeks and reaching a maximum of 104° to 105° F. Myositis and "rheumatic pains" are especially noticeable at this time. In severe infections a generalized scarlatiniform rash may occur. During this acute phase differential blood counts reveal a marked eosinophilia. The last stage is characterized by neurotoxic symptoms and possibly myocarditis. In less severe cases the fever begins to subside and a slow convalescence follows. Loss of weight frequently occurs. Some atypical cases may simulate meningitis or encephalitis.

**Diagnosis** An early diagnosis of this disease is difficult or impossible because of the absence of a clear-cut clinical picture. A history of eating raw or undercooked pork is helpful, but as trichinosis is not often suspected, a pertinent history is rarely elicited at the onset. Frequently members of the same family or even several families in one neighborhood will be involved.

Additional presumptive evidence is found in the periorbital edema and fever, coupled with a significant eosinophilia of 20 per cent or more. A positive skin test in three weeks and a positive precipitin or flocculation test in a month, or the formation of precipitates about

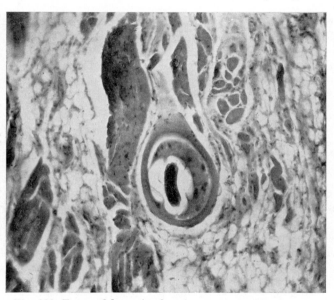

Fig. 222. Encysted larva in chronic stage, myositis absent.

larvae of *T. spiralis* ten to twenty days after infection, are reliable and significant diagnostic aids (see p. 848). False positives when whipworms are present sometimes occur.

Direct evidence of the infection rests upon the demonstration of the parasite. Sometimes this may be accomplished by biopsy of the deltoid, biceps or gastrocnemius muscle, part of which should be compressed between glass slides, and examined under a microscope, part digested and the remainder sectioned. Occasionally in the stage of migration larvae may be demonstrated in the sediment of centrifuged blood or spinal fluid; the methods are described on p. 817. *Trichinella* larvae may be recovered from the spinal fluid of young children with severe trichinosis.

It is necessary to make a differential diagnosis, especially in the initial stages, to exclude food poisoning and diarrhea or dysentery of other etiology. Later, cardiac disease and other causes of fever associated with generalized body pains must be suspected.

The prognosis is good in light infections but becomes grave when heavy parasitization is evident.

**Treatment** The treatment of trichinosis is principally supportive. However, ACTH has been shown to be effective in many diseases in which an antibody-antigen reaction participates in the mechanism. Limited clinical trials indicate that this preparation may terminate dramatically the toxic febrile stage of the disease.

**Prophylaxis** Infection is due largely to the ingestion of raw or insufficiently cooked pork. The larvae of *T. spiralis* are readily killed by thorough cooking of meat or by freezing it for thirty-six hours at —27° C. (—16.6° F.) for twenty-four hours at —30° C. (—22° F.), or for forty minutes at —35° C. (—31° F.). It should be remembered that the United States Government *DOES NOT INSPECT MEAT* for the presence of this parasite.

# 46   The Schistosomes

**Introduction** The blood flukes of man, commonly known as schistosomes, are the most important human trematodes. There are three species which infect man—*Schistosoma haematobium, S. mansoni* and *S. japonicum*—each producing its characteristic disease. Other species, such as *Schistosoma bovis*, a parasite normally of cattle, have been reported as occasional human parasites, but these will be only briefly mentioned.

## Morphology of the Schistosomes

**Schistosome Structure** These parasites differ from other trematodes of man in that they are dioecious (i. e., exist as males and females) (cf. p. 474). They range in length between 6.5 and 26 mm.; the females are longer and more slender than the males. In both sexes the *oral sucker* and the *acetabulum* are approximate. In the females they are of equal size, while in the males the acetabulum is larger. The integument may be partly or completely tuberculate or spined in the males, while such structures are usually found only near the extremities of the females. The most characteristic feature of the males is their ventrally infolded margins, beginning behind the acetabulum and forming a groove or *gynecophoral canal* in which the more slender female lies during copulation and oviposition. A bulbous cluster of glands occurs in the esophageal region in both sexes. The alimentary canal passes into an *esophagus* and soon divides into *intestinal crura* which fuse near the center of the worm to form a single, serpentine trunk extending to a blind terminus near the posterior body tip. The gut frequently appears reddish black owing to the presence of ingested blood. The male reproductive system consists of four to nine *testes* while in the female only a single *ovary* exists. The *yolk glands* are located in the posterior half of the females and the uterus usually contains between one and fifty eggs.

**Schistosome Eggs**    These differ from the eggs of all other trematodes in the absence of an operculum or lid and the presence of a spine or knob on the shell (see Fig. 237, p. 486). In addition all schistosome eggs contain a fully developed *miracidium* when they leave the host. Table 41 summarizes some of the more important characteristics.

*Table 41    Characteristics of Schistosome Eggs*

| SPECIES | LENGTH (MICRONS) | BREADTH (MICRONS) | DIAGNOSTIC FEATURES |
|---|---|---|---|
| S. haematobium | 112–170 av. 150 | 40–70 av. 60 | Terminal spine |
| S. mansoni | 114–175 av. 150 | 45–70 av. 60 | Lateral spine |
| S. japonicum | 70–100 av. 89 | 50–70 av. 66 | Small incurved spine which often is not seen |

**The Generalized Cycle of the Schistosomes**

**Oviposition**    After maturing, the female schistosome enters and remains in the gynecophoral canal of the male until ready to discharge eggs, at which time the pair moves against the current of the portal blood stream into the smaller venous radicles. Here the female may partially or entirely leave the gynecophoral canal of the male in order to migrate further into the venule. The eggs are deposited in a beadlike row, the female retreating gradually with the current, allowing the venule to contract to its original size thus embracing the eggs. As these eggs occlude the venules they are subjected to the pressure of the blood stream which, together with the movements of the surrounding tissues, and perhaps aided by the spines (in *S. haematobium* and *S. mansoni*) accounts for their passage through the capillary walls. It is probable that the process of penetration is aided by lytic substances secreted by the miracidium within the egg. Most eggs eventually reach the lumen of the gut, except those of *S. haematobium*, which typically penetrate the urinary bladder. The eggs reach water in urine or feces and soon hatch, liberating a free-swimming miracidium.

**Development in the Snail**    The miracidia of all three species are actively swimming organisms and are somewhat larger than the eggs from which they emerge. They remain viable for about sixteen hours after hatching, during which time they must reach and penetrate the proper species of snail if further development is to occur (see Table 53, p. 627, for the known snail hosts). In the snail the miracidium becomes transformed into a *mother sporocyst* which in turn produces a second generation of *sporocysts*. After a suitable developmental period, typical apharyngeal fork-tailed *cercariae* are produced. In *S. haematobium* four to eight weeks elapse from the penetration of the miracidium to the liberation of cercariae; in *S. mansoni* under optimum conditions only four weeks are necessary while *S. japonicum* requires five to seven weeks for the production of cercariae (Fig. 223).

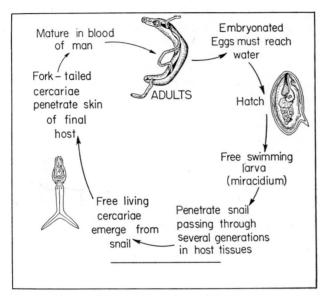

Fig. 223. Trematode cycle—schistosome type.

**Penetration of Cercariae** Upon emerging from the snail the cercariae swim about vigorously tail-first and, after reaching the surface of the water, gradually sink to the bottom. This behavior is repeated many times although some cercariae (especially *S. japonicum*) may remain temporarily attached to the surface film by their suckers.

Persons washing themselves, clothes or vehicles, bathing, wading in, or drinking infested water may acquire schistosomiasis. As the water on the skin evaporates the cercariae penetrate the epidermis by forcing the anterior end of the body through the skin usually after casting off the tail. Penetration occurs within thirty minutes and is aided by the lytic action of secretions of the penetration glands. By the end of twenty-four hours the larvae have worked their way through the epidermis to the peripheral venules; they are then carried through the blood stream to the right side of the heart and thence to the pulmonary capillaries where the larvae are delayed for several days while squeezing through the lumen of the capillaries into the veins. The parasites then journey back through the left side of the heart into the systemic circulation. The majority of these growing larvae are carried into the aorta and it is believed that only those survive which reach the mesenteric capillaries and complete the circuit to the portal circulation. The remainder are filtered out and destroyed. The larvae grow into males and females as they lie in the intrahepatic portion of the portal circulation. These developing parasites become adolescent about three weeks after penetration, and soon pass out of the liver through the portal radicles and anastomosing vessels to become lodged in the walls of the intestine or bladder. *Schistosoma haematobium* reaches these locations between one and three months after penetrating the skin. On or before reaching these plexuses the worms have matured, mated and the fertile females have started to produce eggs.

The penetration and early development of cercariae of *S. mansoni* parallels that of *S. haematobium* but requires an incubation period of only seven weeks before the female begins to produce eggs. The developing *S. mansoni* may complete the circuit of the circulatory system several times before reaching the portal venules. The males hold the females in the gynecophoral canal and both work their way into the upper branches of the superior and inferior mesenteric veins where the females deposit eggs.

*Schistosoma japonicum* follows the same route of invasion until the systemic circulation is reached. From this point on, evidence seems to indicate that only those cercariae reaching the intrahepatic circulation via the mesenteric arteries and capillaries are able to survive. After a period of growth the worms migrate into the venules of the superior mesenteric vessels and mate, and eggs are deposited in their smaller branches.

**Reservoir Hosts**   Man serves as the principal host for both *S. haematobium* and *S. mansoni*. Although monkeys have been found to be naturally infected with both species, it is believed that they do not play an important role as reservoir hosts. *Schistosoma japonicum*, however, is not so specific, for in addition to infecting man, it parasitizes also water buffalo, horses, imported cattle, dogs, cats, and field and other mice.

Several other species of schistosomes have been reported infrequently as potential parasites of man. One is *S. spindale* Montgomery 1906, a parasite of native cattle, sheep, goats, horses and antelopes of India, South Africa and Sumatra. Some workers mention *S. intercalatum* Fischer 1934 from the upper Congo as an additional species parasitizing man but others believe this to be identical with, or a variety of, *S. bovis* or *S. haematobium*. A third species, *S. incognitum* Chandler 1926, was reported from human feces from Bengal; this trematode is probably a parasite of swine.

### Host Response

**General Pathology**   All stages of the parasite in man can produce pathologic changes by the combination of mechanical effects, toxic secretions or excretions, or disintegration products. The host response to these stimuli include the formation of pseudotubercles, papillomas, bilharzial granulomas and verminous phlebitis and arteritis. Eggs deposited in the tissues remain viable for about three weeks. Approximately nine to ten days are required for development to maturity, after which the contained miricidium has an additional ten days to escape from the host. Failing this, the eggs degenerate and may become calcified.

Ectopic lesions may be produced in various parts of the body outside the limits of the portal and inferior vena cava systems. Formerly, these were attributed to embolic localization of eggs. More recently, available evidence indicates that they are produced, in part at least, by adult schistosomes which reach these areas through arteriovenous anastomoses in the lungs and liver or through the superior vena cava and the vertebral venous system to deposit their eggs in situ. Such lesions occur most frequently in the central nervous system, the conjunctiva, the skin and the lungs.

In the central nervous system the lesions are usually multiple pseudotubercles consisting of one or more eggs surrounded by giant cells, epithelioid, mononuclear and plasma cells and numerous eosinophile leukocytes, or granulomatous lesions often containing foci of caseation. In *S. japonicum* infections the brain is involved predominantly, particularly the frontal, parietal and occipital lobes, while in infections by *S. mansoni* and *S. haematobium* involvement of the spinal cord rather than the brain is the rule.

Symptoms of central nervous system involvement may appear as early as two to six weeks after the onset of illness, or they may be delayed for three or more years. The clinical syndromes include disorientation, incontinence, paralyses, epilepsy, unconsciousness, signs of an expanding intracranial tumor and acute or chronic myelitis. Permanent sequelae are twice as frequent in surgically treated cases as in those receiving one or more full courses of tartar emetic.

Lesions of the conjunctiva, commonly single or multiple nodules or polypoid masses, occur in the course of infections by *S. haematobium*, and bilharzial cutaneous nodules may occur in *S. haematobium* and *S. japonicum* infections. Localization of eggs in the lungs causing multiple pseudotubercles may produce a radiologic picture suggestive of miliary tuberculosis, Egyptian Ayerza's disease. However, the nodules are less uniform in size and distribution.

The classic cirrhosis of the liver occurring in the chronic and late stages of schistosomiasis in the presence of heavy infections is periportal in type without generalized fibrosis and is not associated with splenic enlargement. There is increasing evidence to suggest that the form of splenomegaly and cirrhosis frequently observed in schistosomiasis in Egypt and the Orient, which resembles Banti's disease clinically, is in fact of nutritional origin.

**General Symptomology** The general clinical phenomena produced by the three schistosomes may be divided into three stages. The initial phase, occurring from four to ten weeks after infection, is characterized by fever and toxic and allergic phenomena. The intermediate stage appears from two and a half months to several years after infection. The clinical picture is predominantly that of pathologic changes in the intestinal and urinary tracts and the presence of eggs in the excreta. The final stage is that of complications involving the gastro-intestinal, the renal or other physiologic systems.

There are marked similarities in the clinical syndromes produced by each of the three parasites in the initial stage. Remittent or intermittent fever is common and frequently accompanied by urticaria, abdominal pain, bronchitis, enlargement of the liver and spleen, and diarrhea. The terms Yangtze River fever and Katayama disease have been applied to this stage in China and Japan, respectively.

### Diagnosis

**General Considerations**   Specific diagnosis of schistosomiasis depends upon the demonstration of the characteristic eggs, typically from the feces or urine (see 822, 831 for details). In cases of schistosomiasis mansoni or japonica, rectal or sigmoidoscopic biopsies have proved to be equally efficacious. In schistosomiasis haematobia, biopsied material may be obtained through the cystoscope. Other diagnostic aids include the complement fixation and intradermal tests. Both procedures have given highly accurate results in the hands of some workers. Further refinements appear necessary. An euglobulin precipitation test is also suggestive. Some workers recommend comminuting the stool in a flask and checking the liquid for miracidia.

### Treatment

**General Considerations**   Organic compounds belonging to two chemical groups are the most effective drugs for the treatment of schistosomiasis. The first, trivalent compounds of antimony, include potassium antimony tartrate (tartar emetic), sodium antimony tartrate, sodium antimony gluconate, Fuadin, and anthiomaline. These preparations vary in their effectiveness, toxicity, indications and contraindications. The initial effects of antimony compounds upon the parasites are to cause degeneration of the yolk glands in the female worms, degeneration of the ovaries and shrinkage of the whole worm. Some degeneration of the testes of the male worms occurs as well. Effective treatment by these preparations decreases oviposition and finally leads to death of the parasite.

Recently a thioxanthone derivative, lucanthone hydrochloride (Nilodin, Miracil D) has been added to the list of useful therapeutic agents.

**Criteria of Cure**   Radical cure of schistosomiasis is difficult to accomplish. Clinical cure with disappearance of symptoms and of eggs from the excreta, however, is more readily achieved, but relapses (even in the absence of re-exposure) are common. The minimum follow-up period for evaluation of treatment must be not less than one year. In general each successive course of treatment may be expected to decrease the number of living worms. The necessity for continued therapy of minimal residual asymptomatic infections is contro-versial.

### Prophylaxis

**General Considerations**  In most areas where schistosomiasis is endemic, therapeutic prophylaxis has not been highly successful owing largely to re-exposure and the difficulty of administering mass treatments. In some areas, but by no manner of means all, the use of a molluscicidal chemical which destroys the snail intermediate host holds considerable promise of achieving practical control of the dis-ease (see p. 626). This is especially true of some endemic areas of schistosomiasis japonica in Japan and of schistosomiasis mansoni in other regions. Copper sulfate has been used in Egypt, while sodium pentachlorophenate (Santobrite) has proved its usefulness in test areas of Japan. The use of these and related compounds must be weighed against the temporary destruction of proteins such as fish which are often sought to supplement the dietary. Actually any such measures must be supplemented with a long range educational pro-gram concerning the proper use of human nightsoil as fertilizer. In the case of *S. japonicum* there are a number of other mammals which serve as reservoir hosts of this parasite.

### Schistosomiasis Haematobia

**Synonyms**  Urinary bilharziasis, schistosomal hematuria, endemic hematuria, vesical schistosomiasis.

**Definition**  Schistosomiasis haematobia is due to the presence of the blood fluke, *Schistosoma haematobium* in the vesical and pelvic venous plexuses of man. The disease is frequently accompanied by severe hematuria and cystitis.

**Distribution**  Schistosomiasis haematobia occurs throughout much of Africa, the Middle East and in isolated areas of southern Europe (Spain and Cyprus). The Nile Valley is one of the chief endemic centers of the disease. The infection also occurs across North Africa to Morocco, and down the eastern side (Italian Somaliland, Uganda, Kenya, Tanganyika, Mozambique, Nyassaland, North and South Rhodesia, Union of South Africa and the islands of Madagascar, Mauritius and Reunion). The disease occurs extensively in the Gold Coast and parts of the Belgian Congo. In the Middle East schisto-somiasis haematobia is endemic in parts of Palestine, Northern Syria, Arabia, Iran (Khuzistan province) and Iraq (mostly along the Tigris and Euphrates valleys). Recently the disease was reported from Yemen and India (Bombay state) (Fig. 224).

**Etiology**  MORPHOLOGY. The etiologic agent of schistosomiasis haematobia is the blood fluke, *Schistosoma haematobium* (Bilharz 1852) Weinland 1858, which inhabits the vesical and pelvic plexuses of the venous circulation. The parasites are dioecious, the male being shorter and stouter than the female and measuring 10 to 15 mm. and occasionally 18 mm. in length and about 1 mm. in its greatest diameter. The cuticle of the male is covered with small tubercles while that of the female possesses minute papillae which are limited to either extremity of the worm. Like related species the male possesses

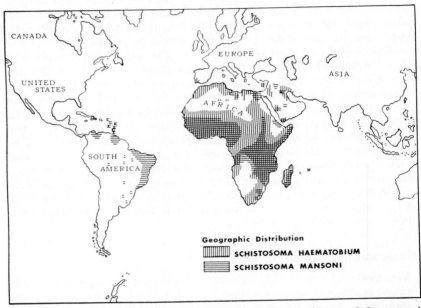

Fig. 224. Geographic distribution of *Schistosoma haematobium* and *S. mansoni.* (Courtesy of History of the Medical Department in World War II. From Ferguson and Bang's chapter on Schistosomiasis.)

two suckers and a well-formed gynecophoral canal. Four to five large testes may be seen grouped just posterior to the acetabulum. The female is darker in color, longer and more slender than the male and measures approximately 20 mm. in length, the suckers being smaller and weaker than those of the male. Eggs range between 112 and 170 microns and possess a terminal spine. For other details of schistosomal morphology see page 461.

DEVELOPMENT. The life cycle does not differ markedly from the generalized life history outlined on page 462, except that the eggs are discharged principally in urine rather than in feces.

*Epidemiology* Man is the main reservoir for *S. haematobium.* While monkeys have been found infected in nature, it does not appear likely that these constitute an important source of infection. Embryonated eggs hatch when the urine becomes diluted with water.

The ciliated miracidia penetrate snails of the genera *Bulinus, Planorbis* and *Physopsis,* in whose tissues mother and daughter sporocysts are formed. The latter produce characteristic brevifurcate (short, fork-tailed) cercariae that penetrate the exposed skin of man.

In endemic regions practically the entire population may be infected. Between 11 and 75 per cent of the population of lower Egypt and 33 to 94 per cent of those examined in Tanganyika harbor this fluke. The distribution of the disease is increasing due to the transfer of snails from infected foci to other areas as new irrigation projects are completed. The proper snail host when present in non-endemic localities may become infected from eggs discharged into canals, streams, or pools by persons harboring the parasite. Transmission in certain Mohammedan countries is facilitated by the religious stipulation that the anal and urethral orifices be washed with water after urination or defecation. This custom is usually carried out in a near-by river or canal. Another epidemiologic factor is that the species of snails serving as intermediate hosts for the parasite thrive in sewage.

The chief intermediate hosts for this parasite in North Africa and Egypt are snails of the genus *Bulinus.* In one region of the Belgian Congo members of the genus *Physopsis* serve as hosts. Other data on the snail hosts appear in Table 53 on page 627.

**Pathology**  The pathologic changes resulting from the presence of *S. haematobium* in man are produced chiefly by eggs of the fluke. The adults themselves probably cause less damage, while the cercariae, upon piercing the skin, give rise usually to no more than a mild and transient local irritation.

With the beginning of egg production in the vesical venules, tissue changes in the bladder wall supervene. These are both hypertrophic and atrophic and result from the penetration of eggs into the muscularis and the mucosa. There is marked round-cell infiltration about the eggs, and whole clusters of such foreign bodies may be encapsulated by fibrotic tissue. This leads on one hand to the formation of calcific bodies and on the other to cysts which rupture into the bladder leaving small ulcerations. The mucosa in such regions proliferates, occasionally forming polyps and sometimes undergoing malignant changes (Figs. 225, 226).

In cases of prolonged and severe infection with *S. haematobium* the entire bladder wall may be involved. The mucosa may become totally deranged, large calculi may be formed, and involvement of the ureteral orifices or the ureters themselves leads to dilatation of these channels and of the renal pelves. Pyogenic sequelae may result. Involvement of the urethra may result in interference with lymphatic return from the penis as well as elephantiasis of that organ. Fistulae of the urethra opening through the perineum or posterior surface of the scrotum may also develop.

The adult flukes uncommonly invade the venules of the rectum and large bowel; when they do eggs appear in the feces. In women

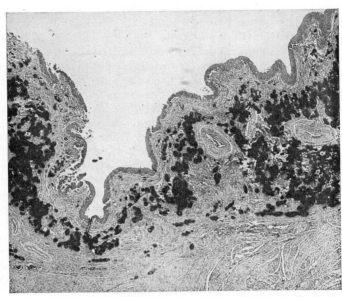

Fig. 225. Schistosomiasis: calcified eggs of *S. haematobium* in wall of urinary bladder; early papilloma formation.

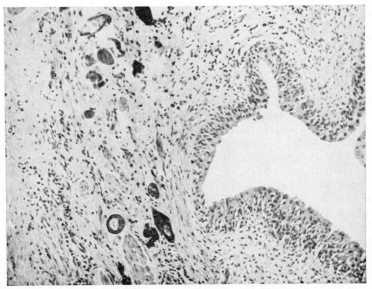

Fig. 226. Schistosomiasis: fibrosis of bladder wall, eggs of *S. haematobium*.

tne cervix, vagina or vulva may be involved. In general, however, cystitis and hematuria constitute the chief pathologic features of this disease.

Ectopic lesions occur occasionally in the central nervous system, particularly the spinal cord, the conjunctiva, the skin and the lungs. These may be caused by migration of adult worms and deposition of eggs in situ, or by embolic distribution of eggs by the blood stream. Pseudotubercle formation in the pulmonary tissues may produce a radiologic picture resembling miliary tuberculosis.

**Clinical Characteristics**    Urinary frequency is a common early symptom and may be accompanied by a scalding sensation along the course of the urethra during and after voiding. Hematuria is frequently gradual in onset, at first microscopic, later becoming gross as frank ulceration of the bladder mucosa develops. Usually it is terminal in character. With extensive ulceration the whole specimen may be bloody and clots may be present. Pain is variable and is usually referred to the suprapubic region or the perineum. Often it is aggravated by distention of the bladder and is most intense at the end of micturition.

Pyogenic cystitis is a frequent complication and carcinoma of the bladder occurs not infrequently in advanced cases. The prostate gland and the seminal vesicles may likewise be involved in this form of schistosomiasis.

**Diagnosis**    The finding of terminal-spined eggs in the urine is pathognomonic of this disease. These are passed with the last few drops of the urine at the end of micturition. The eggs are easily seen under low power of the microscope.

When laboratory confirmation of the disease is lacking, it is necessary to differentiate between schistosomiasis and other forms of cystitis. In typical cases, however, the terminal hematuria is so characteristic that in regions where schistosomiasis haematobia is endemic, it is not difficult to arrive at an early diagnosis.

In severe infections and late cases it may be necessary to resort to cystoscopy, which frequently reveals multiple minute calcific bodies or "sandy" excrescences covering the less gravely involved areas of the bladder mucosa.

**Treatment**    Intravenous administration of potassium or sodium antimony tartrate is generally accepted as the most effective treatment. The less toxic compound, sodium antimony gluconate, will bring about clinical cure and temporary disappearance of eggs from the urine in many cases of vesical schistosomiasis.

Lucanthone hydrochloride (Nilodin, Miracil D) has the advantage of being administered orally. Although it is a gastro-intestinal irritant and not infrequently causes unpleasant side effects, these are not dangerous and rarely require termination of treatment. Other recommended drugs include Fuadin and Anthiomaline.

For the details of treatment see pp. 541–545.

**Prophylaxis**    Control of schistosomiasis is difficult since drinking, wading in or bathing in infected water in endemic regions results in almost certain infection. In some regions all water should be regarded as a potential source of infecton, while in other regions infected snails occur only in specific areas where sewage enters a given body of water.

The chief problem from the biological point of view is to prevent infection of the snails. This may be accomplished, theoretically at least, by educating the population in endemic areas to use latrines.

Control of the snail population through the use of molluscicides is desirable. Copper sulfate (15 to 50 ppm) or copper carbonate (12 to 50 ppm) left to act for three to four days has markedly reduced the snail population. In most areas of the world this alone will not give control. Sodium pentachlorophenate and other related compounds hold considerable promise of being effective molluscicidal agents (see p. 626).

Alternate emptying and filling of canals and ditches may be helpful but is not entirely satisfactory, since many of the snails are able to burrow into the mud and so survive. Recently it has been suggested that control may be effected by clearing vegetation from the distributing ditches and placing the drainage canals beneath the ground, thus eliminating the breeding areas for the snails.

## Schistosomiasis Mansoni

**Synonyms**   Manson's intestinal schistosomiasis, bilharziasis mansoni, intestinal bilharziasis, bilharzial dysentery, schistosomal dysentery.

**Definition**   Schistosomiasis mansoni is an endemic disease with abdominal and dysenteric symptoms and occasional splenomegaly caused by the blood fluke, *Schistosoma mansoni*.

**Distribution**   Schistosomiasis mansoni originally was an African disease which was subsequently imported into the West Indies and South America by the slave trade. It is now known to occur commonly in the inhabitants of the Nile Delta, much of the East Coast of Africa, parts of West Africa, the Congo River basin, South Africa and the island of Madagascar. It is also present in North Africa (Libya), in Eritrea, and in Asia (Arabia and Yemen). In the Western Hemisphere schistosomiasis mansoni is known in parts of Brazil, Venezuela, Dutch Guiana as well as numerous islands in the Caribbean including Puerto Rico, the Dominican Republic and Martinique but not Cuba. The distribution may be seen on the map on p. 468.

**Etiology**   MORPHOLOGY. *Schistosoma mansoni* Sambon 1907 superficially resembles *S. haematobium*. The male *S. mansoni* measures between 6 and 10 mm. and the female between 7 and 14 mm. in length. The cuticula of the male is drawn into larger and more distinct tubercles than those found on the cuticula of *S. haematobium* (Fig. 227). The testes of the male, 6 to 9 in number, though relatively large and conspicuous, are smaller than those of *S. haema-tobium*.

DEVELOPMENT. The life cycle of *S. mansoni* conforms to the generalized description on page 462. The mother sporocysts develop in the head-foot region of the snail while the daughter sporocysts subsequently migrate to the digestive gland.

**Epidemiology** The epidemiology of schistosomiasis mansoni is essentially similar to that of schistosomiasis haematobia except that (1) different species of snails serve as intermediate hosts (see Table

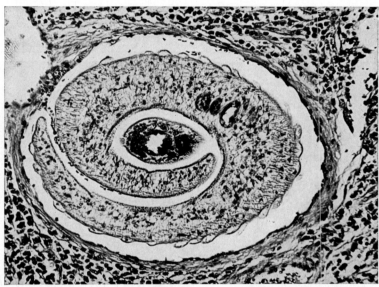

Fig. 227. Schistosomiasis: male and female *S. mansoni* in lumen of mesenteric vein showing tuberculate cuticula of male.

53, p. 627) and (2) defecation rather than urination by infected persons contaminates the water with schistosome eggs. Untreated sewage emptying into ditches, streams or lakes constitutes an ever-present menace to the populations in endemic regions (Fig. 228).

A large number of molluscan intermediate hosts are known to carry *S. mansoni*. Nearly all such *Australorbis* are related to the *Planorbis* group, while members of the genera *Physopsis* and *Isidora* are believed also to serve in this capacity. Within a period of about four weeks after penetration by the miracidium, infective cercariae emerge from the snail and are infective for man.

Although monkeys have been found to be naturally infected, it is not believed that these constitute an important natural reservoir. It is possible that some rodents may be capable of serving as reservoir hosts, since mice, hamsters and rice rats have been infected experimentally and a wild rodent was found in Egypt infected with sexually immature *S. mansoni*.

**Pathology** The pathologic changes occurring in schistosomiasis mansoni are due principally to the irritative effects of the eggs deposited in the tissues. They cause a variety of inflammatory, infiltrative, hyperplastic, ulcerative, and even cirrhotic reactions. The

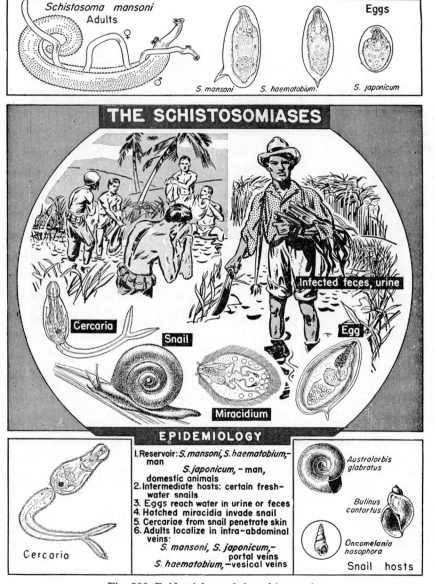

Fig. 228. Epidemiology of the schistosomiases.

eggs lodged in the venules of the submucosa and mucosa of the intestinal wall act as irritating foreign bodies and as such set up an inflammatory reaction, inciting proliferation of the epithelial cells, the formation of pseudotubercles, and subsequently small abscesses. Occlusion of small vessels, together with the local inflammatory foci, leads to necrosis and ulceration. In other areas thickening of the mucosa and epithelial hyperplasia are followed by the development of papillomata which may subsequently undergo carcinomatous change.

In early stages of the infection a marked leukocytosis with high eosinophilia may be present. This is commonly followed by leukopenia.

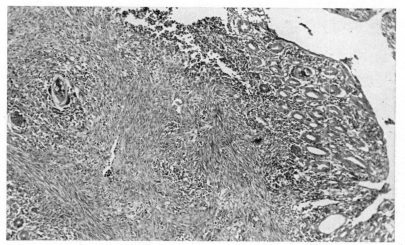

Fig. 229. Schistosomiasis: ulceration and fibrosis of colon, eggs of *S. mansoni* in submucosa.

In the intestinal type of schistosomiasis mansoni the entire digestive tract may be severely affected, since the worms are found throughout the portal system. However, the sigmoid and rectum are the sites of greatest damage, while the stomach and small intestine rarely give evidence of serious involvement. The lower ileum may reveal papillomata and slightly thickened walls, but the large intestine, and especially the sigmoid and rectum, show a variety of lesions including congestion, infiltration, papillomata, ulcers, rugosities, and around the anal opening cutaneous schistosomal tumors (Fig. 229). The peritoneum, omentum and mesenteries may also be affected.

Many eggs which fail to lodge in the capillaries are swept back into the liver, where they may be found in great numbers producing a foreign-body and scarring type of lesion. In chronic cases there is often a periportal type of cirrhosis which when severe is accompanied by ascites and dilatation of the collateral venous channels. The spleen is frequently considerably enlarged, in small part as the result of eggs lodging within it but commonly as the expression of chronic passive congestion secondary to the periportal cirrhosis of the liver.

Sometimes eggs are carried to other regions such as the lungs, kidneys, adrenals, pancreas, spleen, myocardium or spinal cord, where they may at first produce localized inflammatory reactions and later become encapsulated and calcified (Fig. 230).

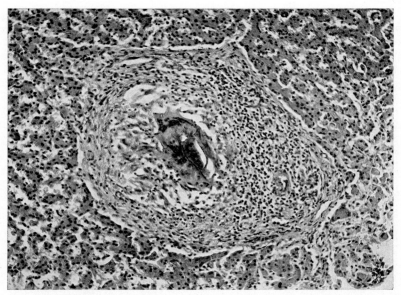

Fig. 230. Schistosomiasis pseudotubercle in liver: foreign-body reaction, cellular infiltration and early connective tissue proliferation about egg of *S. mansoni.*

**Clinical Characteristics**   Penetration of the skin may be accompanied by tingling of the affected skin areas in certain cases. In some instances this may be followed by local dermatitis. The incubation period varies from four to ten weeks. In the latter part of this period there is frequently diarrhea, probably of toxic or irritative origin, accompanied by fever, anorexia, abdominal pain, and sometimes urticaria and pulmonary symptoms.

Oviposition in the radicles of the portal vein begins about six to eight weeks after infection. The intestinal wall, the liver and the spleen are principally affected. The predominant symptoms are abdominal pain, diarrhea with blood, mucus and pus in the feces— the classic schistosomal dysentery. The liver and spleen become tender and progressively enlarge, and embolism of the eggs into other regions may produce special symptoms referable to the particular localization.

The later stages are characterized by the clinical phenomena of cirrhosis of the liver, extensive damage to the colon and multiple fistulae, and are complicated in some instances by the development of carcinoma.

*Egyptian splenomegaly* is now classed as a syndrome attributable to malnutrition.

**Diagnosis**  The clinical picture is so variable that demonstration of the characteristic lateral-spined eggs is necessary to establish the diagnosis. Lesions which may often be seen through the proctoscope or the sigmoidoscope are significant since they are usually discrete nodules or ulcers separated by normal mucous membrane, in this respect resembling the lesions produced by *E. histolytica*. Biopsy of a nodule or scrapings from the base of an ulcer will reveal the etiology. Even in the presence of light infections direct microscopic examination of a small biopsy specimen of rectal mucosa crushed in saline solution under a cover glass will frequently reveal the characteristic eggs.

About six to eight weeks after infection the eggs may be found in the feces on direct examination or after concentration. If the patient has symptoms suggestive of dysentery no concentration methods for the eggs will be necessary. However, in other cases negative direct smears should be followed by the AMS III (acid–sodium sulfate–Triton–ether) sedimentation technique. Sedimentation and centrifugation are also useful methods for concentrating the eggs. In cases of hepatic schistosomiasis mansoni, eggs may not be demonstrable in the stool and other diagnostic aids must be utilized. The complement fixation reaction and intradermal test are helpful. An increase of serum euglobulin is suggestive but is not characteristic of this disease alone. For details on techniques see p. 847.

**Treatment**  The most effective treatment for *S. mansoni* infections is the intravenous administration of potassium or sodium antimony tartrate. Fuadin (Fouadin, Stibophen) and Anthiomaline are less effective but none the less valuable therapeutic agents (see pages 541–545). Because of greater involvement of the liver in many cases of schistosomiasis mansoni an intolerance to the drugs may develop. Furthermore, it is not always possible to effect a cure with a single course of treatment. Advanced chronic cases may prove refractory and it often happens that the liver may be damaged beyond repair.

**Prophylaxis**  The prophylaxis of infection by *S. mansoni* does not differ from that for schistosomiasis haematobia (cf. p. 471).

## Schistosomiasis Japonica

**Synonyms**  Oriental schistosomiasis, eastern schistosomiasis, Katayama disease, Yangtze River fever.

**Definition**  Schistosomiasis japonica is a grave, chronic disease endemic in the Far East, with abdominal and dysenteric symptoms caused by *Schistosoma japonicum*. Man and domestic animals are affected.

**Distribution**  Schistosomiasis japonica is found only in the Far

East in parts of China, Japan, Formosa, the Philippines and Celebes, where its distribution is co-extensive with that of the intermediate snail host, *Oncomelania* spp. In China large portions of the Yangtze Valley and coastal areas from the Yangtze delta to Hong Kong con-

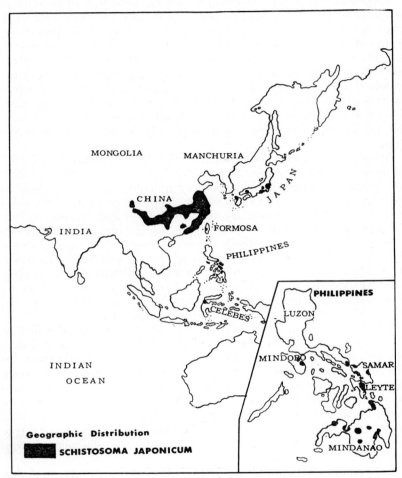

Fig. 231. Geographic distribution of *Schistosoma japonicum*. (Courtesy of History of the Medical Department in World War II. From Ferguson and Bang's chapter on Schistosomiasis.)

stitute one of the principal endemic areas. Other regions include districts above Canton and parts of Yunnan Province (Fig. 231).

In Japan the disease is limited to five distinct loci. These areas and the peak incidence in the several communities surveyed follow: (1) The Tone River Valley northeast of Tokyo (10 to 14 per cent); (2) the Numazu coastal area southwest of Tokyo (less than 4 per cent in a single village); (3) the highly endemic Kofu valley west of Tokyo

(0.2 to 65.9 per cent on a single stool examination of 3055 persons and over 90 per cent when multiple stools were examined); (4) the Katayama area of Hiroshima Prefecture (20 to 33 per cent); and (5) the Kurume-Tosu area of Saga and Fukuoka Prefectures on Kyushu Island (29 to 73 per cent for single stool examinations).

In Formosa the intermediate snail host, *Oncomelania formosana*, is more widely distributed than the disease in man, who seldom seems to pass eggs. Reservoir hosts appear to be important in maintaining the disease.

Schistosomiasis japonica occurs in the Philippines on the southern tip of Luzon, on the northeast side of Mindoro (40 per cent infected), in coastal and inland foci on Samar, in the eastern coastal area of Leyte (up to 90 per cent in children), and in every province on Mindanao except Misamis Oriental (Fig. 231).

In the Lake Lindoë region of the Celebes 50 per cent of the population examined in three villages were positive.

**Etiology** MORPHOLOGY. Adult *S. japonicum* Katsurada 1904 can be distinguished from adults of the other two human species by the absence of the tuberculated integument. Instead, the cuticula of both sexes is covered with minute spines. The esophagus is surrounded by two contiguous clusters of glands. Males are broader and shorter than the females and measure 12 to 20 mm. in length compared with the average 24 to 27 mm. for the female. The male possesses seven testes that are arranged lineally, while the female is characterized by a long uterus which may contain as many as fifty eggs. Those which are passed in the feces of the host measure 70 to 90 by 50 to 70 microns and may be distinguished by the enclosed miracidium and the rarely detectable small knob, or reduced spine, on the lateral aspect of the shell (Fig. 237, p. 486).

DEVELOPMENT. *Schistosoma japonicum* follows the pattern of development described for *S. haematobium* and *S. mansoni* except that the snail hosts differ and *S. japonicum* infects many other mammals as well as man.

Snails of the genus *Oncomelania* serve as intermediate hosts for *S. japonicum* from southern Japan through Formosa to Canton, China (see Table 53, p. 627).

**Epidemiology** Schistosomiasis japonica results from the pollution of soil and water by human or animal feces containing the eggs of *S. japonicum*. Amphibious snails of the genus *Oncomelania* that normally inhabit the banks of irrigation ditches and canals, or marshes and quiet fresh-water, serve as the intermediate hosts of *S. japonicum*. Canals, irrigation ditches, marshes, overflow areas, slow-flowing streams and shallow ponds or pools are often seeded with eggs in human feces from defecation sites or as nightsoil boats or buckets are emptied or rinsed in or near water along, or in which, these snails live.

Human infection results from wading in the shallow water along irrigation ditches, canals, rice fields or rice seedling beds containing cercariae which have emerged from infected snails. The infection may also be acquired by bathing, washing clothes or vehicles, or drinking the contaminated water.

*Schistosoma japonicum* has a wide variety of reservoir hosts in addition to man. Dogs, cats, horses, imported cattle, water buffalo, deer, field and other mice and rats may become infected in endemic areas. Some of these serve also as an additional source of contamination of the water. Schistosomiasis japonica becomes more widespread following floods which facilitate the dissemination of the snails.

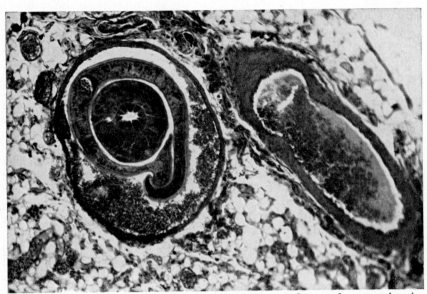

Fig. 232. Schistosomiasis: male and female *S. japonicum* in lumen of mesenteric vein.

Schistosomiasis japonica in China occurs largely as the result of the wet cultivation of rice. Actually, infection by *S. japonicum* may be regarded as almost an occupational disease of the rice farmers. Irrigation ditches to the rice fields are also important in the epidemiology.

**Pathology**    Schistosomiasis japonica, like schistosomiasis mansoni, may present lesions of the intestine as well as of the liver. A period of incubation is followed by one of egg extrusion which in turn provokes tissue proliferation and repair. In cases of heavy infection, lung lesions may develop during the passage of the parasites through this organ. The stomach and kidneys may also be affected if young parasites break out of the blood vessels and enter the tissues. Congestion of the liver, spleen and duodenum may result during the period when the parasites are maturing (Fig. 232).

As the parasites liberate eggs the characteristic lesions develop.

The intestines, peritoneal serosa and liver show the severest reactions. The small intestine is most extensively involved as a rule, particularly in the ordinary case (Fig. 233). In late chronic cases, however, lesions are frequently encountered from the cecum to the rectum. Many of the appendices epiploicae fuse and the wall becomes irregularly thickened. The mucosa is usually swollen and congested and there are areas of superficial erosion caused by necrosis and sloughing of the mucosal layer. Eggs are abundant in such regions

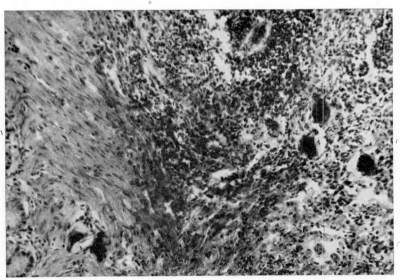

Fig. 233. Schistosomiasis: eggs of *S. japonicum* and inflammatory reaction in wall of intestine.

(Fig. 234). Occasionally fibrous nodules occur on the peritoneal surface, often containing nests of eggs and sometimes showing central necrosis. Various areas of the peritoneum show chronic inflammation. The mesocolon may reveal fibrosis, with eggs appearing singly or in nests, resulting in a hardened and thickened structure. Ectopic lesions consisting of pseudotubercles or granulomas occur occasionally in the central nervous system, particularly in the frontal, parietal and occipital lobes of the cerebrum, frequently giving rise to serious symptoms. Metastatic lesions may likewise be produced in other distant areas such as the skin, the lungs and the myocardium.

Many of the eggs are swept back into the liver; there they break through the walls of the blood vessels and reach the parenchyma where abscesses may be produced. These enlarge and often are encapsulated, forming pseudotubercles. Marked liver damage results from the presence of numerous eggs (Fig. 235). This is followed by connective tissue proliferation and a progressive portal cirrhosis with parallel enlargement of the spleen and the development of ascites.

Leukocytosis with eosinophilia which may reach 30 to 60 per cent is usual during the acute phase. Later anemia, leukopenia and reduction of the eosinophilia occur.

**Clinical Characteristics** The incubation period of approximately one month includes the interval between infection and the onset of symptoms. The early toxic stage of the disease (Yangtze River fever) is ushered in by malaise, anorexia, loss of weight and intermittent or remittent fever which may persist for from one to eight

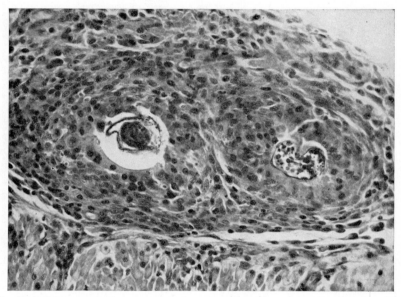

Fig. 234. Schistosomiasis: eggs of *S. japonicum* in subserosal fibrous nodule of intestine.

weeks. Upper abdominal and epigastric pain is common and soreness and stiffness of the neck, myalgic in type, elicited by lateral rotation of the head is very frequent. Harsh unproductive cough is often present. Diarrhea is relatively infrequent in this stage and blood is rarely present in the stools. Urticaria and angioneurotic edema occur in something over half of the cases. In the great majority of instances there is slight to moderate enlargement of the liver, with tenderness on palpation and often splenomegaly. Neurologic symptoms including coma and paralyses occur in approximately 9 per cent of the cases. Sigmoidoscopic examination may show only evidence of congestion of the venules, or may reveal nodules in the mucous membrane. Eggs may frequently be demonstrated by biopsy or aspiration of these areas.

The second stage of the disease coincides with deposition of the eggs in the venous channels of the intestinal wall and is frequently accompanied by profuse dysentery and the discharge of eggs in the stools. During this period embolic phenomena may occur. Fever, toxemia, abdominal pain, and enlargement of the liver and spleen are usual. The acute symptoms commonly terminate within two to three months but recur periodically thereafter.

The final stage, which appears three to five years after infection, is dominated by the clinical picture of progressing hepatic cirrhosis

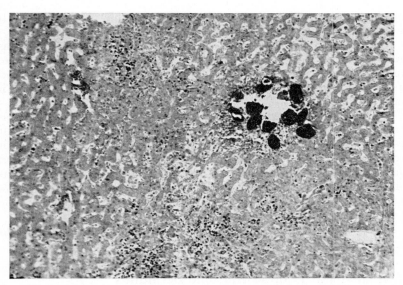

Fig. 235. Schistosomiasis: small abscess in liver containing calcified eggs of *S. japonicum.*

with shrinkage of the liver, enlargement of the spleen and the appearance of ascites. Chronic intestinal symptoms are frequent in response to fibrosis of the wall and chronic ulceration or abscess formation.

In severe infections the prognosis is unfavorable unless treatment is given early.

**Diagnosis** A diagnosis of schistosomiasis japonica can be made upon recovery of characteristic eggs from the stool or lower bowel (Fig. 237, p. 486). The recommended method consists of: (1) The AMS III method (hydrochloric acid–sodium sulfate–Triton–ether concentration technique) for the recovery of eggs from three to five specimens (see p. 822). (2) If the stools are negative, proctoscopic biopsy or aspiration should be attempted. Other methods include sedimentation with washing in 10 per cent alcohol, or sedimentation of screened samples in 0.5 per cent glycerinated water. Sedimentation should not be prolonged beyond four hours, as the eggs soon begin to hatch. A search for miracidia by the inexperienced worker is not recommended, as recognition of species as well as contaminants is difficult. A positive intracutaneous skin (1:10000), or complement fixation test, euglobulin precipitation test, marked eosinophilia, together with the clinical findings and a history of having resided in endemic areas, are all suggestive of schistosomiasis. The differential diagnosis in early cases must include consideration of a variety of acute infections, and urticaria due to other causes. Later various types of dysentery must be distinguished from schistosomiasis japonica, and in advanced cases of cirrhosis of the liver this infection must be considered.

**Treatment**    The intravenous administration of sodium or potassium antimony tartrate is the most effective treatment for schistosomiasis japonica. Fuadin, even when given to the limit of tolerance and in repeated courses, frequently fails. Anthiomaline is useful in some instances.

The serious and not infrequently fatal cerebral complications constitute an imperative indication for the use of tartar emetic intravenously unless the administration of antimony is absolutely contraindicated. This will usually alleviate the central nervous system pathology and should always be used in preference to surgical intervention. Permanent sequelae are twice as common in operated cases as in those receiving one or more courses of tartar emetic. For details of treatment see pp. 541–545.

**Prophylaxis**    Prophylaxis does not differ materially from that described for other schistosomiases.

## "Swimmer's Itch" or Schistosome Dermatitis

Several species of non-human schistosomes are known to penetrate the skin of man and there produce a dermatitis variously designated as "swimmer's itch," "schistosome dermatitis," "sawah itch," or "koganbyo." In the Americas it has been reported from persons bathing in fresh-water lakes from Seattle, Washington, to the east coast, with highly endemic areas in Canada, Minnesota, Wisconsin and Michigan. It has also been reported from Mexico and Colombia. Elsewhere outbreaks have occurred in Wales, Germany, France, Mayala, New Zealand and Japan.

Until recently it was known only from fresh water, but now it has been shown to occur in the coastal waters along the Atlantic seaboard and the Gulf Coast. Schistosome dermatitis producing cercariae have also been reported from the waters off southern California, Lower California and Hawaii.

Dermatitis results from the active penetration of human skin by fork-tailed cercariae of species closely related to, but not identical with, the human schistosomes. In most instances it is believed the parasites are destroyed while they are still in the skin. Characteristic papular lesions are produced, which should not be confused with other types of dermatitis (see p. 404) (Fig. 236). It should be borne

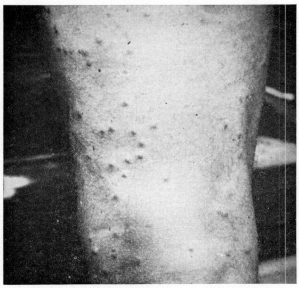

Fig. 236. Schistosome dermatitis—papular eruption on leg. (Courtesy of Dr. D. B. McMullen, Army Medical Service Graduate School.)

in mind that severe reactions occur in persons sensitized through repeated exposures.

Control of the snail host is possible in some areas by treating infested regions with 1 lb. of 10 per cent fresh lime and 2 lbs. of copper sulfate snow per 1000 square feet of bottom.

# 47 Trematodes Exclusive of Schistosomes

## Morphology

**Introduction** The similarity in pattern, structure, and physiology of most trematodes exclusive of the schistosomes, considered on p. 461, warrants their consideration as a group. Despite individual differences in their life cycles these trematodes all gain entrance to man through the digestive tract. Each first parasitizes a snail, then encysts on vegetation or in some aquatic animal, which is ingested by man.

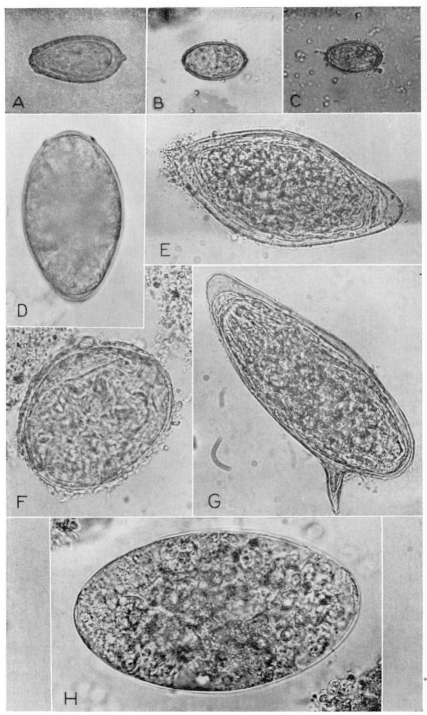

Fig. 237. *See opposite page for legend.*

**Morphology of Adults**   All trematodes of man are nonsegmented, bilaterally symmetrical, and with the exception of the schistosomes, hermaphroditic. As a rule these parasites are leaflike, flattened dorso-ventrally, range in length from a few millimeters to several centi-meters and possess two suckers with which they attach themselves to the mucosa or other tissues of their host. The anterior or *oral sucker* surrounds the mouth while the ventral one or *acetabulum* is merely a holdfast device. The body surface is covered by a thin noncellular cuticle secreted by the underlying cells. In some species this cuticula may be spined.

The *digestive tract* opens through the oral sucker into a muscular *pharynx*, followed by an *esophagus* which bifurcates to form the two lateral *intestinal ceca* or *crura*. In some species, such as *Fasciola hepatica*, the crura may be highly branched. The excretory system has two main lateral ducts which empty into a posterior, terminal *excretory bladder*, which in turn opens externally through an excre-tory pore. The *nervous system* is also bilaterally symmetrical.

The *reproductive systems* are extremely complex. The male system usually consists of two *testes* drained by *vasa efferentia* into a single *vas deferens*. This empties through a ventrally situated *genital pore* near, and usually anterior to, the acetabulum. The terminal portion of the male system is modified to form a muscular copulatory device, or *cirrus*.

The female reproductive system includes a single *ovary* which gives rise to the *oviduct*. The oviduct complex includes a blind *seminal receptacle* which sometimes drains to the exterior through a dorsal *Laurer's canal*, ducts from the laterally situated yolk glands or *vitellaria*, and a *shell gland* which empties into the coiled *uterus*. This latter structure stores the eggs until they are discharged through a genital pore beside that of the male system into the common genital sinus. The lower portion of the uterus serves as a *vagina*. Fertiliza-tion takes place in the oviduct. In rare instances (as in the HETERO-PHYIDAE) the genital pore is surrounded by a muscular sucker-like structure.

**Trematode Eggs**   Eggs of all the trematodes, except those of the schistosomes which are spined or knobbed, possess a lid or *operculum* which opens to allow the ciliated, free-swimming *miracidium* to emerge. As a rule the eggs, when passed in a stool, are undeveloped, containing only the fertilized zygote and a yolk mass. However, in

---

Fig. 237. Some trematode eggs: *A*, Chinese liver fluke, *Clonorchis sinensis. B*, *Heterophyes heterophyes. C*, *Metagonimus yokogawai. D*, Lung fluke, *Paragonimus westermani. E*, Vesical blood fluke, *Schistosoma haematobium. F*, Oriental blood fluke, *Schistosoma japonicum. G*, Manson's blood fluke, *Schistosoma mansoni. H*, Large intestinal fluke, *Fasciolopsis buski.* All figures 500× except *A*, which is 830×. (Fig. *A* courtesy of Dr. E. C. Faust, in Brenemann: Practice of Pediatrics, W. F. Prior Co. Figs. *B* and *C* courtesy of Lt. L. W. Shatterly, MSC, School of Aviation Medicine, Gunter AFB, Alabama. All others courtesy of Dr. R. L. Rouda-bush, Ward's Natural Science Establishment, Rochester, New York; photos by T. Romaniak.)

some species such as *Clonorchis* and *Heterophyes*, each egg contains a fully developed miracidium when evacuated by the host (Fig. 237).

**Group Characteristics**   Because of the morphologic similarity displayed by the various trematodes a brief summary of their group characteristics may prove more useful than a key.

Members of the FASCIOLIDAE infecting man are large trematodes averaging more than 25 mm. in length and producing eggs 150 by 90 microns; their cercariae encyst on vegetation. In members of the genus *Fasciola* (*F. hepatica* and *F. gigantica*) the dendritic testes are arranged in tandem; these, together with the intestinal ceca and vitellaria, are profusely branched, almost entirely filling the posterior two-thirds of the worm with their ramifications.

*Fasciolopsis buski*, which bears a superficial resemblance to *F. hepatica*, belongs in a different taxonomic subdivision of the FASCIOLIDAE. *Fasciolopsis buski* possesses dendritic testes, but has straight, unbranched intestinal crura. The eggs of the FASCIOLIDAE are undeveloped when laid and are approximately the same size. However, the operculum on the ovum of *Fasciolopsis buski* is smaller than that on the egg of *F. hepatica*.

The HETEROPHYIDAE are all small, ovoidal, pyriform or elongate trematodes. They are intestinal parasites which produce minute, embryonated eggs. The chief human representatives of this family are *Heterophyes heterophyes* and *Metagonimus yokogawai*.

*Clonorchis sinensis*, the Oriental liver fluke, is classified in the OPISTHORCHIIDAE which includes also other liver flukes of carnivores. This slender trematode of man ranges between 18 and 40 mm. in length. It is further characterized by the dendritic testes arranged posteriorly in tandem and by the unbranched intestinal crura which extend to the posterior tip of the worm. Another member of the OPISTHORCHIIDAE, *Opisthorchis felineus*, is reported from man.

The Oriental lung fluke, *Paragonimus westermani*, of the family TROGLOTREMATIDAE, is thicker than the others, broader and more generally ovoid. While the intestinal crura are straight, the lobate testes are roughly opposite one another in the posterior third of the body. The ovary is in the mid-region and to one side of the acetabulum. The American species, *P. kellicotti*, is believed by some workers to be identical with *P. westermani* which, if true, would indicate that this fluke is well established in the mammals of North America.

Other parasites of man which might be encountered in some areas include the spiny-collared or echinostome group and *Gastrodiscoides hominis*.

## Generalized Cycle

**Oviposition**   The trematodes mentioned above have similar life cycles. The eggs are discharged in the feces except those of *Paragonimus westermani* the majority of which are eliminated in the sputum, the remainder being passed in the stool. All the eggs are undeveloped when laid except those of *Clonorchis sinensis, Heterophyes* spp., *Metagonimus yokogawai* and *Opisthorchis felineus,* which contain ciliated embryos. All must reach water and, in the case of undeveloped eggs, must undergo a period of growth before hatching of the miracidium.

**The Snail Host**   Eggs or hatched miracidia must reach a specific snail host within a given period if the parasite is to survive. In the tissues of this host the miracidium becomes transformed into a *mother sporocyst* which then produces *rediae* and in some cases *daughter rediae.* Finally free-living *cercariae* develop and emerge;

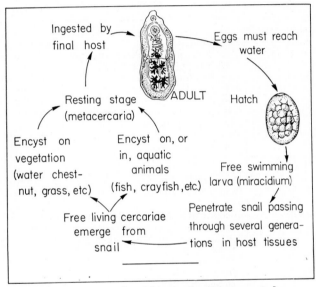

Fig. 238. Life cycle of hermaphroditic trematodes.

these, in turn, must reach a suitable plant or animal host if they are to survive.

**The Resting or Metacercarial Stage**   Encystment occurs if the liberated cercariae are successful in reaching a suitable resting place. In cases when cercariae penetrate tissues of such hosts as fish or crustacea there is a marked host reaction. Typically, all encysting cercariae produce an inner cyst wall from secretions of their own cystogenous glands, which is soon surrounded by an outer cyst wall of host tissue. After varying intervals of time a reorganization or growth of these larvae leads to the formation of resting stages, or *metacercariae,* which soon are ready to infect man (Fig. 238).

The cercariae of *Fasciola hepatica* seek various grasses, while those of *Fasciolopsis buski* encyst on water chestnuts, caltrops, hyacinths and the like. In the case of the liver fluke, *Clonorchis sinensis,* and the intestinal flukes, *Heterophyes heterophyes* and *Metagonimus yokogawai,* the cercariae seek certain species of fish and most of them penetrate beneath their scales and reach the musculature before encysting. The cercariae of the lung fluke, *Paragonimus westermani,* enter fresh-water crabs and crayfishes and encyst throughout their bodies.

**The Final Host**    In all cases, infection of man results from the ingestion of raw or inadequately cooked vegetation, fish or crustaceans

*Table 42    Reservoirs of the Intestinal, Liver and Lung Trematodes*

| SPECIES OF TREMATODE | HOSTS | TYPICAL LOCATION IN HOST |
|---|---|---|
| Intestinal Flukes | | |
| *Fasciolopsis buski* | Pig and man | Duodenum, jejunum |
| *Echinostoma ilocanum* | Dogs, cats, rats, monkeys and man | Small intestine |
| *Echinochasmus perfoliatus* | Dogs, cats, pigs, fox and man | Small intestine |
| *Heterophyes heterophyes* | Cat, dog, fox and man | Small intestine |
| *H. katsuradai* | Man | Small intestine |
| *H. brevicaeca* | Man | Small intestine |
| *Metagonimus yokogawai* | Cats, dogs, pigs, mice (experimental infection), pelicans and man | Small intestine |
| *Gastrodiscoides hominis* | Pigs, "mouse deer" (*Tragulus napu*), man | Cecum and colon |
| Liver Flukes | | |
| *Clonorchis sinensis* | Dogs, cats and man | Biliary passages |
| *Opisthorchis felineus* | Dogs, cats and man | Biliary and pancreatic passages |
| *Fasciola hepatica* | Sheep, cattle and other herbivores, and man | Liver and biliary passages |
| *F. gigantica* | Cattle, water buffalo, other herbivores, man | Biliary passages |
| *Dicrocoelium dendriticum* | Cattle, goats, horses, donkeys, deer, hares, rabbits, pigs, dogs, coypu, camels and man | Biliary passages |
| Lung Flukes | | |
| *Paragonimus westermani* | Tigers, cats, wild cats, panthers, foxes, wolves, dogs, rats, pigs, weasel (*Mustela melampus*), *Lutreola itatsi itatsi,* pencilled cat (*Nyctereutes procyonides*) and man | Lungs |
| *P. kellicotti* | Mink, pigs, dogs, muskrats, cats, wild cats, goats and man | Lungs |

which serve as the "transfer agents" or intermediate hosts for these parasites.

LOCATION IN MAN. *Fasciolopsis buski, Heterophyes heterophyes, Metagonimus yokogawai* and *Echinostoma ilocanum* are intestinal parasites of man. *Clonorchis sinensis, F. hepatica, Opisthorchis felineus* and *Dicrocoelium dendriticum* localize in the bile ducts, while *P. westermani* after migrating through the body usually reaches the lungs where it becomes encapsulated.

Many mammals other than man serve as reservoir hosts for the intestinal, lung and liver flukes. These are summarized in Table 42.

## Diseases Caused by Intestinal Trematodes

### Fasciolopsiasis

**Synonym** *Fasciolopsis buski* infection.

**Definition** Fasciolopsiasis is due to the presence of the giant intestinal fluke, *F. buski*, in the duodenum or jejunum, and more rarely in the pylorus or the colon of man. The parasites may produce local areas of inflammation and sometimes ulceration and hemorrhage.

**Distribution** *Fasciolopsis buski* occurs commonly in pigs and man in certain areas of eastern Asia, particularly in Central and South China, extending as far north as the Yangtze Valley. It is highly endemic in the Chinese provinces of Kwangtung and Chekiang. The disease has also been reported in French Indo-China, India, Siam, Assam and the neighboring Malay archipelago and Sumatra.

**Etiology** MORPHOLOGY. *Fasciolopsis buski* (Lankester 1857) Odhner 1902, the large intestinal fluke, measures 50 to 75 mm. in length when extended. It is fleshy, often broadly ovate and possesses a spined integument. A cephalic cone such as occurs in the genus *Fasciola* is lacking although the oral sucker and ventral sucker (acetabulum) are close together (see p. 493). The latter is about four times as large as the oral sucker and measures 2 to 3 mm. in diameter. The intestinal ceca are unbranched and the dendritic testes lie in the posterior half of the body arranged in tandem.

DEVELOPMENT. Although the adult parasite produces eggs ranging from 67 by 43 to 181 by 95 microns the majority are large eggs measuring between 130 and 140 microns in length and 80 and 85 microns in breadth. These are undeveloped when passed and are capped by a small operculum. Upon reaching quiet fresh water the egg develops a miracidium in three to seven weeks. After hatching, the miracidium must reach a snail of the genus *Hippeutis* or *Segmentina*, which it penetrates. It then transforms into a mother sporocyst; this in turn produces two generations of rediae. The daughter rediae produce free-living cercariae thirty to fifty days after the miracidium has penetrated the snail.

The cercariae encyst on almost any aquatic plant although water caltrops, hyacinths, chestnuts and bamboos usually serve as "transfer hosts." As many as 1000 metacercariae have been found on a single nut or root. The metacercariae are very resistant and will survive for a year or more if kept moist; desiccation, however, soon destroys them. When an infected root or bulb is eaten and the metacercariae are ingested by the definitive hosts, the parasites excyst in the intestine and develop into mature flukes within a month.

**Epidemiology** Infection by *F. buski* results from the ingestion of viable metacercariae on the uncooked stems, bulbs, or fruits of edible water plants. The more important plants and the areas where they are particularly important appear in Table 43.

The red water caltrop, *T. natans*, is probably the most heavily infested since it is cultivated for market in artificial ponds fertilized by nightsoil or by defecation directly into the water. The plants growing wild in the canals and rivers are less heavily infested. Both the water caltrops and so-called water chestnuts are sold fresh in the Chinese markets during the summer months and it is then that man becomes infected. It is a common practice to peel off the external covering with the teeth and eat the succulent inner parts raw. Many

*Table 43    Species of Plants Carrying* Fasciolopsis buski
*Listed by Countries*

| COUNTRY | SPECIES OF PLANT |
|---|---|
| China | |
| Chekian Prov. | Red water caltrop, *Trapa natans* |
| Kwangtung Prov. to Yangtze R., South China | Water chestnut, *Eliocharis tuberosa* |
| India | Water caltrop, *Trapa bicornis* |
| Formosa | Water caltrop, *Trapa bispinosa* |
| | Water chestnut, *Eliocharis tuberosa* |
| | Water hyacinth, *Eichhornia crassipes* |

metacercarial cysts may be ingested in this way. Since desiccation destroys the parasites only fresh plants are dangerous and infection is less frequent when these have been allowed to dry. However, in the markets, vendors of caltrops and nuts often maintain the freshness of their wares by sprinkling them with water, a custom which prevents the drying of the cysts (Fig. 239).

Many different species of snails serve as first intermediate hosts for *F. buski*, the principal ones being *Segmentina hemisphaerula* and *Hippeutis schmackeri* (= *S. umbilicalis*). As developmental stages have been found in *Hippeutis cantori* and *Gyraulus saigonemis*, it is possible that these should be added to the above list.

**Pathology**    The parasites are usually attached to the mucosa of the duodenum or jejunum; less often they are found in the region of the pylorus or in the colon. Localized inflammation followed frequently by ulceration occurs at the site of attachment and when deep erosions are produced hemorrhage may occur. As many as 3721 adult specimens have been recovered from one patient at autopsy and more than 10,000 by anthelmintic medication. The metabolic prod-

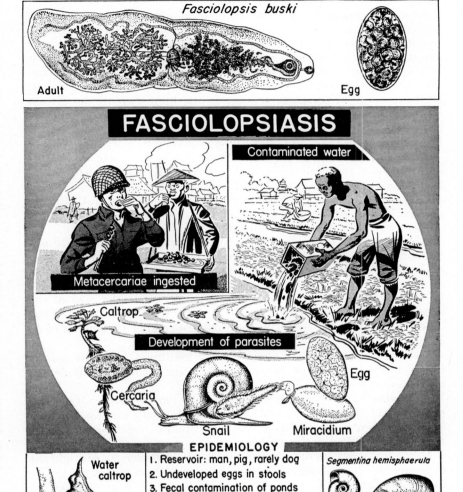

Fig. 239. Epidemiology of fasciolopsiasis.

ucts of the worm are probably toxic and capable of being absorbed by the host. Many patients show a leukocytosis with an eosinophilia up to 34 per cent; in others there may be a lymphocytosis.

**Clinical Characteristics**    The incubation period of fasciolopsiasis lasts thirty to forty days. In cases of light infection it may be asymptomatic or there may be diarrhea and abdominal pain which may simulate duodenal ulcer. The diarrhea often alternates with periods of constipation. Later the stools become greenish yellow and contain much undigested food while ascites, anorexia, nausea and vomiting may occur in severe infections. In the final stage of the disease edema of the face, abdominal wall or lower extremities usually appears. The skin becomes dry and death occurs from cachexia or intercurrent disease.

**Diagnosis**    The clinical picture is not distinctive; hence diagnosis depends upon recovery and identification of the adult worm passed in the feces or demonstration of the eggs in the stool.

The adult may be confused with *Fasciola hepatica* and *Fasciola gigantica* from which it is distinguished by lack of a cephalic cone, suckers of unequal size and unbranched intestinal crura.

The eggs of *F. buski* are large, ranging between 130 and 140 microns in length by 80 to 85 microns in breadth. They may be differentiated with difficulty from the eggs of *Fasciola hepatica* by means of the smaller operculum on the former. Eggs of *F. buski* can usually be distinguished from those of *Fasciola gigantica* as the eggs of the latter are longer, ranging from 160 to 190 microns in length. Most other operculate eggs found in the stool are smaller than those of *F. buski*.

**Treatment**    The drug of choice in the treatment of fasciolopsiasis is Crystoids anthelmintic administered as for ascariasis. For details of treatment see p. 545.

**Prophylaxis**    Prophylaxis is based upon two measures: (1) The proper cooking of all roots and "nuts" which might serve as possible "transfer agents" for *F. buski*. (2) Education of foreigners to avoid sampling uncooked native dishes.

Other measures include sufficiently prolonged storage of nightsoil to insure the destruction of eggs, and the education of natives in the use of privies.

### Heterophyiasis

**Definition**    Heterophyiasis is an infection by the minute intestinal fluke, *Heterophyes heterophyes* (v. Siebold 1852) Stiles and Hassall 1900, in the small intestine of man.

**Distribution**    It is common in the Nile Delta and in Japan, southern Korea, Formosa, Central and South China and the Philippines.

**Morphology**    The parasites are small, less than 2 mm. in length.

**Pathology**    They live attached to the mucosa of the small intestine where they may produce a mild irritation or a superficial necrosis of the mucosa. Eggs may be deposited in the tissues and because of their minute size be carried by the blood stream to other areas, especially the brain, the spinal cord and the heart muscle.

**Clinical Characteristics** Symptoms include abdominal pain frequently associated with mucous diarrhea. When eggs are distributed by the blood stream serious clinical disease may result with evidence of organic changes in the central nervous system and often cardiac insufficiency.

**Diagnosis** Diagnosis is based upon the recovery from the stool of characteristics eggs, which are difficult to differentiate from those of other heterophyid trematodes (see p. 822). They are small, operculate, ovoid, light brown in color and measure 29 by 16 microns.

Transmission of the disease occurs through the eating of raw or salted fish containing the infective metacercariae. In Egypt, the first intermediate snail host is *Pirenella conica* Blainville; in Japan it is *Cerithidea cingulata microptera* Kiener.

A second species, *H. katsuradai* Ozaki and Asada 1925, has been recovered from patients suffering from diarrhea in Japan. The parasite is distinguished from *H. heterophyes* by its relatively enormous acetabulum. The eggs are slightly smaller, measuring 25 to 26 by 14 to 15 microns. Transmission occurs by the eating of infected raw mullet flesh.

A third species, *H. brevicaeca* Africa and Garcia 1935, was reported from man in the Philippines. In some cases heart lesions in man have been caused by the liberation of eggs of the heterophyids into the blood stream.

**Treatment** Tetrachloroethylene as for hookworm, or treat as for fasciolopsiasis (see pp. 545, 552).

## Metagonimiasis

Metagonimiasis is due to the presence of a small trematode, *Metagonimus yokagawai* Katsurada 1912, attached to the intestinal mucosa of man. Other animals such as dogs, cats, pigs, mice and pelicans may serve as reservoir hosts. It is believed to be the most common heterophyid fluke of man in the Far East, being found in parts of China, Japan, the Maritime Provinces of the U.S.S.R. and the northern provinces in Siberia. It also occurs in man in Spain and various Balkan states. The parasite is small, usually less than 3 mm. in length, and resembles *H. heterophyes* in size and shape, but differs in morphologic details. Infection is acquired when the flesh of improperly cooked oriental fresh-water trout or other fresh-water fishes is ingested. The most common intermediate snail hosts of *Metagonimus* in the Orient are *Thiara granifera* Lamarck, *Semisulcospira libertina* Gould and *S. amurensis* Gerstfeld.

**Pathology** These flukes may actually invade the intestinal mucosa, producing inflammation and occasionally ulceration; they ultimately become encapsulated. Rarely eggs deposited in the tissues may be carried by the blood stream and deposited in other regions.

Infection by this parasite usually causes few symptoms. In heavy infections, however, especially when eggs have lodged in other tissues, serious disease may result. The clinical picture in such instances will vary in accordance with the distribution and severity of the pathologic changes.

**Diagnosis** The diagnosis is based upon the recovery from feces of characteristic eggs, which are similar to those of *Clonorchis sinensis* and are almost indistinguishable from those of *H. heterophyes*. They contain a fully developed embryo when passed in the stool and measure 26.5 to 28.0 microns by 15.5 to 17 microns.

**Treatment** Treat as for heterophyiasis (see pp. 545, 552).

## Echinostomiasis

Echinostomiasis is a general term applied to infection by several related genera and species of spiny-collared flukes which parasitize man. Their distribution is limited to the Philippines, Indonesia, Assam and Japan.

About ten species have been reported from man, of which *Echinostoma ilocanum* from the Philippines and Java, *E. lindoensis* from Celebes, and *E. perfoliatus* from Japan are among the more important. Although varying in size and morphologic details, all members of the group are slender and flattened, the majority measuring less than 25 mm. in length. Identification is based on morphologic characteristics, especially the arrangement and number of spines comprising the collar and the size of the eggs. Infection is acquired by eating raw, or improperly cooked, fresh-water snails and clams, many of which serve as the second intermediate host; these snails belong to such genera as *Pila, Gyraulus, Lymnaea* and *Thiara*.

**Pathology** The echinostomes are found attached to the mucosa of the small intestine and their presence ordinarily does not appear to be associated with marked pathologic changes. Heavy infections, however, may be accompanied by abdominal pain and diarrhea. This infection has not been thoroughly studied.

**Diagnosis** Diagnosis depends upon demonstration of the eggs in stools from the infected individual. Echinostome infections may be differentiated from fascioliasis and fasciolopsiasis by the size of the egg since echinostomes have smaller eggs.

**Treatment** The following drugs are recommended for the treatment of echinostomiasis: oleoresin of aspidium for *E. ilocanum;* tetrachloroethylene for *E. lindoensis;* although no drug is known for *E. perfoliatus* it appears probable that Crystoids anthelmintic would prove to be efficacious (p. 545).

## Gastrodisciasis

Gastrodisciasis is an infection by the trematode *Gastrodiscoides hominis* (Lewis and McConnel 1876) Fischoeder 1902 in the cecum and ascending colon of man. It has been reported from India, China and the Malay states and is a relatively common parasite of man in Assam. The pig appears to be the common reservoir host.

**Diagnosis**  The parasite may be identified readily by its pyriform shape, reddish orange color and huge acetabulum which occupies the ventral posterior portion of the worm. The acetabulum bears a characteristic notch at its posterior extremity. Parasites range from 5 by 4 mm. to 10 by 6 mm. in size with a conical anterior portion about 2 mm. in length. The eggs are ovoidal, immature when passed and measure about 150 by 65 microns in length and breadth respectively.

**Clinical Characteristics**  Infection of man by this parasite is associated with diarrhea but other details of the clinical picture are unknown.

**Treatment**  Treat as for heterophyiasis (see pp. 545, 552).

## Diseases Caused by Liver Flukes

### Clonorchiasis

**Synonym**  Chinese liver fluke disease.

**Definition**  Clonorchiasis is caused by the presence of the Oriental liver fluke, *Clonorchis sinensis,* in the biliary passages. It may be associated with proliferation of the biliary epithelium, connective tissue hyperplasia and, in severe cases, fatty degeneration and cirrhosis of the liver.

**Distribution**  This fluke occurs in the Far East as a common parasite of fish-eating mammals. The highly endemic regions of human infection are Japan, Korea, China and French Indo-China. Clonorchiasis is especially important in Okayama Prefecture in Japan, Southern Korea, Kwangtung Province in South China and the Red River Delta in Tonkin, French Indo-China (Fig. 240). Infection by this parasite has been recorded likewise in Chinese inhabitants of the United States, Cuba, India and in native Hawaiians.

**Etiology**  MORPHOLOGY. *Clonorchis sinensis* (Cobbold 1875) Looss 1907 is a slender, attenuated trematode ranging from 10 to 25 mm. in length and 3 to 5 mm. in breadth. The oral sucker is clearly larger than the ventral, or acetabular sucker. Unstained specimens of *Clonorchis sinensis* placed between two slides and held to a strong light reveal the characteristic deeply lobulated testes lying in tandem in the posterior third of the worm. Anterior to the testes is the ovarian complex, while the uterine mass, typically appearing brown due to the presence of numerous eggs, fills the middle third of the worm. Laterally in the same region lie the vitellaria.

DEVELOPMENT. The operculate eggs of *C. sinensis* contain fully developed miracidia and are among the smallest passed by man. The eggs measure 27 to 35 microns in length, appear light brown and are ovoid in shape. The edge of the convex operculum or lid fits down into a swollen lip which surrounds the lid, this portion of the shell

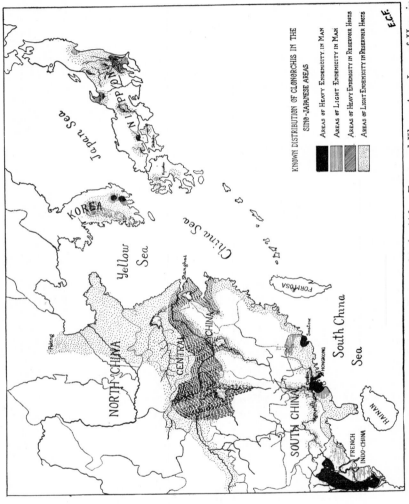

Fig. 240. Geographical distribution of clonorchiasis. (After Faust and Khaw, Am. Jour. of Hyg. in Faust: Human Helminthology, Lea & Febiger.)

being markedly "shouldered." There is also a definite knob or boss at the anopercular end.

The eggs, laid in the smaller bile passages, are carried down the common bile duct to the duodenum and passed in the stools. The eggs must reach water and are believed to hatch when ingested by appropriate species of snails: *Parafossarulus manchouricus* (= *P. striatulus*), *Bulimus fuchsianus, Alocinma longicornis* (= *Bythnia longicornis*) and *Hua ningpoensis*. Development within the snail requires four to five weeks and includes the production of mother sporocysts, followed by a generation of rediae. At the end of this interval typical lophocercous (tail with fin-holds) cercariae break out of the rediae and emerge from the snail. These cercariae penetrate beneath the scales and into the musculature of fresh-water fish where, after a developmental period of several weeks, they produce cysts which are infective for the definitive host.

After ingestion by man or other suitable mammalian host the cysts in the fish muscle are digested and the contained parasites are released in the duodenum where they become attached to the mucosa. They soon migrate through the papilla of Vater into the common bile duct and then into the smaller biliary radicles, especially those of the left lobe of the liver. The entire cycle requires approximately three months.

**Epidemiology**    *Clonorchis sinensis* is found principally in the bile passages of dogs, cats and man, although other fish-eating mammals may be infected. The infective or metacercarial stage occurs in the musculature of over forty species of fresh-water fish belonging to the Cyprinidae, Gobiidae, Anabantidae and Salmonidae. Fish ponds or canals in China are often the chief source of human infection. These pondlike areas are filled with water much of the time and consequently afford ideal habitats for snails and fish serving as intermediate hosts for this parasite. Man acquires the infection from the ingestion of raw, inadequately cooked, or even from dried, salted or pickled flesh of infected fresh-water fish (Fig. 241).

It appears likely that Hawaiians become infected through shipments of infected frozen, dried or pickled fish from China or Japan.

**Pathology**    Adult *C. sinensis* tend to localize in the distal bile passages, especially those of the left lobe of the liver, since passage to this lobe is more direct. One result of infection is proliferation, sometimes desquamation, of the biliary epithelium, while in the larger ducts progressive dilatation, thickening of the wall and crypt formation occur. It is believed by some workers that toxic secretions of the parasite may be responsible for some of the pathologic changes which are found in ducts too small for the worm to penetrate. Liver damage, however, depends upon the number of parasites present, the age of the infection and the number of reinfections that have occurred. In endemic areas surprisingly large numbers of parasites have been found at autopsy, as many as 21,000 having been recovered from a single individual.

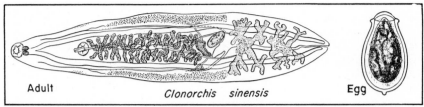

Adult      *Clonorchis sinensis*      Egg

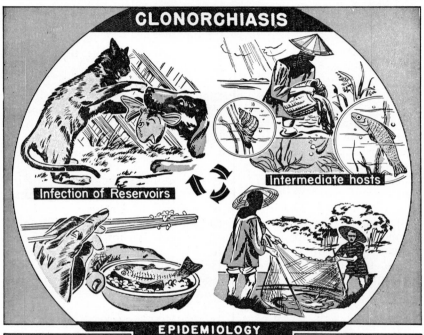

## CLONORCHIASIS

Infection of Reservoirs

Intermediate hosts

### EPIDEMIOLOGY

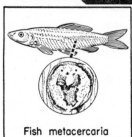

Fish metacercaria

1. Reservoir: man, dog, cat
2. Intermediate hosts: certain fresh-water snails & fish
3. Eggs from feces infect snail
4. Cercariae from snail infect fish
5. Metacercariae in muscles of fish
6. Raw fish ingested by man, dog, cat
7. Parasites localize in bile ducts

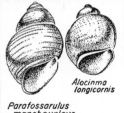

*Alocinma longicornis*

*Parafossarulus manchouricus*
**Snail hosts**

Fig. 241. Epidemiology of clonorchiasis.

Frank cirrhosis is rare although increase of periportal tissue in varying degree and infiltration with eosinophils often occur. In the parenchyma fatty changes in the liver cells and atrophy of cells in the center of the lobule are not unusual. Even in light infections significant histologic changes are usually present in the liver (Fig. 242).

**Clinical Characteristics** Three typical stages in the development of clonorchiasis are recognized. (1) Early stages of the disease are mild and asymptomatic, even though histologic changes in the liver

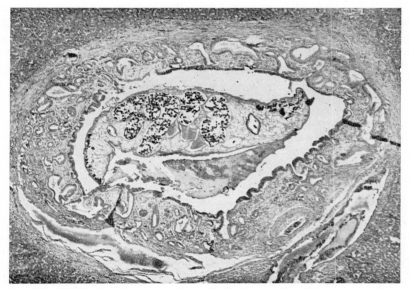

Fig. 242. *Clonorchis sinensis* in dilated biliary duct: adult with eggs in uterus.

may be taking place. (2) The second stage is characterized by edema, diarrhea and progressive hepatomegaly. (3) The most advanced cases are associated with cirrhosis of the liver, anasarca, cachexia and occasionally extreme jaundice.

It should be borne in mind, however, that in endemic areas the majority of infected individuals harbor few worms and do not show significant symptoms.

Prognosis is good in cases of light infections. Patients rarely die from this disease alone; death, however, may occur in heavy infections of long standing when the parasites have caused serious impairment of liver function.

**Diagnosis** Diagnosis depends upon the detection of the characteristic eggs in the feces, or in bile or fluid obtained by a duodenal intubation. Differentiation from eggs of closely related heterophyid flukes, especially those of *Metagonimus yokagawai* and *H. heterophyes*, is necessary. Eggs of *M. yokogawai* are yellowish in color and lighter than those of *H. heterophyes*, the lighter color being due to the thinner shell. The eggs of *C. sinensis* become narrower toward the operculate end and the shell is more distinctly "shouldered" where the operculum occurs (Fig. 237, p. 486). Eggs of *Opisthorchis felineus* are elongate, ovoidal and about three times as long as broad. Adults must be distinguished from the broader, heavier, more ovate members of the *Fasciola* group.

At autopsy the bile ducts should be examined carefully for the presence of this and other parasites of the biliary passages and liver proper.

**Treatment**   Gentian violet medicinal administered orally in 1½ hour enteric coated tablets is clonorchicidal and is the drug of choice. It is believed to be curative in early infections and may be beneficial even in advanced cases. Sodium antimony tartrate administered intravenously tends to reduce the number of worms in the bile passages (see pp. 545, 547).

**Prophylaxis**   The prevention of clonorchiasis in persons occupying an endemic area can be accomplished effectively by insistence upon the thorough cooking of all fresh-water fish. Foreigners should be discouraged from sampling native dishes. Other measures include the storage and treatment of nightsoil with ammonium sulfate, and the education of the population to use privies.

## Opisthorchiasis

This disease is due to the presence of the trematode, *Opisthorchis felineus* (Rivolta 1884) Blanchard 1895, in the bile ducts of man.

**Distribution**   The parasite occurs frequently in cats and dogs in central and western Europe and is the common trematode infection of man in Prussia and in parts of Siberia. It also has been reported from man in India, Japan and French Indo-China and is believed to be present in other areas of the Far East.

**Etiology**   MORPHOLOGY. *Opisthorchis felineus* resembles *C. sinensis* in general shape and arrangement of the organ systems. It is a slender worm measuring 7 to 12 mm. in length and 2 to 3 mm. in breadth, tapering anteriorly and rounded posteriorly. The oral sucker and acetabulum are about of equal size (250 microns), whereas in *C. sinensis* the oral sucker is the larger. In *O. felineus* the testes are lobate and arranged obliquely while in *C. sinensis* they are more deeply lobed and are arranged in tandem. The small, elongate, ovoidal eggs are roughly three times as long as broad (measuring about 30 by 11 microns) and contain a miracidium when the egg is laid. The operculum fits into a thickened rim of the shell; eggs may be distinguished from those of *C. sinensis* by their smaller diameter and less pronounced shouldering at the margin of the operculum.

The eggs are believed to be ingested by the snail *Bulimus tentaculatus*, where they hatch and develop, producing lophocercous cercariae in about two months. These penetrate several fresh-water cyprinoid fish, which after a suitable developmental period for the metacercariae are infective for man and other hosts when their raw infected flesh is ingested.

**Pathology and Clinical Aspects** The pathology and clinical aspects of opisthorchiasis are not thoroughly understood although in general they resemble those of clonorchiasis. The degree of damage to the liver and bile ducts depends upon the mass and duration of the infection. Local injury may be expected in the distal bile capillaries and surrounding liver tissue when large numbers (several hundred) are present. In severe infections and in heavy and long continued reinfection, painful enlargement of the liver, jaundice and congestion of the spleen are not uncommon. In such cases invasion of the pancreas may occur.

**Treatment** is similar to that of clonorchiasis (see pp. 545, 547).

### Fascioliasis

**Synonyms** Fascioliasis hepatica, "liver rot," or sheep liver fluke disease.

**Definition** Fascioliasis is a disease caused by the presence of the sheep liver fluke, *Fasciola hepatica*, in the bile ducts or liver paren-

*Table 44 Distribution of Fascioliasis in Man by Countries*

| Africa | Europe | South America |
|---|---|---|
| Algeria | Corsica | Argentina |
| French Somaliland | France | Chile |
| | Hungary | Venezuela |
| Asia | Italy | |
| China | Rumania | West Indies |
| Turkestan | Salonika | Cuba |
| | U.S.S.R. | Puerto Rico |
| Asia Minor | Scotland | |
| Syria | | |
| Turkey (especially near the Dardanelles) | | |
| Australia | | |
| Queensland | | |

chyma. The disease is characterized by hyperplasia of the biliary epithelium, dilatation of biliary passages, leukocytic infiltration and periductal fibrosis. The disease is one essentially of sheep in which it produces "liver rot." Man is occasionally infected.

**Distribution** *Fasciola hepatica* is widely distributed in sheep throughout the world wherever the proper snail host is present (see Table 44).

**Etiology** MORPHOLOGY. *Fasciola hepatica* Linneaus 1758 is a large, brownish, flat fluke measuring about 25 mm. in length and

13 mm. in breadth. The integument of the anterior portion of the worm is covered with scalelike spines. A cephalic cone extends 4 to 5 mm. anteriorly, beyond the ovoid body proper. Oral and ventral suckers measuring 1 and 1.6 mm. in diameter, lie at the distal and basal portions of the cone respectively. Posteriorly this parasite is broadly pointed. Nearly all organs, especially the testes, vitellaria, ovary and the two main intestinal crura, are highly branched and widely distributed throughout the parenchyma. In adult specimens the uterus, which is confined to the anterior third of the worm, is filled with large operculate eggs usually a light brown color, ranging between 130 and 150 microns in length and 63 to 90 microns in breadth; they are undeveloped when deposited.

DEVELOPMENT. The eggs, which must reach water after leaving the host, require a developmental period of nine to fifteen days. Undeveloped eggs remain viable in moist feces up to nine months. Upon hatching, the miracidia may penetrate many different species of snails where each parasite becomes a mother sporocyst. The next generations are known as rediae and daughter rediae respectively. The latter produce free-living cercariae which emerge from the snail about thirty days after penetration by the miracidium and encyst upon aquatic vegetation, debris, or even free in shallow water to become metacercariae. In the absence of freezing or desiccation, the cysts remain viable for months.

Upon ingestion by the final host the parasites excyst in the intestine and migrate through the intestinal wall. Some reach the liver by the hepatic portal circulation; others pass into the peritoneal cavity and penetrate the liver capsule, ultimately reaching the bile ducts where they mature. Adult parasites have survived three years in rabbits and at least five years in sheep.

**Epidemiology** Numerous ruminants, especially sheep, goats, cattle, horses and camels, as well as some carnivores such as dogs, may harbor the adult *F. hepatica*. Numerous snails including species of *Lymnaea* of the subgenera *Pseudosuccinae* and *Fossaria*, also the genera *Bulinus*, *Succinea*, *Praticolella* and *Ampullaria* serve as intermediate molluscan hosts. The infective, or metacercarial, stage is so readily acquired in endemic areas through the ingestion of vegetation, such as water cress and possibly water containing the cysts, that infections of many host species including man occur.

Fascioliasis is geographically widespread. The parasite does not require large bodies of water for its development. Consequently pasture land with small or temporary ponds and sluggish brooks are a frequent source of infection. Three factors are concerned primarily in the epidemiology of fascioliasis: (1) Many different species of snails may serve as the initial host. (2) Almost any green vegetation furnishes the necessary surface upon which the cercariae may encyst. (3) The feeding proclivities of sheep and cattle make them ideal reservoir hosts.

**Pathology** Infection of sheep by *F. hepatica* is characterized by extensive liver damage. Fascioliasis of man is usually a mild disease, although in the rare case of heavy infection the biliary passages are the site of hyperplasia, necrosis and cystic dilatation accompanied by leukocytic infiltration. The young larvae usually enter the liver from the peritoneal cavity by penetration of the capsule. In subsequent migrations they destroy liver parenchyma and produce more or less extensive necrosis and fibrosis. In very heavy infections the parasites may wander back into the liver parenchyma to deposit their eggs, causing additional liver damage and fibrosis. Eosinophilia as high as 68 per cent has been recorded (Fig. 243).

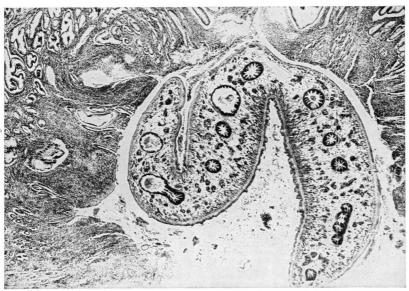

Fig. 243. *Fasciola hepatica* in biliary duct—note marked proliferation of bile ducts.

**Clinical Characteristics**    The symptoms include vomiting, coughing and generalized abdominal pain. Occasionally jaundice, urticaria, diarrhea, and irregular fever are present. A pharyngeal type of fascioliasis is known among the peoples of the Lebanon region of Syria owing to the ingestion of infected raw livers of sacrificial goats and sheep. In such cases the worms often are lodged on the mucosa of the pharynx. These exotic infections result in dyspnea, dysphagia or deafness.

**Diagnosis**    Diagnosis depends upon finding the large operculate eggs, 130 to 150 microns in length, in the feces or in material obtained by duodenal or biliary drainage. False diagnoses may be made in areas where infected livers are eaten raw. In such instances eggs from these livers appear in the stools after passing through the intestinal tract. A differential diagnosis can be made by placing the patient on a liver-free diet for a few days. If eggs continue to be passed, the infection is genuine.

Infections by *F. hepatica* must be differentiated from those caused by other worms (both liver and intestinal) as well as other liver ailments accompanied by jaundice and hepatomegaly. Eosinophilia is suggestive.

The liver and its ducts should be examined carefully at postmortem for the presence of this and other liver inhabiting parasites.

**Treatment**   Intramuscular injections of emetine hydrochloride have been recommended in fascioliasis. For details of dosage see p. 556.

**Prophylaxis**   Drainage of pastures and perhaps the elimination of the snail host through the use of derris, copper sulfate or some other molluscicides may control this disease in limited areas. In regions where sheep livers are eaten they should be thoroughly cooked before being consumed.

### Fascioliasis Gigantica

Fascioliasis gigantica is due to the presence of the giant liver fluke. *Fasciola gigantica* Cobbold 1856, in the liver tissues and ducts of man. Human infections have been reported occasionally from Africa and Asia. The fluke is more lanceolate and has a shorter cephalic cone, a larger acetabulum and more anterior testes than *F. hepatica.* The eggs range from 160 to 190 microns in length and 70 to 90 microns in breadth. The biologic and pathologic picture is similar to that described for *F. hepatica.* Treat as for *F. hepatica* infections (p. 556).

### Dicrocoeliasis

Dicrocoeliasis is due to the presence of *Dicrocoelium dendriticum* (Rudolphi 1818) Looss 1899 in the biliary passages of man, a condition which may be confused with fascioliasis. The small, fully embryonated eggs measure 38 to 45 microns in length by 22 to 30 microns in breadth. They are ingested by various species of land snails in which the eggs hatch and develop. Cercariae are released from the snail in slime balls; these are eaten by ants in which the cercariae develop into metacercariae. The parasites mature following ingestion of the ant by herbivorous definitive hosts. Infections in man, while recorded in Europe, North Africa, U.S.S.R., China and Syria, are not commonly encountered. No treatment appears to be satisfactory. It is suggested that this infection be treated as for *C. sinensis* (see pp. 545, 547).

## Diseases Caused by Lung Flukes

### Paragonimiasis

**Synonyms**   Pulmonary distomiasis; endemic hemoptysis; oriental lung fluke disease.

**Definition**   Paragonimiasis is a disease of man caused by the presence of the oriental lung fluke, *Paragonimus westermani*, encapsulated in the parenchyma of the lung.

**Distribution** *Paragonimus westermani* is widely distributed, being especially prevalent in the Far East. The distribution of the disease is summarized in Table 45, which also lists the important foci of human infection.

*Table 45   Distribution of Paragonimiasis by Countries*

| Africa | Far East | India |
|---|---|---|
| Belgian Congo | *Central China | Assam |
| British Cameroons | French Indo-China | Bengal |
| French West Africa | *Japan | Malabar |
| Tripoli | *Korea | Madras Presidency |
| | Manchuria | |
| | *Formosa | South America |
| | Samoan Islands | Brazil (Matto Grosso area) |
| | Malay Peninsula | Peru |
| | *Philippines | Ecuador |
| | Indonesia | Venezuela |
| | New Guinea | |

* Indicates important endemic foci in man.

**Etiology**   Morphology. *Paragonimus westermani* (Kerbert 1878) Braun 1899 is a plump, ovoid fluke lacking definitely attenuated extremities. In life it is reddish brown in color and measures 8 to 20 mm. in length by 5 to 9 mm. in breadth. Microscopic examination reveals the presence of scalelike integumental spines. The two, approximately equal, well-defined suckers are about 0.8 mm. in diameter, the ventral or acetabular sucker lying just anterior to the equatorial plane on the ventral surface. Unstained specimens do not readily reveal the irregularly lobed testes situated side by side in the posterior half of the body. The long slender excretory bladder extends from the posterior tip to the region of the pharynx. Owing to the thickness of the worm most morphologic details can be detected only after the worms have been carefully flattened, preserved and stained. Then the eccentric, centrally located, lobate ovary can be seen to one side of the acetabulum. At the lateral margins extending from the oral sucker to the posterior tip are the yolk glands while the uterus occupies the central portion of the worm opposite the ovary. Anteriorly are the globose pharynx and short esophagus which divides to form the two unbranched intestinal crura.

A closely related or identical species, *P. ohirai*, has been reported from Japan, while *P. kellicotti* has been described from North American mammals. Opinion is still divided as to the synonymy of these forms with *P. westermani*.

Development. The mature adults produce eggs which range between 80 and 118 microns in length by 48 and 60 microns in width, averaging 85 by 53 microns. These eggs are slightly broader at the operculate end and show some shouldering where the operculum originates. Posteriorly the shell is thicker than in the anterior half. The undeveloped eggs are passed up the respiratory tree and either expectorated in the sputum or swallowed and passed in the feces. Under satisfactory conditions they hatch in water after seventeen to twenty-one days, liberating characteristic miracidia. These penetrate various species of snails. The most important species are *Semisulcospira libertina* Gould, *S. amurensis* Gerstfeldt (and its subspecies *gottschei* von Martens and *nodiperda* von Martens), *Thiara (Tarebia) granifera* Lamarck, and *Hua toucheana* Heude. *Paragonimus* has also been recorded in *Oncomelania nosophora* Robson and *Syncera lutea* A. Adams (= *Assiminea*). *Pomacea luteostoma* needs confirmation as the host in Venezuela. *Pomatiopsis lapidaria* is the known host for the so-called *P. kellicotti* of North America.

Three to five months are required to produce the successive generations of mother sporocyst, rediae and finally the stumpy tailed, or microcercous, cercariae within the tissues of the snail.

The cercariae attack crayfish and fresh-water crabs, the second intermediate host, invading the muscles and viscera where they become metacercariae infective for man after a developmental period of several weeks. The following crustaceans serve as hosts for the metacercariae of *P. westermani* in the Orient: *Cambaroides japonicus; C. similis; Eliocheir japonicus; E. sinensis; Potamon (Goethelphusa) dehaani; Potamon (Potamon) rathbuni; P. (P.) denticulatus; Parathelphusa sinensis; Sesarma (Holometopus) dehaani; Sesarma (Sesarma) intermedia (=S.(S.) sinensis)*. In Venezuela the cercariae encyst in *Pseudothelphusa iturbe* while *P. kellicotti* in North America encysts in members of the genus *Cambarus*.

Infection of man and other reservoir hosts results when the crustacea containing metacercariae of *P. westermani* are eaten raw. The metacercariae excyst in the duodenum and migrate through the wall of the alimentary canal into the peritoneal cavity. Some are destroyed in their wanderings. Most migrate through the diaphragm and penetrate into the parenchyma of the lungs where the parasites are finally encapsulated by the host. About three weeks are needed for this migration, even though the diaphragm may be reached in three to four days. Maturity is attained five to six weeks after ingestion.

**Epidemiology**    The following carnivores and omnivores in addition to man serve as reservoir hosts for both species of *Paragonimus:* tiger, cat, wild cat, leopard, fox, wolf, dog, panther, rat(?), hog, beaver, wolverine, civet cat (*Viverra zibetha ashtoni*), Chinese lesser civet cat (*Viverricula malaccensis pollida*), pencilled cat (*Nyctereutes procyonides*), mongoose (*Herpestes urva*) and Indian mongoose (*Mungos mungo*). All acquire the metacercariae through the ingestion of infected, raw fresh-water crabs or crayfishes. In addition man secures the infection by eating salted or wine-soaked parasitized crustacea. While the wine kills the crabs the metacercariae survive for several hours (Fig. 244).

The disease is limited to areas where such dishes are common;

roasting or heating the crustacea in water at 55° C. for five minutes will kill the metacercariae, thus preventing infection.

Pollution of water by the eggs of the parasites, especially those from reservoir hosts other than man, serves as the principal source

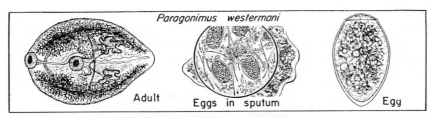

*Paragonimus westermani*

Adult     Eggs in sputum     Egg

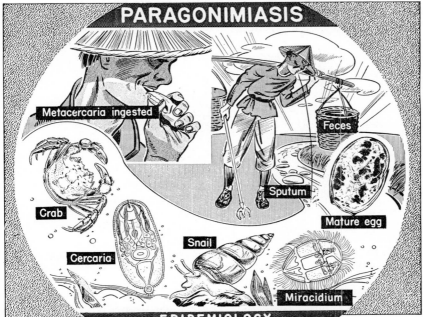

PARAGONIMIASIS

Metacercaria ingested

Feces

Crab

Sputum

Mature egg

Cercaria

Snail

Miracidium

EPIDEMIOLOGY

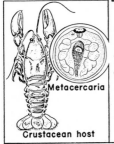

Metacercaria

Crustacean host

1. Reservoir: man, various omnivores and carnivores
2. Intermediate hosts: certain fresh-water snails, crayfish, crabs
3. Undeveloped eggs in sputum and stool
4. Contamination of water
5. Miracidia infect snails
6. Cercariae from snail infect crayfish and crabs
7. Ingestion of metacercariae from crayfish and crabs
8. Parasite migrates from intestine through body cavity
9. Adult in lung and other tissues

*Semi-sulcospira libertina*

Snail host

Fig. 244. Epidemiology of paragonimiasis.

of infection for the snails which in turn produce the cercariae that invade the crustacean hosts.

**Pathology**    The young flukes migrate through the peritoneal cavity and penetrate the diaphragm to reach the lungs. Many never reach their destination but become encapsulated and sometimes destroyed in other locations such as the peritoneum, intestine, liver, mesenteric lymph nodes, brain, testes and muscles. Parasites encysted in the intestinal mucosa elicit an inflammatory reaction which sometimes terminates in ulceration resulting in passage of eggs in the feces.

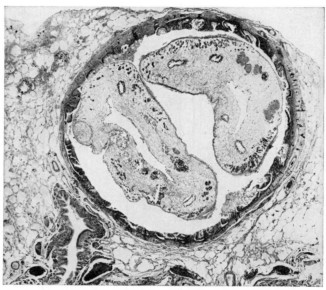

Fig. 245. *Paragonimus westermani* in the lung of a Bengal tiger. (Courtesy of Dr. T. W. M. Cameron, Macdonald College of McGill University.)

The most characteristic and significant pathologic changes are found in the lungs (Fig. 245). These have been divided by some into four categories, as follows: (1) nonsuppurative, with eggs infiltrated in host tissue, leading to round-cell and connective tissue reaction and usually to abscess formation; (2) tubercle-like, in which the abscess may contain caseous material; (3) suppurative; and (4) ulcerative, in which healing is only partially successful.

On arrival in the pulmonary tissue the parasites produce a surrounding inflammatory reaction with leukocytic infiltration, necrosis of parenchyma, and the formation of an enclosing fibrous tissue capsule. The resulting cysts, which may reach 2 cm. in diameter, are more frequent in the deeper portions than at the periphery of the lung. In other instances tunnels or burrows lined with fibrous tissue are formed from damaged and dilated bronchioles and bronchi, and larger cysts may be formed by break-down of adjacent tunnel walls. The lesions are often directly connected with radicles of the bronchial tree.

The cysts characteristically have a reddish or chocolate brown color while the cystlike burrows often have a bluish tint. Each cyst contains one or more living or dead worms, together with quantities of brownish, necrotic, frequently purulent exudate composed of eggs, debris, and Charcot-Leyden crystals (Fig. 246).

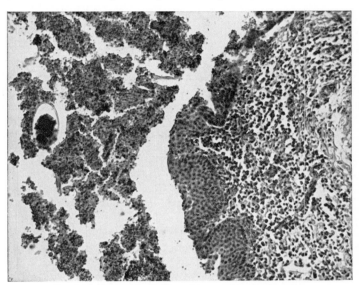

Fig. 246. Egg of *P. kellicotti* in exudate in bronchus.

Leukocytosis with eosinophilia may occur but is frequently absent. In highly endemic areas such as parts of Korea and Japan, cerebral paragonimiasis with its attendant complications is fairly common.

**Clinical Characteristics** The clinical picture of paragonimiasis is predominantly that of a chronic bronchitis or bronchiectasis with morning cough productive of variable amounts of gelatinous tenacious sputum which characteristically is brownish or reddish in color. Exertional dyspnea is common. The term "endemic hemoptysis" is due to the frequency with which hemoptysis occurs. When cysts are localized in close proximity to the pleura, pleural pain may be troublesome, or pleural effusion may occur. In other instances the clinical phenomena indicate a nonresolving bronchopneumonia. In heavy infections lung abscess may occur.

Abdominal symptoms occur when considerable numbers of parasites have localized in this region. They include pain, tenderness, rarely muscle spasm, and diarrhea sometimes bloody with mucus and eggs in the stools.

The cerebral type of the disease occurs only when wandering

parasites lodge in the brain. The local lesions in these cases resemble those of cysticercosis, and epilepsy is a frequent clinical manifestation.

Rarely, localization in the skin or subcutaneous tissues leads to abscess formation.

The prognosis is good in light infections; in heavy infections, however, it is grave.

**Diagnosis**    The clinical picture of pulmonary paragonimiasis and especially the brownish or reddish purulent sputum may be suggestive.

A positive diagnosis is made by detecting the characteristic eggs in the sputum, feces and, more rarely, cutaneous lesions. By using the AMS III technique (acid–sodium sulfate–Triton–ether) on stool specimens nearly 80 per cent of a known positive series were positive by stool. While this egg is sometimes confused with that of the fish tapeworm, a careful comparison of the two makes differentiation possible. The sputum may contain egg masses appearing as rusty-brown flecks, or may be tinged with blood. A specimen containing much mucus should be diluted with an equal amount of 3 per cent solution of sodium hydroxide and shaken thoroughly before centrifuging at a high speed to concentrate the eggs These, if present, are found in smears of the centrifuged sediment. Leukocytes, especially eosinophils, and Charcot-Leyden crystals also appear in the sputum (see p. 832).

It is necessary to differentiate paragonimiasis from such other pulmonary diseases as lobular pneumonia, tuberculosis, bronchial spirochetosis and bronchiectasis.

The abdominal form of the disease may be confused with a variety of intestinal infections, new growth, and certain surgical lesions. The cerebral type likewise may produce a varied clinical picture. These unusual localizations seldom permit etiologic diagnosis from the clinical findings. Intradermal tests, using antigen made from adult worms (1:10000) gives 90 to 95 per cent correlation with known positives in Japan.

**Treatment**    No satisfactory treatment is known. Emetine hydrochloride given intramuscularly or subcutaneouly has been recommended. However, its efficacy is doubted. Emetine hydrochloride has also been administered concurrently with prontosil. Various antibiotics as well as other new compounds such as Hetrazan and chloroquine, have been tested without being able to demonstrate marked evidence of cure.

**Prophylaxis**    Human infection may be avoided easily by thorough cooking of all fresh-water crustaceans used for food. The relatively large number of reservoir and intermediate hosts in many endemic areas renders effective control by other measures impracticable or impossible at present.

# 48  Cestodes

## Introduction

### Biology of the Cestodes

**Introduction**  The cestodes, or tapeworms, include several divergent groups which may be separated not only on the basis of their morphologies but also on clear-cut biologic criteria. The latter distinctions become evident as the life cycles of the parasites are studied. The various epidemiologies also are modified by these specific biologies. On such criteria the cestodes may be divided into two large groups. In the first the eggs must reach water while in the second this is not necessary. The broad tapeworm of man, *Diphyllobothrium latum,* is the only important human parasite in the first group.* All the remaining common tapeworms of man fall in the second category. One cestode of man, *Hymenolepis nana,* requires no intermediate host, but passes directly from person to person, while other species must have at least one intermediate host to complete the cycle. While the members of these two groups will not be segregated as their morphology is discussed, their biology is sufficiently distinct to warrant separate consideration of their development (Fig. 247).

### Morphology of the Cestodes

**The Adults**  The tapeworms, Cestoda or cestodes, as they are commonly called, range in size from the small *Hymenolepis nana* of 40 mm. or less to the huge *Taenia saginata* and *Diphyllobothrium latum* which may measure up to 10 or 12 meters in length. Members of this entire class have morphologic and biologic characteristics which differentiate them from the other helminths.

All tapeworms have a mechanism for attaching the *scolex* or "head" to the host's intestinal wall. In the case of *Diphyllobothrium latum* and related species the scolex bears two sucking grooves or *bothria* which serve in this capacity. Other common human tapeworms possess four round and highly muscular sucking cups located on the scolex. These in turn may be supplemented further by a terminal, sometimes retractile protruberance, known as a *rostellum.* The rostellum in a given species of tapeworm is characteristic and is often armed with small hooks, the number, the length and the arrangement of which serve as further differential aids (Fig. 248).

Behind the scolex is a short, unsegmented narrow *neck* which is the region from which the partially segmented young *proglottids* develop. This region of immature proglottid formation is succeeded by a region of fully developed proglottids each of which contains

* The eggs of *Diplogonoporus grandis* are not considered here as only a few cases of human infection are known.

a full complement of mature reproductive organs. This gives way
to a distal group of *gravid segments* which are frequently little more
than sacs of eggs and which, exclusive of the scolex, represent the
oldest portion of the worm. As new segments are continuously being

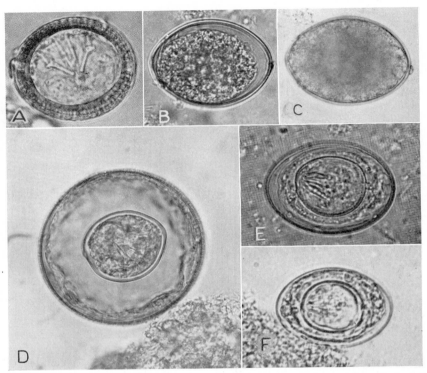

Fig. 247. Some cestode eggs: *A*, Human tapeworm, *Taenia* sp. 750×. *B*, Broad
tapeworm of man, *Diphyllobothrium latum*. 500×. *C*, Broad tapeworm of man,
*Diphyllobothrium latum*. 500×. *D*, Rat tapeworm, *Hymenolepis diminuta*. 650×.
*E*, Dwarf tapeworm, *Hymenolepis nana*. 750×. *F*, Dwarf tapeworm, *Hymenolepis
nana* (note polar filaments) 750×. (Figs. *B* and *F* courtesy of Lt. L. W. Shatterly,
School of Aviation Medicine, Gunter AFB, Alabama. All others courtesy of Dr.
R. L. Roudabush, Ward's Natural Science Establishment, Rochester, New York;
photos by T. Romaniak.)

formed at the neck, the old proglottids are pushed farther and farther
from the scolex thereby increasing the length of the parasite. The
entire worm from the scolex to, and including, the gravid proglottids
is termed the *strobila*.

Tapeworms differ from most other helminths in that they have
no alimentary canal. Each mature proglottid possesses nerve trunks,
excretory canals, a well-developed musculature and a complete set
of male and female reproductive organs. The gravid proglottids
should be studied when making a diagnosis, since the human species

are differentiated by the position of the genital pore and the branchings of the uterus (Fig. 248).

**Eggs**  Tapeworm eggs are either operculate or nonoperculate. The former are adapted for development in water (*D. latum*) while the latter must reach the soil (as in the *Taenia* group). Representatives of the first or *D. latum* type are undeveloped when passed. Their lid or operculum permits the subsequent hatching of a free-swimming larva or *coracidium*. Eggs of all tapeworms in the *Taenia* group

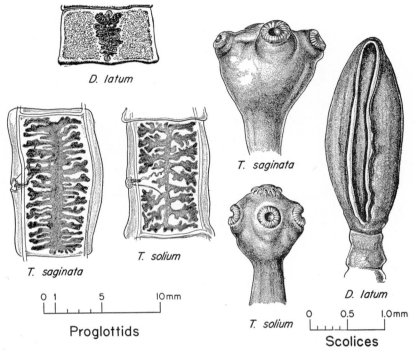

Fig. 248. Scolices and gravid proglottids of some tapeworms of man.

contain an inner, developed, six-hooked embryo or *onchosphere*. This is surrounded by an outer protective layer or layers, the nature and arrangement of which are frequently diagnostic of the species (Fig. 247).

**Developmental Stages**  Tapeworm eggs or larvae that are ingested by a proper host soon develop into typical stages. Upon ingestion by a copepod, coracidia of the *D. latum* group produce a procercoid larva which may retain the embryonic six hooks and show developing holdfast devices or bothria. This is followed by the infective stage, called a plerocercoid larva, found in the flesh of fish (Fig. 249).

Embryos of the *Taenia* group may develop several types of cysts. If the onchosphere gives rise to a single cyst containing but one scolex it is called a *cysticercus* (Fig. 250), or in the case of members of the genus *Hymenolepis*, a *cysticercoid*. On the other hand if a single

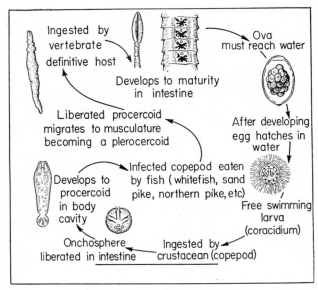

Fig. 249. Cestode cycle—*D. latum* type.

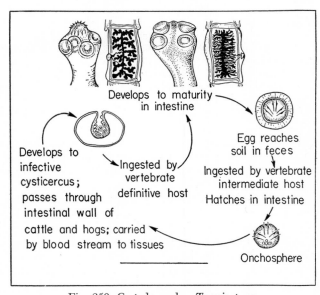

Fig. 250. Cestode cycle—*Taenia* type.

onchosphere produces a single cyst containing many scolices it is called a *coenurus* as in the larvel stage of *Multiceps multiceps* in sheep. In instances when daughter cysts, each containing many scolices, are elaborated, a *hydatid,* or echinococcus cyst, is said to result (Fig. 251).

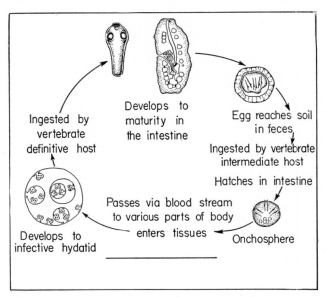

Fig. 251. Cestode cycle—hydatid type.

### The Generalized Cycle

The development characteristics of the two groups mentioned earlier will be considered separately.

**Nonembryonated Eggs**    *Diphyllobothrium latum* is the human representative of greatest importance in this group. The undifferentiated, operculate eggs of parasites in this category develop in water, hatch, and liberate a free-swimming ciliated larva or coracidium. This organism is ingested by a copepod (a minute crustacean), the first intermediate host, and metamorphoses into a procercoid larva. The next intermediate host is a fish in which the plerocercoid stage, infective for man, develops. Infection occurs when insufficiently cooked fish containing this parasite is eaten.

**Embryonated Eggs**    All the human tapeworms considered in this category retain the eggs *in utero* until they are embryonated, at which time the six hooklets, diagnostic of such tapeworm eggs, become apparent. These worms may or may not require an intermediate host for the completion of development. In the case of *Hymenolepis nana* none is necessary as infection is direct, the only requirement being the introduction of viable eggs into a susceptible definitive host. Eggs of the others, after reaching the ground, are ingested by the intermediate host where development to the infective stage, usually a cysticercoid, cysticercus or hydatid cyst, takes place. When these larvae in the infective stage are ingested raw by man or other final hosts the parasites reach maturity in the digestive tract.

## Diphyllobothriasis

**Synonyms**   Broad tapeworm infection, fish tapeworm infection.

**Definition**   Diphyllobothriasis is the infection of man by adult *Diphyllobothrium latum*. Its presence is sometimes associated with debility, anemia and loss of weight.

**Distribution**   *Diphyllobothrium latum* is common in persons living in the Baltic countries, western Russia, Finland, parts of Scandinavia and in certain endemic foci in the United States and Canada. In the latter regions the parasite occurs in northern Wisconsin, Minnesota, Michigan, and in provinces of Canada bordering on those states. In these populations the incidence varies between 2 and, rarely, almost 100 per cent. Recently cases have been reported also from Florida. The parasite occurs in the lake regions of Italy, Switzerland, parts of Germany, and in the valley of the Danube, particularly in Rumania. It has been reported in Manchuria, Japan, and portions of Siberia, and has also been found in scattered areas of Africa.

**Etiology**   MORPHOLOGY. The broad tapeworm of man, *D. latum* (Linnaeus 1758) Lühe 1910, lives with its scolex attached to the mucosa of the small intestine. It may reach a length of ten meters or more. The spatulate head is small and bears a deep sucking groove on either surface. Posterior to the scolex is the narrow unsegmented neck measuring 5 to 10 mm. in length; the remainder of the worm consists of segments or proglottids which total 3000 or more.

The chief diagnostic feature of *D. latum* is the rosette-shaped, egg-filled uterus of the gravid proglottids. The finding of the genital pore on the flattened surface in the anterior third of the proglottid is also helpful. Gravid segments are normally retained as part of the strobila, being sloughed off only as they degenerate. It has been estimated that a fully developed strobila will produce about 1,000,000 eggs a day. These eggs average 70 by 45 microns in size and like some trematode eggs have a lid, or operculum; they are undeveloped when laid.

DEVELOPMENT. The eggs must reach water where after approximately two weeks at the optimum temperature the egg hatches, liberating a free-swimming coracidium consisting of a typical six-hooked onchosphere invested by ciliated epithelium. The larva must be ingested by species of *Cyclops* or *Diaptomus* (copepods). About eight species are believed to act as hosts for this tapeworm. Within the alimentary tract the larva loses its ciliated epithelial layer and immediately penetrates to the body cavity of the copepod where it develops into a procercoid larva in ten to twenty days. The cycle is continued when the infected copepod is ingested by any of twenty-two or more species of fresh-water fish capable of serving as the second intermediate host. The larva migrates from the alimentary canal to the flesh where it coils between the muscle fibers as a plerocercoid, often reaching a length of 16 mm. or more. It becomes infective in one to four weeks, the time varying with the temperature. It is believed that often two fish, one of which becomes infected by eating the other, may serve as intermediate hosts. When a viable parasite is ingested by man the larva develops to maturity in the intestine. The complete cycle requires eight to fifteen weeks.

**Epidemiology**   In the United States the wall-eyed pike, sandpike, great northern pike and burbot have been implicated as second intermediate hosts. In Africa it is the barbel, while in Europe the pike, perch, salmon, Miller's thumb, trout, lake trout, grayling, white fish, ruff and eel are known hosts. Comparable species of trout or salmon serve in Japan. Transmission of the parasite to man is accomplished by the eating of insufficiently cooked fish containing viable plerocercoid larvae. Housewives who sample "ludefisk" or "gefüllte" fish while it is being prepared are often infected, as well as persons eating the fish (Fig. 252).

It is believed by many that bears, mink, foxes, cats, mongooses, walruses, seals, sea-lions, pigs and dogs serve as reservoirs in endemic areas.

**Pathology**   In most infections with *D. latum* there is scant evidence of significant pathologic change. The presence of the adult worms in the intestine causes no distinct lesions although sometimes the mucosa may undergo mechanical injury at the point of attachment, or the worms may cause obstruction.

Although not incontrovertibly established, it appears possible that occasionally infection with *D. latum* is productive of anemia or toxemia.

**Clinical Characteristics**   Infection with *D. latum* is asymptomatic in many people. Others, however, experience hunger pains, diarrhea, abdominal pain, and may suffer a loss of weight. In general the clinical picture is not clear.

**Diagnosis**   Diagnosis depends upon the recovery of the characteristic operculate eggs in the stool. These must be differentiated from eggs of other parasites such as the lung fluke, *Paragonimus westermani*, occurring in the Orient, and a closely related tapeworm, *Diplogonoporus grandis*, which has been reported only from the Japanese. Diagnosis may be confirmed following the administration of a saline purge which usually results in the recovery of some proglottids of the worm. These should be examined to determine the arrangement of the reproductive system, since the rosette-shaped uterus lying medially in each proglottid is diagnostic, while there is a bilateral set in *D. grandis*.

**Treatment**   The accepted anthelmintic for intestinal tapeworm infection is oleoresin of aspidium (male fern or filix mas). If this drug is contraindicated, hexylresorcinol or Atabrine may be tried (see pp. 545, 551, 555).

**Prophylaxis**    The prevention of *D. latum* infection is readily accomplished by thorough cooking of fish before consumption. Freezing

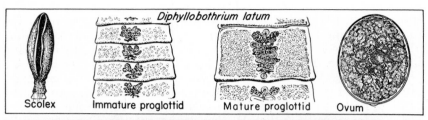

Scolex    Immature proglottid    Mature proglottid    Ovum

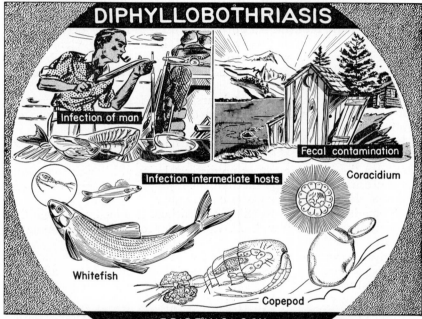

# DIPHYLLOBOTHRIASIS

Infection of man

Fecal contamination

Coracidium

Infection intermediate hosts

Whitefish

Copepod

## EPIDEMIOLOGY

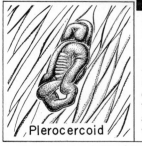

Plerocercoid

1. Reservoir: man, carnivores
2. Intermediate hosts: copepods, fresh-water fish
3. Undeveloped ova in stool
4. Fecal contamination of water
5. Coracidia ingested by copepods
6. Infected copepods eaten by fish
7. Plerocercoids in muscles of fish
8. Ingestion of undercooked fish
9. Adults in small intestine

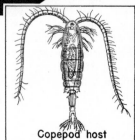

Copepod host

Fig. 252. Epidemiology of diphyllobothriasis.

the fish for twenty-four to forty-eight hours at 14° F. (—10° C.) will also effectively destroy the plerocercoid larvae. Other measures which might be practiced under favorable conditions include sewage treatment in endemic areas and the education of Scandinavian and Jewish housewives against sampling "ludefisk" and "gefüllte" fish while preparing it.

## Sparganosis

**Synonym**   Sparganum infection.
**Definition**   Sparganosis is caused by the presence of migrating larvae or sparganum of several species of tapeworms related to *D.*

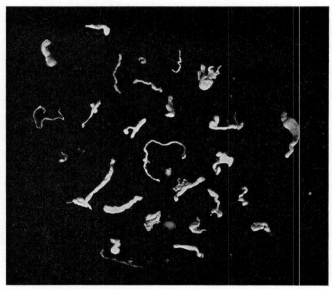

Fig. 253. *Sparganum proliferum:* excised larvae. (Courtesy of Dr. J. F. Mueller, Syracuse University Medical School.)

*latum* but requiring final hosts other than man. Localization occurs primarily in the subcutaneous tissue and muscle fascia.

**Distribution**   The greatest number of cases of sparganosis has been reported from Japan, China, Indo-China and Indonesia, while scattered instances are known from other areas of the world including Holland, British Guiana and the United States.

**Etiology**   Sparganosis is a disease caused by the migration of several species of closely allied parasites which accidentally infect man. These parasites normally mature in other mammals such as dogs and cats. Morphologically indistinguishable sparganum occur in subcutaneous tissue and between the muscles of frogs, snakes, birds and mammals in endemic areas. It has been shown in the case of

*Diphyllobothrium mansonoides* that the eggs hatch in water and the coracidium is ingested by a copepod. Following ingestion of the infected copepod, spargana develop in mice and rhesus monkeys, while adult worms mature in the definitive or final hosts, the dog, cat or bobcat (Fig. 253).

*Sparganum proliferum* (Ijima 1905) Stiles 1908 is a proliferating type of larva which is unknown in the adult stage. In the tissues of man it appears as an elongate mass with branched and sometimes proliferating processes. Some of these may become separated from

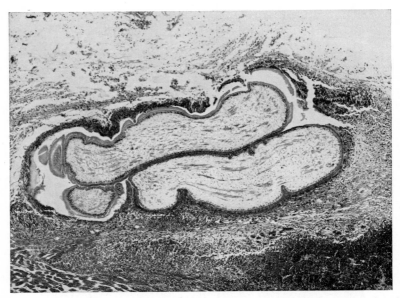

Fig. 254. Sparganosis: larva of *Diphyllobothrium mansonoides* in tissues showing surrounding inflammation and foreign body reaction. (Courtesy of Dr. J. F. Mueller, Syracuse University Medical School.)

the parent worm and develop individually. These parasites invade not only the subcutaneous tissues and intermuscular fasciae but also the viscera and brain.

**Epidemiology**  Human sparganosis results from either of two causes: (1) the ingestion of infected copepods containing the infective larvae, or (2) the local application of infected vertebrates to the skin as poultices from which the larvae migrate into human tissue.

**Pathology**  The larvae invade primarily the subcutaneous tissues where they develop and produce considerable inflammation, swelling and fibrosis. When opened, the lesions may be characterized by a shiny matrix within which the living larvae contract and elongate. Sometimes the parasite has degenerated and only a caseous mass remains (Fig. 254).

In China, where infections occur in the eye owing to the application of infected frogs as poultices, edematous conjunctivitis and corneal ulceration are seen.

**Clinical Characteristics** Symptomatology depends upon the number of larvae present and their location. Many cases of light infection remain asymptomatic. When the number of larvae is high, the infected cutaneous tissues become edematous and extremely painful to the touch. Ocular sparganosis results in redness, nodule formation, edema in the conjunctiva, excessive lachrymation, toxemia, and in cases of penetration of the retrobulbar region, corneal ulceration. Lesions limited to the skin reveal acne-like nodular pustules frequently surrounded by tissue honeycombed with parasites. Invasion of the lymphatics may cause elephantiasis.

**Diagnosis** Infections due to sparganosis are extremely difficult to diagnose except in areas where they are common. Consequently they often remain undiagnosed until after surgical removal of the worm.

**Treatment** The lesion may be injected with 2 to 4 cc. of 40 per cent ethyl alcohol with Novocain (epinephrine free) to kill the worms *in situ*, thus permitting ultimate resorption. Other workers recommend 0.3 to 0.45 gm. per dose of novarsenobenzol intravenously for adults. This drug is given every four to five days for two to six administrations. In some instances excision may prove more satisfactory.

**Prophylaxis** Infection by this parasite can be avoided in endemic areas by the use of boiled or adequately filtered water. Education of the public against the application of freshly killed vertebrates as poultices is essential if ultimate control is to be achieved.

## Taeniasis Solium

**Synonyms** Pork tapeworm infection, *Taenia solium* infection, cysticercosis.

**Definition** Taeniasis solium is due to the presence of the adult pork tapeworm, *T. solium*, in the intestine of man; cysticercosis is caused by the cysticerci in the tissues of man.

**Distribution** The pork tapeworm has a cosmopolitan distribution, being found throughout the world wherever raw or inadequately cooked pork is eaten. Infection is rare in England, Canada and the United States. In Mexico and parts of Central and South America the infection rate is somewhat higher. In Europe the Slavic groups are most heavily infected, while in Russia the rates vary from 0.2 to 1.5 per cent.

**Etiology** MORPHOLOGY. The adult "measly pork" tapeworm, *Taenia solium* Linnaeus 1758, attains a length of 2 to 7 meters. It lives attached to the intestinal wall of man. The scolex is about 1 mm. in diameter and has been described as being "roughly quadrate." Anterior and central to the four suckers is a prominent terminal rostellum which bears two circular rows of hooklets. These hooklets number between twenty-two and thirty-two in an upper and lower row. The neck is short. Posterior to this structure are the immature, mature and gravid proglottids. The mature proglottids are nearly square, and while the gravid ones are longer than broad they do not attain the length of the corresponding proglottids of *T. saginata*. Morphologically the mature proglottids of *T. solium* are in general similar to those of *T. saginata* except that the testes in the former number between 150 to 200 compared with the 300 to 400 in *T. saginata*. In addition the ovary is trilobed instead of bilobed as in *T. saginata*. The uterine sac runs up the middle of the proglottid with the ovarian complex in the posterior third of the segment. In the more elongate gravid proglottids the reproductive organs degenerate, with the exception of the uterus, which has seven to thirteen, with an average of nine, main lateral branches on a side. The complete strobila of *T. solium* usually consists of less than 1000 distinct proglottids.

Eggs are spherical to subspherical in shape, measure 31 to 43 microns in greatest diameter and cannot be differentiated from those of *T. saginata*. The terminal proglottids often become separated and are passed entire. Occasionally they migrate actively from the anus when the host is not at stool.

Development. The eggs burst from the gravid proglottids either before or after the proglottids have become detached from the strobila. Eggs reaching the soil remain viable for weeks, and when ingested by hogs or man hatch immediately. The liberated onchosphere penetrates the intestinal wall and reaches the lymphatic or circulatory system. These embryos are distributed throughout the body, most localizing in the musculature or subcutaneous tissues. Within sixty to seventy days they become metamorphosed into infective bladder worms, or *Cysticercus cellulosae*, which measure about 5 mm. in length by 8 to 10 mm. in breadth.

In the usual course of events, cysticerci reach man when he ingests raw or inadequately prepared "measly pork." The larvae are digested out of the cysts, become attached to the intestinal wall and grow to maturity in five to twelve weeks. *Taenia solium* adults are believed to have survived as long as twenty-five years in the intestine of man.

**Epidemiology**    Man is the only known definitive host of *T. solium* and the hog is the usual intermediate host. Two forms of human infection occur. When man serves as the definitive host the adult tapeworm is present in the intestine. Such infection is acquired only by the ingestion of raw or insufficiently cooked "measly pork" containing viable cysticerci (Fig. 255).

In cysticercosis man serves as the intermediate host and the larval stages, cysticerci, are present in his tissues. Human infection results usually from the ingestion and subsequent hatching of viable eggs. They reach the alimentary canal in food or drink contaminated by feces from a person harboring the adult worm. Autoinfection may occur when eggs are carried from feces to the mouth on the hands of infected persons. It is believed to occur also, however, when reverse peristalsis brings eggs back to the stomach or duodenum where they hatch. Occasionally other primates, dogs and sheep are infected with cysticerci.

Taeniasis solium, infection with the adult worm, is not found

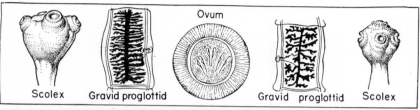

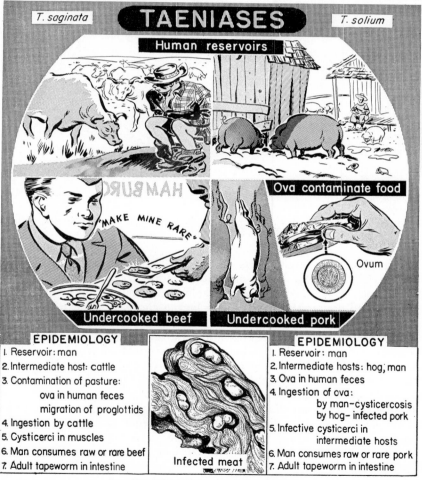

Fig. 255. Epidemiology of the taeniases.

among such groups as the Jews and Mohammedans since they rarely eat pork; cysticercosis, on the other hand, may occur.

The infection is maintained in nature by improper disposal of human feces which permits ingestion of the eggs by the normal intermediate host, the hog.

**Pathology** THE ADULT WORM. The mature tapeworm in the intestine seldom causes significant pathologic changes. A moderate eosinophilia may be present.

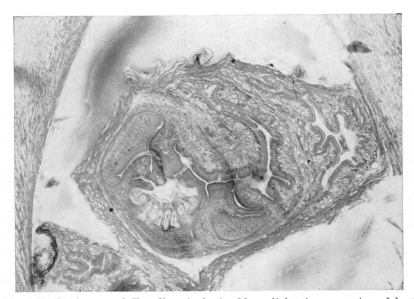

Fig. 256. Cysticercus of *T. solium* in brain. Note slight tissue reaction of host, rostellar hooks and laterally placed suckers of parasite.

CYSTICERCUS CELLULOSAE. The cysticerci may be lodged in any tissue of the body. They are most frequently found in the subcutaneous tissues, brain, eye, skeletal musculature, heart, liver, lungs, and abdominal cavity. The larvae cause, at first, a local surrounding inflammatory reaction with infiltration by neutrophils, eosinophils, and lymphocytes and a stimulation of fibroblast production. Subsequently the larvae become enclosed within a fibrous capsule or necrosis may occur followed by caseation and calcification. Giant cells may be found about the lesions. The resulting cysts may vary from 0.5 to 2 or even 3 cm. in diameter.

**Clinical Characteristics** THE ADULT WORM. No untoward symptoms other than digestive disturbances, hunger pains, and diarrhea sometimes alternating with constipation, have been noted.

CYSTICERCUS CELLULOSAE. The clinical picture of cysticercosis is extremely variable and depends upon the location and the number of cysticerci in the host. When these are few and restricted principally to the subcutaneous tissues, symptoms may be negligible or absent. When they localize in the brain, the spinal cord, the eye or the heart muscle, serious effects are common. The phenomena associated with tumor formation in the particular anatomic region are then noted. Localization in the fourth ventricle or in the cerebral cortex is frequent and in these instances there may be epileptiform convulsions, mental changes and other phenomena which accompany brain tumor irrespective of type (Fig. 256). Eosinophilia is not reported in this infection.

Cysts may be palpable as firm nodules in the superficial tissues.

**Diagnosis**    THE ADULT. As noted on p. 524 differentiation between *T. saginata* and *T. solium* infections on the basis of their eggs is not possible. Therefore, it is important to differentiate between the mature proglottids, which may be pressed between two slides and held to the light. The uterus may be injected with India ink to facilitate the determination of the number of main lateral uterine branches, which range between seven and thirteen in *T. solium*.

CYSTICERCUS CELLULOSAE. The occurrence of epilepsy or the clinical picture of brain tumor developing in a previously healthy individual who is known to have been in a hyperendemic area should arouse suspicion and lead to careful search of the entire body surface for the characteristic nodules in the subcutaneous tissues. Soft tissue roentgen examination of the extremities will often reveal characteristic calcific shadows.

The differential white blood count is not of assistance in view of the lack of eosinophilia, and skin and precipitin tests are not specific. Definitive diagnosis depends upon recovery of the larva by excision of a cyst and identification of species by the presence of two rows of hooks of unequal size on the inverted rostellum.

Since cysticercosis may be due to autoinfection, stool examinations should be made for the presence of eggs.

**Treatment**    Oleoresin of aspidium (male fern or filix mas) is the drug of choice for intestinal infections (see p. 555 for details). The drug is contraindicated in very old or very young persons. Hexylresorcinol administered as for ascariasis, or preferably by duodenal intubation of an emulsion of this drug in water, is quite effective (see p. 545). Atabrine appears to be quite efficacious (see p. 551) and may prove to be the drug of choice.

There is no specific treatment for cysticercosis. Individual cysts which are causing pressure symptoms may be amenable to surgical excision.

**Prophylaxis**    Intestinal infection by *T. solium* is prevented by proper cooking of all pork products. Cysticerci present in pickled or salted pork may be viable; they are destroyed, however, by freezing. United States Government meat inspection provides a safeguard but not complete protection.

Sanitary disposal of human feces prevents infection of the hog and is the essential procedure in the control of taeniasis solium.

Cysticercosis may often be prevented by prompt and effective therapy of the individual harboring the adult worm, efficient methods of personal cleanliness to prevent autoinfection, and protection of food and drink against possible contamination by human feces containing eggs of *T. solium*.

## Taeniasis Saginata

**Synonyms**   Beef tapeworm infection, *Taenia saginata* infection.

**Definition**   Taeniasis saginata is caused by the presence of the adult beef tapeworm, *T. saginata*, in the intestine of man.

**Distribution**   The beef tapeworm is cosmopolitan in distribution. It is endemic in parts of Africa, especially Abyssinia, Northern Syria, probably Tibet and in the Mohammedan countries where *T. solium* is virtually unknown.

**Etiology**   MORPHOLOGY. *Taenia saginata* Goeze 1782 is a large tapeworm usually measuring 5 to 10 meters in length and consisting of 1000 to 2000 proglottids. The scolex appears quadrate in cross section and carries four round suckers. The rostellum and hooks which are typical of *T. solium* are lacking in *T. saginata*. The neck is short, being about half as broad as the head and several times its length. Then follow the immature, mature and gravid proglottids respectively. The mature proglottids are broader than long and contain about twice as many testes (300 to 400) as comparable proglottids of *T. solium*. The gravid proglottids are longer than broad, measuring 5 to 7 mm. in width by about 20 mm. in length. There are fifteen to twenty main uterine branches on either side of this median saclike structure which virtually fill the entire proglottid.

The spherical to ovoid eggs measure 31 to 43 microns in greatest diameter and cannot be differentiated from the eggs of *T. solium*. The onchosphere, containing six characteristic hooklets, is surrounded by a narrow space filled with a transparent material. This clear area in turn is surrounded by a thick outer shell heavily marked by radial striations. The delicate, hyaline, thin outer envelopes which surround these eggs *in utero* are rarely present when the eggs are detected in the stool.

DEVELOPMENT. Eggs develop in cattle, giraffes, llamas and buffaloes, while sheep and other herbivorous animals are recorded as experimental intermediate hosts. After ingestion the outer shell membrane is digested, thus setting the embryos free in the upper part of the small intestine. These larvae migrate through the intestinal wall of the intermediate host, reach the blood or lymph streams and are carried about the body until filtered out in the striated muscles. Here they metamorphose into cysticerci. Man, the only definitive host, acquires the infection upon ingesting infected meat containing viable *Cysticercus bovis*. An incubation period of eight to twelve weeks is required for maturation of the parasite and the appearance of eggs in the stool.

*Epidemiology* Infection results from the ingestion of infected raw or poorly cooked beef (Fig. 255). Among certain religious groups, such as the Mohammedans, who merely sear the outside of large chunks of beef before eating it, the infection rate is particularly high. In the United States only about 0.37 per cent of the federally inspected cattle has been found infected. Soil may be contaminated directly by eggs in feces or indirectly by viable proglottids which sometimes migrate through the anus even when the infected individual is not at stool, and subsequently wander about on the ground.

*Pathology* No significant pathologic phenomena usually occur, although an eosinophilia up to 34 per cent has been reported. Leukocytosis is sometimes present in the early stages. Human infection with *Cysticercus bovis* is very rare.

*Clinical Characteristics* Many cases of taeniasis saginata are asymptomatic. Some persons may experience diarrhea, hunger pains and sometimes loss of weight.

*Diagnosis* Diagnosis depends upon (1) the detection of characteristic *Taenia*-like eggs in the stool and (2) the finding of gravid proglottids, since species identification cannot be made on eggs alone. The proglottids may be pressed between two glass slides and the number of main lateral uterine branches counted under a dissecting microscope or with a hand lens. These range in number from fifteen to twenty and average eighteen or nineteen. In *Taenia solium* there are only seven to thirteen with an average of nine.

*Treatment* Atabrine is the drug of choice; hexylresorcinol administered by duodenal intubation is reported to give good results. These have largely replaced oleoresin of aspidium. (See pp. 545, 551, 555 for details of treatment.)

*Prophylaxis* Beef tapeworm infections may be prevented in the United States by avoiding all beef that does not bear a proper inspection label. Adequate freezing or salting of uninspected meat is efficacious. The eating of raw beef and the drinking of raw beef juice should be discouraged. Thorough cooking of beef prevents infection of man and the sanitary disposal of human feces prevents infection of the intermediate host.

## Hydatid Disease

*Synonyms* Echinococciasis, echinococcosis, echinococcus disease.

*Definition* Hydatid disease is an infection by the larval form of *Echinococcus granulosus* in man or other intermediate host. It is characterized by the formation of single or multiple expanding cysts which may be unilocular or alveolar in character.

*Distribution* Hydatid disease is prevalent in sheep-raising countries where man is closely associated with heavily infected sheep dogs. Such regions are mainly temperate or subtropical. In certain localities the exogenous or alveolar type of cyst is produced more often than in others. Table 46 shows the distribution of hydatid disease by continents and countries.

**Etiology** THE ADULT. Adult *Echinococcus granulosus* (Batsch 1786) Rudolphi 1805 (= *Taenia echinococcus*) occur mainly in carnivores such as dogs, wolves, jackals and foxes. These are small tapeworms ranging from 3 to 6 mm. in length and consisting of four parts: (1) The pyriform scolex is only about 0.3 mm. in diameter and carries four suckers and a rostellum which bears two circular rows of hooklets varying in total number but ranging from twenty-eight to fifty (usually thirty to thirty-six). The scolex is continued without evidence of segmentation into a narrow neck. (2) Be-

*Table 46   Distribution of Hydatid Disease*

| Africa | Asia | Australasia |
|---|---|---|
| *Algeria | *Palestine and Syria | *South Australia |
| Tunisia | North China | *Tasmania |
| Liberia | Mongolia | *New Zealand |
| *Egypt | Japan | Europe |
| Abyssinia | Tonkin | *Central |
| *Cape Colony | Philippine Islands | Northern |
| | Siberia | North America |
| | Arabia | U. S. (occasional) |
| | India (Punjab area) | Canada |
| | | South America |
| | | *Argentina |
| | | Chile |
| | | *Uruguay |
| | | *Paraguay |

*Regions of higher incidence in man.

hind this occurs an immature proglottid. (3) More posteriorly is the single mature proglottid which is nearly twice as long as the preceding one and contains a complete set of reproductive organs. (4) The terminal or gravid proglottid may reach 2 mm. in length. It consists principally of a uterus with lateral evaginations; these become so distended with eggs that the uterus finally bursts, liberating the eggs either before or after detachment from the strobila. The eggs are indistinguishable from other *Taenia* eggs found in dogs or man. They possess thick brown shells which surround the six-hooked onchospheres. Maximum diameter of the eggs is 30 to 38 microns.

THE HYDATID CYST. Human infection results from the ingestion of the eggs of *E. granulosus*. These hatch in the duodenum and most of the liberated onchospheres then penetrate its wall. The larvae are carried throughout the body, most being filtered out in the liver and lungs and the remainder in other tissues where many of them are destroyed by phagocytic cells. Probably 60 to 70 per cent of the surviving larvae reach maturity in the liver. Growth at first takes place quite rapidly; on the fourth day the parasite is only 40 microns in length, but in three weeks it is 0.25 mm. long, and at the end of five months has grown to about a centimeter in size. Cysts subsequently grow more slowly and frequently come to the notice of a physician as late as twenty years after the initial infection.

Two main types of hydatid cyst may result from the ingestion of eggs, a unilocular type and the more dangerous alveolar variety; the latter may develop from the former secondarily. If a young developing cyst is comparatively uninfluenced by pressure the following structural characteristics of the growth may be noted:

(1) An external laminated cuticula produced by the host.

(2) An interior germinative membrane which buds off the daughter cysts or brood capsules.

(3 The hydatid fluid which fills the hydatid cyst and gradually produces considerable distention.

(4) The germinative membrane which lines the new budding daughter cysts.

(5) The daughter cysts free in the hydatid fluid which in turn may produce granddaughter cysts within them.

(6) Some of the brood capsules become separated from the wall and settle to the bottom together with liberated scolices as a fine "hydatid sand."

Not all of the germinal epithelium that lines the hydatid cyst is fertile, nor are all the daughter cysts fertile.

Two types of development may occur in hydatid cysts—endogenous and exogenous. In the former a cyst buds internally into or towards the cyst cavity; this is the usual method of reproduction. In the case of exogenous development the budding occurs in an outward direction. Exogenous buds may be produced by a herniation of the germinal layer through the laminated outer layer of the hydatid, directly from transplanted scolices, or from cells of the germinative layer of the brood capsules. In most cases this exogenous budding arises as the result of intracystic pressure or traumatic rupture.

The alveolar type of cyst is a malignant, metastasizing tumor which resembles a sponge in section. The surrounding tissue is infiltrated by parasitic elements which have usually arisen by exogenous budding. At the same time the central portion of the mass undergoes necrosis.

The cycle is completed when the hydatid cysts are ingested, usually by a carnivore such as a sheep dog feeding on the discarded viscera of an infected sheep, or of a wolf preying upon a flock. The hydatid cyst contains many scolices, each of which may develop to a mature, adult tapeworm in the intestine of the carnivorous host.

***Epidemiology*** Hydatid disease is important in many parts of the world. The dog is the common definitive host and the chief reservoir of infection, although other wild CANIDAE have been reported as carrying the adult. The common intermediate hosts are sheep, cattle, hogs and occasionally man. Eggs are deposited in the feces of the hosts carrying the adult parasites and thus contaminate the range or pasture. Herbivores grazing over this seeded area ingest the eggs. After a variable period these intermediate hosts develop characteristic hydatid cysts which will produce adults when they, in turn, are ingested by a suitable definitive host. Human infection results from ingestion of eggs of *Echinococcus granulosus*. Such eggs reach the mouth of man by hands, food, drink or containers contaminated with feces of infected dogs (Fig. 257).

When living in sheep-raising countries the sheep dogs should be

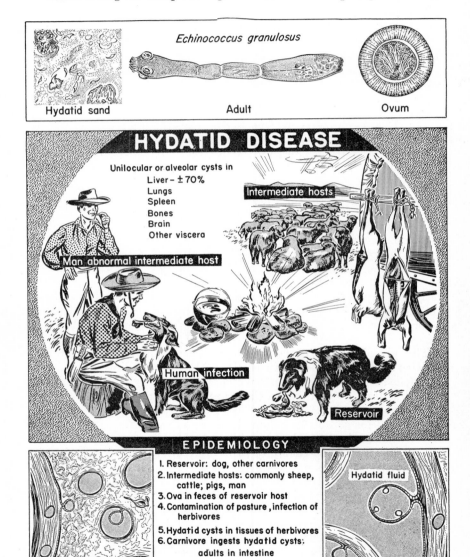

Fig. 257. Epidemiology of hydatid disease.

regarded with suspicion, since many carry the adult tapeworms. Dogs in Iceland were formerly heavily infected (28 per cent) while human infections ran as high as 16 per cent. In recent years both the human and dog infections have been controlled. Other areas, such as the sheep-raising districts of Australia, report a high infection rate in dogs (up to 50 per cent) while only 3 per cent of the human population is infected. In New Zealand about 120 human cases with about 14 per cent fatality are seen each year.

In northern Canada "sylvatic echinococciasis" exists. Wolves are highly infected and so seed areas with eggs. These are ingested by such wild herbivores as the caribou and moose, and the cycle is completed when these herbivores are killed by wolves. This sylvatic cycle breaks into the domestic picture because the wild herbivores are slaughtered in large numbers for food. The viscera are fed to the dogs, which become infected with the adult parasite. By infecting his

*Table 47   Intermediate and Definitive Hosts of* Echinococcus granulosus

| DEFINITIVE HOSTS | COMMON INTER-MEDIATE HOSTS | RARE INTERMEDIATE HOSTS | |
|---|---|---|---|
| Dog | Sheep (optimum) | Monkey | Squirrel |
| Wolf | Cattle | Asiatic Elephant | Mongoose |
| Jackal | Pigs | Moose | Deer |
| Domestic cat | Horses | Caribou | Giraffe |
| | Camels | Argali | Tapir |
| | Goats | Antelope | Dog |
| | Man | Zebra | Leopard |
| | | Kangaroo | Rabbit |
| | | Cat | Wart hog |

dogs man initiates a cycle in which he assumes the role of inter-mediate host, and so many eventually develop echinococciasis.

A variety of final or definitive as well as intermediate hosts is known. These are summarized in Table 47.

**Pathology**   The unilocular hydatid cyst produces a characteristic reaction on the part of the host. This consists at first of a localized surrounding inflammatory reaction with infiltration by eosinophils, round cells and giant cells. This is followed by fibroblast prolifera-tion, the appearance of new-formed blood vessels and the gradual formation of an enclosing fibrous capsule. As progressive growth of the cyst takes place, pressure necrosis and absorption of adjacent tissue occur (Figs. 258, 259).

Alveolar hydatid cysts, on the other hand, are characterized by a partial discontinuity or rupture of the surrounding connective tissue capsule. The germinal epithelium of the cyst is in direct contact with the parenchyma of the organ and consequently new cysts are con-tinuously budded off and set free in the surrounding tissue of the host, thus rendering successful surgical intervention virtually impos-sible. Frequently the liver tissue surrounding these large alveolar cysts is replaced largely by scar tissue. The small daughter cysts which have already been budded off contain a jelly-like matrix which is said to be characteristic of this type of cyst. The freed daughter cysts in the blood or lymph stream or body cavities often metastasize to other sites.

Hydatid cysts may develop in bone, causing extensive destruction,

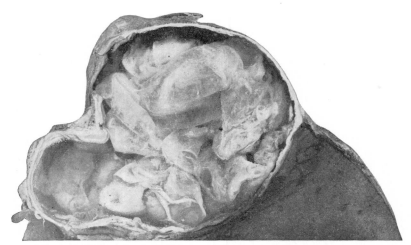

Fig. 258. Unilocular hydatid cyst of liver containing daughter cysts.

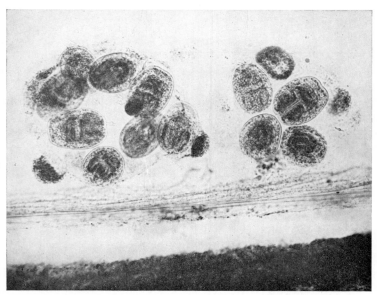

Fig. 259. Wall of hydatid cyst: two daughter cysts budding from germinal epithelium of wall. Note contained scolices. (Courtesy Dr. A. C. Chandler, Rice Institute.)

and spontaneous fractures and non-union are not unusual. The subsequent invasion of the soft tissues is typically associated with the deposition of calcium.

Since the onchospheres are distributed through the body by the blood stream, hydatid cysts may develop in any region. They are most commonly found, however, in the liver, lungs, omentum and mesentery (Fig. 260).

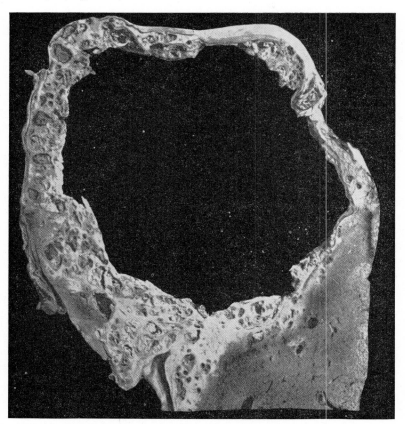

Fig. 260. Alveolar hydatid cyst invading liver. (From Craig and Faust: Clinical Parasitology. Lea & Febiger, Phila., 1943.)

**Clinical Characteristics**    Hydatid cysts frequently cause no symptoms during early stages, especially if localized in the liver, but later as the tumor increases in size it may give rise to both subjective and objective signs due to pressure. When large cysts are situated on the convex surface they may be mistaken for a pleural effusion. Infected cysts will give the symptoms of abscess. Spontaneous rupture into the peritoneal cavity, lung or pleura usually produces a violent and sometimes fatal reaction. Anemia, emaciation and general weakness may be noted.

When the cyst is located in bone, pain, spontaneous fracture and deformity may result, while if the brain is the site of the infection, epilepsy and blindness may become apparent. In about 12 per cent of the cases the lungs may be involved. Such cases are characterized by cough, hemoptysis and sometimes fever.

**Diagnosis** A history of signs indicative of an expanding tumor in an individual who has been in an endemic area may be suggestive. Eosinophilia, however, occurs in only 20 to 25 per cent of the cases. Hydatid thrill may be demonstrable over large intra-abdominal cysts; when present, it is a specific diagnostic sign of unilocular hydatid. Roentgen examination may likewise be of assistance. If cysts of the lung have ruptured into a bronchus, examination of the sputum may reveal hydatid sand. Exploratory puncture is not advised because of the hazard of contaminating uninjured tissues.

The clinical picture of alveolar hydatid, on the other hand, may be confused with that of metastatic carcinoma. In such instances the presence of eosinophilia may be of great assistance in differential diagnosis.

Intradermal, precipitin, and complement fixation tests are reasonably specific and valuable diagnostic aids.

**Treatment** The only effective treatment is complete excision of the cyst. Whether or not this is practical depends upon the location and type of cyst. Surgical intervention should be considered only in cases of unilocular cysts. In many cases the cyst may be removed intact, but such a procedure is difficult as the fibrous capsule surrounding the cyst proper gradually gives way to normal tissue. Two procedures have been commonly used: (1) aspiration of 10 to 15 ml. of the fluid and replacement with 10 per cent Formalin. This kills the scolices and brood capsules and renders the contents of the cyst harmless in the event they are accidentally scattered during removal. (2) Marsupialization, in which case the cyst, after sterilization with 10 per cent Formalin, may be stitched to the abdominal wall and allowed to heal by granulation.

**Prophylaxis** Prophylaxis of the disease on a wide scale entails elimination of the infection in the common definitive host. Proper disposal of carcasses on sheep ranges or of entrails leaving slaughter houses will prevent dogs from gaining access to them. Prophylaxis, so far as sporadic human cases are concerned, involves care in the detection of infected pets and caution against the contamination of hands, food or drink with dog feces.

## Other Tapeworms Infecting Man

There are records in the literature of infection of man by many other tapeworms. A few of these parasites are briefly mentioned because of the necessity of differentiating them from more important species.

## Bertielliasis

*Bertiella studeri* (Blanchard 1891) Stiles and Hassall 1902 has been reported occasionally from man. The scattered records of human infection from Mauritius, India, Sumatra, St. Kitts in the British West Indies and the Philippines suggests a more cosmopolitan distribution than is now known. The parasite reaches approximately 30 cm. in length; the scolex possesses four large suckers that measure about 220 by 150 microns and a small, poorly developed, unarmed rostellum.

**Diagnosis** depends upon the recovery and identification of proglottids which measure about 6 mm. in breadth by 0.75 mm. in length and are passed in the feces in short chains. The eggs also are quite characteristic, measuring 45 by 50 microns. The thin outer shell is irregularly oval; in addition the inner envelope which incloses the onchosphere has a diagnostic "U" shaped notch at one side.

Related species occur in primates and more rarely in man.

## Dipylidiasis

The dog tapeworm, *Dipylidium caninum* (Linnaeus 1758) Railliet 1892, may be readily identified by its mature and gravid proglottids. It has been infrequently found in man in the United States, most European countries, the Philippine Islands, China and Southern Rhodesia. Infection is due apparently to the ingestion of infected dog fleas or lice which serve as intermediate hosts.

**Diagnosis** depends upon the recovery of double-pored proglottids or upon the recognition of embryonated eggs or the ovoid to spherical egg capsules each of which encases several eggs. The spherical outer shells are brick red in color thus giving the gravid proglottids a pinkish tinge.

## Raillietiniasis

The parasite, *Raillietina madagascariensis* (Davaine 1869) Joyeux and Baer 1929, is known more commonly as the Madagascar tapeworm. Cases in man have been reported from Madagascar, Siam, British Guiana, the Philippine Islands, Mauritius, Island of Niossi-Be and Cuba. In northern Formosa it occurs also in rats.

**Diagnosis** is based on characteristics of the eggs, namely the thick, ovoid or ellipsoidal outer shells and the lancet shaped onchospheral hooklets. It is believed that the cockroach, *Periplaneta* spp., serves as the intermediate host.

Other species of *Raillietina* have been found in man occasionally.

## Hymenolepiasis Nana

**Synonym** Dwarf tapeworm infection.

**Definition** Hymenolepiasis nana is caused by the presence of *Hymenolepsis nana* in the alimentary canal of man.

**Distribution** This small tapeworm has a cosmopolitan distribution. It is known to occur most frequently in temperate and tropical climates, being especially abundant in the European countries bordering the Mediterranean Sea, as well as in Egypt, Sudan, India, Siam and Japan. In South America it has been reported from Brazil and Argentina, while in the southern part of the United States *H. nana* has been the commonest tapeworm encountered in fecal surveys, being found in about 1 per cent of the stools examined. In South America (Argentina) eggs have been reported in 9 per cent of the small children and in 2.3 per cent of the adults.

**Etiology**   MORPHOLOGY. *Hymenolepis nana* (V. Siebold 1852) Blanchard 1891 measures 25 to 40 mm. in length by 1 mm. in

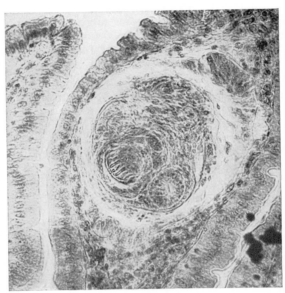

Fig. 261. Cysticercoid of *H. nana* in intestinal villus of mouse. (Courtesy Dr. Arne V. Hunninen, U. of Tennessee Medical School.)

breadth. The scolex bears four small suckers and a short rostellum armed with twenty to thirty hooks arranged in a single ring. The rostellum and the hooks may be invaginated into the tip of the scolex.

DEVELOPMENT. This tapeworm requires no intermediate host. Eggs are infective for man and mice. Hatching occurs in the small intestine where each onchosphere penetrates a villus and develops into a cysticercoid. Eventually the minute parasites break out into the lumen of the gut, pass further down the tract and attach themselves between the villi, where they reach maturity. There is experimental evidence which indicates that insects may serve as nonobligatory intermediate hosts (Fig. 261).

**Epidemiology**   The worm is especially prevalent in children. Infection is acquired by ingestion of the infective eggs passed in the stools. Since the murine strain is probably seldom acquired by man, the important reservoir is the human one.

**Pathology**    There are no characteristic pathologic changes. Eosinophilia, ranging between 8 and 16 per cent, sometimes accompanies a heavy infection.

**Clinical Characteristics**    Infection by *H. nana* differs from other human tapeworm infections in that many adults are often present in a single host. Patients infected by these parasites are usually asymptomatic except when worms are present in large numbers. In such cases nervous manifestations, abdominal pain, and diarrhea may occur.

**Diagnosis**    Diagnosis is based upon the following characteristics of the eggs (Fig. 247): (1) *shape*—usually ovoid; (2) *size*—30 to 47 microns in diameter; (3) *shell*—hyalin with clear area between shell and inner envelope; (4) *six-hooked embryo*—enclosed in an inner envelope; (5) *filaments*—four to eight threadlike filaments arising from each of the two polar thickenings of the inner envelope.

**Treatment**    Crystoids anthelmintic is the drug of choice although Atabrine has given good results in a small series. Oleoresin of aspidium is also effective. (See pp. 545, 551, 555 for details of treatment.)

**Prophylaxis**    Prophylaxis depends upon sanitary disposal of human feces. Domestic rodent control and proper protection of food will prevent infection originating from mice.

## Hymenolepiasis Diminuta

**Synonym**    Rat tapeworm disease.

**Definition**    Hymenolepiasis diminuta is due to the presence of *Hymenolepis diminuta* in the alimentary canal of man.

**Distribution**    This parasite occurs most commonly in persons residing in the U.S.S.R., the southern United States (especially Georgia, Tennessee and Texas), India, Italy and Japan. It is found likewise in Belgium, China, the Philippine Islands, Argentina, Brazil and the West Indies.

**Etiology**    MORPHOLOGY. The rat tapeworm, *Hymenolepis diminuta* (Rudolphi 1819) Blanchard 1891, is a parasite of the rat, mouse, and more rarely, of man. The strobila ranges from 20 to 60 cm. in length. The scolex carries four suckers and an unarmed retractile rostellum. Mature proglottids are wider than long; each contains a central ovary flanked on one side by two testes, on the other by one. Eggs are nearly spherical, measuring 60 to 86 microns in greatest diameter. The yellowish outer membrane is distinct and is clearly set off from the inner membrane which invests the six-hooked onchosphere. The space between the outer and inner membranes is filled with a gelatinous substance.

DEVELOPMENT. Since the gravid proglottids disintegrate after detachment from the strobila, eggs appear in the feces of the definitive host. Numerous insects such as fleas, cockroaches and meal worms serve as intermediate hosts for this tapeworm. These animals become infective for the final hosts as soon as the cysticercoid larvae have completed their intermediate development (Fig. 262).

**Epidemiology**   Infection in man occurs through the ingestion of parasitized insect hosts which are often encountered as larvae in grains and cereals. In many instances the parasites remain viable during metamorphosis of the insect.

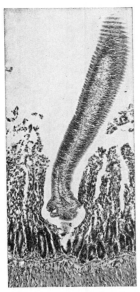

Fig. 262. *Hymenolepis diminuta* attached to intestinal mucosa of rat.

**Pathology**   No pathologic changes are recognized.

**Clinical Characteristics**   The alleged symptoms include indefinite gastro-intestinal complaints, diarrhea and abdominal pain.

**Diagnosis**   Diagnosis depends upon detecting eggs with the following characteristics (Figs. 247, 248): (1) *shape*—roughly spherical; (2) *size*—moderately large, 60 to 86 microns; (3) *shell*—transparent yellowish outer membrane lines shell, clear area between this zone and inner envelope; (4) *six-hooked onchosphere*—within inner envelope, the latter sometimes bearing polar thickenings but never polar filaments.

**Treatment**   Same as for taeniasis solium (see pp. 545, 551, 555).

**Prophylaxis**   The ingestion of infected insects, especially those occurring in processed grains and cereals, to which rodents have access, should be guarded against. Education and provision for adequate sanitation with reference to rodent control and food storage are important preventive measures.

# 49  The Drug Therapy of Helminth Infections

A given anthelmintic drug is specifically deleterious or lethal for only certain helminth parasites, depending on the biologic response of the worms to the drug, on the possible routes of drug administration and on the position of the parasites within the host. Thus in dealing with a given infection by helminths, one must first accurately diagnose the species present and then select the drug which gives most promise of eradicating the parasites. In some cases no medication has yet been found which is fully or even partially efficacious. Furthermore several drugs, originally advocated as desirable, have subsequently been found to have serious drawbacks. The modes of action of these drugs, whether vermicidal or only anesthetic, are in many instances not fully understood.

Helminths may be regarded as highly resistant to drug therapy. It is often true, therefore, that highly toxic substances must be used in combating them. As a result, effective dosage against the parasites sometimes approaches the toxic dose for man and great caution must be exercised during anthelmintic treatment.

The following pages list some of the more efficacious drugs commonly used in therapy (see Table 48). A number of them should be considered as distinctly dangerous and many have recently been replaced by safer forms of medication, which are also listed. The dangers and contraindications, as well as toxic manifestations and treatment of such complications, are briefly outlined.

Anthelmintic procedures other than drug therapy are discussed in connection with each helminthic disease (see Chapter 41 to 48).

## Antimony Compounds

### Anthiomaline

**Synonyms**  Lithium antimony thiomalate; 110L.

**Composition** $\left\{ \begin{array}{l} \text{LiO·CO·CH—S} \\ \text{LiO·CO·CH}_2 \end{array} \right\}_3 \text{Sb·9H}_2\text{O}$ contains 15 per cent antimony; a trivalent salt. Anthiomaline is supplied in a 6 per cent solution and contains 15 per cent antimony; therefore 1 ml. of the proprietary solution (6 per cent) contains 60 mg. Anthiomaline or 9 mg. of antimony.

**Pharmacology**  The pharmacology resembles that of the other antimony drugs.

**Toxicology**  Local or general reactions are uncommon following the administration of this drug. Intramuscular injections are not attended by pain although rheumatic pains have been reported subsequently in some instances. When toxic reactions do occur they are seldom severe; symptoms include headache, epigastric and joint pain,

*Table 48    Drugs Used for the Eradication of Helminth Infections*

| SPECIES | DRUG | | REFERENCE FOR PRIMARY CHOICE |
| --- | --- | --- | --- |
| | PRIMARY CHOICE | SECONDARY CHOICES | |
| **NEMATODES** | | | |
| *Trichuris trichiura* | Leche de higuerón | Crystoids anthelmintic Tetrachloroethylene with oil of chenopodium Emetine hydrochloride | 553 |
| *Enterobius vermicularis* | Oxytetracycline (Terramycin) | Crystoids anthelmintic Phenothiazine | 556 |
| *Ascaris lumbricoides* | Crystoids anthelmintic Hetrazan syrup | Oil of chenopodium | 545 |
| *A. lumbricoides* with hookworm | Crystoids anthelmintic followed by tetrachloroethylene if many hookworms persist | Tetrachloroethylene with oil of chenopodium | 547 |
| Hookworm | Tetrachloroethylene | Crystoids anthelmintic | 552 |
| *Strongyloides stercoralis* | Gentian violet medicinal | | 547 |
| *Ancylostoma braziliense* in skin | Hetrazan | Ethyl chloride spray Carbon dioxide snow Fuadin | 548 |
| *Gnathstoma spinigerum* | Hetrazan | | |
| *Wuchereria bancrofti* and *W. malayi* | Hetrazan | Suramin | 548 |
| *Onchocerca volvulus* | Suramin | Hetrazan | 551 |
| *Loa loa* | Hetrazan | | 548 |
| *Dracunculus medinensis* | Phenothiazine in olive oil | | 550 |
| *Trichinella spiralis* | ACTH | | |
| **TREMATODES** | | | |
| *Schistosoma haematobium* | Tartar emetic (potassium antimony tartrate) | Sodium antimony tartrate Sodium antimony gluconate Nilodin Fuadin Anthiomaline | 544 |
| *S. mansoni* | Tartar emetic | Sodium antimony tartrate Fuadin Anthiomaline | 544 |
| *S. japonicum* | Tartar emetic | Sodium antimony tartrate Fuadin Anthiomaline | 544 |
| *Fasciolopsis buski* | Crystoids anthelmintic | | 545 |
| *Heterophyes heterophyes* | Tetrachloroethylene | Crystoids anthelmintic | 552 |
| *Metagonimus yokogawai* | Tetrachloroethylene | | 552 |
| *Gastrodiscoides hominis* | Tetrachloroethylene | | 552 |
| *Echinostoma ilocanum* | Oleoresin of aspidium | | 555 |
| *Clonorchis sinensis* | Gentian violet medicinal | Sodium antimony tartrate | 547 |
| *Fasciola* spp. | Emetine hydrochloride | | 556 |
| *Opisthorchis felineus* | Gentian violet medicinal | Sodium antimony tartrate | 547 |
| *Dicrocoelium dendriticum* | Gentian violet medicinal | Sodium antimony tartrate | 547 |
| *Paragonimus westermani* | Emetine hydrochloride | | 556 |
| **CESTODES** | | | |
| *Diphyllobothrium latum* | Oleoresin of aspidium | Hexylresorcinol by duodenal intubation Atabrine | 555 |
| *Taenia solium* | Oleoresin of aspidium | Hexylresorcinol by duodenal intubation Atabrine Hexylresorcinol crystoids | 555 |
| *Taenia saginata* | Atabrine | Hexylresorcinol by duodenal intubation Oleoresin of aspidium | 551 |
| *Hymenolepis nana* | Crystoids anthelmintic | Atabrine Oleoresin of aspidium | 545 |
| *Hymenolepis diminuta* | Oleoresin of aspidium | Hexylresorcinol by duodenal intubation | 555 |

substernal oppression, salivation, nausea and vomiting. There may be slight albuminuria.

**Indications** This drug appears to be somewhat less effective than Fuadin. However, it has proved useful for the treatment of schistosomiasis haematobia, mansoni and japonica, although reports are not uniformly favorable.

**Treatment** Intramuscular or intravenous injections of 2 ml. of a 6 per cent solution every other day are recommended until ten doses have been completed (total 20 ml. or 1.20 gm.; total dosage should not exceed 1.38 gm.). Intravenous injections are preferable.

**Contraindications** None recorded.

## Fuadin

**Synonyms** Fouadin; neoantimosan; antimony pyrocatechin sodium disulfonate; pyrostib; stibophen.

**Composition** $C_{12}H_4O_{16}SbS_4Na_5 \cdot 7H_2O$. Antimony content 13.5 per cent. A trivalent salt. It is supplied in the form of an isotonic solution containing 6.3 per cent of the drug; 1 ml. of the solution contains 8.5 mg. of trivalent antimony.

**Pharmacology** The action is typical of antimony compounds, although Fuadin is less toxic and less irritant than the tartrates of antimony.

**Toxicology** This is a safer drug than tartar emetic but it is less efficacious. Local irritation, necrosis, nausea, bronchial irritation or marked liver damage do not occur following its judicious administration. However, when used for intensive treatment or in high dosage, electrocardiographic changes including low, diphasic or inverted T waves are produced. These are reversible.

**Indications** Although less effective than potassium or sodium antimony tartrate, Fuadin is recommended for the treatment of all forms of schistosomiasis. However, it frequently fails to cure infections by *S. japonicum*.

It has been recommended for the treatment of creeping eruption due to infection by *A. braziliense* (see p. 403).

**Treatment** For Schistosomiasis. Intramuscular injections of the 6 per cent solution are recommended. On the first day give 1.5 ml. (12.75 mg. trivalent antimony), on the second 3.5 ml. (29.75 mg.), on the third 5.0 ml. (42.5 mg.), repeating the latter dosage every other day for seven injections.

For children the total dosage in one course is from 15 to 25 ml., beginning with 0.5 ml. and increasing to 3.5 ml.

Treatment may be repeated after an interval of one to two weeks.

For Creeping Eruption Due to *A. braziliense*. Treat as for schistosomiasis.

**Contraindications** Since the toxicity is low this drug is safer to use intravenously than are antimony preparations used as anthelmintics other than Anthiomaline. See comments on potassium and sodium antimony tartrates.

### Potassium Antimony Tartrate

**Synonyms** Antimonyl potassium tartrate; tartar emetic.

**Composition** $K(SbO)C_4H_4O_6 \cdot \frac{1}{2}H_2O$. Antimony content approximately 36 per cent.

**Pharmacology** The absorption and excretion of this drug resemble those of arsenic. It is more irritating than arsenic but is absorbed more slowly. If injected hypodermically potassium antimony tartrate causes deep suppuration and sloughing. A cumulative action is uncommon due to the rapid excretion of the drug in the urine, 30 per cent being recovered forty-eight hours after ingestion.

**Toxicology** Potassium antimony tartrate is irritating to the stomach, causing vomiting if sufficient is ingested. The drug acts as a capillary poison. Chronic poisoning is rare and may be associated with dermatitis, nausea, gastro-intestinal upsets, anorexia, headache, cardialgia and albuminuria. Transient electrocardiographic changes including prolonged Q-T interval, depressed S-T segment, and inverted T waves have been reported, and in toxic dosage circulatory collapse and sudden death may occur. Antimony may be detected in the stool. Larger doses are tolerated better by vein than by mouth. The trivalent compounds are more toxic than the more recently introduced pentavalent forms.

**Indications** It is the drug of choice for the treatment of all three forms of schistosomiasis, and should be used in preference to surgical intervention for the treatment of complications involving the central nervous system.

**Treatment** FOR SCHISTOSOMIASIS. Because of the irritating effect on the tissues it must be given by intravenous injection. A freshly prepared 0.5 per cent solution in 5 per cent glucose in physiologic saline solution, isotonic sodium chloride solution, or sterile distilled water should be used. It may be sterilized by gentle boiling for five minutes but solutions of tartar emetic *MUST NOT BE AUTOCLAVED.*

The initial dose for an adult should be 8 ml. (0.04 gm. tartrate). If no untoward reaction occurs subsequent injections are given on alternate days, increasing each dose by 4 ml. (0.02 gm.) until an individual dose level of 28 ml. (0.14 gm.) is reached. Unless contraindicated by toxic reactions, a total of 18 doses is recommended (444 ml. of 5 per cent solution containing 0.799 gm. antimony). The patient should remain recumbent for a minimum of an hour after treatment in order to avoid respiratory complications.

**Contraindications** If toxic reactions occur the time interval between doses should be increased, or treatment temporarily withheld. The use of potassium antimony tartrate is contraindicated in diseases involving febrile, cardiac, respiratory, renal, hepatic and central nervous system disturbances, except for the central nervous system complications of schistosomiasis. The drug should not be given concurrently with other metals or potential cardiac depressants.

## Sodium Antimony Tartrate

*Synonym* Antimonyl sodium tartrate.

*Composition* A much less stable compound than the potassium salt.

*Pharmacology* Essentially similar to that of potassium antimony tartrate.

*Toxicology* Slightly less toxic than potassium antimony tartrate.

*Indications* Some workers believe this is the preferred drug in the treatment of schistosomiasis (see comments under potassium antimony tartrate). It may be used in the treatment of liver fluke diseases but its efficacy is not established.

*Treatment* For SCHISTOSOMIASIS. Intravenous injection of a 1 to 2 per cent solution in sterilized water is recommended. Follow the dosage as outlined for potassium antimony tartrate.

For CLONORCHIASIS AND OTHER LIVER FLUKES. Treat as for schistosomiasis.

*Contraindications* Contraindications are the same as for potassium antimony tartrate.

## Sodium Antimony Gluconate

*Synonym* Triostam.

*Composition* A trivalent salt containing 30 per cent antimony.

*Pharmacology* The action is similar to that of other trivalent antimony compounds.

*Toxicology* Sodium antimony gluconate is less than one-third as toxic as potassium antimony tartrate and less than one-half as toxic as sodium antimony tartrate.

*Indications* This drug has been recommended particularly for the treatment of schistosomiasis haematobia. Although reports of its usefulness are conflicting, it appears that it will accomplish clinical cure in many cases of vesical schistosomiasis.

*Treatment* For SCHISTOSOMIASIS HAEMATOBIA. Six daily intravenous injections of 225 mg. for an adult of 60 kilograms body weight, dissolved in 3.5 ml. of cold sterile water immediately before use, are recommended. The dosage for children is in proportion to body weight.

*Contraindications* None reported. The general contraindications to the use of antimony salts should be observed.


# Hydrocarbons

## Crystoids Anthelmintic

*Synonyms* Hexylresorcinol Crystoids, Caprokol.

*Composition* 1, 3-hydroxy-4-hexylbenzene. $C_6H_{13} \cdot C_6H_3(OH)_2$

**Pharmacology**    About one-third of the dose is absorbed from the intestine and is subsequently eliminated by the kidneys as an inert compound which is formed in the blood. The remaining two-thirds are passed in the feces.

Crystoids anthelmintic kills many intestinal nematodes outright, although the drug does not usually reach them all. As a result repeated treatments may be necessary.

**Toxicology**    This is a relatively nontoxic drug. If the capsules are chewed (as sometimes happens with children) superficial erosion of the buccal mucosa occurs. This drug occasionally acts as a gastro-intestinal irritant and upsets the stomach, although no untoward effects are usually experienced after swallowing. Its low toxicity permits the treatment of ambulatory patients.

**Indications**    This is the drug of choice in the treatment of uncomplicated ascariasis or of mixed *Ascaris lumbricoides* and hookworm infections. It is less effective against whipworm, hookworm, pinworm and *Fasciolopsis buski* infections. Crystoids anthelmintic may be given also to remove other species of intestinal trematodes, although it is not the drug of choice. It is recommended for *Hymenolepis nana* infections and appears to be quite effective against *Taenia solium*.

Hexylresorcinol in solution, administered by duodenal tube, is useful in most other intestinal cestode infections, while the use of retention enemas has been recommended for the treatment of enterobiasis and trichuriasis.

**Treatment**    For Ascariasis, Hookworm, Fasciolopsiasis and Hymenolepiasis nana. Prepurgation the previous evening with Glauber's salt (sodium sulfate) is helpful but not necessary. Adults receive five 0.2 gm. capsules (children 0.1 gm. per year of age up to 10 years) on an empty stomach. Glauber's salts should be given two hours after the administration of the drug and no food should be taken for five hours. The treatment may be repeated in three days. Patients may remain ambulatory.

For Intestinal Tapeworms. Greater success is obtained in the treatment of intestinal cestode infections when 1.0 gm. of the drug dissolved in 20 ml. of water is introduced into the duodenum by tube. Care should be taken to be certain that the tip of the tube has passed through the pylorus. A saline purge should be given two hours later.

For Pinworm and Whipworm Infections. The drug should be given by mouth as indicated above and by retention enemata for the treatment of *E. vermicularis* infections. In the evening of the day of oral treatment, following a cleansing soapsuds enema, from 500 to 1000 ml. of a 1 to 1000 solution of hexylresorcinol crystals in water should be given as a retention enema and held for fifteen to thirty minutes. Three days later the retention enema should be repeated. Several courses of treatment may be necessary.

Similar treatment is recommended for trichuriasis.

**Contraindications**    Because of its low toxicity there are no contraindications. A few persons, however, experience swelling and itching of the buccal mucosa or epigastric distress following the ingestion of normal therapeutic doses.

## Crystoids Anthelmintic and Tetrachloroethylene

Mixed infections by *Ascaris lumbricoides* and hookworm should be treated with Crystoids anthelmintic as for ascariasis (*vide supra*). If large numbers of hookworms remain, tetrachloroethylene may be administered a week following the last dose. Adults receive 3 ml. For details of treatment see p. 552.

## Gentian Violet Medicinal

**Synonyms** Methylrosaniline, methylrosanilinum, N.F.; methyl violet; crystal violet.

**Composition** A mixture of pentamethylpararosaniline and hexamethylpararosaniline chlorides.

**Pharmacology** This drug readily penetrates the tissues and is irritating to the gastric mucosa but not to the intestinal mucosa. The highest safe blood level in man is 7 mg. per kilogram of body weight. Intravenous injection causes a temporary bluish tint to the skin.

The action on intestinal parasites is not understood.

**Toxicology** Dizziness, nausea, vomiting, diarrhea and headache following administration are experienced by about 15 per cent of patients. Sometimes anorexia and abdominal cramps occur. Allergic reactions have also been noted.

**Indications** This is the drug of choice in the treatment of strongyloidiasis, clonorchiasis, opisthorchiasis and dicrocoeliasis. It may be used in treating children.

**Treatment** For STRONGYLOIDIASIS. For strongyloidiasis administer two 0.5 gr. 1½-hour enteric-coated tablets t.i.d. with meals for sixteen days. Two courses of treatment may be necessary. Children receive daily dosage of 9 mg. for each year of age. In refractory cases transduodenal intubation of 25 ml. of a 1 per cent aqueous solution may be effective. In pulmonary strongyloidiasis 25 ml. of sterile 0.5 per cent aqueous solution given intravenously is recommended.

For CLONORCHIASIS, OPISTHORCHIASIS AND DICROCOELIASIS. In clonorchiasis 1½ hour enteric-coated tablets or intravenous injections may be given. The drug does not reach the flukes directly but acts following its absorption and later secretion in the bile. Encapsulated worms (probably) escape the anthelmintic effects.

**Contraindications** These have not been fully defined, but it is stated that gentian violet medicinal should be avoided in moderate or severe cardiac, hepatic, renal and gastro-intestinal disease and alcoholism. Hospitalization is desirable for intravenous administration.

## Diethylcarbamazine

**Synonyms** Hetrazan, Banocide.

**Composition** 1-diethylcarbamyl-4-methylpiperazine.

**Pharmacology** Hetrazan is nonirritating, mildly diuretic and analgesic. It is rapidly excreted in the urine.

**Toxicology** Side reactions following the administration of Hetrazan are common but usually not serious or of sufficient intensity to require termination of therapy. The symptoms include malaise, headache, vertigo, lassitude, nausea, vomiting and, rarely, skin rash. These appear to be due to the interaction of the drug and the helminthic parasite and the products of metabolism or of disintegration. In certain individuals who appear to have become sensitized to their parasites severe allergic reactions may occur accompanied by giant urticaria and angioneurotic edema. These are particularly apt to occur in onchocerciasis and loiasis. In the former disease when there is involvement of the eye serious focal reactions involving permanent damage may occur.

**Indications** Diethylcarbamazine is the drug of choice for the treatment of filariasis bancrofti and malayi and for loiasis, and is recommended for creeping eruption due to infection by *Ancylostoma braziliense* or *Gnathostoma spinigerum*. Hetrazan syrup is the preparation of choice for the treatment of ascariasis in young children who cannot swallow Crystoids anthelmintic.

**Treatment** For FILARIASIS BANCROFTI. Administer 2 mg. per kilogram of body weight three times daily after meals if treatment is directed to possible cure. For mass treatment designed to reduce microfilariae to subinfective levels for mosquitoes, use 2 mg. per kilogram of body weight three times daily after meals for seven days (100 to 200 mg. per dose for adults and 50 to 100 mg. per dose for children over five years of age).

For FILARIASIS MALAYI. Administer 0.3 to 2 mg. per kilogram of body weight three times daily after meals for two to three weeks.

For LOIASIS. The first course of diethylcarbamazine treatment is accompanied by allergic reactions in approximately 70 per cent of cases. For this reason the first course should be as follows: first day, 0.1 gm.; second day, 0.2 gm.; third day, 0.3 gm.; fourth day and daily through the tenth day, 0.4 gm. In the presence of a heavy infection it is desirable to administer an antihistaminic drug prior to the initial dosage and to continue it through the fourth day. It is recommended to give more than a single course of treatment. Since severe reactions are uncommon following the first course the daily dosage may be 0.4 gm. for ten days.

For ONCHOCERCIASIS. Diethylcarbamazine is not the drug of choice for the treatment of onchocerciasis. The maximum dose is 0.1 to 0.2 mg. per kilogram of body weight, daily, for two to three weeks.

For ASCARIASIS. Syrup of Hetrazan is the medication of choice for the treatment of ascariasis in children although it cannot be depended upon to eliminate all the parasites. The syrup contains 30 mg. diethylcarbamazine per milliliter.

Give 12 mg. per kilogram of body weight once a day for four days, or 6 to 10 mg. per kilogram of body weight three times daily after meals for seven to ten days. Pretreatment fasting and pre- or post-treatment purgation is not required.

CAUTION. Such high doses should not be used in areas where onchocerciasis is endemic.

FOR CREEPING ERUPTION CAUSED BY HOOKWORM LARVAE. Give 2 mg. per kilogram of body weight three times daily after meals for ten to twenty-one days, or until larvistasis and cure have been obtained.

FOR GNATHOSTOMIASIS OR LARVA MIGRANS. Administer 0.5 to 0.7 gm. per kilogram of body weight three times daily after meals for five to seven days.

TREATMENT OF ALLERGIC REACTIONS. Benadryl, Pyribenzamine, or other antihistamine drug, 10 to 50 mg., according to weight and age, can be given every two hours until relief is obtained. Thereafter the intervals between doses should be lengthened.

**Contraindications**   Diethylcarbamazine should not be used in the presence of onchocerciasis with active involvement of the eyes.

### Lucanthone Hydrochloride

**Synonyms**   Miracil D, Nilodin.

**Composition**   A thioxanthone compound, 1-diethylaminoethyl-amino-4-methylthioxanthone hydrochloride.

**Pharmacology**   It is a yellow powder moderately soluble in water. It is administered by mouth and excreted in the urine. It is generally well tolerated in therapeutic dosage although transient side effects are common. It is a gastro-intestinal irritant, and, in toxic doses in experimental animals, produces pathologic changes in the liver, kidney and heart. When injected intramuscularly inflammation and necrosis result.

**Toxicology**   At therapeutic levels evidence of gastric irritation is not infrequently observed, characterized by nausea, abdominal pain or discomfort and occasional vomiting. These effects are usually transitory and may be controlled by administration after meals and by the taking of small feedings between meals. Less frequently there may be light-headedness, insomnia, restlessness, muscular twitching and yellow staining of the skin.

**Indications**   Miracil D is recommended particularly for the treatment of schistosomiasis haematobia. It appears to be less effective in schistosomiasis mansoni and relatively ineffective in schistosomiasis japonica.

**Treatment**   FOR SCHISTOSOMIASIS HAEMATOBIA. Since the drug is administered by mouth hospitalization is not required and it has proved useful for mass treatment. The optimal total dosage is considered to be about 75 mg. per kilogram of body weight. It should be given in divided doses, taken after meals, over a period of five or six days.

**Contraindications**    None reported.

### Phenothiazine

**Synonym**    Thiodiphenylamine.

**Composition**    Dibenzo-1,4-thiazine. $C_6H_4N\text{-}C_6H_4S$. A close chemical relative of methylene blue.

**Pharmacology**    Probably in man, as in animals, as much as 50 per cent of the ingested dose may be absorbed. Once absorbed the degradation products are excreted relatively rapidly in urine, milk or sweat. Such excretions turn red upon exposure to air, owing to the dyes formed by oxidation of the precursors in the excretions. Judging from the action in animals the presence of conjugated phenothiazine in the blood stream appears to enhance the action of a substance, lysolecithin, which is a hemolytic agent normally present in serum. As a result of this change acute toxic hemolysis may occur.

This drug is believed to kill intestinal nematodes by inhibiting cell respiration.

**Toxicology**    Phenothiazine may be a highly toxic drug. Effective anthelmintic doses may reach the toxic level in many patients. Toxicity is manifested principally by nausea, vomiting and hemolysis and later by pallor and hematuria as well as damage to the bone marrow and kidneys. Keep the bowels open, as only the constipated seem to be poisoned.

**Indications**    Phenothiazine may be tried in refractory cases of enterobiasis or in patients who are intolerant to gentian violet. It has been recommended also in olive oil emulsion for dracunculiasis (p. 454 or below).

**Treatment**    For Enterobiasis. Adults and children, six years or over, may receive 1 gm. per day for six days; rest for eight days, and repeat. Children two to six may be given 0.5 gm. doses for the same period.

For Dracunculiasis. Preparation of a phenothiazine emulsion: Triturate 2 gm. of phenothiazine with 0.35 gm. of lanolin in a sterile mortar with 15 ml. of sterilized olive oil (heated to 150° C. for one hour). The addition of 5 ml. of sterile water produces an emulsion. Add another 20 ml. of sterile olive oil, pour the emulsion into a sterilized 2 oz. bottle, seal and autoclave at 115° C. for 30 minutes.

Injection. (1) Assuming the lesion is on the dorsum of the left foot proceed as follows: Inject the limb with a 3 per cent solution of Novocain as follows: 2 ml., into the vastus medialis muscle of the left thigh just lateral to its center. Make two similar injections, one in the calf muscles in the upper third of the leg and the other in the dorsum of the foot. (2) Shake the phenothiazine emulsion vigorously. Inject 20 ml. of the emulsion into the vastus medialis muscle and 10 ml. of the remaining 20 ml. into each of the other sites into which the novocain was injected. (3) Massage the injection sites firmly for 5 minutes.

It is important to inject half the emulsion as near the buried worm as possible. As much as 4 gm. of phenothiazine may be injected at one time if needed.

This preparation should be made and sterilized just before use.

**Contraindications**   This drug should not be used in treating persons with hepatic, renal, gastro-intestinal or cardiac diseases, or in infants less than two years of age.

## Quinacrine Hydrochloride

**Synonyms**   Atabrine, mepacrine.

**Composition**   Quinacrine is a yellow acridine dye.

**Pharmacology**   The drug is soluble in water, absorbed rapidly and is deposited in the tissues, especially the liver and the gallbladder. When administered over prolonged periods of time there is yellowish discoloration of the skin. It acts as a gastro-intestinal irritant and may cause nausea, vomiting and diarrhea.

**Toxicology**   There is little or no significant toxic effect. In rare instances when the drug is taken for malaria suppression over prolonged periods dermatitis may occur and there may be leukoplakia or pigmentation of the buccal mucous membrane.

**Indications**   Quinacrine hydrochloride has given good results in some cases of cestode infections. However, the effective dose is large and not infrequently causes vomiting. The drug seems to be particularly effective against *Taenia saginata* and probably *T. solium*. It may be used against *Hymenolepis nana* and *Diphyllobothrium latum*.

**Treatment**   FOR TAPEWORMS. It is desirable to give a saline purge the night before treatment and the following morning to give phenobarbital 0.03 gm. to 0.09 gm. depending upon the weight and age of the patient. One hour later 0.2 gm. Atabrine is given every ten minutes for four or five doses (total dose 0.8 to 1.0 gm.). Sodium bicarbonate 0.6 gm. should be given with each dose to minimize nausea and vomiting. A saline purge should be administered approximately two hours later.

**Contraindications**   None reported.

## Suramin

**Synonyms**   Naphuride Sodium, Bayer 205, Antrypol, Fourneau 309, Germanin.

**Composition**   A highly complex carbamide compound.

**Pharmacology**   This organic chemical combines with the plasma proteins and remains in the blood for considerable periods of time. It is excreted through the kidneys and frequently acts as a renal irritant.

*Toxicology* Side reactions which occur occasionally include fever, nausea, headache, muscle and joint pains, abdominal pain and hyperesthesia of the soles of the feet.

Troublesome allergic reactions occur in certain persons with filarial infection who appear to have become sensitized to their parasites.

*Indications* Suramin is the drug of choice for the treatment of onchocerciasis and has been used in filariasis. Suramin causes death of the adult worms and slow disappearance of the microfilariae. For this reason severe allergic reactions are much less frequent than after treatment by Hetrazan, which causes rapid death of large numbers of microfilariae.

*Treatment* FOR ONCHOCERCIASIS AND FILARIASIS. Eight weekly doses should be administered intravenously dissolved in 10 ml. of sterile distilled water. For an adult of average size the initial dose should be 0.5 gm. and the succeeding doses 1.0 gm.

Dosage should be reduced proportionately for children.

*Contraindications* Renal disease.

### Tetrachloroethylene

*Synonyms* Ethylene tetrachloride; perchlorethylene.

*Composition* $Cl_2C = CCl_2$. A liquid.

*Pharmacology* This drug is much less toxic and is almost as effective an anthelmintic as carbon tetrachloride. In experimental animals there is no evidence of absorption, as the drug is almost entirely excreted from the alimentary canal. Absorption is facilitated by fats and alcohol.

It is believed that this drug acts as a narcotic on intestinal parasites.

*Toxicology* If absorbed, this drug produces vertigo, headache and nausea. Alcohol and fats should be withheld for forty-eight hours preceding treatment and a saline purge should be given following its administration.

*Indications* This is the drug of choice in the treatment of hookworm infections uncomplicated by ascariasis and for such intestinal trematodes as *Heterophyes heterophyes, Metagonimus* spp. and *Gastrodiscoides hominis.*

*Treatment* FOR UNCOMPLICATED HOOKWORM INFECTIONS, HETEROPHYIASIS, METAGONIMIASIS AND GASTRODISCOIDIASIS. Withhold alcohol and all fats including milk for two days prior to the administration of the drug. The patient should remain in bed throughout the period of treatment. The preceding evening purge with Glauber's salts. Administer tetrachloroethylene orally in three 1 ml. soft gelatin capsules on an empty stomach the following morning. Children receive 0.2 ml. per year of age. Follow in two hours or less with a saline purge and allow no food until the bowels have moved. Do not repeat for three weeks. This will remove about 90 per cent of the worms and the balance will usually do the patient no harm provided an adequate diet is maintained.

For Mixed Infections of Hookworms and Ascaris. In cases of mixed infections by hookworms and ascarids, treat first with Crystoids anthelmintic as for ascariasis (p. 545). If numbers of hookworms remain after such treatment, tetrachloroethylene may be administered in one week (*vide supra*).

**Contraindications** If *Ascaris lumbricoides* is concomitantly present, this worm should be removed before hookworm therapy is instituted, as tetrachloroethylene stimulates the ascarids and may cause the formation of obstructive boli of intertwined worms. Severely anemic patients should be prepared for treatment by a week or more of appropriate measures including adequate diet and iron ammonium citrate or blood transfusions.

### Tetrachloroethylene and Oil of Chenopodium

**Administration and Dosage** For Trichuriasis and Mixed Hookworm and Ascaris Infections. Tetrachloroethylene in conjunction with oil of chenopodium is used for the treatment of trichuriasis and mixed infections by hookworms and ascarids. It is used as follows: tetrachloroethylene, 2.7 ml.; oil of chenopodium, 0.3 ml.; given orally on an empty stomach together with pre- and post-treatment with Glauber's salts for thorough purgation. In trichuriasis, the patient is given a pretreatment high cleansing soapsuds enema.

See "Oil of Chenopodium," p. 554.

### Tetrachloroethylene and "Crystoids" Anthelmintic

See "Crystoids anthelmintic and Tetrachloroethylene," p. 547.

## Semi-Refined Plant Products

### Leche de Higerón

**Synonyms** None.

**Composition** The crude sap or latex of the bastard fig, *Ficus laurifolia*, and of certain other wild fig trees in Central and South America. The active ingredient is a proteolytic enzyme, ficin.

**Pharmacology** This vermifuge ferments rapidly unless stored in refrigerators or preserved with 1 per cent sodium benzoate. The latter procedure is not entirely satisfactory.

The enzyme permits digestion of the parasites within the intestine of the host.

**Toxicology** Gastro-intestinal irritation; diarrhea in some cases.

**Indications** This is the drug of choice in the treatment of trichuriasis. It is available, however, chiefly in the American tropics, its use being therefore limited geographically.

**Treatment** For Trichuriasis. Administer a saline purge the preceding evening. Give no food the following morning and administer 60 ml. orally. Follow with saline purge in two to four hours.

**Contraindications** Gastro-enteritis.

## Oil of Chenopodium

**Synonym** Oil of American wormseed.

**Composition** A volatile oil extracted from the plant, *Chenopodium ambrosoides* var. *anthelminticum*. The active principle, ascaridol ($C_{10}H_{16}O_2$), is present to the extent of 65 per cent. It is an unstable organic peroxide.

**Pharmacology** Oil of chenopodium is readily absorbed from the stomach and intestines, especially in the presence of alcohol and fats. It is partly excreted by the lungs.

In therapeutic dosage this drug only paralyzes the worms; consequently prompt postpurgation is necessary. The oil is highly effective against *Ascaris lumbricoides* and whipworms and has been used in treating enterobiasis and clonorchiasis. It is not effective against tapeworms.

**Toxicology** Oil of chenopodium is toxic and the margin of safety is small. Toxic effects may be delayed in their appearance for as long as seven to ten days. Toxicity is evidenced by headache, nausea, dizziness, blurred vision and paresthesia. More severe complications that may occur are depressed respiration, lowered blood pressure, stupor, prostration and collapse. Damage to the liver and kidneys usually accompanies such untoward effects and fatalities have occurred. Absorbable fats as well as alcohol should be withheld for two days prior to treatment. Purgation following therapy is essential in preventing absorption of the drug and resultant toxic effects.

**Indications** Ascariasis and trichuriasis respond to this drug. Its use in intestinal infections by other nematodes is less successful.

**Treatment** For Ascariasis and Trichuriasis. Withhold fats and alcohol for two days prior to treatment. Put the patient to bed the preceding evening and give purgation with Glauber's salts the following morning. Adults receive 1 ml. of the oil in gelatin capsules on an empty stomach. Follow in two hours with purgation by Glauber's salts, the patient remaining in bed until the bowels have fully moved. Do not repeat this drug for three weeks. An alternative method is to give 30 ml. of castor oil containing 2 ml. of chloroform as the post-treatment purge. Allow no food until this has acted. The therapeutic dose approaches the minimum lethal dose, 3 ml. or less, and should never be administered except under careful supervision.

**Contraindications** Oil of chenopodium is contraindicated in various renal, hepatic and cardiac ailments, in pregnancy and in patients with intestinal ulcers. Even in healthy subjects this remedy is not recommended because of its toxicity, especially since safer preparations are available. It should not be utilized in the treatment of children.

## Oleoresin of Aspidium

**Synonyms** Male fern; filix-mas.

**Composition** Aspidium, U.S.P., filix-mas, B.P., is extracted from the green rhizomes and stipes of *Dryopteris filix-mas*. The active constituents, among them filicic acid, consist of several related methane derivatives of phloroglucin and its homologues, with butyric radicles in ketone combination.

**Pharmacology** The absorption of this drug is enhanced by alcohol and absorbable fats. Individual variations in absorption and susceptibility occur. Filicic acid decomposes in the body, forming trimethylphloroglucin.

Oleoresin of aspidium is believed to paralyze the musculature of parasites without affecting their nervous systems.

**Toxicology** Oleoresin of aspidium is irritating to the intestinal mucosa and if absorbed may give mild or severe symptoms. The former include headache, dizziness, diarrhea, colic, dyspnea, yellow vision and temporary blindness. Severe reactions consist of violent muscular cramps, delirium, tonic convulsions and coma which may be associated with glycosuria, albuminuria and casts, and icterus. The patient recovers slowly. Permanent blindness and death due to respiratory paralysis have been reported.

**Indications** This is the drug of choice for *Diphyllobothrium latum*, *Taenia solium*, *Hymenolepis diminuta*, and *Echinostoma ilocanum*.

**Treatment** FOR DIPHYLLOBOTHRIASIS, TAENIASIS SOLIUM, HYMENOLEPIASIS DIMINUTA, AND ECHINOSTOMIASIS ILOCANUM. Oleoresin of aspidium should be administered orally or transduodenally. The night preceding treatment give a saline purge, preferably Glauber's salts. The following morning allow the patient to drink only black coffee or plain tea. Keep the patient in bed and at half-hour intervals administer three doses containing 1 ml. each of the drug in gelatin capsules. Follow in two hours with another purge of Glauber's salts. Allow no food until the bowels have thoroughly moved. Children should be given a dose based on 0.06 ml. for each year of age up to twelve years.

Complete rest before, during and after treatment reduces the likelihood of complications. Alcohol and fats should be withheld for two days preceding treatment.

All stools passed for forty-eight hours should be carefully examined for the scolex of the worm.

**Contraindications** The drug is contraindicated in marked anemia, in pregnancy and in renal, hepatic and cardiac diseases, as well as in the very young or old.

## Alkaloids

### Emetine Hydrochloride

**Synonyms**   None.

**Composition**   An alkaloid, $C_{29}H_{40}O_4N_2 \cdot 2HCl$, plus water of crystallization, from the dried root of *Cephaelis ipecacuanha*.

**Pharmacology**   The emetic action of emetine is greater following oral than parenteral administration. There is a local action in the stomach as well as a central reflex action on the vomiting center. It is irritating to mucous membranes. It is absorbed slowly from the gastro-intestinal tract. Emetine hydrochloride should not be injected intravenously. The action of the drug is cumulative, as it is only slowly excreted in the urine.

**Toxicology**   Emetine is a general protoplasmic poison. Toxic doses cause muscular relaxation, especially of vascular organs, with resultant fall in blood pressure, weakened cardiac tone and occasionally myocarditis.

**Indications**   The drug is used in fascioliasis, trichuriasis and paragonimiasis. Prontosil has been administered concurrently in cases of paragonimiasis.

**Treatment**   FOR FASCIOLIASIS, PARAGONIMIASIS, AND TRICHURIASIS. Emetine hydrochloride should be given intramuscularly, as follows: 1.0 mg. per kilogram of body weight daily for a period of seven to ten days. Do not repeat this course of treatment for two or three weeks because of the slow excretion of the stored drug.

**Contraindications**   Chronic cardiac disease. Since this protoplasmic poison does not effect a permanent cure, it cannot be highly recommended.

## Antibiotics

### Oxytetracycline

**Synonym**   Terramycin.

**Composition**   A crystalline antibiotic isolated from broth cultures of the actinomycete *Streptomyces simosus*. It is prepared as the amphoteric or hydrochloride salt.

**Pharmacology**   Oxytetracycline is rapidly absorbed from the gastro-intestinal tract, producing effective concentrations in plasma and tissues. It is excreted in the urine and feces. It is a broad spectrum antibiotic with an unusually wide range of action against gram-positive and gram-negative bacteria, certain viruses, rickettsiae and protozoa, and likewise against *Enterobius vermicularis*.

**Toxicology**   Although oxytetracycline is generally well tolerated it may act as a gastric irritant causing nausea and vomiting. As with all the broad spectrum antibiotics, administration should not be long continued because of the inhibitory effect on the normal intestinal flora and the possible development of secondary moniliasis.

**Indications**  It is the drug of choice for the treatment of *Enterobius vermicularis* infections, in which its efficiency approaches 100 per cent.

**Treatment**  FOR ENTEROBIASIS. Oxytetracycline should be administered orally in a single daily dose for seven days in accordance with the following schedule:

Children under 5 years .......... 1.0 gm. daily for 7 days.
Children between 5 and 10 years . 1.5 gm. daily for 7 days.
Age 10 years and over .......... 2.0 gm. daily for 7 days.

## 50  Introduction

The science of nutrition is concerned with food and the ingredients of food necessary for health, with the physiologic action of these nutrients and with the consequences of lack of effective concentrations of the fifty or sixty known specific substances. The same essentials are provided by many different staples. It is possible therefore, to provide protective diets by utilizing a variety of foods. In fact, variety of diet constitutes one of the cardinal principles of nutrition practice. Except in the case of milk for infants there is no single food which, of itself, is essential for good nutrition, and even in this instance a "soybean milk" provides a satisfactory substitute.

An adequate diet must contain sufficient amounts of protein, fat, carbohydrate, water, the numerous essential minerals and vitamins. The absolute requirements for these substances cannot be stated, since many have interrelated physiologic functions. The amount of protein required in the diet depends upon the calories furnished by carbohydrate and fat. The requirement for the B vitamin niacin is based upon the available amount of the amino acid tryptophan and, similarly, the need for iron is related to the ascorbic acid content of the diet.

However, we do know the relative amounts and ranges of many of the specific factors required for good health. The caloric content must meet the basal metabolic need in order to maintain weight equilibrium and it must provide for the activity of the individual. The range for an adult may vary from 2000 to 5000 calories per day. Generally, carbohydrate provides 60 to 75 per cent of the required total, fat 10 to 40 per cent, and protein 5 to 15 per cent. Excluding pregnant and lactating women, the protein requirements of adults approximate 30 gm. per day but in practical nutrition twice this

*Table 49   Desirable Ranges for Daily Intake of Certain Nutrients*

| | SEDENTARY | MODERATELY ACTIVE | VERY ACTIVE |
|---|---|---|---|
| Calories.......................... | 1800–2000 | 2200–3200 | 3200–5000 |
| Protein, gm....................... | 50– 100 | 50– 100 | 50– 100 |
| Calcium, gm....................... | 0.4– 1.0 | 0.4– 1.0 | 0.4– 1.0 |
| Iron, mg.......................... | 12– 15 | 12– 15 | 12– 15 |
| Sodium, gm........................ | 1– 5 | 1– 5 | 1– 5 |
| Vitamin A, I.U.................... | 3000–5000 | 3000–5000 | 3000–5000 |
| Thiamine (vitamin $B_1$) mg............ | 1– 2 | 1– 2 | 1– 2 |
| Riboflavin (vitamin $B_2$) mg............ | 2– 3 | 2– 3 | 2– 3 |
| Niacin, mg........................ | 10– 20 | 10– 20 | 10– 20 |
| Ascorbic acid, mg................. | 40– 75 | 40– 75 | 40– 75 |

amount or more is desirable. Therefore the recommended daily allowances of the more important food constituents are based on the theoretical minimal requirements with a substantial increment to provide for special needs and to afford a factor of safety (Table 49).

## Effect of Tropical Climate on Nutritional Requirements

The opinion is frequently expressed that tropical climates cause unusual changes in nutritional requirements. Except in the matter of calories and water, there is little evidence to support this. The widely prevalent malnutrition is largely an expression of insufficient supplies of protective foods, selectivity of diet determined by the cultural and religious backgrounds of the people and the direct and indirect effects of infection. Many people in tropical climates are unable to obtain the basic foods essential for a good diet. The problems are basically agricultural and economic rather than climatic. Other groups because of religious beliefs or social practices avoid available animal protein. Still others prefer polished to unpolished rice. Parasitic or other gastro-intestinal infections may interfere with the absorption of specific food factors or utilize those available for their own economy at the expense of the host. Systemic infections, by their effect on the metabolism or the tissues of the host, may greatly increase the daily requirements for particular nutrients. Thus the essential problem will vary from region to region depending upon the practices of man and only secondarily upon the effects of climate.

**Calories**   Energy requirement is decreased in the tropics since the higher environmental temperatures diminish the need for heat production. The relative importance of temperature has, however, often been overemphasized. Observers have been unduly impressed by the temporary anorexia which frequently follows sudden passage from the temperate to tropical climates. An investigation of calorie requirements was conducted during World War II using United States and Canadian troops stationed in various parts of the world. All of the groups retained their usual food habits and all were engaged in the same types of duty. Under these conditions a linear correlation was observed between voluntary calorie intake and climatic environment, with the daily intake decreasing by 16 calories for each degree of increase in mean Fahrenheit temperature, or 29 calories for each degree centigrade. For ordinary populations, the Calorie Requirement Committee of the United Nations Food and Agriculture Organization estimated that there is a decrease in caloric requirements of 5 per cent for every 10° C. increase in mean annual temperature.

**Protein and Fat**    Available evidence indicates that high environmental temperatures introduce no change of practical importance in human protein requirements. Attention has been called to the low fat consumption in many tropical areas. This appears to be due essentially to local economic conditions. A low fat diet may also have been found empirically to be of value where conditions causing impaired liver function are widespread.

**Vitamins**    While it has been claimed that requirements for thiamine and for ascorbic acid are increased by heat, the evidence in support of this assertion is unconvincing. Similarly, claims that tropical climates *per se* predispose to rickets are obscured by lack of control of other factors, such as the availability of calcium and phosphorus. The great preponderance of evidence indicates that vitamin requirements of healthy persons are essentially the same in temperate and in tropical climates.

**Water and Minerals**    Water requirements are increased roughly in proportion to the amount of sweat secreted. They may increase from 2.0 or 3.0 liters per day in a temperate climate to 13 liters or more during work in a hot environment. Under extreme conditions, the need for water may actually outstrip thirst. Wartime studies demonstrated that the best level of performance is obtained when the water lost in sweat is replaced hour by hour. While loss of minerals, sodium chloride in particular, is increased in individuals first exposed to hot climates, acclimatization is accompanied by decreased salt concentration in sweat so that salt requirements are increased only slightly. The trend in recent practice is against the need, or advisability, of providing salt to men working in the heat as tablets or as salinized drinking water, except possibly in the case of unacclimatized individuals or of unusual extremes of activity and temperature.

## Foods as Sources of Nutrients

Rice is the single most important food of many tropical regions because it is usually more plentiful, but other predominantly carbohydrate foods such as corn, millet, other grains, and root vegetables such as taro are widely used. Unfortunately, these are low in vitamins, minerals, and protein. When refined, as they usually are by preference and for stability, they contain even less of these nutrients. Vegetable proteins are incomplete since they lack sufficient amounts of one or more of the essential amino acids, particularly lysine. On the other hand, the proteins of legumes, the germ of grains, and of nuts are more complete. These foods are also better sources of vitamins and minerals. Hence rice diets can be improved by including supplements of some of these "superior" vegetable and grain foods.

Animal foods such as meat, fowl, fish, eggs, milk and milk products provide complete protein and are generally excellent sources of minerals and vitamins. They are often unavailable in adequate quantity to many peoples in the tropics. However, inclusion of even small amounts significantly improves the dietary since they supplement the "weak links" of the incomplete vegetable diet.

Poor quality protein is probably the single greatest cause of nutritional ill health in the tropics. Although it may be difficult if not impossible to provide certain peoples with adequate protein, qualitatively and quantitatively, it is usually possible to improve conditions by more effective use of indigenous foodstuffs. Even in the absence of refrigeration, excess meat can be preserved for reasonable periods of time if it has been smoked, dried or pickled and is protected against flies. Invertebrates and other lower animals are often valuable protein sources and the proteins of cereals can be supplemented with legumes, nuts and preparations of whole grains.

Milk is of special importance in nutrition. In many areas it is unobtainable or available only in limited supply, in part because of lack of a dairy industry and in part because of the problems associated with conservation and distribution. In the hot climates, in the absence of refrigeration, canning or drying provide the only safe means for storage and transport.

The problem of providing a satisfactory milk substitute is crucial in many regions, particularly where animal milk is not available. In some areas soybean milk, and powdered small fish rich in protein and calcium, have been used with considerable success.

Enrichment of foods with one or more key nutrients may offer a partial solution. The enrichment of salt with iodine, milk with vitamin D, margarines with vitamin A, and white flour and corn meal with thiamine, riboflavin, niacin and iron have been outstanding advances in public health nutrition. Similar addition of thiamine to rice in the Philippines has resulted in a dramatic decrease in the prevalence of beriberi. Comparable improvement in the nutritional qualities of rice may be achieved by modern methods of milling, by parboiling brown rice and by making "converted" rice. However, manufacturing facilities for the latter are expensive, and parboiled rice may not be acceptable to indigenous populations because of altered flavor, color, and consistency. Acceptability of food and local dietary customs are necessarily determining factors in the development of any practical nutrition program. At present it appears that enrichment with synthetic vitamins is the most realistic approach to the problem of the predominantly rice diet. Similarly, addition of synthetic amino acids may prove to be practical in the future for supplementing the deficient proteins in regions where the complete proteins of animal origin are unobtainable in sufficient amounts.

Diets typical of the tropics commonly provide only a limited choice of foods. Selection is still further restricted by the hazard of contamination by parasitic or other infectious agents. However, the daily diet should be as varied as local conditions permit. It should include animal products, fruits, greens and vegetables, particularly beans, in addition to the carbohydrate staple rice, corn or millet. Scalding of fruits which are eaten raw and light boiling of greens will afford protection against infection without impairing nutritional values. The chemical treatment of foods, such as washing in permanganate solution, is not a dependable safeguard.

## General Physiologic Effects of Inadequate Diet

Investigation of the various deficiency diseases of man indicates that they are the resultant of the action of a variety of factors having a complex interrelationship, and not the expression of single specific deficiencies. This is to be anticipated, since it is very doubtful that a defective diet is ever lacking in only one factor.

The water-soluble vitamins, namely the whole B complex and vitamin C, are not stored in large amounts within the body and are rapidly depleted in the absence of dietary sources. The fat-soluble vitamins A and K, however, appear to be stored in considerable amounts and prolonged periods of dietary deficiency are required to deplete them.

Present indications of the roles of the vitamins in intracellular metabolism and of their probable interactions strongly suggest that lack of various of these substances may produce similar disturbances of normal physiology. It seems probable that any deficit below the physiologic requirements is associated with impairment of function and, if sufficiently great, with the appearance of symptoms. Later, if the deprivation is severe and long continued, this disturbance of function is accompanied by alteration of structure and consequently the deficiency is then expressed clinically by the presence both of symptoms and of physical signs. It follows, therefore, that the responses to a defective diet may be protean and are the resultant of (*a*) multiple deficiencies in the diet, (*b*) the degree to which each essential substance is deficient, and (c) the duration of the particular deficits.

The ultimate clinical expression of inadequate diet will, therefore, vary in accordance with the type of deficiency of the diet with respect to its content of calories, biologically complete protein, mineral constituents and the various vitamins. The clinical picture will vary further in accordance with the magnitude of the deprivation, its duration and the level of energy output of the individual. Thus, under certain conditions, the indications of sodium chloride deficit may be acute and appear within a very brief period of time. The expression of vitamin B complex deficiency will appear much earlier than those clinical syndromes depending upon lack of the fat-soluble factors; and a diet providing inadequate protein may require a prolonged period before its effects become clinically evident.

Finally, in the presence of a definite clinical syndrome functional changes occur in the small intestine which interfere with normal utilization of the diet and consequently operate still further to augment existing deficiencies. Thus, there is created a vicious progressive spiral in which both a primary dietary deficit and a secondary disturbance of normal physiology causing impaired absorption contribute to progression of the deficiency state.

The operation of these varied factors upon population groups is well illustrated by studies of the nutritional status of the inhabitants of Madrid during the Spanish Civil War. These observations can be used likewise to predict with a reasonable probability of accuracy the status of groups subjected to famine or near-famine if the approximate duration of the period of deprivation is known. During the siege of Madrid the available dietary consisted mainly of starches. Animal protein and good sources of the vitamin B complex were both seriously restricted. The first noticeable effects of this deficient dietary were indicative of lack of adequate amounts of the B complex vitamins. Thus, functional neurologic disturbances appeared early. Later a marked increase in the incidence of pellagra occurred particularly during the spring seasons of the second and third years. Famine edema, however, did not appear until the third year of the war.

During World War II internees in areas of the Far East developed beriberi because the limited food available to them was polished rice devoid of thiamine and other B vitamins. Internees in Western Europe were fed on whole grain breads and potatoes, reasonably good sources of the water-soluble vitamins, and few cases of the classic vitamin deficiencies developed. In Western Holland, for example, during the last six months of the war severe starvation was frequent, but not vitamin deficiencies because, with little food to metabolize, the need for the B-complex vitamins which function in various metabolic reactions is minimal.

Although the most striking clinical phenomena occurring in the specific nutritional diseases may indicate a marked deficit of one particular substance or group of substances, other important deficiencies exist as well. Immediate institution of a completely adequate diet becomes, therefore, the essential procedure in the treatment of this whole group of conditions. It is frequently necessary, however, to supplement dietary therapy by administration of pharmacologic preparations of certain of the vitamins, and of ample amounts of particularly rich crude sources. Additional amounts of certain minerals and an excess of biologically complete protein are likewise often required to obtain the most complete and most rapid response to treatment.

## Tropical Malnutrition

No striking deviation from temperate zone requirements, except for water, is thus characteristic of tropical conditions. The significance of tropical nutritional diseases lies in fields other than human physiology. An obvious and well known factor is the prevalence of parasitic and infectious diseases. These will often contribute to decreased intestinal absorption, sometimes to increased requirements, and usually to some degree of anorexia. Another and more important factor is the agricultural, economic and social status of many tropical populations. Many such peoples subsist on a diet based almost exclusively on one principal starchy staple food—rice, millet or corn, for example. The classic deficiency diseases characteristic of such diets could perhaps best be termed "diseases of society" rather than "tropical diseases," despite their geographic localization.

Pathologic conditions associated with malnutrition and found in the tropics may be classed in four categories:

1. Syndromes which are essentially of dietary origin, even though they may be complicated by parasitic and infectious conditions, for example beriberi, pellagra and kwashiorkor.

2. Conditions which are probably of nutritional origin such as tropical ulcer, sprue, pernicious anemia and certain urolithiases.

3. Conditions of unknown etiology in which nutritional factors appear to be important, such as primary carcinoma of the liver, and certain pancreatic fibroses.

4. Diseases, the primary causes of which are non-nutritional, but in which nutritional factors affect directly the response to the pathogenic agent or which indirectly contribute to the development of complicating malnutrition.

Important examples of the first two categories only will be considered in this section. The recognized clinical syndromes present one part of the picture of malnutrition. Nutritional diseases characteristically develop as multiple deficiencies. The signs and symptoms characteristic of several nutritional syndromes commonly appear simultaneously or in succession.

# 51 Pellagra

**Synonyms**  Mal de la rosa, mal del sole, psilosis pigmentosa, Alpine scurvy, chichism (northern South America).

**Definition**  Pellagra is the principal manifestation of a severe deficiency of niacin, generally complicated by deficiencies of other B vitamins. It is characterized clinically by a red, sore tongue, disturbances of the alimentary tract, symmetrical dermatitis and changes in the central and peripheral nervous systems.

**Distribution**  The disease has a world-wide distribution. It is generally associated with the consumption of diets containing an excessive proportion of corn (maize). The disease is more prevalent during the spring that at any other season.

**Etiology**  Endemic pellagra is due to prolonged ingestion of a low protein diet containing small amounts of nicotinic acid. The amino acid tryptophan can be converted to niacin by the human organism, so that low levels of both of these nutrients must generally be present for pellagra to appear. Diets high in corn and containing little or no meat, milk, fish or other good sources of protein are pellagragenic. The importance of the amino acid composition of the diet is illustrated by the fact that wheat diets are not pellagragenic in spite of a niacin content often lower than that of corn diets.

Lack of niacin interferes with the formation and the function of two essential respiratory enzymes, the di- and tri-phosphopyridine nucleotides. The effects of this deficiency can therefore be expected to be widespread. Less severe deficiencies of niacin produce milder symptoms.

While the lack of nicotinic acid and tryptophan in the diet are essential etiologic factors of endemic pellagra, certain organic diseases which interfere with the ingestion, assimilation or utilization of pellagra-preventing food factors contribute to the prevalence. Among such diseases, amebic dysentery, hookworm infection, malaria and cirrhosis of the liver are of particular importance in tropical regions. Secondary pellagra is one of the secondary deficiency diseases sometimes associated with chronic alcoholism.

As in other deficiency diseases, the phenomena characteristic of pellagra are usually accompanied by a relative lack of other essential nutrients. Cheilosis responding to riboflavin administration and peripheral neuritis responding to thiamine treatment are frequently seen as complications. In South Africa, the clinical picture and the probable etiology of infantile pellagra and of kwashiorkor are often closely associated.

**Pathology**  No characteristic or constant pathologic changes are observed. In acute cases there is active inflammation of certain skin areas and of the mucosa, particularly of the mouth and pharynx. Repeated attacks lead to atrophy and pigmentation of the affected skin regions.

**Clinical Characteristics**   The clinical picture is variable and the disease may be acute, subacute or chronic. The onset is usually gradual with asthenia, loss of weight, mental depression, and a sore red tongue.

Dermatitis may or may not occur. Characteristically it is symmetrically distributed, affecting areas which are exposed to irritation such as the dorsum of the hands and wrists, the elbows, face, neck, the skin beneath the breasts, the perineal region, the patellar areas and the dorsum of the feet. In most instances it is restricted to parts exposed to the sun. In the early stage there is erythema resembling

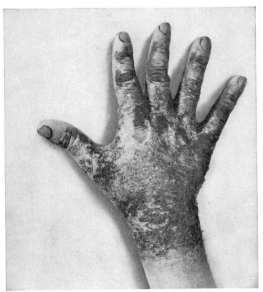

Fig. 263. Acute pellagra—dermatitis of hand and wrist. (Courtesy of Dr. Julian Ruffin, Duke Hospital.)

sunburn. This may be followed by vesiculation and bulla formation. The skin becomes thickened and roughened and as the acute inflammation subsides brownish pigmentation remains. Repeated attacks lead to marked atrophy of the skin (Figs. 263, 264).

Lesions of the tongue and mouth are usual. Acute glossitis and stomatitis may progress to extensive ulceration. Simultaneously there is fissuring at the angles of the mouth. The tongue is swollen, denuded of its papillae, often painful, and extremely sensitive (Fig. 265).

Hypochlorhydria or achlorhydria are common and there may be diarrhea or alternating periods of diarrhea and constipation. The stools are not abnormal in color and contain no excess of fat.

Pellagra is accompanied by a variety of symptoms referable to the nervous system. In the early stages the picture is that of neu-

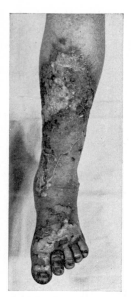

Fig. 264. Acute pellagra—dermatitis of exposed areas of leg and foot. (Courtesy of Dr. Julian Ruffin, Duke Hospital.)

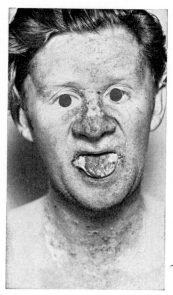

Fig. 265. Acute pellagra—characteristic dematitis of exposed skin of face and neck, acute glossitis. (Courtesy of Dr. Julian Ruffin, Duke Hospital.)

rasthenia which increases in severity with progression of the disease. In advanced and long-standing cases true psychoses occur. In these cases peripheral neuritis, spastic gait and other indications of organic involvement are not uncommon.

**Diagnosis** The four cardinal symptoms—dermatitis, glossitis, gastrointestinal symptoms and psychic disturbances—are characteristic of the well-developed acute case. There is no specific diagnostic procedure.

Diagnostic difficulties may be encountered in the early stages of the disease or in advanced chronic cases in which the characteristic acute phenomena are lacking. The combination of pigmentation and atrophy of exposed skin areas, smooth atrophy of the tongue, and the picture of neurasthenia should arouse suspicion.

**Treatment** 1. High-protein, high-vitamin diet.

2. Nicotinic acid or nicotinic amide, 300 to 500 mg., daily in divided doses.

3. Therapeutic doses of the B-complex vitamins, in particular thiamine chloride, 5 to 10 mg. daily as indicated.

**Prophylaxis** The prophylaxis of pellagra is based upon subsistence on an adequate diet.

# 52  Beriberi

**Synonyms** Polyneuritis endemica; barbiers; kakke (China and Japan); maladie des sucreries (French Antilles); hinchazon (Cuba); inchacao or perneiras (Brazil); maladie des jambes (Louisiana); alcoholic neuritis.

**Definition** Beriberi is a nutritional disease due to deficiency of vitamin $B_1$ (thiamine) and other vitamins. It exhibits acute and chronic forms characterized by peripheral neuritis and in severe cases by congestive heart failure. It may occur in all age groups.

**Distribution** Beriberi has been widespread in the past in the Orient and in areas of the tropics where polished rice is an important dietary staple. It has also been prevalent in Labrador, Newfoundland and Iceland where the winter dietary is restricted largely to white flour and other non–vitamin-bearing foods.

**Etiology** Primary beriberi is the result of prolonged subsistence on a deficient diet. Secondary beriberi may occur as a complication of other disease states attended by deficient absorption, incomplete utilization or unusual requirements for thiamine such as occur with elevated levels of metabolism.

**Epidemiology** The incidence of beriberi varies with the dietary habits and the availability of foods providing adequate amounts of essential food factors. It is seen most commonly in men and there is evidence to indicate that hard physical labor is a precipitating factor. Among women the disease occurs particularly during pregnancy and lactation. Infantile beriberi is a frequent cause of death among breast-fed infants in the endemic areas. Although it is not an infectious disease "epidemics" have been noted when outbreaks of diarrheal disease have occurred in populations subsisting on borderline diets, since diarrhea increases the physiologic requirements of the individual and diminishes the utilization of specific food factors.

**Pathology** The heart and the nervous system are involved primarily. The cardiac changes are predominantly hypertrophy and subsequent dilatation. The weight of the heart is frequently considerably increased. No specific lesions have been identified and the observed pathologic changes are often insufficient to account for the deaths from cardiac failure. The effects on tissues other than those of the nervous system are those of congestive heart failure.

Degenerative lesions without evidence of inflammation may be found throughout the nervous system. They occur in the peripheral nerves, the spinal cord, spinal ganglia, the nuclei of the medulla and pons, and in the structures of the autonomic nervous system. In the spinal cord the changes predominate in the posterior columns and in both the anterior and posterior nerve roots. There is destruction of myelin sheaths which may or may not be accompanied by fragmentation of the nerve fibers and atrophy of the nerve cells. Usually these changes affect only part of the fibers constituting a nerve trunk. The extent of these changes depends upon the duration and the severity of the disease. Of the peripheral nerves the sciatic is most frequently involved and evidence of this appears early. Of the cranial nerves the vagi and the phrenics are most frequently affected. With the disturbance of nervous innervation there is secondary atrophy of the muscles.

**Clinical Characteristics** Four clinical types of the disease are recognized: dry beriberi, wet beriberi, infantile beriberi and atypical beriberi.

There are no specific phenomena which are necessarily common to all types. The clinical manifestations of the disease fall into three general categories: those referable to degenerative lesions of the nervous system, those resulting from cardiac hypertrophy and dilatation, and the secondary effects of edema and anasarca. The onset may be rapid or gradual, the condition may become chronic, and recurrences of the acute form are frequent. The disease is commonly ushered in by the development of muscle weakness, anorexia and neurasthenia. Tachycardia and cardiac enlargement usually become evident early. There is often slight anemia. As the disease becomes established progressive peripheral nerve palsies appear.

DRY BERIBERI. The onset is usually gradual and the outstanding symptom is progressive weakness of the muscle groups which are most used. This most commonly appears in the extensor muscles of the thighs, and a significant early symptom in many instances is inability to rise from a squatting position. With the weakness there is atrophy of the muscles. Sensory disturbances appear at the same time but are usually less prominent. These may take the form of paresthesias, hyperesthesias or hypesthesias. In severe cases many muscle groups may be affected and the clinical picture is that of flaccid paralysis, muscular atrophy with or without evidence of cardiac enlargement, and tachycardia.

WET BERIBERI. In wet beriberi the clinical picture is predominantly that of acute congestive failure with relatively little evidence of nervous system involvement. Signs of neuropathy, however, can be elicited in most instances. The onset is frequently rapid and acute and the marked edema may mask the presence of significant muscle atrophy.

Electrocardiographic changes are common and characteristically consist of alterations in the T waves and prolongation of the electrical systole (Q–T). Sudden collapse is not infrequent. The exact mechanism of this form of the disease is uncertain but it seems probable that both the heart and the peripheral vascular system are concerned.

INFANTILE BERIBERI. Breast-fed infants of mothers subsisting on a diet deficient in thiamine develop an acute condition differing markedly from the disease of adults. In the usual type the onset is preceded by a period of diminished urine secretion accompanied by progressively increasing edema. If treatment is withheld acute cardiac failure suddenly supervenes and death may rapidly follow. With the appearance of the acute phenomena the child cries constantly and meningismus and convulsions may occur.

In the more uncommon dry type of infantile beriberi, edema and circulatory disturbances are not prominent. There may be vomiting, constipation, anorexia, loss of weight, pallor, fretfulness, and a characteristic plaintive cry or aphonia. The muscles are hypersensitive but there is usually little definite evidence of nervous system disease.

ATYPICAL BERIBERI. The clinical picture of the disease may be modified by other nutritional disorders such as scurvy, pellagra, or nutritional edema. So-called ship beriberi and land scurvy fall in this category.

**Diagnosis**   The essential diagnostic features are signs and symptoms of peripheral neuritis with weakness of the most used muscle groups. Hyperesthesia of muscles, particularly the plantar muscles and the gastrocnemius, is common and significant. An important and early physical sign is reduction or loss of vibratory sensation over the distal portions of the affected extremities with diminution or loss of distal proprioceptive sense. Tendon reflexes are later diminished and then lost. In severe cases marked muscle atrophy occurs. Measurement of thiamine excretion in the urine may provide confirmatory evidence. The range, considered to be normally 100 to 200 micrograms daily, is markedly reduced in clinical cases of beriberi.

The occurrence of diminished urinary secretion with edema in a breast-fed infant should immediately arouse suspicion and lead to prompt institution of specific therapy.

Beriberi must be differentiated from other types of peripheral neuritis, tabes dorsalis, postdiphtheritic paralysis and acute heart failure due to other causes.

The following eight criteria have been suggested to differentiate cardiac disease due to other causes from that of beriberi:

1. Enlarged heart with normal sino-auricular rhythm.
2. Dependent edema.
3. Elevated venous pressure.
4. Peripheral neuritis.
5. Nonspecific changes in the electrocardiogram.
6. Lack of other recognized cause of heart failure.
7. Grossly deficient diet for at least three months.
8. Clinical improvement with reduction of heart size after specific treatment.

**Treatment** 1. Thiamine chloride, 5 to 10 mg. parenterally twice daily.

2. High vitamin diet supplemented by rich sources of the B complex, such as vitamin preparations, or if these are not available, brewer's yeast 180 gm. daily, or tiki tiki (extract of rice polishings) 90 gm. daily.

The wet form of beriberi must be treated by absolute rest and heavy dosage of thiamine, which should be administered both intravenously and subcutaneously. The appropriate measures for the management of acute congestive failure should be used as they may be indicated.

Infantile beriberi should be treated by appropriate alteration of the mother's diet and the infant should receive heavy doses of thiamine parenterally.

**Prognosis** Deaths from the acute form of wet beriberi are not infrequent. The chronic form may leave permanent disability such as muscle weakness or flaccid paralysis due to nerve cell degeneration. Recovery from the disease in adults is slow, the muscle weakness and neuritis frequently persisting for months. Infantile beriberi, on the other hand, responds very rapidly and completely when treatment is adequate.

# 53 Sprue

*Synonyms*   Psilosis, Ceylon sore mouth, Cochin-China diarrhea.

*Definition*   Sprue is a chronic afebrile relapsing disease characterized by sore tongue, flatulence, steatorrhea, progressive emaciation, cachexia, and anemia. The latter is at first hypochromic, becoming hyperchromic and, in the terminal stages of untreated cases, occasionally aplastic.

*Distribution*   It occurs predominantly in the Far East in India and Ceylon, and in the Western Hemisphere in Puerto Rico. It occurs sporadically in the United States and other parts of the world with the exception of Africa, where it is extremely rare.

*Etiology*   The exact etiology is unknown. The fully developed syndrome is the expression of mixed multiple nutritional deficiencies, among which folic acid deficiency appears to play the dominant role. The fact that daily administration of pteroylglutamic (folic) acid relieves the symptoms of sprue might be interpreted to indicate that sprue is a specific deficiency disease. The etiology is confused, however, and some of the epidemiologic data have suggested that the primary mechanism may be of infectious origin. Despite this, nutritional considerations dominate both the etiologic and the therapeutic aspects of the disease.

Digestion of protein, carbohydrate and fat is normal but there is incomplete absorption of fatty acids and glucose. This dysfunction is associated with flatulence and bulky, gaseous, acid stools which contain large amounts of unabsorbed fatty acid crystals. There is likewise excessive loss of calcium in the form of insoluble calcium soaps in the feces. Hypochlorhydria is the rule and achlorhydria occurs occasionally.

It has been suggested that the basic defect—loss of ability to absorb fatty acids, glycerol and glucose—is due to failure of phosphorylation and to loss of phosphorus as the result of failure of phospholipid formation.

*Epidemiology*   It has not been possible adequately to explain the geographic distribution of the disease. Its incidence is not associated with any particular type of diet or dietary deficiency. It is a disease characteristically of the white race, affecting especially individuals in the upper economic levels and persons long resident in endemic areas.

*Pathology*   There is no specific or characteristic pathology. The findings at postmortem are limited essentially to wasting and atrophy of the various organs and of the body as a whole.

In the advanced stage showing macrocytic anemia the bone marrow is characteristically hyperplastic as in pernicious anemia. In still later cases the marrow may be aplastic and contain little active hemopoietic tissue.

*Clinical Characteristics*   The clinical picture varies greatly and

**573**

the onset is gradual and insidious. In the majority of cases, however, the three cardinal symptoms—sore tongue and mouth, flatulent indigestion and diarrhea—are present when the disease is fully established. These features appear simultaneously or in succession in any order.

Mouth lesions are prominent in most instances and usually precede the appearance of diarrhea. At first they consist of small, painful, aphthous ulcers on the tongue and buccal mucosa. Later the tongue becomes acutely inflamed and denuded. Extension of the lesions into the pharynx and the esophagus may cause severe dysphagia. Salivation may be troublesome.

Flatulence, at first mild and intermittent and frequently relieved by evacuation of a stool, gradually becomes continuous and increasingly severe. Eventually extreme and persistent abdominal distention may be a source of much distress to the patient.

In the early stages the diarrhea is usually intermittent and frequently mild. The stools tend to come in the early morning accompanied by urgency, and gradually become increasingly voluminous, gassy, foul and light yellow or gray in color. At first there may be only one evacuation each day; later the number increases and they become more fluid and irritating.

Spontaneous remissions of symptoms are characteristically followed by increasingly severe relapses. The latter result in progressive papillary atrophy of the tongue, weight loss and increasing asthenia. In the early stages of the disease there is commonly a moderate microcytic anemia.

In advanced cases emaciation is often extreme. The tongue is characteristically smooth, fiery red, painful and extremely sensitive to heat and condiments. There is marked mental depression and severe anorexia. Paresthesias of the extremities may be present. The patient often complains of epigastric distress and flatulence. The skin, especially of the face and the flanks, frequently exhibits muddy pigmentation. The abdomen is markedly distended and individual coils of intestines are visible. In some instances there may be evidence of subacute combined degeneration of the cord. Stools are frequent, liquid, white or yellowish white in color, abnormally bulky and gassy. Evacuation may be painful owing to excoriation of the anus. At times severe tetany may occur and in some instances there may be bleeding due to lack of vitamin K.

In the advanced case the anemia is macrocytic and may be severe. Gastric analysis will reveal hypo-acidity or anacidity but not achylia. There is a large excess of fat and fatty acids in the stools but no evidence of failure of fat splitting or of incomplete digestion of starch and protein. The fecal nitrogen is not elevated. The blood calcium is frequently low and the phosphorus is normal or somewhat low. Hypoproteinemia is common in severe cases. The glucose tolerance test after the ingestion of 1.5 gm. of glucose per kilogram of body weight reveals a flat blood sugar curve with the maximum rise seldom exceeding 40 mg. per 100 ml. Intravenous administration of

0.2 gm. of glucose per kilogram of body weight, however, gives a normal blood sugar curve. Vitamin A tolerance tests reveal a flat curve indicative of poor fat absorption.

Roentgen examination of the small intestine reveals characteristic functional disturbances. The barium tends to accumulate in dilated coils. The mucosal pattern is much coarser than normal and the progress of the opaque meal is slow and intermittent. Barium enema may reveal a markedly dilated and atonic colon.

**Diagnosis**    The characteristic case with glossitis, hyperchromic anemia and steatorrhea presents little diagnostic difficulty. The typical clinical phenomena, however, may not all be present, a feature which has led to the clinical classification of "complete" and "incomplete" sprue. The *differential diagnosis* entails differentiation from chronic pancreatitis, carcinoma of the pancreas, pernicious anemia, gastro-jejuno-colic fistula and regional enteritis. The following features are characteristic of sprue:

1. Steatorrhea with normal splitting of fat and normal digestion of starch and protein.

2. Flat glucose tolerance curve on oral administration.

3. Normal glucose tolerance curve on intravenous administration.

4. In severe cases, macrocytic anemia with megaloblastic arrest of the bone marrow.

**Treatment**    1. High-protein, high-vitamin, low-fat diet. In cases with marked flatulence it may be necessary to restrict starches and sugars.

2. Daily intramuscular injection of 15 mg. of folic acid, followed by maintenance dosage of 5 mg. by mouth when the patient's condition permits.

3. Parenteral administration of vitamin K, or oral administration of a water-soluble vitamin K preparation.

4. If folic acid is not available, brewer's yeast 60 gm., or tiki tiki extract of rice polishings, 30 gm. should be given daily by mouth, and concentrated aqueous liver extract 5 ml. intramuscularly each day.

When treatment is effective it is followed by rapid healing of the mouth lesions and progressive improvement in the intestinal features. Stools become less frequent, the volume is diminished, the consistency improved, the color returns toward normal, and the amount of unabsorbed fatty acids decreases. Lack of gastrointestinal and of hematologic response to folic acid should lead to doubt of the diagnosis. The response to vitamin $B_{12}$ should then be tested.

**Prognosis**    The prognosis depends to a large extent upon the duration and severity of the disease prior to the institution of adequate therapy. Mild cases may ultimately be able to resume a normal diet without medication. More commonly fats in the diet must be restricted permanently and parenteral injections of liver continued at intervals of one to two weeks. The character of the stools, the amount of unabsorbed fatty acids in the feces and the presence or absence of flatulence provide satisfactory guides to therapy.

peared in mass outbreaks, especially in India, often accompanied by the neurologic symptoms and signs of beriberi and by erythematous skin lesions, followed by pigmentation of exposed areas suggestive of endemic pellagra.

# 56   Osteomalacia

**Synonym**   Adult rickets.

**Definition**   Osteomalacia is a calcium-phosphorus deficiency disease characterized by a negative balance of calcium and phosphorus and by deficient calcification of all osteoid tissue. It is a disease primarily of women, particularly during pregnancy and lactation, increasing in severity with each successive pregnancy.

**Distribution**   It is widely endemic in North India, China, and Japan, and occurs sporadically in Central Europe.

**Etiology**   Osteomalacia and rickets are the same disease. Continuous resorption and new bone formation occur and there is failure of calcification of newly formed osteoid tissue because of insufficient absorption of calcium and phosphorus from the diet.

Failure of calcium-phosphorus absorption may be due to deficient diet, abnormal dietary calcium-phosphorus ratio, steatorrhea, or vitamin D deficiency. Usually several of these factors are operative, particularly lack of calcium and phosphorus in the diet and insufficient vitamin D. The elevated mineral demands of pregnancy and lactation upon the maternal organism are important factors in the progression of the disease.

**Pathology**   The abnormal ossification produces gross progressive skeletal deformities, especially of the pelvis, thorax, spine and long bones. The bones become soft and flexible and the deformities are more frequently the result of bending than of fracture. The bone cortex is thin and the trabeculae are greatly reduced in number or may be absent.

Microscopic examination reveals deficient calcification. Osteoclasts are present in normal numbers while osteoblasts are very numerous.

**Clinical Characteristics**   The symptom picture is dominated by weakness, bone pains, and often generalized aching. Bony tenderness is common and severe tetany may occur. Symptoms are particularly acute during pregnancy and lactation. The process characteristically remains relatively stationary in intervals between pregnancies.

Progression of the disease leads to great deformity and disability. Distortion of the bony pelvis causes difficult labor or makes parturition impossible.

**Diagnosis**   The marked deformities, particularly of the lower extremities, the thorax and the spine, are suggestive in endemic areas.

X-ray examination of the skeleton reveals generalized osteoporosis and the vertebrae often show biconcave deformity, the so-called "fish vertebrae." The diagnosis is established by blood chemistry findings. In severe cases the serum calcium and phosphorus are low and the serum phosphatase increased. In mild cases the calcium may be normal or only slightly reduced while the phosphorus is below normal levels and the phosphatase slightly increased.

*Differential diagnosis* entails differentiation from other osteoporotic diseases; especial difficulty is encountered with the osteoporotic form of hyperparathyroidism. The blood chemistry findings in the latter condition are distinctive, however. The serum calcium is elevated, the phosphorus low and the phosphatase above normal levels.

**Treatment** Treatment of the disease can protect only against further deformities. It consists of the institution of a diet high in calcium and phosphorus and the administration of 10,000 to 50,000 units of vitamin D daily.

# 57 Vitamin A Deficiency and Tropical Macrocytic Anemia

## Vitamin A Deficiency

**Distribution** Vitamin A deficiency is widely prevalent in the tropics, especially in those regions where the other nutritional deficiency conditions are common.

**Etiology** It usually occurs as a primary response to a diet which provides an insufficient supply of the vitamin, or, less frequently, it may be a secondary complication of diseases which are associated with defective absorption of fats.

**Clinical Characteristics** Vitamin A deficiency is characterized by skin changes, reduced dark adaptation, eye lesions and lesions of the nervous system. In many regions of Africa and India a majority of children present skin changes which respond to vitamin A administration, while a large proportion of hospitalized patients show evidence of xerophthalmia. The characteristic signs of vitamin A deficiency are as follows:

SKIN CHANGES. Synonyms: toad skin, phrynoderma, shark skin, keratosis pilaris, lichen pilaris, lichen spinulosis, Darier's disease.

The usual changes in the skin include dryness and roughness which is followed by eruption of hyperkeratotic papillae. The hair becomes dry and brittle and the nails develop transverse or longitudinal ridges.

EYE CHANGES. Dark adaptation is impaired, producing so-called "night blindness." There may be photophobia and xerosis, Bitot's spots and, in extreme cases keratomalacia may lead to corneal ulceration, panophthalmitis and loss of the eyes.

NERVOUS SYSTEM CHANGES. The susceptibility of the nervous system to vetches (*Lathyrus* sp.) is increased by vitamin A deficiency. The clinical syndrome lathyrism is common in parts of India and has been reported from other regions of the world. It is characterized by a spastic paraplegia.

**Treatment** Effective treatment of the conditions due to lack of vitamin A requires daily administration of large doses, from 50,000 to 100,000 International Units.

## Tropical Macrocytic Anemia

Tropical macrocytic anemia appears to be a response of the hematopoietic system to a nutritional deficiency. Although it may resemble certain aspects of sprue there is no interference with intestinal absorption. Like sprue, it responds satisfactorily to treatment with folic acid.

## 58   Epidemic Hemorrhagic Fever

**Synonyms**   Songo fever, Far East hemorrhagic fever, endemic hemorrhagic nephroso-nephritis, Kokka disease, Korin fever, Nidoko disease.

**Definition**   Epidemic hemorrhagic fever is an acute infectious disease of still unproven etiology, characterized by fever, purpura, peripheral vascular collapse, and acute renal failure.

**Distribution**   The disease has been recognized in the Amur River basin of Siberia and Manchuria since 1935. It first appeared among United Nations forces in Korea in the summer of 1951 (Fig. 266).

Other hemorrhagic fevers of Western Siberia, European Russia and the Balkans appear to be different entities.

**Etiology**   It has been established that the etiologic agent is filtrable; that it is transmissible by inoculation of blood, urine, or tissues obtained early in the disease; and that neutralizing antibodies appear in the serum in convalescence. There is evidence to suggest that the agent is maintained as a natural infection of field rodents and is spread to man by mites or "chiggers." No susceptible experimental animal has been found.

**Epidemiology**   The lack of a susceptible laboratory animal and of a specific diagnostic laboratory test limits epidemiologic study, since dependence must be placed on those human infections which are

**581**

recognizable clinically. The disease occurs throughout the year in certain endemic foci, with two distinct peaks of incidence, one in May-June, the other in October-November (Fig. 267). The disease occurs in rural environments, and 90 per cent of infections are isolated events as regards time, place, and person. The remaining 10 per cent, however, consists of sharply defined outbreaks limited to a

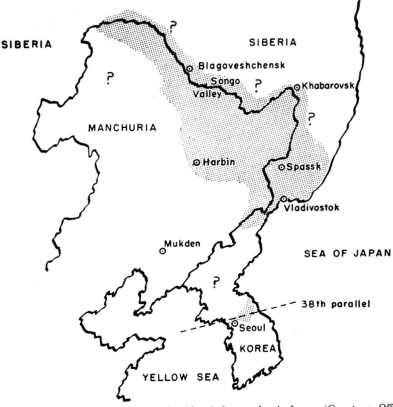

Fig. 266. Geographic distribution of epidemic hemorrhagic fever. (Courtesy, Office of the Surgeon General, Dept. of the Army, TB Med. 240.)

company, platoon, or squad. In such instances it is possible to trace the exposure to a limited period of time and a geographic focus. Current studies strongly support the concept that trombiculid mites are probably the vectors. The disease is not communicable from person to person by ordinary contacts.

**Pathology**   Three-fourths of all deaths occur within the first ten days of the disease. Shock is the most common cause of death, particularly in the early period although not limited to it. Later in the disease, acute renal failure, hemorrhage into vital centers, or pulmonary edema are also responsible for fatal outcome. The basic morphologic changes observed are (*a*) evidence of capillary dysfunction, (*b*) necrosis probably resulting from ischemia, and (*c*) a mononuclear cellular response. The kidney is invariably involved, the medulla being congested or frankly hemorrhagic. Necrosis in the same region varies from involvement of tubular epithelium only to extensive necrosis of all pyramids. The heart characteristically shows a hemorrhagic right atrium, focal myocarditis, and cellular infiltra-

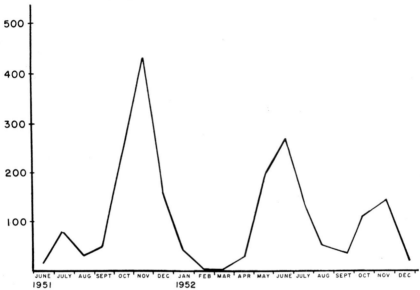

Fig. 267. Hospitalized cases of epidemic hemorrhagic fever in United Nations forces in Korea, 1951–52. (Courtesy, Office of the Surgeon General, Dept. of the Army, TB Med. 240.)

tion of the endocardium. Focal necrosis is common in the anterior pituitary and adrenal glands. Retroperitoneal edema is marked early but disappears later in the disease. Edema of areolar tissue, particularly in the retroperitoneum, is striking early in the disease.

**Clinical Characteristics**    The incubation period is usually about fourteen days, with extremes of nine days to five weeks. The disease varies widely in its severity, the greater number of cases taking the form of a mild febrile illness with proteinuria, and minimal symptoms of infection. One-fourth of clinically recognized cases can be classed as moderate or severe and in these the progression of symptoms is relatively uniform. For descriptive purposes this relatively typical clinical picture may be divided into phases each arbitrarily named for an obvious clinical feature. Although such phases are recognizable, in their progressive appearance there is often some degree of overlap.

Febrile Phase. The onset is acute, with fever, anorexia, thirst, and malaise. The temperature rises rapidly to 103 to 105° F., persists for three to seven days, and usually falls by rapid lysis about the sixth day. During this period there is often a distinct flush of the face and neck, the throat is similarly flushed but *not* sore, and the conjunctivae are suffused. Evidence of increased capillary permeability or frank leakage of plasma may be manifested by chemosis, periorbital edema, and proteinuria. Abdominal or lumbar pain may possibly indicate developing retroperitoneal edema. Petechiae may be found in the axillary folds, the conjunctivae, or elsewhere, and their appearance is thought to reflect varying degrees of trauma. Hematuria is common; Rumpel-Leede's test is positive, and thrombocytopenia may be present. The blood count, which earlier was normal or slightly leukopenic, often shows a leukemoid leukocytosis by the third day. Hemoconcentration results from the capillary leakage and is manifested by a rising hematocrit.

HYPOTENSIVE PHASE. At the time of defervescence, hypotension appears. In severe cases faintness, anxiety and apprehension are signals of the approach of medical shock in which the pulse may rapidly become imperceptible and the blood pressure undemonstrable. The finding of warm extremities, indicating arteriolar dilatation, suggests that this picture is a composite of the pre-existing hypovolemia from plasma leakage and a collapse of peripheral resistance. This period, characterized chiefly by hypotension, lasts from several hours to a few days. Shock merges with the phase of renal failure, but is not established as a causal factor.

RENAL FAILURE PHASE. Hematuria continues, proteinuria is pronounced and even in the absence of preceding shock some signs of renal failure appear, heralded by a diminishing urinary output and rising levels of nitrogenous products in the blood. The degree to which each of these basic functions is impaired is variable, and not necessarily parallel. Oliguria of some degree is common in severe cases, and even anuria may develop. Mild azotemia or severe uremia may be seen. During this oliguric period hypotension disappears, arterioles apparently regain their tone, capillary leakage ceases, extravasated plasma returns to the vascular compartment, and the elevated hematocrit falls. Apparently the dilated capillary channels which were packed with erythrocytes during the period of shock do not rapidly return to a functional state. The restoration of blood volume combined with the reduced capillary space produces a "relative hypervolemia."

At this time blood pressure rises, sometimes to hypertensive levels, peripheral veins are distended despite normal venous pressure, circulation time is reduced but renal plasma flow is diminished, hemorrhages become more frequent or marked, and symptoms appear which are ascribed by some to "relative hypervolemia" and considered by others to be typical of uremia. Furthermore, there appears to be a hemodynamic inflexibility in which minor variations in fluid balance result in pulmonary edema, or dehydration and shock.

RECOVERY PHASE. Following a one- to five-day period of mild or marked urinary suppression, diuresis occurs. Concomitantly, capillaries obstructed by sequestered red cell masses are cleared. There follows a relatively rapid readjustment of hemodynamics, fluid balance, electrolyte equilibrium, and azotemia. Urinary excretion may reach 6 or even 8 liters per day, but the specific gravity remains low, indicative of residual impairment of tubular function.

CONVALESCENCE. Symptoms and signs rapidly disappear, except polyuria, and concentrating functions of the kidney return more slowly to normal over the next few weeks. Residua are rarely seen, and long-term sequelae are unknown.

**Diagnosis** The diagnosis is suspected with the acute onset of a high fever in a person who has been exposed to rural conditions in a known endemic area. No single early finding is diagnostic, but the appearance of the flush, petechiae, hematuria, proteinuria, and leukemoid leukocytosis offer strong supporting evidence. Progressive defervescence, shock, and renal failure in the absence of other obvious causes establish the diagnosis.

DIFFERENTIAL DIAGNOSIS. At various stages before the full progression of the disease is apparent there may be confusion with leukemia, thrombocytopenic purpura, infectious mononucleosis, leptospirosis, acute glomerulonephritis, scarlet fever, the typhus fevers, encephalitis, purpura variolosa, and an acute surgical abdomen.

**Prognosis** With close observation and sound supportive care the case fatality rate can be held to 5 per cent. Recovery is usually rapid and apparently complete, although rarely a case may show evidence of persistent renal tubular damage. Sequelae are unknown.

**Treatment** No specific chemotherapeutic agent is known to date. Sulfonamides, antibiotics, vitamins, antihistaminics, pituitary and adrenal hormones, convalescent serum and whole blood have had little or no effect on the course of the disease. At present, treatment is primarily supportive, as follows:

1. *Early hospitalization* is recommended, since the severity of the disease cannot be prophesied on the basis of early symptoms. The tendency toward hemorrhage and shock is reduced by gentle handling, avoidance of trauma and physical activity, and institution of early bed rest.

2. *Maintenance of fluid balance* must begin early to avoid the overhydration which can result from the patient's attempts to satisfy the thirst which is prominent early in the disease. In fact, if hospitalization is delayed and careful intake-output records have not been kept it is often wise to allow only minimal fluid requirements. Until convalescence begins, it is of prime importance to set fluid requirements on the basis of the volume lost in urine and vomitus plus an allowance of 500 to 700 ml. per day for insensible loss. The maintenance of fluid balance is of such importance that routine use of an indwelling catheter is advisable in moderate and severe cases. Fluids above minimal requirements leak through the damaged endothelium, accentuating the clinical symptoms in the early phases

and precipitating pulmonary edema or hemorrhages in later stages. At the same time dehydration must be avoided. When intravenous administration of fluid is required because of severe nausea and vomiting, 5 per cent dextrose is recommended. Saline solutions are contraindicated because of their potential oncotic effect.

3. *Hypotension* must be watched for by recording periodic blood pressure readings early in the disease in order to avoid the insidious and often sudden appearance of severe shock. Mild degrees of medical shock may be handled by the simple but effective measures of the Trendelenburg position and elastic bandaging of the extremities. If shock is more severe, continuous intravenous pressor therapy is usually required. For this purpose *l*-arterenol (*l*-nor-epinephrine, Levophed) is the drug of choice, and administration in 5 per cent glucose using an indwelling catheter in the femoral vein is recommended. The diastolic pressure should not be raised to 90 mm. of mercury or above, since such pressures result in reduced blood flow through the kidney. When plasma volume has been greatly reduced as indicated by hematocrit levels above 55 to 60 per cent, the administration of salt-free albumin is indicated. After capillary leakage has ceased, albumin probably serves no useful purpose and may even be harmful. With the hypertension of the late renal phase, a phlebotomy of 500 ml. may be effective in relieving the uremic or "hypervolemic" symptoms, particularly if improvement has been noted on a preceding trial of bloodless phlebotomy using pneumatic cuffs about the extremities.

4. *Electrolyte imbalance* must be corrected where possible by replacement of deficits. Cautious administration of insulin and 5 per cent dextrose in water may alleviate hypercalcemia; retention enemas of cation exchange resin have also been useful, but care must be taken to avoid inspissation and impaction in dehydrated patients.

5. *Sedation* is effective in allaying or reducing many of the symptoms which disturb the patient or aggravate the physiologic imbalance. Barbiturates may be sufficient, but there should be no hesitation to employ meperidine hydrochloride (Demerol) if required. In the presence of severe shock and impaired circulation, repeated intravenous doses of 10 mg. of this drug are more effective than larger doses by other routes and are less likely to result in overdosage.

6. Close *medical observation* and good nursing care are essential.

7. *Ambulation* during convalescence should be based on return of renal tubular function as determined by concentration tests. When a concentration to 1.012 is reached, bathroom privileges are permitted; free ambulation on the ward is allowed with a concentrating power of 1.014; and full activity when specific gravity reaches 1.023.

**Prophylaxis and Control**   In view of the suggested implication of trombiculid mites as vectors of the disease, the control measures applicable to scrub typhus should be effective. These have been applied in Korea, but their evaluation is pending at this time. These methods include impregnation of clothing with miticides, use of mite repellents on exposed body surfaces, rodent control measures, and burning or bulldozing of camp-sites (see Table 69, p. 751).

# 59   Bartonellosis

**Synonyms**   Verruga peruana, Oroya fever, Carrión's disease, enfermedad de Carrión.

**Definition**   Bartonellosis is a specific infection caused by *Bartonella bacilliformis*, presenting two clinical types of disease. The severe form, Oroya fever, is characterized by fever, a rapidly developing, macrocytic anemia, and frequently intercurrent infection with high mortality. The cutaneous form, verruga peruana, is characterized by a verrucous eruption of hemangioma-like nodules and by a negligible mortality.

**Distribution**   The disease is restricted to the western portion of South America between latitudes 2° North and 13° South, occurring especially in Peru, Ecuador and Colombia. Its distribution is further restricted to narrow river valleys and canyons at altitudes between 800 and 3000 meters above sea level. It has been reported from both sides of the Andes.

**Etiology**   *Bartonella bacilliformis* is a minute gram-negative, rod-shaped or rounded organism found in varying numbers within both the red blood cells and cells of the reticulo-endothelial system, especially those of the lymph nodes, spleen, liver, and kidney. In the past there has been divergence of opinion with respect to the classification of these intracellular bodies. This genus is now considered as standing apart from true bacteria, rickettsiae and filterable viruses.

In stained preparations of blood both rod-shaped and rounded forms are seen. The rods are often slightly curved, occurring singly or end-to-end in pairs or in chains. Frequently they lie parallel or arranged in V's or Y's. The rod forms stained by Giemsa's method commonly show a deep red or purplish granule at one end suggestive of chromatin, the remainder taking a bluish stain (Fig. 269).

They may be cultivated best in semisolid nutrient agar containing 10 per cent rabbit serum and 0.5 per cent rabbit hemoglobin.

**Epidemiology**   The disease is endemic in certain arid river valleys of the Andes region and is coextensive with the distribution of the sandflies, *Phlebotomus noguchii* and *P. verrucarum* in Peru. However, the former does not bite humans and only rarely enters houses. At the present time only *P. verrucarum* has been incriminated as a vector. Other species are reported from the endemic areas in Colombia. The disease is especially prevalent at the close of the rainy season when these flies are most numerous.

Proboscis infections with *Bartonella* have been found in wild-caught female *Phlebotomus*. The source of these infections is unknown since there is no known reservoir host.

The disease in children is often mild, and latent infections without significant symptoms have been observed in adults. Immunity is believed to follow upon both Oroya fever and verruga peruana.

**Pathology** In the acute disease the lymph nodes and the spleen are enlarged, the latter containing melanin-like pigment and sometimes showing areas of infarction. The liver is likewise increased in size, contains pigment, and may present areas of degeneration.

On microscopic examination the reticulo-endothelial cells of the lymphatic system and of the viscera are seen to be packed with organisms. The bone marrow is megaloblastic and hyperplastic.

The chronic disease, verruga peruana, is characterized by hemangiomatous nodules in the skin and subcutaneous tissue. The early lesion consists of newly formed blood vessels within edematous connective tissue. There are marked proliferation of the endothelial lining and pronounced capillary dilatation. Late lesions may resemble fibrosarcomas. The causative organisms are often demonstrable in the endothelial cells although they are usually much less numerous than in the reticulo-endothelial cells in acute Oroya fever.

**Clinical Characteristics** Bartonellosis presents four stages, incubation, invasion, the pre-eruptive, and the eruptive. An incubation period of from 19 to 30 days, rarely up to 100 days, precedes the gradual onset of Oroya fever.

OROYA FEVER. The early symptoms are frequently vague and indefinite. In the invasive period fever is usually moderate and is accompanied by the characteristic progressive anemia and slight jaundice. Although the organisms are commonly not demonstrable microscopically early in the course, they can be recovered by blood culture. Subsequently great numbers of the bacillary forms appear in the erythrocytes.

The anemia progresses with great rapidity. Within two weeks the hemoglobin may fall to 20 or 30 per cent and the erythrocyte count to one to two million. There is marked evidence of new blood formation with reticulocytosis, at times up to 50 per cent. The erythrocytes are macrocytic, frequently hypochromic, and normoblasts and megaloblasts may be numerous. Leukocytosis is variable, apparently depending upon the presence or absence of intercurrent infection.

The "critical stage" is characterized by the apparent beginning of convalescence. The *Bartonella* change from bacillary to coccoid forms, the parasitized red cells become less numerous and there are fewer organisms within the cells. Macrocytosis diminishes, the erythrocyte and reticulocyte counts rise; lymphocytosis and reappearance of monocytes and eosinophils occur, and there is a shift of the polymorphonuclear series to the right.

Intercurrent infections accompanied by high fever, diarrhea, splenomegaly and marked leukocytosis are prone to occur at this time. They are associated with mortality rates well above 50 per cent. It is thought that *Bartonella* anemia predisposes to fatal septic invasion by organisms from the gastro-intestinal tract. In the presence of *Salmonella* and *Endamoeba histolytica* infections and of pulmonary tuberculosis the prognosis is very grave. Deaths likewise occur from complicating thrombocytopenic purpura.

Although malaria is the commonest intercurrent infection, it is less serious. The clinical picture is usually atypical. Fever is absent or lacks the characteristic periodicity. Profuse sweating, intermittent

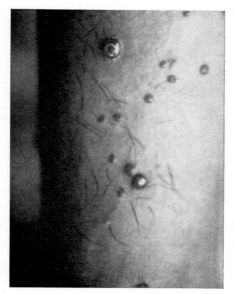

Fig. 268. Miliary hemangiomatous lesions of verruga peruana.

fever, splenomegaly and monocytosis, none of which occur in *Bartonella* anemia, are usual.

VERRUGA PERUANA. This is the chronic eruptive or cutaneous form of bartonellosis. It usually runs a course of two to three months and is characterized by miliary and nodular hemangiomatous lesions which have a definite tendency to hemorrhage and occasionally to ulceration; in the absence of intercurrent infection it is almost never fatal.

The incubation period is thought to be thirty to sixty days. The onset is usually accompanied by joint pains and fever seldom exceeding 100° F. The fever commonly subsides shortly after the onset of the eruptive stage.

The miliary type of eruption is more common and is most abundant on the face and the extensor surfaces of the extremities, appearing first as pink macules, later becoming bright red, nodular and bleeding easily. The mucous membranes of the eye, nose and throat may be involved. The eruption disappears without scar formation (Fig. 268).

The nodular subcutaneous lesions develop slowly and may reach 1 to 2 cm. in diameter. Not infrequently they break down, producing an ulcerating and fungating process which may be a source of danger from hemorrhage. They do not occur in the mucous membranes and are commonly confined to the regions of the appendicular joints. They tend to appear in successive crops. Scarring varies with the extent of tissue destruction.

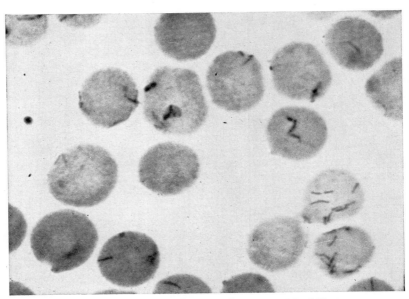

Fig. 269. *Bartonella bacilliformis* in stained blood film.

**Diagnosis**    The strictly limited geographic distribution and the distinctive clinical features of the infection tend to obviate diagnostic difficulties. Definitive diagnosis depends upon the demonstration of *Bartonella* in Giemsa-stained blood films or on culture (Fig. 269).

**Treatment**    Although there is no certain specific treatment for bartonellosis, preliminary reports indicate that chloramphenicol (Chloromycetin) may be of definite value, particularly in the presence of intercurrent infection. Transfusions of whole blood are helpful in the stage of acute anemia.

**Prophylaxis**    The prophylaxis of bartonellosis consists of control of or protection against *Phlebotomus*. Residual spraying of buildings and adjacent potential breeding areas with 5 per cent DDT in kerosene gives excellent results which persist for several months. Temporary individual protection may be obtained by the use of insect repellents.

# 60 Tropical Ulcer

**Synonyms** Ulcus tropicum, Naga sore, tropical sloughing phagedena.

**Definition** A chronic, often progressive, sloughing ulcer, usually occurring on the lower extremities. It may extend deeply with destruction of underlying muscles, tendons, periosteum and bone. Numerous spirochetes and fusiform bacilli as well as other bacteria are generally present in the lesions.

**Distribution** It is widespread throughout the tropical areas of the world and is particularly prevalent in the wet tropics.

**Etiology** Tropical ulcer is a clinical entity of uncertain etiology. Spirochetes and fusiform bacilli are often present in the developing lesion. It is improbable that they can penetrate the unbroken skin. The ulcer commonly develops at the site of an injury or abrasion.

Both the spirochetes and the fusiform bacilli are obligate anaerobes which can be cultivated on artificial media. The spirochetes, which are morphologically identical with *Treponema (Spirochaeta) vincenti (S. schaudinni)*, are slender and delicate and present a variable number of shallow irregular turns. *Bacillus (Fusobacterium) fusiformis* is a coarse, plump, banded or beaded gram-negative rod with tapered ends.

Other bacteria which may be present include staphylococci, streptococci, and various gram-negative organisms.

Recent studies indicate that malnutrition, especially deficiency of vitamins, may be important in the etiology of tropical ulcer and that the infection is secondary.

**Pathology** The pathologic change in tropical ulcer is essentially a coagulation necrosis of the skin and subcutaneous tissues in which many micro-organisms are demonstrable. The process tends to extend by continuity to adjacent structures. The walls and base are composed of infected indolent granulation tissue, in chronic cases bounded by dense fibrous scar (Fig. 270).

**Clinical Characteristics** Tropical ulcer may occasionally develop in the absence of visible abrasion of the skin. In such instances it is preceded by vesicle formation or it may appear first as an inflamed papule which breaks down to produce a rapidly extending phagedenic ulcer.

The process may be associated with pain, fever and toxemia. In most instances it rapidly enlarges and may reach a diameter of 5 to 10 cm. The base of the ulcer is composed of necrotic tissue and unhealthy granulations. The edges are not greatly indurated or raised but may be undermined. It is commonly attended by marked disability.

**Diagnosis** Laboratory examination is required to exclude cutaneous diphtheria, oriental sore and other specific ulcerations.

**Treatment** General measures, particularly complete bed rest and a full diet, are important. Specific treatment falls into two phases: (1) the control of infection and (2) the subsequent promotion of healing.

For the control of infection large intramuscular doses of penicillin combined with local mild antiseptic dressings, such as a 1/1000 watery solution of acriflavine, should be used. The local application of penicillin is not recommended and in any case it should not be so employed for more than five days because of the great risk of sensitization.

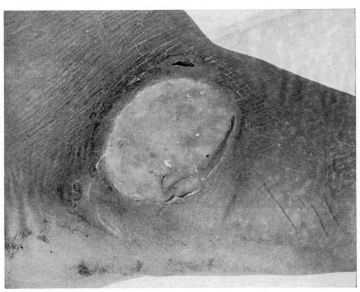

Fig. 270. Tropical ulcer. (Courtesy of Dr. Hardy A. Kemp, Baylor University.)

The newer antibiotics such as bacitracin, aureomycin and neomycin are probably of value applied locally although their status is not as yet fully known.

When gross infection is controlled the ulcer should be covered with soft paraffin gauze and the parts immobilized by a plaster of paris cast or, less effectively, by adhesive tape. Skin grafting by "pinch" grafts is of great value and if used should be combined with immobilization.

**Prophylaxis**  Prophylaxis against tropical ulcer consists of cleanliness of the skin, adequate protection against minor injuries, early and proper treatment of minor trauma such as scratches, small abrasions or insect bites, and subsistence upon an adequately balanced diet.

# 61 Desert Sore

**Synonyms**  Veld sore, Barcoo rot.

**Definition**  A form of ulcer of uncertain etiology occurring usually on the face, dorsum of the hands and forearms, or on the lower extremities. Its relationship to tropical ulcer is not established.

**Distribution**  It occurs in various desert regions of Australia, Africa and the Near East.

**Etiology**  Lack of personal cleanliness, local trauma and infection are important. Desert sore is often associated with impetigo of the face and is considered to be related to this condition as well as to ecthyma. The lesion characteristically develops at the site of a scratch, an insect bite or an abrasion. Staphylococci, streptococci, or both are frequently present. The role of diet is unknown.

**Clinical Characteristics**  Desert sore begins as a small vesicle containing thin sero-pus surrounded by a narrow zone of hyperemia. The vesicle extends rapidly to a diameter of 1 to 3 cm. and after rupture of the roof a purulent ulcer is revealed. Undermining of the edges with burrowing of the infection leads to irregularity of shape. The edge of the ulcer is not raised and the base of exuberant granulations may be flush with the skin. In the *chronic* stage the ulcer is covered by a dry brownish crust, from the edges of which pus oozes periodically.

In the *acute* stage the lesion is frequently painful and tender and it may be accompanied by regional adenitis, slight fever and malaise. Complete healing may require a period varying from weeks to months. A pigmented scar remains.

The condition may spread rapidly among groups under desert conditions.

**Diagnosis**  Desert sore must be distinguished from oriental sore, cutaneous diphtheria and tropical ulcer. It differs from the latter in being more superficial and more purulent, and in the absence of phagedenic sloughing.

**Treatment**  The treatment of desert sore is similar to that of tropical ulcer.

# 62  Cutaneous Diphtheria

**Distribution**  This infection has been reported especially from Palestine, North Africa, India and Burma.

**Clinical Characteristics**  Cutaneous diphtheria may be primary or secondary. Secondary invasion by the diphtheria bacilli may occur in wounds, wound diphtheria, and in any other skin lesion such as a burn, insect bite, tropical ulcer or even an eczematoid rash. The clinical features are pleomorphic. The infection should be watched for, even in the absence of flare-up of the primary lesion, necrosis or membrane formation.

Primary cutaneous diphtheria, on the other hand, is rather characteristic. It affects the extremities principally although it is not confined to them, and there may be a history of mild trauma. The most typical lesion is a round or oval ulcer measuring 1 to 3 cm. in diameter. Vesicles or pustules are sometimes seen in early stages.

The ulcer is shallow with rolled, blueish, tender edges and characteristically is covered by an adherent membrane or, more often, by a hard, dark scab (eschar). An adjacent bulla may be present. After a week or more the eschar separates, leaving a shallow punched-out ulcer with flat unhealthy floor. Multiple lesions are common.

Pain is generally present at first but later there may be anesthesia, a helpful point in diagnosis. Healing is from the periphery and is exceedingly slow. The resulting scar is thin and depressed. It may break down repeatedly before healing is complete.

Infection (or the carrier state) in the throat or nose may be associated but are not invariable.

During the prolonged course of four months or more, neurologic and cardiac complications must be watched for. Regular electrocardiographic tracings should be made if possible.

**Diagnosis**  Diagnosis depends upon bacteriologic examinations with culture on selective media. The inoculum must be taken from the deep aspect of the eschar or membrane. Virulence tests are usually necessary for confirmation of cultures.

**Treatment**  Immediate isolation, bed rest and proper nursing care in hospital for at least five weeks are essential. After previous intracutaneous testing for sensitivity and desensitization if required, diphtheria antitoxin should be given intramuscularly in doses of 20,-000 to 40,000 units. Palliative measures include use of the antibiotics and simple antiseptics locally for control of secondary pyogenic infections.

**Prophylaxis**  Schick-positive contacts should be immunized using antitoxin. Others who are Schick-positive should be immunized using diphtheria toxoid.

# 63 Granuloma Inguinale

**Synonyms**  Granuloma venereum, ulcerating granuloma of the pudenda.

**Definition**  Granuloma inguinale is usually a venereal infection characterized by destructive, granulomatous, ulcerated and painful lesions generally involving the pudenda and adjacent tissues. Occasionally invasion of the lymphatics and the blood stream produces metastatic foci accompanied by serious systemic disturbances which may lead to fatal outcome. There is little tendency to spontaneous healing.

**Distribution**  The disease is widespread in the tropics of Africa, the West Indies, South America, in the Pacific Islands, New Guinea, North Australia, Southern China and India. It is not uncommon among Negroes in the Southern United States.

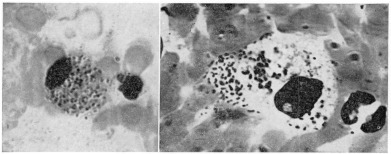

Fig. 271.                    Fig. 272.

Fig. 271. Granuloma inguinale: Donovan bodies in large mononuclear phagocytic cell in stained smear from lesion. (Courtesy of Dr. Donald C. A. Butts, University of Miami, Florida.)

Fig. 272. Biopsy of lesion: Donovan bodies in large mononuclear phagocytic cell. (Courtesy of Dr. Donald C. A. Butts, University of Miami, Florida.)

**Etiology**  The etiologic agent is an encapsulated bacillus, *Donovania granulomatis*, the Donovan body. It occurs intracellularly in large mononuclear phagocytic cells and is constantly present in the lesions. It can be cultivated only in embryonated eggs or embryonic yolk medium. Isolated capsular material gives positive precipitin tests and fixes complement with sera of patients suffering from the disease (Figs. 271, 272).

**Epidemiology**  Granuloma inguinale occurs in both sexes but is more common in the female. It has not been observed before puberty and is transmitted by sexual contact. The disease is common in young Negroes.

**Pathology**  The pathologic changes are essentially those of a granulomatous lesion of the skin with superficial ulceration extending by continuity to adjacent areas, especially on the genitalia, the

**595**

groins and the thighs. Although the disease is usually restricted to the genital region, involvement of the face, mouth, nose, neck, back and legs has been reported. In these regions it is probably the result of autoinoculation or metastasis. Metastatic lesions may occur in the bones or internal organs. Healing is accompanied by extensive fibrosis.

Histopathologic examination reveals a prominent round-cell infiltration of the corium with swelling, degeneration and ultimate disappearance of normal connective tissue elements. A surrounding infiltration of polymorphonuclear leukocytes, lymphoid and plasma

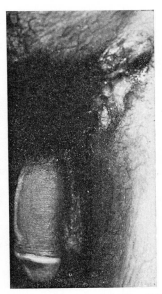

Fig. 273. Granuloma inguinale: involvement of skin of inguinal region. (Courtesy of Dr. Donald C. A. Butts, University of Miami, Florida.)

cells and reticulo-endothelial cells occurs. Many swollen mononuclear phagocytes containing numerous Donovan bodies are present in the lesion. There is marked formation of new connective tissue in which focal areas of inflammation and necrosis are commonly seen.

**Clinical Characteristics** The incubation period is variable, extending from a few days to two to three months. The initial lesion may be a vesicle, papule or nodule commonly on the penis or the labia minora. This becomes eroded and superficially ulcerated with new nodule formation at the periphery as the lesion extends.

In severe cases there may be extensive superficial destruction of the genitalia and the skin of the groins and thighs. Severe involvement of the vagina is followed occasionally by rectovaginal fistula. Concurrently with extension of the process there is marked scar tissue formation and epithelization often presenting areas of secondary involvement and breakdown (Fig. 273).

**Diagnosis** The diagnosis is based upon demonstration of the characteristic Donovan bodies. These are found within large mononuclear phagocytes in smears of scrapings from the margins of the lesions, stained by Wright's or Giemsa's stains.

**Treatment** Streptomycin is the drug of choice. It should be given intramuscularly for a period of 5 to 10 days depending upon the severity of the case. Marked relief of pain may be anticipated within twenty-four to forty-eight hours accompanied by evidence of healing. *Dosage:* 4 gm. daily in divided dosage administered intramuscularly every four hours. While toxic effects are uncommon, they should be watched for, particularly evidence of eighth nerve involvement.

Aureomycin, likewise, has given good results and has proved useful in streptomycin-resistant cases; minimal dosage, 250 mg. four times daily.

Chloramphenicol (Chloromycetin) also is effective. *Dosage:* It should be given by mouth in divided doses each 250 mg. to a total of 20 gm. in the course of 5 to 10 days.

Intensive antimony therapy has been widely used but is not to be recommended because of the limited margin of safety between therapeutic and toxic doses. Although the antimonials cause regression of the disease and healing of the lesions, in many instances treatment must be prolonged. Lithium antimony thiomalate (Anthiomaline) and stibophen (Fuadin) are preferred because of the greater stability and lesser toxicity. *Dosage:* Anthiomaline should be administered intramuscularly in doses of 3 ml. six times a week for four weeks. Fuadin likewise should be administered intramuscularly daily or three times a week to a total of 40 ml. of the solution. The recommended initial dose is 1.5 ml., the second 3.0 ml. and subsequent doses 5.0 ml.

Local treatment of the lesion with podophyllin for 5 to 7 days has given dramatic results. It is usually followed by prompt healing as in any simple uncomplicated ulcer. As originally used, a 20 per cent suspension of the resin in olive oil is gently smeared over the lesions once or twice daily. This commonly produces a secondary inflammatory process with pronounced local pain. Much of the irritation is avoidable if a varnish composed of a suspension of the resin in compound tincture of benzoin is substituted for the olive oil suspension, and if surrounding skin areas are protected by petroleum jelly. In either case secondary bacterial infection should be reduced to a minimum before the institution of podophyllin therapy.

# 64 Scabies

**Synonyms**  The itch, seven-year itch, Norwegian itch, sarcoptic acariasis; gale (French).

**Definition**  Scabies is an irritation of the skin of certain mammals caused by *Sarcoptes scabiei*. Species or varieties of this mite specifically infest the epidermis of man and several domestic animals. It is probable that slight physiologic variations in the host-parasite relationship operate to prevent the survival of ectopic varieties of *S. scabiei* in foreign hosts, i.e., the cat variety does not successfully establish itself in man. Human scabies, therefore, is produced almost exclusively by the human variety of this ectoparasite. Scabies in other mammals is referred to as sarcoptic mange.

**Distribution**  This is coincident with the distribution of man. Clinical scabies may be common among crowded populations with low standards of sanitation; it occurs sporadically under a wide range of environmental conditions.

**Etiology**  *Sarcoptes scabiei* is a minute arthropod classified among mites of the Family SARCOPTIDAE, Order ACARINA, Class ARACHNIDA. Its entire existence is passed in or on the skin of the host mammal. The life cycle is outlined in the section on Medical Entomology (p. 682).

**Epidemiology**  Transmission of the mites occurs most readily through close bodily contact. Cohabiting or sleeping with an infested person is the commonest means of acquiring the disease. Owing to the frequency of interdigital lesions, shaking hands is also a ready method of transfer; this is especially true in the case of children who play games requiring the prolonged clasping of hands. It is now well-recognized that clothing and bedding of infested individuals play only minor roles in the spread of the infection, for although the mites under optimal conditions can survive for several days apart from their original host, they do not readily find a new one.

The stage or stages accounting for most cases of successful transmission are in dispute. Some workers believe this to be the young newly impregnated female, while others name the larvae or the nymph.

**Pathology**  The pathologic responses to the presence of scabies mites are those characteristic of previous sensitization. Waste products or other substances liberated into the epidermis by the parasites promote erythema and edema. The regional tissues become water-logged and eosinophils tend to infiltrate the lesion. Vesiculation eventually occurs. Following rupture of the vesicle secondary infection is the rule. Since the burrows are in most instances very superficial, healing of the lesions occurs without scar formation (Fig. 274).

Some patients exhibit a mild eosinophilia during acute stages of the infestation.

**Clinical Characteristics**  An initial attack of scabies is asymptomatic for the first few weeks. After sensitization takes place, the initial attack resembles subsequent attacks. The cardinal symptom then occurring is severe itching. This is most intense shortly after the patient has gone to bed, the gradual warming of the body inducing greater activity among the mites. Loss of sleep resulting from scabies has at times been a cause of many lost man-days during military operations.

Scratching serves to kill some of the parasites and to inoculate others into new sites. The swelling induced by scratching also destroys some of the mites in their burrows; however, the most serious

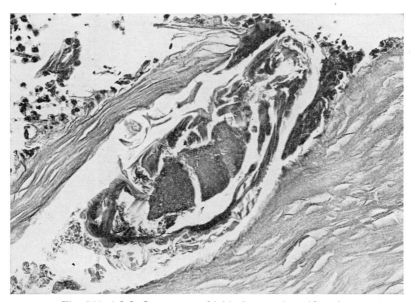

Fig. 274. Adult *Sarcoptes scabiei* in burrow in epidermis.

sequel is the development of secondary infection, usually of a pyogenic nature. This is a common complication.

An untreated case of scabies usually terminates spontaneously after several months. This seems to be due to the development of sufficient sensitization to interfere with the processes of reinoculation, each new colonist being at once surrounded by transudates which interfere with its normal activity. Some cases, however, progress into a chronic state in which the actual number of parasites is much smaller than was true in the acute stage of the disease. These cases constitute the reservoir of infection.

**Diagnosis** Definitive diagnosis of scabies is based on demonstration of the parasite. This, however, may be difficult to accomplish in many cases. In attempting to do so the physician should first study the lesions minutely with a hand lens. A typical burrow is a tortuous channel a few millimeters in length appearing as a fine line on the patient's skin. Its orifice may be marked by a black plug of crusted serum and mite feces. Toward the blind extremity the skin is erythematous and frequently a small vesicle is found even closer to the inner end of the tunnel. The adult female mite is situated at the end of the burrow itself. This region should be incised with a fine-pointed scalpel or sharp needle and the contents placed on a glass slide. Ten per cent potassium hydroxide solution may be added to clear the cutaneous scales and other débris that may be present. After adding a coverslip the operator should then examine the

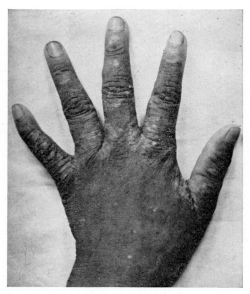

Fig. 275. Scabies—showing advanced lesions and characteristic distribution.

preparation with a strong lens or low-powered microscope. The finding of a mite in any stage of the life cycle is diagnostic.

Lacking success in demonstrating the parasite, one may make a dermatologic diagnosis on the characteristic distribution of the lesions in adult patients. The classic sites are the interdigital spaces, wrists, extensor aspects of elbows, axillae (particularly the axillary folds), abdomen and belt-line (especially the umbilical region), scrotum, penis and areolae of the nipples. In severe cases lesions may extend around the trunk to the small of the back. The upper back as well as the face, scalp, palms and soles are rarely involved in adults. However, in infants all parts of the body seem equally susceptible to invasion (Fig. 275).

The history of the infection is likewise often of value, since the occurrence of the primary lesion between the fingers is suggestive of scabies. Furthermore, a history of close contact with persons having characteristic symptoms, especially members of the family group, may be highly significant.

Although several other dermatologic conditions may superficially resemble scabies, in general it is safe to rely on the characteristic distribution of scabies lesions. This distribution is mimicked only rarely by other diseases (see Table 50).

**Treatment** When secondary infection of the scabetic lesions is present, this should be treated first with a sulfonamide or neomycin ointment. To kill the scabies mites one of the following regimens is recommended.

1. Eurax cream, 10 per cent N-ethyl-*o*-crotontoluide in vanishing cream, should be rubbed into the skin of the entire body except for the face and scalp unless these areas are involved. Preliminary bathing is unnecessary. After twenty-four hours the treatment should be repeated. This will give almost 100 per cent cures.

*Table 50   Differentiation of Pediculosis and Scabies*

| CRITERION | PEDICULOSIS | SCABIES |
|---|:---:|:---:|
| Lesions in scalp...................... | + | − |
| Parallel scratches, upper back........... | + | − |
| Lesions on hands and wrists............ | − | + |
| Burrows and parasites in skin........... | − | + |
| Nits................................ | + | − |
| Parasites commonly in clothing......... | + | − |

This preparation is valuable in the presence of secondary pyoderma since it exerts a bacteriostatic action on both staphylococci and streptococci. It is also an efficient antipruritic, and does not cause irritation, sensitization or systemic toxicity.

2. Kwell ointment, 1 per cent gamma isomer of benzene hexachloride in a vanishing cream base, should be used similarly for two applications to the entire body at intervals of twelve hours. Care must be taken to avoid contact with the eyes. It is said to be effective in approximately 95 per cent of cases.

This preparation is likewise nonirritating and may be used in the presence of secondary skin infection.

3. Benzyl benzoate is less effective and is an irritant to the skin in certain cases. It is most conveniently used in the form of Topocide, an aqueous emulsion containing in each 100 ml. benzyl benzoate 12.5 gm., benzocaine 2 gm. and DDT 1 gm.

Following a soapy bath, the emulsion should be applied to the dry skin of the entire body with gauze sponges, rubbed in gently and allowed to dry. It should be reapplied to the hands only after each washing. Bathing must be avoided for twenty-four hours and the eyes protected from the lotion. A second treatment should not be given for from ten to fourteen days.

The use of sulfur has been largely superseded. It is an undesirable method of treatment since dermatitis not infrequently follows.

**Prophylaxis**   Personal cleanliness and avoidance of close contact with crowded and infested populations will prevent the acquisition of scabies. Treatment of cases is an obvious necessity but equally important is the treatment of case-contacts. These will often include members of the patient's family or rooming house or his close occupational associates. In time of war or famine the inmates of prisons or the members of entire military units or other population groups must occasionally be treated *en masse* regardless of their infestation or noninfestation in order to check the spread of this disease. Sterilization of clothing and bedding has limited value.

# 65   Effects of Heat

## Physiology of Heat Regulation

Body temperature is the resultant of the rates of heat production within the body and of heat loss by the body. These processes are controlled by the nervous system, the main center being in the hypothalamus. Exposure to high environmental temperature initiates

*Table 51   Physical Mechanisms of Heat Loss from the Body at Ordinary Temperatures\**

|  | Percentage of Total Heat Loss |
|---|---|
| Radiation, convection and conduction | 70 |
| Evaporation of sweat | 14.5 |
| Vaporization of water from lungs | 8 |
| Liberation of dissolved $CO_2$ in lungs | 3–4 |
| Warming of inspired air | 2–3 |
| Urine and feces | 1–2 |

\* Adapted from Best, C. H., and Taylor, N. B.: The Physiologic Basis of Medical Practice. Baltimore, William Wood & Company, 1937.

a combination of physiologic processes serving to increase the dissipation of heat through physical mechanisms. The relative importance and effectiveness of each of these mechanisms is determined in part by the relative humidity.

Loss of heat by radiation, convection and conduction are the most important of these mechanisms. The quantity of heat eliminated varies with such factors as the environmental temperature, the relative humidity, the clothing and the rate of heat production. Loss by radiation from the body surface is accomplished by cutaneous vasodilitation, increased blood volume and increased circulation rate. Loss by conduction varies inversely with the amount of subcutaneous fat. Further dissipation of heat is accomplished by convection currents created between the layer of warm, moisture-laden air in contact with the clothed body and the surrounding atmosphere when the latter is cool and dry.

Loss by radiation and convection ceases when the environmental temperature approaches that of the body. When the relative humidity is high, dissipation of heat by evaporation of sweat is reduced to a minimum.

Significant amounts of heat are dissipated through the evaporation of sweat secreted from the skin. Sweat is a weak solution of sodium chloride varying in concentration from 0.2 to 0.5 per cent, containing traces of urea and inorganic salts. A rise in blood temperature acts upon the nervous centers providing the normal stimulus to perspire. Heavy muscular work and profuse sweating over a prolonged period increase the sodium chloride content of the sweat. Thus the combination of severe exertion in high temperatures with a large intake of water leads to depletion of chloride stores and lowered concentration of salt in the blood and tissue fluids (Table 51).

In man, the vaporization of water from the lungs is less effective than sweating as a mechanism for heat dissipation. However, when the efficiency of dissipation of heat through the skin is impaired, there may be an increase in the respiratory rate with some corresponding increase of heat loss through the lungs.

## Physiologic Response to Heat

The physiologic responses to exposure to high temperature are vasodilatation, acceleration of the pulse and respiration, profuse sweating, and a reduced capacity for muscular work. Acclimatization to hot environments is essentially an adaptation of the heat-regulating mechanisms. One of the most important features of acclimatization is the development of an increased capacity for sweating without undue loss of sodium chloride. In most individuals this adjustment is fairly well established within one week and is effected mainly by the adrenal cortex.

## Effects of Heat

The ill effects of heat are expressions or resultants of the excessive loss of chlorides and water and of failure of the heat regulatory mechanisms. The clinical syndromes are not sharply defined; intermediate and mixed types are frequent. The principal syndromes have been designated as (1) heat pyrexia, (2) heat cramps, (3) heat exhaustion and (4) anhidrotic asthenia (anhidrotic heat exhaustion). Miliaria rubra, a disease of the skin, is a fifth effect of heat.

### Heat Pyrexia

**Synonyms**   Heat stroke, sunstroke, heat hyperpyrexia, thermic fever, sun traumatism, siriasis.

**Definition**   Heat pyrexia is a response to exposure to excessive heat and humidity characterized by high fever, circulatory collapse and, in severe cases, coma, convulsions and death. It probably arises from a profound disturbance or failure of the central nervous heat-regulating mechanism. After recovery from the acute episode a fairly prolonged period of instability of the heat control mechanism is usual. In some instances there is permanent loss of ability to adapt to high temperature and humidity.

**Etiology**   Heat pyrexia usually occurs after prolonged exposure to an excessively high temperature, often accompanied by high humidity and lack of air movement. Predisposing factors are hard physical work, heavy tight clothing and lack of ventilation. Alcohol is an important immediate cause. Cessation of sweating often precedes the onset.

**Pathology**   Although there are no specific lesions, edema, congestion and petechial hemorrhages are often seen in the brain, meninges, serous membranes, heart and stomach. The upper intestine may be so severely congested as to create suspicion of poisoning.

Microscopically, the brain shows scattered areas of edema, thrombosis, hemorrhage, degeneration of neurones and gliosis. Comparable pathologic changes are found in the heart, liver, kidneys and adrenals. Massive hemorrhage, edema and inflammation are frequent in the lungs.

**Clinical Characteristics**   Diminution or cessation of sweating and frequency of micturition may occur some hours in advance of the acute attack and constitute important warning signals. Other prodromes are weakness, lassitude, headache, vertigo, anorexia, nausea and increase of body temperature and pulse rate. Muscle cramps may or may not occur.

The onset is often sudden, with vomiting, precordial distress, muscular twitchings and anxiety or even mental derangement. The patient is flushed; the skin, hot and dry; the peripheral vessels are distended, giving the appearance of plethora. The pulse is full and regular and the blood pressure maintained. Dehydration is usually not prominent in the early stages although it may be later. Shortly after the onset there is a rapid rise of body temperature which may reach 105° to 110° F. Delirium appears simultaneously and rapidly progresses to coma. Convulsions and projectile vomiting are not uncommon and are of serious import.

In the later stages the pupils, hitherto contracted, are dilated. Cheyne-Stokes respiration may be present and the tendon reflexes are usually diminished or absent. The pulse gradually becomes weak and irregular, the blood pressure falls and significant grades of dehydration may be encountered. The urine output is diminished or there may be anuria, and the chloride content of the urine is markedly reduced. Moderate amounts of albumin are present. The spinal fluid is clear and under increased pressure. Temperatures above 108° F. may induce irreversible changes in the brain.

When recovery begins the temperature falls rapidly; resumption of sweating is a favorable sign. Relapses on slight provocation are frequent and reflex changes and central nervous system symptoms may persist for three weeks to a month. The individual thereafter is often abnormally susceptible to heat.

**Diagnosis** The *differential diagnosis* from the hyperpyrexial form of *falciparum* malaria and from meningitis and pneumonia may be difficult. Suspected heat pyrexia, however, is an acute emergency, and efficient therapy must not be delayed to permit exact identification of the etiology.

**Treatment** Intensive treatment should be initiated immediately wherever the patient is, the essential problem being to bring down the body temperature as quickly as possible. An air-conditioned room, with temperature at 65° F. and low humidity, is an advantage but not essential. The basic therapy is to place the patient in a water bath cooled with abundant ice. Meanwhile, to assist the circulation, the limbs are briskly massaged towards the heart. Rectal temperatures are taken every ten minutes and when 102 to 103° F. is reached the patient must be removed to a bed and lightly covered. Excessive cooling in or out of the bath is a real danger. Care must be taken to read the correct body temperature uninfluenced by water or environment. Dehydration, if definite, calls for the cautious intravenous infusion of physiologic sodium chloride solution. The indications for spinal fluid drainage are not established.

For milder cases cold sponges or wet packs, combined with fanning, are sufficient. If required, chloral hydrate, light chloroform anesthesia or intravenous Pentothal sodium may be administered. Morphine and atropine are contraindicated. After termination of the acute phase absolute rest and protection against even moderately high temperatures are required. Relapses should be watched for.

**Prognosis** Heat pyrexia constitutes a serious threat to life. The mortality rate ranges from 15 to 50 per cent. The prognosis depends primarily upon the duration of the acute condition prior to treatment and is poor in the older age groups. Cardiac and renal disease and chronic alcoholism minimize the possibilities for recovery.

## Heat Cramps

**Synonyms** Stoker's cramps, miner's cramps, fireman's cramps, cane cutter's cramps.

**Definition** This condition is characterized by the development of painful cramps of the skeletal muscles following exertion in high temperatures.

*Etiology*  Under conditions of high environmental temperature, sweating is profuse and leads to the loss of much water and sodium chloride. When the subject replaces only the water through massive thirst there tends to arise a state of relative hypotonicity and lack of chloride in the tissues. In the case of certain muscles this leads to severe cramp.

*Clinical Characteristics*  Typically the onset is gradual and characterized by mild cramps in the extremities. The cramps are usually symmetrically distributed and transitory but tend to recur at shorter intervals and with increasing severity, gradually involving the major muscle groups of the extremities and abdominal wall. They are disabling and frequently extremely painful. In severe cases they may recur for many hours unless checked by therapy.

*Treatment*  The administration of sodium chloride and water is specific. In mild cases sodium chloride, 1 gm. with large fluid intake, should be given every hour to a total of fifteen doses. The salt should be given dissolved in water since tablets may cause vomiting. In severe cases sterile physiologic salt solution should be given intravenously. Symptomatic relief is rapid.

### Heat Exhaustion

*Synonyms*  Heat prostration, heat syncope, heat exhaustion type I.

*Definition*  This is a type of response to exposure to excessive heat characterized by prostration and varying degrees of circulatory collapse accompanied by little if any rise in body temperature.

*Etiology*  Under conditions of heat stress there tends to occur an excessive loss of water and sodium chloride from the body. The sodium chloride loss is particularly important because imbibed water cannot be stored unless the tissues contain enough sodium chloride to maintain isotonicity.

Sodium chloride deficiency is thus largely responsible for progressive dehydration of the body. This in turn means lowered blood volume and a resultant shocklike form of circulatory collapse which is the chief feature of classic heat exhaustion. In the aged and others with feeble hearts, central cardiac failure may complicate the picture. Associated heat cramps are common.

Those who secrete much chloride in their sweat are particularly prone.

*Clinical Characteristics*  Warning symptoms over a period of two or three days are common. These may consist of undefinable malaise and anxiety or there may be, in addition, headache, vertigo, irritability, dim or disordered vision, shallow respiration, cramps, nausea, and frequently vomiting.

The actual onset may occur during the night. Heat exhaustion may appear in the course of other disease syndromes and may complicate surgery in the tropics, especially after lengthy procedures when the patient has been heavily draped.

The clinical picture is predominantly that of shock with:

1. Low blood pressure and syncope on standing. The blood pressure while lying may be well maintained.

2. Marked reduction of pulse pressure persisting as long as the diastolic pressure is readable.

3. Oliguria.

4. Marked reduction of urinary chlorides.

5. Moderate elevation of rectal temperature even though the mouth temperature may be normal or even subnormal.

6. Profuse sweating and cold clammy skin.

There is usually marked pallor, and, if exposure to undue heat is continued, unconsciousness occurs and death follows from circulatory failure.

Heat exhaustion in the tropics must be differentiated from algid malaria, food poisoning, and chemical poisoning which may produce an almost identical clinical picture.

**Treatment** In planning treatment it is well to keep in mind an important aphorism: "Keep the exhaustion case warm, get the stroke case cool." The essential problem is the correction of the "salt-deficiency dehydration" and the associated acute circulatory failure. If the patient is conscious he should be pressed to drink cool water containing between 0.1 and 1.0 per cent sodium chloride; concentrations at the upper range are more effective providing they do not cause vomiting. In severe cases intravenous infusion of sterile physiologic sodium chloride solution (0.9 per cent) should be used with due regard to volume and speed, especially in those with organically diseased hearts. Intragastric and rectal delivery of saline may be considered for unconscious patients in the lack of intravenous fluids. If facilities are available, fluid and electrolyte balance charts are desirable. Morphine is contraindicated.

## Anhidrotic Asthenia

**Synonyms** Anhidrotic heat exhaustion, thermogenic anhidrosis, heat exhaustion type II.

**Definition** A recently recognized subacute disorder of heat control due to the blockage of many of the sweat glands of the body by miliaria rubra (prickly heat). It is the *most common* heat disorder under military conditions in both the wet and dry tropics.

**Etiology** The sweat glands involved by miliaria remain blocked for some weeks after the acute inflammation subsides. When extensive blockage occurs physiologic adaptation to heat is disturbed. Acute erythematous sunburn may close many pores temporarily and other skin diseases may interfere with the normal function of the sweat glands, thus contributing to the etiologic mechanism in certain cases.

**Clinical Characteristics**    There is usually a history of severe or recurrent miliaria rubra some weeks before onset of general symptoms which characteristically take the form of excessive fatigue responses to physical exertion. The patient notices over a period of a week or more that exercise in the heat of the day, especially in sunshine, causes exhaustion, frontal headache, giddiness, dyspnea, palpitation and, in severe cases, tremor and syncope. With rest in the shade symptoms are largely relieved in one-half to three hours. In between periods of exercise a sense of well-being is largely restored; however, there may be polyuria. The disease lasts a few weeks and

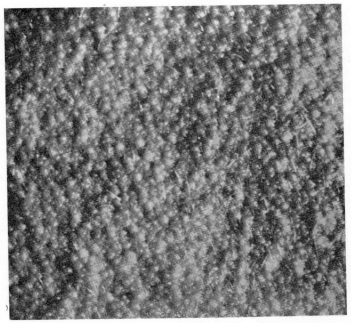

Fig. 276. An enlarged picture of human skin showing miliaria profunda. Notice the gooseflesh-like appearance. (Courtesy of Drs. G. O. Horne and R. H. Mole. Trans. Royal Soc. Tropical Med. & Hygiene, Vol. 44, 1951.)

recovery then gradually takes place.

**Diagnosis**    Anhidrotic asthenia may be readily diagnosed by the following features, provided the patient is examined after exertion:

1. Relative or complete anhidrosis (absence of sweat) on the *covered* parts of the body.

2. The presence of diffuse miliaria rubra or more often, a generalized rash which, although not related to the hairs, looks like "gooseflesh" (Fig. 276). This rash, called miliaria profunda (or mammillaria), and the associated anhidrosis are the cardinal signs. Miliaria profunda is not red, generally not pruritic, and may disappear entirely on resting. In dry desert heat the whole syndrome may

come on more acutely while the skin is still at the miliaria rubra stage.

3. *Excessive* sweating, probably compensatory, of the forehead and face. Palms and soles sweat normally.

4. Marked tachycardia and tachypnea and a slightly raised temperature (average rectal, 100 to 101° F.).

5. Features absent in typical cases: hyperpyrexia, dehydration, salt deficiency, cramps, vomiting, coma, and immediate danger to life.

**Complications**  This disease is likely to precipitate a more acute heat disorder, especially heat pyrexia.

**Treatment**  The patient should avoid exercise and be placed in a cool environment such as an air-conditioned room. Evacuation from the tropics should rarely be necessary. During recovery, exercise tolerance and sweat secretion should be checked regularly.

LOCAL TREATMENT. Inasmuch as the anhidrosis and miliaria *profunda* are due mainly to keratotic plugging of the pores, restoration of sweating sometimes may be hastened by causing desquamation with applications of 10 per cent salicylic acid in 70 per cent ethyl alcohol. First paint a small area to detect any undue reaction. Peeling may need to be repeated. Following desquamation (and between courses of the lotion), inunction of lanolin cream should be used over the treated areas once a day.

If for any reason desquamation is not accomplished in miliaria profunda, it is necessary to await the natural shedding of the obstructive plugs—this may take some weeks. While ample inunction of lanolin may increase sweating (and exercise tolerance) during this period, it is unwise to discharge the patient until sweating is normal without the use of lanolin.

For treatment of acute miliaria rubra see below.

## Miliaria Rubra

**Synonyms**  Prickly heat, miliaria, heat rash, lichen tropicus.

**Definition**  Miliaria rubra is an acute inflammatory disorder of the skin associated primarily with blockage of the pores. It is common throughout the hot, moist tropics.

**Etiology**  A large number of factors are now known to close the sweat pores. In the case of tropical miliaria rubra, the most important are probably maceration of the keratin of the stratum corneum and infection of the pores, especially by staphylococci (Fig. 277A). Lipoid depletion of the stratum corneum may play an ancillary role.

Sudamina (crystallina or miliaria crystallina) is similar to miliaria rubra except that the blockage is more superficial and less prolonged. Many physical factors such as ultraviolet light (e.g., sunburn) may cause it.

**Pathology**  The changes appear to be entirely secondary to the pore blockage. Pressure built up through the continued secretion of sweat causes dilatation and finally rupture of the sweat ducts as they pass through the stratum mucosum (malpighii). Vesicles containing sweat are thus produced in the stratum mucosum (miliaria rubra) (Fig. 277B). Congestion of dermal vessels and leukocytic infiltration occurs.

In the course of approximately ten days the acute vesicles disappear and a parakeratotic reaction, with formation of a plug, produces

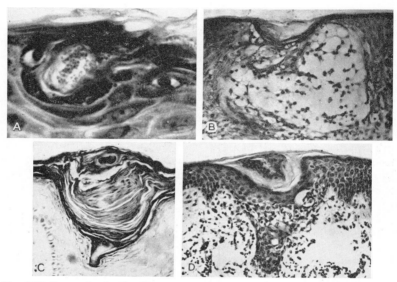

Fig. 277. Stages in the development of miliaria. *A*, Probable staphylococci in a pore from a case of miliaria. This may be the earliest lesion. *B*, Miliaria rubra showing the vesicle in the epidermis. The closed sweat pore is in the surface depression. *C*, At a later stage a large darkly stained parakeratotic plug obstructs the sweat pore. *D*, Miliaria profunda, the final stage, showing the parakeratotic plug on the surface and large empty spaces in the dermis representing extravasation of sweat. (Courtesy of Dr. J. P. O'Brien in (*A*) J. Inves. Dermat., *15:*105,1950; (*B* and *D*) Brit. J. Dermat. & Syph., *59:*125, 1947; (*C*) original.)

*chronic* obstruction. This in turn leads to a deeper vesicle formation because the rupture of the ducts is in the dermis rather than the epidermis, thus producing miliaria profunda (Figs. 276, 277D).

The stage of acute vesiculation (miliaria rubra) is brief but the *profunda* stage is prolonged, persisting for weeks. Characteristically, lesions in all stages of development co-exist. When all the pores of an area of skin are obstructed the area becomes completely dry and the lesions are, for the most part, in the chronic *profunda* stage.

**Clinical Characteristics**    The rash of miliaria rubra is largely confined to the clothed areas. It consists of innumerable tiny vesicles on a red base and is accompanied by intense itching. The early vesicles are succeeded by red papules and these, in turn, by the deep vesicles of the *profunda* stage. These are not red, not pruritic, and resemble closely the white papules of "gooseflesh."

Recurrent episodes of miliaria rubra represent progressive involvement of more and more gland groups. Various pyodermas, chronic dermatitis and anhidrotic asthenia are frequent complications.

**Treatment** Exposure to a cool environment even for part of each day is of great benefit.

After preliminary testing of a local skin area, the following mild antiseptic desquamating lotion should be applied twice daily to the affected skin:

| | |
|---|---|
| Salicylic acid | 3 |
| Glycerol | 5 |
| Ethyl alcohol (70%) | to 100. |

When the rash has disappeared inunctions of a lanolin cream should be used.

In well established cases without erythema, miliaria profunda, the salicylic acid content may be increased to 10 per cent.

When pyogenic complications are present neomycin ointment, 2.5 to 5.0 mg. per gram of base, is helpful.

**Prophylaxis** Clothing should be loose, light, clean and brief. Heavy continuous sweating should be avoided. If facilities exist, the spending of 8 to 12 hours of each day in an air-conditioned atmosphere is helpful. Soap should be used only sparingly. Routine application of powders is not recommended except perhaps in intertriginous areas such as the groin. In susceptible persons occasional inunctions with lanolin cream are probably beneficial.

## Prophylaxis Against Effects of Heat

Prophylaxis against the acute effects of heat consists in the maintenance of normal salt and water balances and avoidance of unnecessary exposure to conditions of high temperature and humidity. Alcohol in a hot humid environment, especially prior to hard physical work, constitutes a serious menace.

Water requirements are subject to great variation; in the desert they may vary from two quarts to three gallons per day. They are directly proportional to the environmental temperature and the amount of physical work performed. At high temperatures a man at rest may lose one pint of water per hour. Under extreme conditions *total* daily chloride needs may reach 30 gm. The following essential rules should be observed:

1. Working hours should be adjusted to permit the maximum amount of sleep. Fatigue is a principal predisposing cause of acute effects of heat.

2. Avoid unnecessary exposure to the sun; the head should be protected and clothing should be light and loose.

3. Drink plentiful amounts of water containing 1.3 gm. of sodium

chloride per quart (450 gm. of sodium chloride per 375 liters of water). A daily urinary volume of *at least* 900 ml. should be maintained and in special instances a watch on body weight and urinary chloride may be advisable.

4. Take fluid despite absence of thirst or presence of nausea.

5. Salt food plentifully.

6. Rest in shade immediately upon the appearance of mild symptoms.

7. Avoid and treat skin disease, especially miliaria (q.v.). Suntanning is desirable but *acute* sunburn is a hazard as it may obstruct many sweat pores.

8. Air conditioning facilities are of great value. Evacuation from the tropics may sometimes be necessary as a prophylactic measure against recurrences.

# 66   Certain Medically Important Animals

**General**   The following discussion covers a miscellaneous group of animals which commonly injure man, either mechanically or otherwise. Except for leeches and vampire bats, it does not include direct parasites or vectors of disease, since these are discussed elsewhere. Arthropods in all categories are omitted for the same reason. Echinoderms are not mentioned because of their relative unimportance as direct agents of harm.

No attempt is made here to furnish keys for the identification of fish and snakes; rather, a few generalizations are offered concerning the recognition and treatment of injuries caused by the dangerous species and the methods of protection against them.

## Coelenterates (Phylum Coelenterata)

Persons bathing in tropical or subtropical oceans may occasionally be stung by a variety of marine animals, certain coelenterates being the commonest of such offending agents. These organisms occur either as free-swimming jellyfish (medusae) or as sessile polyps. The latter resemble plants, since they have stalked bodies and a flower-like crown of tentacles, but they are true animal forms. Both medusae and polyps possess tentacles which bear numerous tiny stinging structures (nematocysts). When a tentacle comes into contact with any organism, each nematocyst discharges a small barb and a minute quantity of toxin into the victim's cuticle or skin. Man responds variably to the attack, depending on the number of stings sustained and the type of toxin injected. There may be a mild local reaction or a profound systemic one. The stings of tropical species are more severe and may rarely result in death.

Jellyfish often occur together in large numbers, being brought close to land or washed ashore by storms and shifting ocean currents in certain seasons. It may then be wise to avoid sea-bathing and to wear shoes while walking along the beach. Sessile polyps are much less of a menace and are annoying chiefly to divers.

**Clinical Characteristics**   The Portuguese man-of-war is a large colonial coelenterate that floats by means of a brightly colored air bladder. The stringlike tentacles of this elaborate assemblage of inter-dependent individuals stretch for many yards around it. A person engaging such a tentacle while swimming at once receives many sharp stings, and soon the exposed part shows a row of circular erythematous patches, spaced a few millimeters apart, where contact with individual nematocysts was made.

Local marks of the stings of jellyfish may be absent in some cases. Pain, swelling and redness of the affected part usually occur, how-ever. Systemic effects following severe stinging appear within an hour, often in a much briefer time, and may consist of anxiety, mus-cle pains and cramps, dyspnea, constriction of the throat, cardiac weakness and prostration. Sensitive individuals may show an anaphy-lactoid type of reaction in which cough, coryza and urticaria are outstanding.

**Treatment**   In untreated cases the systemic signs usually subside within a few hours or days, although an itching dermatitis at the site of the stings may persist for weeks. The intravenous injection of 10 ml. of a 10 per cent solution of calcium gluconate has been found specific for the systemic disturbances. Topical applications of weak alkaline solutions help relieve the cutaneous symptoms.

## Leeches (Phylum Annelida; Class Hirudinea)

These animals have segmented bodies provided with anterior and posterior suckers used in locomotion and attachment. At the center of the anterior sucker is the mouth, which may possess cutting teeth. In sucking blood, leeches secrete an anticoagulant, hirudin, the action of which often continues even after the animals have engorged them-selves and dropped off the host; the lesions bleed for some time, heal slowly and therefore may become infected.

Most leeches inhabit fresh water although a few tropical species have adapted themselves to a moist terrestrial environment. Land leeches are found in South America and in the Far East where they are especially troublesome in Malaya, Assam, Burma, India, Borneo and parts of the Southwest Pacific. They are most abundant during the monsoons. They reach a human host from brush at the edges of overgrown trails or else climb up his legs from the ground, quickly finding openings in clothing and gaining access to the skin. Aquatic leeches affix themselves to bathers or reach the mouth in unfiltered drinking water.

**Clinical Characteristics**  Leeches entering the mouth may migrate to the nasal cavity, pharynx, trachea or bronchi. In such locations their subsequent engorgement leads to mechanical obstruction of the passages. They may be removed by applying strong cocaine to their bodies, the patient first being placed with his head in a lowered position to prevent deeper penetration of the respiratory tract by the dislodged parasites.

Invasion of the urethra and bladder is also known and may be overcome by irrigations with strong salt solution. Leeches reaching the stomach are digested.

The bites of these animals are ordinarily either painless or felt only as a slight irritation. Persons in areas inhabited by land leeches are sometimes unaware that they are carrying them. Travelers occasionally become weakened to the point of exhaustion by loss of blood without knowing the cause of their condition until their clothing is removed and a heavy infestation is discovered. Exsanguination of animals due to numerous bites has been observed, and death in man resulting from this cause is alleged to have taken place on rare occasions.

Ordinarily, however, land leeches are soon discovered by a human victim. This may proceed from the unpleasantness occasioned when an inch-long engorged leech is squashed inside a shoe. At other times the blood-staining of trouser legs, resulting from continued bleeding after leeches have fed and detached, is an indicator of the presence of these animals. Local guides may give warning of a leech-infested forest before permitting travelers to enter. In such a case many leeches can be removed before they have a chance to inflict their wounds, or they may be dislodged before completing engorgement.

Many persons suffer no after effects from leech bites, but those with sensitive skins or allergic tendencies may experience severe local itching for several days.

**Treatment**  A leech attached to the skin may sometimes be dislodged by the simple expedient of pulling it off by hand. Otherwise it can be induced to detach itself by applying cocaine, vinegar, table salt or other strong solutions to it. Touching it with a lighted cigarette will also cause it to let go. Oozing of blood should be controlled with a styptic pencil. Secondary infection and ulceration may occur if the bites are neglected, or if the mouthparts remain in the skin after removing the rest of the leech.

**Prophylaxis**  Recent work with several ordinary mosquito repellents (Indalone, 612 and dimethyl phthalate) has demonstrated that these substances are fairly efficient in repelling leeches, retaining their effectiveness against these animals long after the effect against mosquitoes has been lost. However, newer repellents now under test hold promise of greater efficacy.

## Fish (Superclass Pisces)

Species of both marine and fresh-water fish may injure man by sharp spines which sometimes are associated with underlying poison glands. The salt-water varieties usually wound bathers who step on them, for many of these forms habitually lie half-buried in silt or hidden under marine vegetation or in crevices of coral formations. Sting rays are the most dangerous fish in this category, being found in shoals or bays with sluggish currents and muddy or sandy bottoms. Such elasmobranchs may be very large and possess long slender lashing tails near the base of which one or more stout barbed spines are situated. These are dorsal fin rays, often associated with poison glands, although it has been said that a coating of mucus is the chief agent responsible for the toxic effects of the sting. Rays are especially abundant in Australian and Asiatic seas, often frequenting shallows where they live as scavengers. They may be largely avoided if bathers drag their feet along the bottom, since the fish will usually swim away if not directly trodden upon. Wounds are most frequent on the ankle, the barb sometimes being driven to the bone.

In the Pacific Ocean, stone and scorpion fishes are found on coral reefs. These bony fish have poison spines whose effect may be very severe. The toad fishes of the American tropics are similarly dangerous. These forms may all be easily recognized by their very spiny appearance.

Fresh waters in the tropics, especially the Amazon, also may harbor sting rays as well as large catfish bearing sharp spines. Other species of catfish give painful wounds the world over. They usually inflict their damage while being removed from fishhooks. Poison glands are associated with the spines of many of these. Puncture wounds produced by spiny fish are usually ragged and easily become secondarily infected.

There are also biting fish, some of which secrete poison. The famous piranha of the Amazon and its tributaries is not venomous but is attracted in large schools to any wounded animal, quickly tearing it to pieces. Electric eels and rays represent another dangerous type of fish, large specimens causing transient partial paralysis or possibly fatal shocks in man.

**Clinical Characteristics**    The most severe cases of poisoning due to the stings of venomous fish are confined chiefly to a few marine varieties. There is an immediate painful reaction at the puncture site or sites, followed rapidly by marked swelling and erythema. Systemic effects may include dyspnea, prostration or delirium. Death has occurred rarely. Immediate local treatment as for snake bite, including incision and suction, may be of aid in preventing or retarding the absorption of poison.

The ingestion of spoiled fish containing bacterial toxins will not be considered. Poisoning of man following the eating of certain fresh-caught inherently poisonous marine fish has commonly been noted, however. This has occurred in many parts of the world both in the tropics and elsewhere. The poisonous properties of such fish are not understood, since a given species may be inedible in one coastal region and entirely wholesome in a closely adjacent area. There are also seasonal variations in the edibility of certain species within a given region. Poisonous species rarely if ever occur far at sea.

**Prophylaxis** The best guide to safety in consuming fish is the example set by natives of each region. If such local advice cannot be obtained, one should avoid fish with leathery, bristly, spiny or tuberculated skin. This will exclude the highly poisonous trigger fish, pufferfish and porcupine fish. The pufferfish inflates itself with air when caught. Trigger fishes are brightly-colored; the anterior part of their dorsal fin is modified as a spine resembling a trigger and there is a wide gap between this structure and the posterior unmodified part of the fin. The "trigger" is situated far forward over the eyes. Porcupine fishes have long sharp bristles or spines over the head and back and smaller ones over the belly. The parrot fish and red snapper, normally scaled species, may likewise occasionally be poisonous. Parrot fish have mouths resembling a parrot's beak.

Evisceration preparatory to cooking should be done with meticulous care; fish showing enlarged gonads had best be discarded, since some species are inedible only during their breeding season. Even so there is some danger in consuming unfamiliar species, as not all the harmful varieties are excluded by the above criteria and the poison of dangerous forms is not destroyed by cooking. Unfamiliar fish eggs should never be eaten.

**Treatment** Treatment in the early stages consists of gastric lavage or the administration of an emetic. Later it is necessary to support the circulation if cardiac failure appears. Deaths have been known to occur within two hours of eating unspoiled adequately-cooked poisonous fish. Although inherently poisonous fish exist, all amphibians, reptiles, birds and mammals are edible and may be eaten with safety after thorough cooking.

## Lizards (Class Reptilia; Order Squamata; Suborder Lacertilia)

Lizards the world over are non-poisonous with the exceptions of the gila monster of southern Arizona and New Mexico and the beaded lizard of southwestern Mexico. Even these are rarely harmful since the venom secreted at the base of certain of their lower teeth does not readily enter the shallow wounds produced. They do not often bite man, but when they do they may maintain a firm grasp with their jaws and it is sometimes most difficult to dislodge them. Their tendency to turn over on their backs when biting enables the venom to flow into the lacerations more readily. Paralysis, dyspnea, convulsions and, rarely, death may result. Local treatment as for snake bite should be practiced for removal of the venom. These reptiles may be recognized by their tuberculated skin, stumpy tails and coloration. Gila monsters are mottled salmon-pink and black, attaining a size of about two feet. The slightly larger Mexican beaded lizard is yellow and black.

## Snakes (Class Reptilia; Order Squamata; Suborder Ophidia)

Harmful snakes are widely distributed, especially in warm parts of the world. Large boas and pythons occur strictly within the tropics and, while capable of injuring or killing man by biting and constriction, are rarely encountered. They are nonpoisonous. The chief danger from snakes lies in the effects of bites by venomous species.

Poisonous snakes occur in both the tropics and temperate regions. In Tasmania all the snakes are poisonous and in the rest of Australia they outnumber the nonpoisonous fauna, but elsewhere in the world they take a decidedly minor place both in number of species and in actual number of individuals. In the Amazon valley, for example, snakes are not numerous generally speaking and poisonous ones account for only 3 to 5 per cent of the total snake population. Certain islands, such as Hawaii, New Zealand, New Caledonia, Ireland, Madagascar and many others, as well as the Arctic regions, are entirely free of poisonous land-dwelling snakes; however, tropical islands of the Pacific and Indian Oceans, some of which are terrestrially snake-free, have sea snakes in their fringing surf. The chief poisonous snakes of importance are listed in Table 52.

FANGS. Many venomous snakes possess fangs that are ill-adapted for piercing the human skin. This is especially true of the rear-fanged colubrids in which the fangs not only are set far back in the upper jaw but also are merely grooved rather than hollow. This means that venom, poured from the duct of the venom gland at the base of the fang, must flow along the groove to reach the surface of the wound. In many front-fanged snakes the duct leads directly into the hollow fang itself and venom may be ejected with force through the hypodermic-needle–like tooth deeply into the wound.

Front-fanged snakes may have either of two types of fang, movable or immovable. The immovable type, found in sea snakes and elapids, is relatively less efficient since, due to its permanently erect position, it must be short to permit closing of the jaws. Moreover, this type is invariably grooved rather than hollow. Thus highly poisonous snakes such as cobras, kraits, coral snakes and all the Australian species, are rendered less effective in their attempts to bite. Even cobras must sometimes chew their victims after striking them in order to introduce enough venom to subdue their struggles.

The true vipers and the pit vipers have hollow front fangs solidly attached to movable premaxillary bones. These complex structures are folded back against the roof of the mouth when not in use but are directed forward while the snake is striking. This arrangement permits the fangs to attain greater length; some large species have fangs so long that they can deliver their venom intramuscularly. These snakes strike quickly and immediately withdraw to await the effect of their bites.

The fangs of vipers and elapids when not in use are enclosed in a protective mucous membrane sheath. In examining a specimen to

*Table 52   Important Poisonous Snakes of the World*

| FAMILY AND TYPE OF FANGS | COMMON NAMES | TYPE OF VENOM | DISTRIBUTION | REMARKS |
|---|---|---|---|---|
| COLUBRIDAE; rear, immovable, grooved | Colubrids | Mostly mild | Warm parts of both hemispheres | Over 1000 species, the few poisonous ones not dangerous |
| Example: | Boomslang | Hemorrhagin | South Africa | Arboreal, timid |
| ELAPIDAE; front, immovable, grooved | Elapids | Predominantly neurotoxin | Mostly in Old World | Over 150 species, very poisonous |
| Examples: | Cobras | Mostly neurotoxin | Africa, India, Asia, Philippines, Celebes | Spitting cobra in Africa aims at eyes |
| | Kraits | Strong neurotoxin | India, S.E. Asia, Indonesia | Sluggish, often buried in dust |
| | Mambas | Neurotoxin | Tropical W. Africa | Arboreal |
| | Blacksnake | Neurotoxin | Australia | Large snake, wet terrain |
| | Copperhead | Neurotoxin | Australia, Tasmania, Solomons | Damp environment |
| | Brown snake | Neurotoxin | Australia, New Guinea | Slender |
| | Tiger snake | Strong neurotoxin | Australia | Dry environment; aggressive; very dangerous |
| | Death adder | Neurotoxin | Australia, New Guinea | Sandy terrain |
| | Coral snakes | Neurotoxin | United States, tropical America | About 26 species, 2 in southern U. S. A. |
| HYDROPHIDAE; front, immovable, hollow | Sea snakes | Some mild; others very toxic | Tropical, Indian and Pacific Oceans | Gentle. Rudder-like tail. Over 50 species |
| VIPERIDAE; front, movable, hollow | True vipers | Predominantly hematoxin | Entirely in Old World | About 50 species |
| Examples: | European viper | Hematoxin | Europe (rare), N. Africa, Near East | Dry rocky country |
| | Russel's viper | Hematoxin | S.E. Asia, Java, Sumatra | Mostly open terrain; deadly |
| | Sand vipers | Hematoxin | N. Sahara | Buried in sand |
| | Puff adder | Hematoxin | Arabia, Africa | Open terrain; sluggish |
| | Gaboon viper | Neurotoxin and hematoxin | Tropical W. Africa | Forests; deadly |
| | Rhinoceros viper | Hematoxin | Tropical Africa | Wet forests |
| | Habu viper | Neurotoxin | Okinawa | Caves and dry rocky country |

*Table 52   Important Poisonous Snakes of the World*—(Continued)

| FAMILY AND TYPE OF FANGS | COMMON NAMES | TYPE OF VENOM | DISTRIBUTION | REMARKS |
|---|---|---|---|---|
| CROTALIDAE; front, movable, hollow | Pit vipers | Predominantly hematoxin | Old and New Worlds; none in Africa | Over 80 species; pit between eye and nostril |
| Examples: | Rattlesnakes* | Predominantly hematoxin | N. Central and S. America | South American form neurotoxic |
| | Bushmaster | Hematoxin | Central and S. America | Large. In wet forests |
| | Fer-de-lance | Hematoxin | Central America, N. South America, few West Indies | Common on plantations |
| | Palm vipers | Hematoxin(?) | S. Mexico, Central and South America | Arboreal; small, greenish. Bite face |
| | Copperhead | Hematoxin | United States | Dry stony terrain |
| | Water moccasin | Hematoxin | Southeast U.S.A. to Texas | Swamps |
| | Asiatic pit vipers | Hematoxin | Southeast Asia, Formosa | Most arboreal |

\* All rattlesnakes are poisonous.

detect the fangs it is necessary to draw or dissect away this covering, using appropriate care to avoid direct contact with any of the structures since the severed head of a freshly-killed snake may reflexly go through the actions of biting when thus stimulated.

The *identification* of poisonous snakes may be difficult. There are no simple rules which can be followed to cover all cases. Many venomous snakes resemble typical harmless varieties. When dealing with snake-bite problems in foreign territory, one must be guided by whatever native advice, professional or otherwise, may be available. The discovery of a pair of fangs in the upper jaw of a specimen is certain evidence of its poisonous nature. If several pairs of enlarged teeth are present, the specimen is probably harmless. Other indications, but by no means all-inclusive, are (1) a pit situated between the eye and nostril, (2) a vertical slit-like pupil, (3) a large triangular head with relatively narrower neck, (4) a thick body and stumpy tail (though many poisonous species are whip-like) and (5) a series of unpaired scales immediately posterior to the vent.

The importance of identifying poisonous snakes lies in the different prognosis and course of treatment indicated for different types of venom. Without relation to size, various species of snakes deliver characteristic doses of venom that vary both as to quantity and quality. Hence the bite of one snake may not be markedly dangerous although a fair quantity of venom has been introduced, while in another case a relatively insignificant bite may be fatal.

*Various types of venom* are produced by snakes. These may be divided conveniently into two main classes, namely, those that affect the respiratory and other centers in the brain stem or spinal cord (neurotoxins) and those that affect the tissues at the site of injection and possibly also the blood stream in general (hematoxins). The latter components of snake venom include hemolysins, cytolysins, endotheliolysins and several other lytic, coagulant and anticoagulant substances. A given species of snake usually has venom that is preponderantly of one type or the other, although more or less equal mixtures of the two occur in a few cases.

It is essential, therefore, to know the offending species of snake in evaluating the probable effects of a bite. If it is at all possible the victim or his companions should kill the snake and bring it with him to the place of treatment. In a given region the number of dangerous poisonous species is usually small and may be learned quickly. In submitting a specimen to a distant laboratory or museum for identification it is not necessary to send the entire reptile—its head in a jar of 70 per cent alcohol or 10 per cent Formalin is sufficient.

**Clinical Characteristics**   In a case of snake bite when no knowledge of the offending species can be obtained, one must examine the wound carefully to appraise its importance. Nonpoisonous snakes will often bite man if molested or surprised; the only treatment necessary is the prevention of secondary infection. The bites of nonpoisonous snakes leave uniform rows of teeth marks or scratches on the skin, while the poisonous species show in addition the laterally placed points of entry of the fangs. The latter two marks are of distinctly larger size and the distance separating them is some indication as to the size of the snake concerned. When only one fang punctures the skin, a proportionately smaller quantity of venom enters and the sequelae are correspondingly milder.

If some time has elapsed between the bite and the arrival of the patient at the place of treatment, the victim's condition is a further aid in estimating the seriousness of the situation; grave symptoms appear rapidly following the efficient injection of highly virulent venom but more slowly in less serious cases. However, some neurotoxic venoms are slow to show their effects, especially if the bite is on the lower extremity—the apparently good condition of the patient is *not* a reliable sign in these cases. The bitten part shows little local reaction in the case of neurotoxic venoms but is swollen, discolored and painful when infiltrated by the hematoxic type. Deaths have occurred as late as two weeks after the bite, although such cases are usually complicated by secondary infection. Gas gangrene is a common complication. The most fulminating cases are those in which the patient has been bitten on the face.

The size of the bitten individual determines how much of the venom will be neutralized by natural processes within the body. Children and small adults neutralize less than large persons and are consequently more severely affected by a given quantity of toxin.

Since neurotoxic venom produces little local pain, the layman and the inexperienced physician are often misled into treating the bite too casually. Delayed systemic reactions may supervene acutely twenty-four or forty-eight hours later and lead rapidly to respiratory paralysis and death. *All* bites by poisonous snakes should therefore receive prompt attention regardless of the patient's seemingly favorable condition.

**Treatment** When a person is bitten he should remain quiet if possible, since physical activity accelerates the absorption of venom. If the bite is on an arm or leg, a tourniquet should be applied proximal to the wound. This should not be so tight as to occlude the arterial circulation and should be partially loosened at intervals, not longer than every twenty minutes, to prevent complete venous stasis.

IMMEDIATE. The patient should then walk slowly to the nearest aid station for appropriate treatment, preferably by a physician. Snake-bite kits have been assembled for such emergencies; they contain iodine, rubber tubing, razor blades, a rubber suction bulb, metal suction applicators and sterile dressings. Most authorities recommend that the bite site be incised by multiple deep criss-cross or parallel incisions. The metal suction applicator, inserted into the bulb, is applied to each wound in succession, venom and serum being sucked out.

Others state that suction without incision, using the rubber bulb or the mouth alone, withdraws the venom efficiently along the preformed tracts of the fangs; they believe also that incision increases the area through which venom can be absorbed as well as the surface on which subsequent secondary infection can develop, thereby enhancing dangers which may already be considerable.

In the light of common practice it would seem that incision and suction should be elected. Numerous devices for withdrawing venom may be improvised. Ordinary breast-pump suction bulbs may be applied to the incisions, or heated glass bottles of any size may be used, the cooling of their contained air providing a suitable vacuum. If oral suction is necessary, a square of thin rubber should be placed over the fang marks or surgical incisions to protect the operator's mouth from the venom and to keep the wound as free from bacterial contamination as possible. Swallowed venom is inactivated by the digestive juices; however, significant amounts of it can be absorbed through abrasions or other open lesions of the lips, tongue or buccal mucosa.

Intermittent suction may profitably be continued for fifteen hours, at least three-quarters of each hour being devoted to evacuation of venom and serum. New incisions may be made at the advancing edge of the swelling, especially in regions proximal to the bite, and suction should be applied to these openings also. The tourniquet should be moved toward the body as the swelling progresses.

Two traditional remedies—permanganate crystals and whiskey—are now regarded not only as useless but the latter may produce fatal results in certain cases.

*Antivenins* have been prepared for use in many parts of the world. Some of these sera are polyvalent, so that in the appropriate geographic region their administration neutralizes whatever toxins are present; others are effective only for a particular species, the identity of which must therefore be known to the physician. If the correct antivenin cannot be obtained, however, it is always worth using the one or ones available, since most of the individual components of snake venom have at least a partial antigenic relationship and may therefore be neutralized in part by antivenins that are not strictly homologous. This is not true, however, of widely different venoms, i.e., hematoxins are not inactivated by an antivenin prepared against the neurotoxins of cobras or coral snakes.

Antivenin may both be injected intravenously and infiltrated about and into the site of the bite, subcutaneously and intramuscularly. In serious cases the intravenous route is by far the most important. The amount of antivenin to be injected varies with each case. Children require more than adults, since they neutralize less of the venom with natural substances in their own bodies. The progress of the case will determine how many injections to give; apparently there is no contraindication to giving large quantities in serial dosage —the chief requisite is to neutralize whatever venom still remains active.

Most antivenins consist of serum from immunized horses. An intracutaneous test for hypersensitivity should be made prior to their administration and desensitization performed if indicated. Immediate incision and suction are of vital importance when hours must be lost in desensitizing the patient. Liquid antivenin must be stored in the refrigerator to preserve its potency. Modern antivenin manufactured in the United States is now dehydrated and retains its activity at room temperature.

*Further measures* in treatment are chiefly supportive, being designed to combat paralysis or circulatory failure. Sedatives are contraindicated as a rule, although some authorities permit the use of morphine for cases with severe pain. Donors for transfusion should stand by in case of emergency; repeated blood counts will indicate the need for such treatment if it occurs.

Spitting cobras, of which two species occur in Africa, can spray their poison for a distance of eight to twelve feet. This venom is often directed at the eyes of the cobras' prey, causing local damage that may result in blindness; it is also absorbed slowly through the conjunctivae and may produce delayed systemic reactions. The eyes should be washed out at once with boric acid or Argyrol solution to minimize effects of the venom.

**Prophylaxis** Prophylaxis against snake bite consists in wearing field shoes and leather or heavy canvas puttees in infested areas, since most bites occur on the leg below the knee. However, in the absence of such protection *loose* trouser legs are to be desired in preference to tight-fitting riding breeches. Most snakes are nocturnal, but they are nevertheless somewhat active while basking by day.

Palm vipers, found in Central and South America, and the water moccasin in the Gulf States of U. S. A. are especially dangerous to those who attempt to cut trails through thick jungle or underbrush, since the former snakes are arboreal and the latter often climb small trees in order to bask above ground. They drop from their perches when disturbed and in doing so many inflict bites on the face. As already stated this site permits the most rapid absorption of venom; in addition, the venom of these species is highly toxic. Arboreal species in other parts of the world constitute a similar menace.

Rodent control around camps will remove a source of attraction for snakes. In tropical Pacific waters sea snakes may be a danger to bathers who are tempted to handle these docile and unaggressive creatures; however, they ordinarily have difficulty in inflicting their venomous bites, since their small mouths adapt them to a diet of fish.

Snakes are not nearly as great a menace as is commonly supposed. As a rule they are not aggressive by nature and will try to avoid man rather than attack him. Their relative scarcity in most regions is itself an assurance against being bitten. Many travellers to tropical wildernesses return months later without having seen a single serpent, poisonous or otherwise.

## Crocodilians (*Class Reptilia; Order Crocodilia*)

Among the large reptiles that can injure man mechanically are crocodilians which include the alligators, caymans, crocodiles and gavials. Of these the first three have relatively wide jaws while gavials, found only in Africa and the Far East, have a long narrow snout. All forms, however, possess many sharp teeth in each jaw. These animals inhabit swamps and slow-flowing streams in the tropics and subtropics. There is only one marine member of the group, namely the salt-water crocodile of the Far East and the South Seas. It is very common in the Solomons. The others spend much time basking in the sun on the banks of their native river or swamp. When hungry they enter the water and submerge until only their eyes and nostrils protrude from the surface. An animal swimming or wading too close is seized and dragged to the bottom. The reptile may then revolve rapidly on its long axis, thus twisting off the appendage it has grasped. The prey is then seized at another part and eventually dies as the result of drowning, exsanguination and mutilation.

Large specimens in all the above groups may reach twenty-five feet in length. All except gavials are formidable when attacking man. Employing the tactics already outlined, they can dismember and kill a grown human being. Except in certain regions they do not frequently molest man, however, being dangerous chiefly in the vicinity of their nests along river banks or if surprised by a bather who is equally unaware of the reptile's presence. Once seized, man has only a slim chance of escaping from a large specimen. It is said that gouging the reptile's eye with one's thumb will sometimes cause it to let go. The only possible rescue measure is to attempt to shoot the animal with a rifle, but the creature's activity and submergence make it difficult to get an effective shot that does not further endanger the victim. Those who escape usually sustain ragged wounds and great loss of blood.

Gavials rarely attack man, since their narrow snouts are better adapted for catching fish. Crocodiles are most dangerous along rivers in parts of tropical Africa where they annually kill a significant number of the rural inhabitants. Crocodiles are found throughout the tropics, while caymans and alligators are confined almost exclusively to the Western Hemisphere, the exception being a single species of alligator found in China.

## Vampire Bats (Class Mammalia; Order Chiroptera; Family (Desmondontidae)

Vampire bats occur in tropical parts of Mexico and Central and South America including Trinidad. They are small creatures, only three inches long, having front teeth specially modified for cutting skin. Their biting is said to be painless. They feed exclusively on blood.

These bats are greatly feared because of the wealth of legend that surrounds their blood-feeding behavior. However, they are a menace to man only because they have been shown to be capable of transmitting rabies. In parts of Mexico it is now known that vampire bats transmit a modified form of rabies virus to cattle, causing a disease in these hosts long familiar to the ranchers as derriengue. It is suspected, although not proved, that human beings in the endemic regions also become infected either following bites of vampire bats or the butchering of diseased cattle. The symptoms in alleged cases may be clinically indistinguishable from poliomyelitis, encephalitis or encephalomyelitis, and the clinical course does not lead necessarily to death as in canine rabies.

Screened quarters or bed nets afford protection against the nocturnal visits of vampire bats. Near human habitations or encampments it is often possible to find many of their daytime shelters in caves or hollow trees and destroy them.

# 67  Molluscs and Disease

## Introduction

Certain molluscs have become of increasing medical importance because of direct or indirect injury which they are capable of inflicting, or because of their role as intermediate hosts of helminthic parasites of man or animals. In the great majority of instances the medically important members of this phylum are restricted to the fresh-water snails. The exceptions include: the fatally venomous cone shells of the Indo-Pacific; certain squids and octopi which may inflict a poisonous bite; the marine blue mussels that have been a source of *Gonyaulax* food poisoning; the fresh-water clams which serve as second intermediate hosts of *Echinostoma;* and certain species of terrestrial, pulmonate gastropod snails which serve as intermediate hosts of *Dicrocoelium,* a common parasite of the biliary tract of mammals.

## Role of Molluscs as Direct Agents of Human Disease

Five species of the marine cone shells are known to inflict a venomous sting, in some cases proving to be fatal to man within four hours.

Venomous specimens are known only from the coral reefs of the Indian and Pacific oceans. The venom is injected through a puncture made in the victim's skin by a half-inch long, needle-like, hollow tooth. Care should be exercised in handling live specimens over two inches in length. The cones are heavy, conic shells with a long, narrow aperture, usually of attractive coloration, and covered with a thin or thick, horny periostracum (Fig. 281).

Octopi must be large to be dangerous and such specimens are very infrequently encountered in shallow water. The secretion from the salivary gland of most octopi is a proteolytic ferment, and the bite of the creature can cause considerable pain and local swelling.

Blue mussels and certain other bivalves found along the open coast, especially the West Coast of North America, are likely to cause paralytic poisoning if eaten during the summer months. A number of human deaths have been reported from this source which is due to the bivalve's having ingested certain planktonic organisms (*Gonyaulax*). The toxin is water-soluble and is not destroyed by boiling.

## Role of Molluscs as Carriers of Disease

All species of trematodes parasitic in man have gastropod snails as obligatory intermediate hosts. The various species of trematodes have each become adapted to a single, or at most, a few species of snails. With other species of snails the miracidia either are not attracted, fail to penetrate, or else do not complete their larval development. A few snails are capable of experimental infection, but are not the natural hosts.

The most important human diseases carried by molluscs are listed in Table 53 and the molluscs are illustrated in Figs. 278 to 282.

**Snail Control**   All trematode parasites of man must pass through a snail intermediate host. Interruption of the biologic chain by control of this obligatory intermediate host constitutes one of the important potential methods of eliminating these trematode diseases of man. The application of such control measures, however, is neither easy nor always practical. Consequently other procedures must be utilized as well. Research in the field of snail control by means of molluscicides is still in its infancy and it is doubtful if the optimal agent has yet been developed.

In areas where fresh-water fish and molluscs are important elements in the local dietary, the use of chemical molluscicidal agents may not be permissible because of their lethal effect upon these protein sources and consequent adverse effects upon the diet and the nutrition of the population. Furthermore, such chemical agents must not be toxic for man, domestic animals or plant crops.

Snail-control operations may be concerned with both the amphibious and aquatic species. The semiamphibious prosobranchs (*Oncomelania* and *Pomatiopsis*) are best controlled by spraying

*Table 53   Human Diseases Carried by Molluscs*

| DISEASE | ETIOLOGIC AGENT | FIRST INTERMEDIATE SNAIL HOST | GEOGRAPHICAL RANGE OF MOLLUSC | MOLLUSCAN FAMILY | SECOND INTERMEDIATE HOST |
|---|---|---|---|---|---|
| Schistosomiasis japonica | *Schistosoma japonicum* | *Oncomelania quadrasi* *Oncomelania formosana* *Oncomelania nosophora* *Oncomelania hupensis* *Pomatiopsis lapidaria* | Philippine Islands Formosa Japan and China China U. S. A. (experimental) | Hydrobiidae | none |
| Schistosomiasis haematobia | *Schistosoma haematobium* | *Bulinus truncatus* *Bulinus africanus* *Bulinus forskali* | North half of Africa South half of Africa Mauritius | Bulinidae | none |
| Schistosomiasis mansoni | *Schistosoma mansoni* | *Biomphalaria alexandrina* *Biomphalaria pfeifferi* *Australorbis glabratus* *Tropicorbis havanensis* | Northern Africa Southern Africa South America; West Indies U. S. A. (experimental) | Planorbidae | none |
| Clonorchiasis | *Clonorchis sinensis* | *Hua ningpoensis* *Bulimus fuchsianus* *Alocinma longicornis* *Parafossarulus manchouricus* | China China China and India China and Japan | Thiaridae Hydrobiidae Hydrobiidae Hydrobiidae | Fresh-water cyprinoid fishes |
| Fascioliasis | *Fasciola hepatica* | *Lymnaea auricularia* *Lymnaea ollula* *Lymnaea rubella* *Lymnaea bulimoides* | North Asia; Europe Asia; Hawaii Hawaii U. S. A. | Lymnaeidae | Encysts on grass and herbs |
| Fasciolopsiasis | *Fasciolopsis buski* | *Segmentina hemisphaerula* *Hippeutis cantori* | Eastern Asia Eastern Asia | Planorbidae | Encysts on water plants |
| Paragonimiasis | *Paragonimus westermani* | *Semisulcospira libertina* *Semisulcospira amurensis* *Thiara granifera* | North China; Japan North China; Korea Formosa to Hawaii | Thiaridae | Fresh-water crabs and crayfish |
| Metagonimiasis | *Metagonimus yokogawai* | *Semisulcospira libertina* *Thiara granifera* | North China; Japan S. E. Asia to Hawaii | Thiaridae | Salmonoid, cyprinoid fishes |

their habitat with sodium pentachlorophenate (Santobrite) or dinitro-*o*-cyclohexylphenol (DCHP) at a rate of about 20 to 30 lbs. per acre (lethal to snails at 1 to 2 ppm). Treatment should be repeated *at least* twice a year, if eggs and surviving adult stragglers are to be eliminated.

The fresh-water pulmonates (*Lymnaea, Australorbis, Planorbis,* etc.), aquatic snails, are best attacked by the use of copper sulfate (lethal to snails at 1.0 ppm), sodium pentachlorophenate (Santobrite) 5 to 15 ppm, or other molluscicidal agents. These may be applied in the form of an aqueous spray, by dusting or by immersion of bags or porous balls containing the chemical.

Limited field trials in Japan, Nigeria, the Dominican Republic and South America indicate that effective snail control may be obtained at reasonable cost using sodium pentachlorophenate (Santobrite), or DN-1 (40 per cent dinitro-*o*-cyclohexylphenol). The results reported must be regarded as preliminary until more extensive evaluations have been made.

In some areas successful control operations may require combining chemical treatment with drainage and alteration of the local environment of the snail species under attack.

# 68  Structure, Classification and Biology of Medically Important Molluscs

Field surveys and control operations directed against snails of medical importance require accurate identification of the various species of molluscs which may be encountered. This is frequently difficult. Although several important species of molluscan intermediate hosts are easily identified, there are many unimportant species possessing shells which superficially resemble those of species which carry pathogenic parasites. A further difficulty lies in the fact that there are many major families the systematics and nomenclature of which are still in a state of flux.

However, the problems of identification are diminished by use of animal characteristics such as the size and shape of the *tentacles,* the shape of the *copulatory organ,* the number of gill branches or *lamellae,* and the number and shape of the *radular teeth* (Fig. 278*A* and *B*).

The phylum MOLLUSCA consists of five classes:
1. Gastropoda: snails, slugs, whelks, conchs, etc.
2. Pelecypoda (Lamellibranchia): clams, mussels, oysters.
3. Cephalopoda: squids, octopi.
4. Scaphopoda: tusk shells and dentaliums.

5. Amphineura (Loricata): chitons, or coat-of-mail shells.

All of these possess a fleshy mantle which generally secretes a calcareous shell. The buccal mass, except in the Pelecypoda, contains a radular ribbon of rather hard denticulate teeth.

Molluscs are either bisexual, hermaphroditic or capable of changing sex one or more times during their life span. The eggs may be

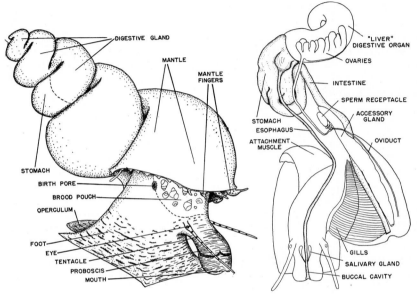

A. EXTERNAL ANATOMY OF THIARA          B. INTERNAL ANATOMY OF ONCOMELANIA

Fig. 278. Gross anatomy of the prosobranch snail. (*A*) *Thiara granifera* (left) is the oriental host of *Paragonimus*, and (*B*) *Oncomelania quadrasi* (right) is the Philippine host of *Schistosoma japonicum*. (Redrawn from Abbott.)

shed freely into the water, laid in capsules or brooded within the parent.

## Class Gastropoda

### Subclass Prosobranchia

The subclass Prosobranchia (Streptoneura) are the operculate snails, which possess a horny or calcareous *operculum* that is usually attached on the upper hind surface of the foot. The visceral nerve loop is crossed, forming a figure 8, and most have lamellate gills attached to the inside of the mantle. The majority are bisexual, but a few are hermaphroditic, parthenogenetic or capable of changing sex. This subclass is generally divided into three orders:

1. Archaeogastropoda (Scutibranchiata): a group of primitive, mainly marine snails of no medical importance.

2. Mesogastropoda (Pectinibranchiata): This subclass contains the majority of the medically important fresh water snails. They are characterized by comblike gills which are attached to the mantle along their entire length.

3. Neogastropoda: marine snails, including the venomous cone shells. They are characterized by one to three transverse rows of strong radular teeth.

**Order Mesogastropoda.** FAMILY HYDROBIIDAE. The family HYDRO-BIIDAE (AMNICOLIDAE, BITHYNIIDAE) comprises two subfamilies, the HYDROBIINAE (Fig. 279) and the BULIMINAE. These are of consider-able medical importance since the former contains the only known intermediate hosts of *Schistosoma japonicum,* and the latter, the ma-jority of the first intermediate hosts of the biliary flukes, *Clonorchis* and *Opisthorchis.*

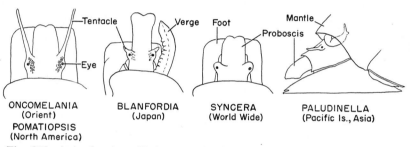

Fig. 279. Animals of small, brown Hydrobid snails with a horny operculum. *Oncomelania* and *Pomatiopsis* are hosts of oriental schistosomiasis; the other genera are not carriers. (Redrawn from Abbott.)

The members of this family are small, aquatic or amphibious gastropods with slender or subspherical shells which rarely exceed a length of 10 mm. The sexes are separate. The males possess an ex-ternal copulatory organ, known as the *verge,* attached to the right side of the body and appearing as a single or multipronged finger. The mantle edge is smooth. The operculum is either horny or cal-careous. Eggs are laid in gelatinous packets and may be covered with mud or tiny pebbles.

SUBFAMILY HYDROBIINAE. Members of the subfamily HYDRO-BIINAE are characterized by: (1) thin, horny and paucispiral oper-cula; (2) males having a fleshy verge which may or may not be frilled along its edge.

*Genus Oncomelania.* This is the only genus known to serve as in-termediate hosts of *Schistosoma japonicum* (Fig. 279). It comprises four species in all of which the outer lip of the aperture is strength-ened by a *varix* or thickening of the rim. Three of the species have smooth, brownish, slender shells; the fourth, *O. hupensis,* has ten to thirty small, axial ribs per whorl and is yellowish brown in color. The verge is a simple prong. The most characteristic feature is a streak of small, yellowish granules over each eye, forming a false "eyebrow." The four species are:

1. *Oncomelania hupensis* Gredler.

SYNONYMS. *Oncomelania schmackeri* Moellendorff, *longiscata* Heude, *elongata* Bartsch, *yaoi* Bartsch, *multicosta* Bartsch, and *anhuinensis* Li.

DISTRIBUTION. This species is common in the canals in the Yangtze River basin in the provinces of Kiangsu, Chekiang, Anhwei, Kiangsi and Hupeh. It is the principal host of *Schistosoma japonicum* in China.

The adults are gray-brown to waxy yellow in color. They are 7 to 10 mm. in length and have six to nine whorls. Each whorl has ten to thirty small axial ribs, and nuclear whorls may be tinged with rose.

2. *Oncomelania nosophora* Robson.

DISTRIBUTION. It is common in or along small creeks, irrigation ditches, rice paddies, or unflooded river bottoms in China, south of the Yangtze, and on Honshu and Kyushu Islands, Japan. It is the only known host of *S. japonicum* in Japan.

The adults are dark to light chestnut brown in color. They measure 5 to 12 mm. in length, are smooth, and have six to nine whorls.

3. *Oncomelania formosana* Pilsbry and Hirase.

DISTRIBUTION. This species is common in rice paddies and irrigation ditches in the western half of Formosa. It is the only host of *S. japonicum* in Formosa.

The adults are light chestnut brown in color, smoothish, and measure 4 to 6 mm. in length. The length of the last whorl is always greater than that of the whorls above.

4. *Oncomelania quadrasi* Moellendorff.

SYNONYM. *O. hydrobiopsis* Rensch.

DISTRIBUTION. This species is common in small creeks and among the vegetation above the waterline of slow-flowing streams in eastern Leyte, eastern Mindoro, Mindanao, Samar and Sorsogon Province, Luzon Island, Philippines. It is the only known intermediate host of *S. japonicum* in these islands.

The adults are translucent chocolate-brown, sometimes covered with a thin, black, encrusting slime, smoothish, and measure 3 to 5 mm. in length. The last whorl is always greater in length than those in the spire. *Oncomelania quadrasi* resembles, and may be confused with, *Syncera.*

*Genus Blanfordia.* Members of this genus are restricted to the Japanese Islands. Despite their close resemblance to *Oncomelania,* they have never been implicated as a carrier of schistosomiasis. There are four species of which *B. simplex* Pilsbry from Honshu is the commonest. The shells are not as slender as those of *Oncomelania* species. The verge is a simple prong with strong serrations on the inner concave edge. There are yellow color granules close to the eyes. The eye peduncles are well developed with a short, stubby, triangular tentacle projecting forward. The gill lamellae are only ten to twelve in number.

*Genus Pomatiopsis.* This is an American genus having shells and bodies that closely resemble those of *Oncomelania.*

DISTRIBUTION. This genus is found in woodland swamps and on low river banks in the United States from Minnesota east to New York, south to Alabama and Texas, and on the Atlantic seaboard from Pennsylvania south to Virginia.

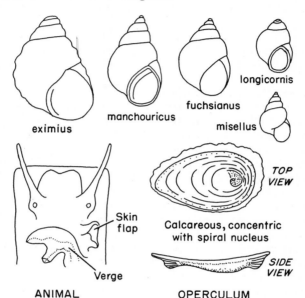

Fig. 280. The Bulimoid snails of the Orient serve as the main hosts of *Clonorchis* and *Opisthorchis.* (Redrawn from Abbott.)

There are ten described species. One, *P. lapidaria* Say, has been shown to be the natural host of *Paragonimus kellicotti,* the North American lung fluke of animals, and it is an experimental intermediate host of *Schistosoma japonicum.*

The shell is brownish, 5 to 8 mm. in length, and resembles that of *Oncomelania nosophora.* The verge is a flat, meat cleaver–shaped prong with a variable number of serrations on the inner, concave edge. There are yellow color granules above the eyes.

*Genus Fukuia.* Two species are known in this Japanese genus, which is not of medical importance. The shells resemble those of *Oncomelania,* but are more ovate, much thicker, glossy, reddish brown and without a thickened outer lip. The spiral sculpturing consists of numerous microscopic, incised lines.

The verge is a single prong bearing a rather large button-like gland on the upper side. The tentacles are very short. Yellow granules are present behind the eyes.

SUBFAMILY BULIMINAE. The subfamily BULIMINAE contains the majority of the first intermediate hosts of the human biliary flukes, *Clonorchis* and *Opisthorchis* (Fig. 280). The following genera, sometimes treated as subgenera of the genus *Bulimus* (formerly *Bithynia*), are all of medical importance:

1. *Bulimus* (north temperate regions);
2. *Alocinma* (India and China);
3. *Parafossarulus* (eastern Asia).

Members of this subfamily are characterized by: (1) a thick calcareous operculum; (2) a verge with a lateral finger-like appendage; (3) a small, cup-shaped skin flap attached to the right side of the head just behind the right tentacle. The genera are distinguished by shell characteristics.

*Genus Bulimus.* 1. *Bulimus fuchsianus* Moellendorff.

DISTRIBUTION. This genus is especially common in southern China where it serves as the principal snail host of *Clonorchis sinensis* (Fig. 280).

The adult shell is greenish brown in color, and about 10 mm. in length. It is rather fragile, smoothish, with a dull finish and fragile outer lip. The whorls are well rounded.

The mantle is black with numerous small, round spots of translucent cream, and the animal is gray with many brilliant orange-red spots.

2. *Bulimus misellus* Gredler. This is a common, medically unimportant Asiatic species (Fig. 280).

The adult shell is 5 to 7 mm. in length with five well rounded whorls. It is distinguished from *B. fuchsianus* by its smaller, more slender shell and its mantle, which is cream-colored with sparse, black, cobwebby mottlings.

3. *Bulimus tentaculatus* Linn.

DISTRIBUTION. This is a common north European species in lakes and ponds, which has become established in the north central and northeastern United States. It is one of the principal snail hosts of the liver fluke, *Opisthorchis felineus*.

The shell is yellowish, greenish or brownish in color, measuring 5 to 11 mm. in length. The operculum is calcareous. The animal is yellowish white with a blackish head and proboscis, and with a few golden yellow spots. The outer marginal radular tooth has approximately sixteen denticles; the inner marginal, approximately twelve; the central, seven at the top edge and approximately six at each lower corner.

*Genus Alocinma.* 1. *Alocinma longicornis* Benson.

DISTRIBUTION. This snail is common in canals and ponds in China, where it serves as one of the intermediate hosts of *Clonorchis sinensis* (Fig. 280).

The adult shell is 5 to 8 mm. in length, smooth, globular, with a short blunt apex. The animal is slate gray, dotted with greenish yellow color granules tending to be yellow near the anterior end.

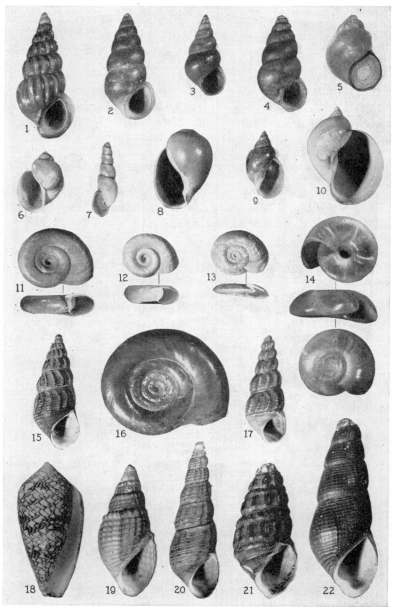

Fig. 281. Medically important molluscs. *1, Oncomelania hupensis* Gredler (China). *2, O. nosophora* Robson (China and Japan). *3, O. quadrasi* Mlldff. (Philippines). *4, Pomatiopsis lapidaria* Say (United States and Canada) (last 4 all 4 ×). *5, Bulimus tentaculatus* L. (United States; northern Europe) (3 ×). *6, Bulinus truncatus* Audouin (Africa and Asia Minor). *7, Bulinus forskali* Ehrenberg (Mauritius; Africa). *8, Bulinus (Physopsis) africanus* Krauss (Africa). *9, Lymnaea ollula*

The tentacles have a black "core," and the mantle is black with large, irregular, chalk white blotches.

*Genus Parafossarulus.* 1. *Parafossarulus manchouricus* Bourguignat.

SYNONYM. *Bithynia striatula* Benson.

DISTRIBUTION. This species is common in ponds in China, Formosa, Korea and Japan (Fig. 280). It is the principal intermediate host of *Clonorchis sinensis* in Japan and the second most important in China. It likewise carries *Opisthorchis felineus* and *Echinochasmus perfoliatus*.

The adult shell is yellowish to greenish brown in color and measures 7 to 10 mm. in length. There are spiral raised ridges of varying strength on the whorls. The calcareous operculum is not withdrawn into the shell.

The animal is slate gray with many fine, bright cream-orange spots, and the top visceral whorls are pinkish tan. The tentacles have an internal black core.

2. *Parafossarulus eximius* Frauenfeld. This largest of all Chinese bulimoid snails is common in lakes and ponds in eastern and central China. It is not of medical importance (Fig. 280).

The shell is reddish brown in color, reaching a length of 17 mm. There are three to four strong spiral cords on each whorl.

FAMILY SYNCERIDAE (ASSIMINEIDAE). This is a large family of small snails found mainly in tropical and subtropical areas, some members of which closely resemble schistosomiasis carriers, such as *Oncomelania*. The group is of little medical importance, although *Syncera lutea* Adams is reported to be a minor host of *Paragonimus westermani* in southern China. These snails are amphibious or terrestrial, with shells less than 8 mm. in length and with a translucent, horny, paucispiral operculum. The animals of *Syncera* (formerly *Assiminea*) have very short, stubby tentacles welded to the eyestalk, and the shell has a single, microscopic, spiral thread just below the suture of the whorls. A similar, terrestrial genus, *Paludinella*, lacks this thread, and its animal has short tentacles and a short cape encircling the upper part of the proboscis.

FAMILY THIARIDAE (MELANIIDAE). The THIARIDAE is a widely distributed and diversified family of operculate snails living in fresh and brackish water. A number of species are the main snail hosts for *Paragonimus, Metagonimus, Troglotrema* (salmon poisoning), *Ha-*

---

Gould (Hawaii and China). *10, Lymnaea auricularia* L. (northern Eurasia). *11, Biomphalaria alexandrina* Ehrenberg (northern Africa). *12, Biomphalaria pfeifferi* Krauss (southern Africa). *13, Hippeutis cantori* Benson (China). *14, Segmentina hemisphaerula* Benson (eastern Asia) (5 ✕). *15, Goniobasis silicula* Gould (northwest United States). *16, Australorbis glabratus* Say (West Indies and South America). *17, Hua ningpoensis* Lea (China). *18, Conus textile* L. (Indo-Pacific reefs). *19, Thiara (Tarebia) granifera* Lamarck (southeast Asia; Pacific Ids.). *20, Thiara (Melanoides) tuberculata* Müller (Africa to S. E. Asia; Pacific Ids.). *21, Semisulcospira amurensis* Gerstfeldt (northern China; Korea). *22, Semisulcospira libertina* Gould (Japan to Formosa). (Numbers *6* to *22* are 1½ ✕, except *14*.)

*plorchis* and *Diorchitrema*. The shells are usually 1 to 3 inches in length, black or brown in color and fairly slender. There are two major subfamilies: the true THIARINAE, in which the young are brooded in a neck pouch and in which the mantle edge is digitate; and the PLEUROCERINAE, whose members lay eggs or brood the young in a uterine pouch and whose mantle edge is smooth or wavy, but never digitate. This family has been generally referred to as ME-LANIIDAE in medical literature.

SUBFAMILY THIARINAE. *Thiara (Tarebia) granifera* Lamarck. This common species lives in fast-flowing streams in Southeast Asia, the East Indies, Formosa, and the western Pacific islands, where it serves as the first intermediate host for *Paragonimus westermani, Metagonimus yokogawai, Diorchitrema formosanum* and *Haplorchis taichui* (Fig. 281). The snail has become established in Lithia Spring, Florida. Adults 6 to 40 mm. in length, elongate-turrite, yellowish to reddish brown; whorls with four to six spiral rows of round to squarish, small beads; outer lip fragile. Mantle edge with several prominent, fleshy digitations, four of which may be seen projecting beyond the shell lip on the left side. Mature specimens with shelled young in brood pouch under skin behind head. Operculum two-thirds the size of the aperture, horny and blackish brown. "*Melania obliquegranosa*" is a synonym.

*Thiara (Melanoides) tuberculata* Müller. Common in warm, sluggish water from Africa to subtropical Asia and the western Pacific islands. Animal similar to that of the above species (Fig. 281). Shell 1 to 2 inches in length, slender, with well-rounded whorls and with sculpturing of numerous axial and spiral threads. Color brownish and sometimes mottled with reddish brown. A host for *Diorchitrema formosanum*, and suspected to be a minor host for *Clonorchis sinensis*.

SUBFAMILY PLEUROCERIINAE. *Semisulcospira libertina* Gould. This species is considered to be the main intermediate snail host of *Paragonimus westermani* in the Orient (Fig. 281). It has an insular distribution which extends from Japan and Korea to Formosa. Shell ¾ to 2 inches in length, somewhat spindle-shaped and with slightly flattened, smoothish whorls. Length of aperture is about half the total length of the shell. Whorls with numerous fine, spiral threads. Color brownish to yellowish brown, but sometimes heavily flushed with greenish blue. Mantle edge smooth. Uterus on inside of mantle may be filled with many, equal-sized, small young. Males without verge.

*Semisulcospira amurensis* Gerstfeldt. Common in fast-flowing streams in northern China and Korea (Fig. 281). It is an intermediate host of *Paragonimus westermani*. This species has many minor races in Korea. Shell ½ to 1 inch in length, dark-brown to greenish brown. Sculpture usually heavy, with two or three very strong cords on the base of the shell. Blunt axial ribs and low nodules sometimes present.

Animal similar to the above species. Operculum opaque brown, horny and paucispiral.

*Hua (Namrutua) ningpoensis* Lea. Very common in canals and small rivers of central and southern China, where it serves as one of the main intermediate hosts of *Clonorchis sinensis* (Fig. 281). It was formerly known as *Melania cancellata* Benson. Operculum translucent, thin, horny and paucispiral. Shell about 1 inch in length and slender; the upper two-thirds of each whorl with even, strong, slightly curved, axial ribs, and with three or four smooth, spiral cords on the base of the shell. Animal lays eggs. Mantle edge wavy, but without digitations.

*Goniobasis silicula* Gould. This is the only known snail host of *Troglotrema salmincola* Chapin, the trematode associated with "salmon poisoning" in northwestern United States (Fig. 281). It is common in lakes and creeks of Washington and Oregon. Shell ½ to 1 inch in length, brownish to greenish, slender, and with rounded whorls. Strong axial ribs are usually present on the first few whorls, and the numerous spiral threads are strongest on the last whorl. It is erroneously listed in the literature as *"Galba plicifera silicula."*

FAMILIES VIVIPARIDAE AND PILIDAE. These are the large "apple snails" of ponds and lakes, and although a number of cercariae have been found in them, no trematodes of medical importance have been associated with either of these families. In *Viviparus* the operculum is horny, with a concentric nucleus near the margin. Females brood pea-sized young in the uterus. In the males the right tentacle is truncate or recurved and serves as the penis. The eyes are on large, bulbous swellings at the base of the tentacles. The central tooth of the radula is quadrate and denticulate only on the top edge. In the PILIDAE, which have similarly large, 3-inch shells, the operculum is calcareous, the tentacles are very long and slender, the penis arises from the right side of the mantle edge, and the females lay clusters of pea-sized, calcareous eggs on reeds just above the surface of the water. The genera *Pila* and *Pomacea* belong in this last family, but are of no medical importance.

## Subclass Euthyneura

**Order Pulmonata. Suborder Basommatophora.** FAMILY PLANORBIDAE. The planorbid pond snails are world-wide in distribution and play an important part in the life cycle of many trematodes. The foot of the planorbs is elongate, truncate in front, and usually tapering to a point behind. Above and in front of the foot is a short, broad, fleshy velum which bears the head and two tentacles. The small, black eyes are situated at the inner bases of the tentacles. The respiratory opening and pseudobranch or false gill are on the left side of the body. The genital openings are also on the left side. There is no operculum. The animals are monoecious and lay gelatinous globs in which the eggs are embedded (Fig. 282).

*Australorbis glabratus* Say. This species and its several minor races are the main intermediate hosts of *Schistosoma mansoni* in the West Indies and South America (Figs. 281, 282). It is the largest species in those areas and reaches a diameter of a little over an inch. The shell is smooth and made up of slowly widening whorls which are either rounded or slightly angular in cross section. The color of the animal is gray or black, and the mantle is mottled with brown or cinnamon. Difficulties arise in separating small specimens from

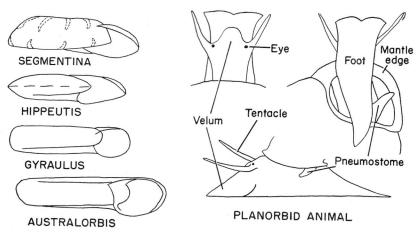

Fig. 282. *Segmentina hemisphaerula* and *Hippeutis cantori* (above) are oriental hosts of *Fasciolopsis buski*; *Gyraulus* is the second intermediate host of *Echinostoma*; *Australorbis glabratus* (above) is the tropical American host of *Schistosoma mansoni*. (Redrawn from Abbott.)

several innocent species, but by comparing a graded growth series it is possible to distinguish *Australorbis* from *Drepanotrema* (which has a V-shaped, black mark on the velum between the tentacles) and *Tropicorbis* by observing the color patterns of the animal and the shape of the shell. Among the synonyms or races of this species are *Planorbis guadaloupensis, P. olivaceus* and *P. antiguensis.*

*Biomphalaria alexandrina* Ehrenberg. This is the main snail host of *Schistosoma mansoni* in the northern third of Africa. It is variable in shape and has been called *Planorbis boissyi* Potiez and Michaud, and *Planorbis ruppelli* Dunker. The shells are typically planorbid. An adult specimen from Egypt has five whorls, a diameter of 17 mm. and a height of 5.5 mm. The upper side of the shell is slightly concave, but almost flat, and the apex is not very deep. The upper part of the aperture is usually arched, and may be a little higher than the next to the last whorl. The aperture is more or less evenly oval in cross-section.

*Biomphalaria pfeifferi* Krauss. This is the main host of *S. mansoni* in central and southern Africa. It is considered a subspecies of the above species by some workers. It is similar to *B. alexandrina,* but is generally not as flat (diameter 12 mm., height 4.2 mm.), and is much more concave at the top with a deep apex. The upper part of the aperture is generally less arched, and the aperture has a tendency to be more pinched or triangular in cross section. In both species, the young shells may have small, whitish teeth or folds within the aperture. The systematic and nomenclatural condition of the genus is still unsatisfactory.

*Segmentina hemisphaerula* Benson. In eastern Asia, this small, common species serves as one of the intermediate hosts of *Fasciolopsis buski* (Figs. 281, 282). Adult shell "fat," with a height of about 3 mm. and a diameter of 7 to 9 mm. Color glossy, reddish brown to light brown; umbilicus very deep. The internal calcareous lamellae are visible through the shell. *Planorbis nitidellus* von Martens is a synonym.

*Hippeutis cantori* Benson. In eastern China, this species is one of the main intermediate hosts of *Fasciolopsis buski* (Figs. 281, 282). The adults are fairly large (8 to 10 mm. in diameter) but rather flat (1 to 2 mm. in height). Spire slightly concave; umbilicus very wide but not very deep. Periphery of the last embracing whorl may be sharp. No internal shell folds. Color a glossy translucent brown. Common in ponds and lakes. A similar species, *H. umbilicalis* Benson, is fatter (6 by 2 mm.), with a neatly indented spire and a much narrower umbilicus. It is of no known medical importance.

FAMILY BULINIDAE. *Genus Bulinus.* Members of this genus are the main intermediate hosts of *Schistosoma haematobium* in Africa. Some authorities consider *Physopsis* as a subgenus of *Bulinus*. *Bulinus* is readily recognized by its glossy, 13 mm. long, left-handed or sinistral shells. Mantle without digitations (Fig. 281).

1. *Bulinus (Bulinus) truncatus* Audouin. This is a widespread species found in most parts of Africa and in Asia Minor. It appears to be the main host of *S. haematobium* in the northern third of Africa (Fig. 281). Probable synonyms of this species are *Bulinus contortus* Michaud, *B. brocchi* Ehrenberg and *B. tropicus* Krauss. Adults about 8 to 13 mm. in length, sinistral, brownish and not very glossy. Microscopic axial growth lines irregular. Columella thin, not rolled back to form a ridge, callus or tube, and not abruptly truncate at the base. Three to four whorls.

2. *Bulinus (Physopsis) africanus* Krauss. This is the main carrier of *S. haematobium* in South, East, West and Central Africa (Fig. 281). It has several races or ecologic types which have been named *globosa* Morelet, *nasuta* von Martens and *ovoidea* Bourg. It is similar to *B. truncatus*, but may reach a length of 19mm., is usually quite glossy, and has a reflected columella which is strongly twisted and truncate below. Microscopic sculpturing of growth lines and very fine, punctate dots or short, crowded, wavy threads. The spire may be high or low. Common.

3. *Bulinus (Pyrgophysa) forskali* Ehrenberg. This species has been shown to carry *S. haematobium* in Mauritius, but the range

extends over the southern half of Africa (Fig. 281). Adult shell about 13 mm. in length, elongate, with a high spire whose five to six whorls usually have flattish sides. Color buff to whitish. Moderately common.

FAMILY LYMNAEIDAE. The genus *Lymnaea*, a group of dextrally coiled pond snails, is of moderate importance, and some of its species, such as *L. auricularia* Linné, *L. ollula* Gould and *L. bulimoides* Lea, serve as the first intermediate hosts of *Fasciola hepatica*. "Swimmer's itch" or schistosome dermatitis is caused by non-human schistosomes; in northern central United States the snail hosts are certain species of *Lymnaea*. Identification of the lymneid molluscs generally requires the services of an expert. The head, tentacles and eyes resemble those of the planorbs, but the genital openings are on the right side of the body. There is no operculum (Fig. 281).

**Suborder Stylommatophora** The slugs and garden snails are characterized by their two pairs of head tentacles, with the eyes at the tips of the second pair. There are many thousands of species of land snails, but only relatively few have been found to serve as snail hosts to trematodes infecting man. The following families and genera have been shown to carry *Dicrocoelium dendriticum:* PUPILLIDAE (*Chondrina* (= *Torquilla*); FRUTICICOLIDAE (*Bradybaena*); HELICIDAE (*Helicella, Cochicella* and *Zebrina*); CIONELLIDAE (*Cionella*). The sheep liver fluke, *Fasciola hepatica*, is carried by *Lymnaea* and the following land groups: SUCCINEIDAE (*Succinea*) and POLYGYRIDAE (*Praticolella*).

# MEDICALLY IMPORTANT
# ARTHROPODS

## 69   Introduction

In the foregoing chapters it has been made apparent that many of the important tropical diseases depend for their dissemination upon various species of arthropods (insects, ticks, mites, etc.) whose behavior and life cycles are intimately involved with the continued existence of the parasites concerned. In addition to their role as *vectors* of disease, the arthropods also include a number of species which hold an important place in medical science by reason of their ability to function *directly* as agents of human disease or discomfort, that is, to serve themselves as etiologic agents of various pathologic conditions. Before proceeding to a discussion of particular groups it will be desirable to consider each of these aspects in an introductory manner.

### Role of Arthropods as Vectors of Disease

Table 54 presents a recapitulation of all important parasitic diseases in which arthropod vectors are concerned. Column 4 shows that at least three classes of the Phylum ARTHROPODA are represented in the list. For example, the CRUSTACEA are represented by the minute *Cyclops*, certain species of which play host to the guinea worm

(*Dracunculus medinensis*) while others transmit *Diphyllobothrium latum,* the broad tapeworm of man. Larger forms, such as crayfish and crabs, harbor infective stages of the lung fluke *Paragonimus.*

A second major group, the ARACHNIDA, is represented by the ticks and mites, proved vectors of certain rickettsial, viral, bacterial and spirochetal diseases.

The third and by far the most important group of arthropods is the Class INSECTA (HEXAPODA), or true insects. Here occur the majority of arthropod vectors. Not all groups of insects, however, are equally fitted to serve in this capacity. Of the thirty or more orders of insects known to science, only five are significantly involved in the distribution of viruses, bacteria, or other disease-producing organisms:

1. The ORTHOPTERA (cockroaches and others)
2. The HEMIPTERA (true bugs, such as *Triatoma*)
3. The ANOPLURA (sucking lice)
4. The SIPHONAPTERA (fleas)
5. The DIPTERA (true flies, including mosquitoes)

Again within each of the above listed orders, only certain families and, in many instances, only certain species, are biologically adapted for the harboring and transmission of pathogenic forms. Such adaptation, however, manifests itself in many ways, as illustrated by the following outline:

Arthropods as Vectors of Disease
1. *Accidental* (e.g., typhoid, by house fly)
    (*a*) On mouth parts
    (*b*) Through alimentary canal
    (*c*) On body, legs and hairs
2. *Obligatory*
    (*a*) Propagative only: parasites multiply, but do not change in form or type (plague bacillus in gut of flea)
    (*b*) Developmental only: parasites grow in size and change in structure but do not multiply (microfilariae in bodies of flies)
    (*c*) Cyclico-propagative: parasites both multiply and undergo developmental changes (*Plasmodium* in body of mosquito)

Special mention should be made also of transovarial transmission, by which the disease organism may pass into the egg of the infected arthropod and is thus capable of being transmitted by the succeeding generation. The vector in this case becomes also a reservoir of the disease, as do ticks in the transmission of Rocky Mountain spotted fever.

## Role of Arthropods as *Direct Agents* of Human Disease or Discomfort

All blood-sucking vectors are more or less important as pests in their own right. If, in addition to these, consideration be given to the blood-suckers which are not vectors, also to the spiders, centipedes and stinging forms, as well as to various groups which live as parasites within tissues and cavities, the list of species capable of acting as direct agents of dangerous or at least annoying conditions in man becomes exceedingly large. Four classes of arthropods are here involved:

1. Class ARACHNIDA (scorpions, spiders, ticks, mites)
2. Class PENTASTOMIDA (tongue worms)
3. Class CHILOPODA (centipedes)
4. Class HEXAPODA (insects, many groups)

It will be noted that two of the above listed classes (ARACHNIDA and HEXAPODA), were also mentioned as containing vectors of disease.

The particular role played by each group (or species) will be treated in its proper place.

Pathological conditions caused by these various arthropods may be classified as follows:

1. Entomophobia
2. Accidental injury to sense organs
3. Envenomization (inclusive of allergies)
    (*a*)  Bites (centipedes, spiders, certain ticks, mites, reduviid bugs)
    (*b*)  Stings (bees, wasps, scorpions)
    (*c*)  Effects of urticating hairs (certain caterpillars)
    (*d*)  Irritation by vesicating fluids (blister beetles)
    (*e*)  Specific types of allergy (Mayflies)
4. Infestation by insect larvae—Myiasis (flies), Canthariasis (beetles), Scholeciasis (lepidopterous species)
5. Dermatoses (fleas, lice, mites, ticks, etc.)

**Entomophobia**   This term refers to any of a number of psychic or nervous states, in which the patient exhibits an abnormal fear or dread of the presence of insect forms. In rare instances the services of a psychiatrist may be required.

**Accidental Injury to Sense Organs**   Many practitioners have had the experience of removing an insect or parts thereof from the eye, ear or nasal passages of a patient. The discomfort is usually mechanical in nature, although in some instances the insect produces an irritating secretion as well. More serious is the presence of fly larvae in the eyes, nose, sinuses. Such larvae (or the eggs from which they hatch) must be deposited in or near the definitive location by the fly. (See Myiasis, p. 793).

**Envenomization**   In a number of ways, insects and other arthropods are known to poison human beings, the degree of discomfort depending upon the susceptibility of the individual as well as upon the species of arthropod concerned. Hemolytic, hemorrhagic, neurotoxic and vesicating effects have been recorded. Specific examples will be considered in connection with the discussion of particular taxonomic groups.

It is not easy to separate the better-known types of envenomization (bites, stings) from reactions manifestly allergic in character. Ordinarily a degree of discomfort more or less common to all exposed individuals is not regarded as allergic in nature. When, how-

*Table 54  Human Diseases Transmitted by Arthropods*

HELMINTHIC DISEASES

| DISEASE | ETIOLOGIC AGENT | GEOGRAPHICAL DISTRIBUTION | VECTOR | RESERVOIR | LOCATION OF ETIOLOGIC AGENT IN MAN | DIAGNOSTIC PROCEDURES |
|---|---|---|---|---|---|---|
| Loiasis | Loa loa | Tropical Africa, especially Congo River basin | Mango flies (Chrysops dimidiata and C. silacea) | Man | Subcutaneous tissues; microfilariae in blood | Clinical picture; worm beneath skin; blood exam., day |
| Filariasis | Wuchereria bancrofti and W. malayi | Tropical Africa, Asia, Australia, South America, Pacific Islands | Mosquitoes (Culex, Aedes, Anopheles and Mansonia spp.) | Man | Lymph nodes and vessels; microfilariae in blood | Clinical picture; worms in lymph nodes; microfilariae in blood or chyle |
| Onchocerciasis | Onchocerca volvulus | Africa, Mexico, Central America, Venezuela | Blackflies (Simulium spp.) | Man | Nodules and tumors; microfilariae in skin, eyes | Puncture of tumors and nodules; biopsy; skin section |
| (1) Mansonella ozzardi and (2) Acanthocheilonema perstans | | (1) Latin America (2) Latin America and Africa | Midges (Culicoides spp.) | Man | Microfilariae in peripheral blood; rarely pathogenic | Blood smear |
| Dracunculiasis | Dracunculus medinensis | Africa, India, U.S.S.R., Middle East | Cyclops spp. | Man | Loose connective tissue | Roentgenograms |
| Diphyllobothriasis | Diphyllobothrium latum | Northern Europe, northern U.S.A., U.S.S.R. | Copepods (Diaptomus and Cyclops) | Man, dog, cat, fox, bear, etc. | Intestine | Fecal examination |
| Sparganosis | Spargana of several species of tapeworms | Asia, scattered areas including Holland, British Guiana and U.S.A. | Cyclops spp. | Man,* frogs, snakes, birds, mammals | Subcutaneous tissues | Excision (?) |
| Dipylidiasis | Dipylidium caninum | Europe, Asia, U.S.A., Africa, Pacific Islands | Fleas, dog louse(?) | Man, dog | Intestine | Fecal examination |
| Hymenolepiasis diminuta | Hymenolepis diminuta | India, U.S.S.R., Japan, Italy, U.S.A. | Fleas, cockroaches, meal worms | Man, rat, mouse | Intestine | Fecal examination |
| Hymenolepiasis nana | Hymenolepis nana | Cosmopolitan | Fleas (?), mealworms (?) | Man, mouse | Intestine | Fecal examination |
| Paragonimiasis | Paragonimus westermani and P. kellicotti | Far East, India, Philippines, Africa, Pacific Islands, North and South America | Fresh-water crabs and crayfish | Man, carnivores | Lungs, intestinal mucosa | Examination of sputum and feces |

* Maturity not reached in man.

## PROTOZOAL DISEASES

| Disease | Organism | Distribution | Vector | Reservoir host | Location | Diagnosis |
|---|---|---|---|---|---|---|
| Malaria | *Plasmodium vivax, P. malariae, P. falci- parum, P. ovale* | Worldwide (see exceptions in certain Pacific Islands, Arctic, Antarctic) | Mosquitoes (*Anopheles* spp.) | Man | Erythrocytes; reticulo-endothelial system | Blood smear |
| African sleeping sickness | *Trypanosoma gambiense, T. rhodesiense* | Africa | Tsetse flies (*Glossina* spp.) | Man, game (?) | Peripheral blood, spinal fluid, lymph nodes | Stained blood smear or fresh preparation; lumbar puncture; lymph node puncture |
| Chagas' disease (South American trypanoso-miasis) | *Trypanosoma cruzi* | South America, Central America, Mexico | Kissing bugs (*Triatoma, Panstrongylus* spp.) | Armadillo, opossum, dogs, cats, rodents, etc. | Peripheral blood, heart muscle, etc. | Blood smear and culture (N.N.N.); complement fixation; animal inoculation; xeno-diagnosis |
| Kala-azar (visceral leishmaniasis) | *Leishmania donovani* | China, India, Mediterranean, South America | Sandflies (*Phlebotomus* spp.) | Man, dogs | Spleen, liver, bone marrow, reticulo-endothelial system | Sternal marrow biopsy, splenic puncture, blood culture (N.N.N.) |
| Oriental sore (cutaneous leishmaniasis) | *Leishmania tropica* | Mediterranean, Asia Minor, India, China | Sandflies (*Phlebotomus* spp.) | Man | Skin lesions | Smear and culture of lesions (N.N.N.) |
| South American cutaneous and mucocutaneous leishmaniasis (uta, espundia) | *Leishmania braziliensis* | Latin America | Sandflies (*Phlebotomus* spp.) | Man | Skin and mucous membrane lesions | Smear and culture of lesions (N.N.N.) |

## SPIROCHETAL DISEASES

| Disease | Organism | Distribution | Vector | Reservoir host | Location | Diagnosis |
|---|---|---|---|---|---|---|
| Relapsing fever, louse-borne | *Spirochaeta recurrentis*(?) | Europe, Asia, Africa | Human body louse (*Pediculus humanus* var. *corporis*) | Man | Peripheral blood | Direct and darkfield exam., and animal inoculation of blood |
| Relapsing fever, tick-borne | *Spirochaeta duttoni*(?) | Africa, America, Europe, Asia | Soft ticks (*Ornithodoros* spp.) | Ticks, rodents and other mammals | Peripheral blood | Direct and darkfield exam., and animal inoculation of blood |
| Yaws | *Treponema pertenue* | Tropics | Eye gnat (*Hippelates* sp.) | Man | Skin lesions | Clinical picture, Kahn test |

## BACTERIAL DISEASES

| Disease | Organism | Distribution | Vector | Reservoir host | Location | Diagnosis |
|---|---|---|---|---|---|---|
| Bubonic plague | *Pasteurella pestis* | Pandemic | Rat fleas, especially *Xenopsylla cheopis* | Rats and wild rodents | Blood stream, lymph nodes | Lymph node puncture, blood culture |
| Tularemia | *Pasteurella tularensis* | United States, Canada, Japan, Europe, Turkey | Hard ticks (*Dermacentor andersoni* and *D. variabilis*); deer fly (*Chrysops discalis*) | Rabbit and other wild animals | Blood stream, lymph nodes, skin lesions | Clinical picture, agglutination, animal inoculation |

*Table 54  Human Diseases Transmitted by Arthropods—Bacterial Diseases—Continued*

| DISEASE | ETIOLOGIC AGENT | GEOGRAPHICAL DISTRIBUTION | VECTOR | RESERVOIR | LOCATION OF ETIOLOGIC AGENT IN MAN | DIAGNOSTIC PROCEDURES |
|---|---|---|---|---|---|---|
| Verruga peruana (Oroya fever, bartonellosis) | *Bartonella bacilliformis* | Peru, Colombia, Ecuador: altitude 1700–10,000 ft. | Sandflies (*Phlebotomus* spp.) | Man | Erythrocytes, reticulo-endothelial system | Clinical picture, blood smear and culture, perhaps biopsy of skin lesion |
| Catarrhal conjunctivitis | Koch-Weeks bacillus (?) | Tropical and temperate regions, especially Egypt | Eye gnats (*Hippelates, Siphunculina,* spp.); mechanical transmission | Man | Conjunctiva | Clinical picture, smear of exudate |
| RICKETTSIAL DISEASES | | | | | | |
| Epidemic typhus (Brill's disease) | *Rickettsia prowazekii* | All Continents except Australia | Human body louse (*Pediculus humanus* var. *corporis*) | Man | Intracellular (intra-cytoplasmic) | Clinical picture, Weil-Felix test, specific complement fixation and agglutination |
| Murine typhus | *Rickettsia typhi* | All Continents | Rat fleas, especially *Xenopsylla cheopis,* also *X. astia* and *Nosopsyllus fasciatus* | Rats | Intracellular (intra-cystoplasmic) | |
| American spotted fever | *Rickettsia rickettsii* | Canada, United States, Mexico, Panama, Colombia, Brazil | Ticks: *Dermacentor andersoni, D. variabilis, Amblyomma americanum.* In Mexico, *Rhipicephalus sanguineus* and *A. cajennense.* In South America, *A. cajennense* principally | Rodents (?), ticks | Intracellular (intranuclear) | Clinical picture, Weil-Felix test, complement fixation |
| Fièvre boutonneuse (including Kenya typhus, South African tick-bite fever, and Indian tick typhus) | *Rickettsia conorii* | Mediterranean, Crimea, Africa, India | Ticks: *Rhipicephalus sanguineus, R. evertsi, Amblyomma hebraeum, Haemaphysalis leachi* and probably others, in appropriate geographic areas | Ticks, dogs (?), wild animals (?) | Initial lesion and lymphatics. Endothelial cells | Clinical picture, Weil-Felix test |
| North Queensland tick typhus | *Rickettsia australis* | Queensland | *Ixodes holocyclus* (?) | Unknown | Intracellular (intranuclear) | Clinical picture; Weil-Felix test; complement fixation |

| Disease | Agent | Distribution | Arthropod vector | Reservoir | Location in body | Diagnosis |
|---|---|---|---|---|---|---|
| Siberian tick typhus | *Rickettsia* sp. | Central and Eastern Siberia | Ticks: *Dermacentor silvarum*, *D. nuttalli*, *Haemaphysalis concinna* | Ticks, rodents (?) | Blood (and probably tissues) | Clinical picture, Weil-Felix test |
| Scrub typhus (tsutsugamushi disease) | *Rickettsia tsutsugamushi* | Various Asiatic-Pacific areas | Trombiculid mites (chiggers): *Trombicula akamushi* et al. | Mites, field rats and other small mammals | Intracellular | Clinical picture, Weil-Felix test |
| Q fever | *Coxiella burnetii* | Australia, North America, Panama, Europe, Middle East, Africa, China (?) | Rickettsiae present in certain ticks but no proved instance of tick transmission to man | Ticks, cattle, sheep, goats, and probably certain wild animals | Intracellular | Isolate rickettsiae; complement fixation and agglutination with Q rickettsial antigen; no Weil-Felix |
| Rickettsialpox | *Rickettsia akari* | Northeastern United States | Mite: *Allodermanyssus sanguineus* | House mice (*Mus musculus*) | Intracellular (intranuclear) | Clinical picture; isolate rickettsiae; complement fixation |
| Trench fever | *Rickettsia quintana* | Europe | Human body louse (*Pediculus humanus* var. *corporis*) | Man | Blood, urine | Clinical picture, no Weil-Felix |
| VIRUS DISEASES | | | | | | |
| Yellow fever—urban | Virus | Central and South America, Africa | Mosquitoes (*Aedes aegypti*) | Man | Blood in early stages, liver parenchyma | Clinical picture in severe cases; autopsy findings; in mild cases isolate virus; neutralizing antibodies |
| Yellow fever—jungle | Virus (same as above) | Central and South America, Africa | Mosquitoes (*Haemagogus spegazzinii* et al. in S.A. *Aedes simpsoni* et al. in Africa) | Monkeys and other animals, as yet undetermined | Blood in early stages, liver parenchyma | |
| Dengue | Virus | Tropics and subtropics | Mosquitoes (*Aedes* spp.) | Man? | Blood in early stages | Clinical picture; leukopenia important |
| Sandfly fever | Virus | Tropics and subtropics | Sandflies (*Phlebotomus papatasi* and others) | Sandflies, man? | Blood in early stages | Clinical picture; leukopenia, differential W. B. C. |
| Rift Valley fever | Virus | Africa | Mosquitoes (*Eretmapodites* spp. and *Aedes* spp.) | Cattle? | Blood | Complement fixation and neutralization tests |
| Colorado tick fever | Virus | United States | *Dermacentor, Amblyomma* spp. | Ticks? | Blood? | Complement fixation and neutralization tests |
| Bwamba fever | Virus | Uganda, Africa | ? | ? | ? | Neutralization tests |

*Table 54 Human Diseases Transmitted by Arthropods—Virus Diseases—Continued*

| DISEASE | ETIOLOGIC AGENT | GEOGRAPHICAL DISTRIBUTION | VECTOR | RESERVOIR | LOCATION OF ETIOLOGIC AGENT IN MAN | DIAGNOSTIC PROCEDURES |
|---|---|---|---|---|---|---|
| Western equine encephalomyelitis | Virus | United States, South Canada, Argentina | Mosquitoes (*Culex tarsalis* and others) | Probably wild and domestic mammals and birds | Central nervous system | Isolate virus, complement fixation, neutralizing or hemagglutination-inhibition antibodies, pathology |
| Eastern equine encephalomyelitis | Virus | United States, Canada, Mexico, Cuba, Panama, Dominican Republic | Mosquitoes (*Aedes sollicitans, Mansonia perturbans*) | Horses, pheasants, probably others | Central nervous system | |
| California encephalomyelitis | Virus | San Joaquin Valley, California | Mosquitoes (*Aedes dorsalis, Culex tarsalis*) | Horses and other mammals | ? | |
| Venezuelan equine encephalomyelitis | Virus | N. South America, Trinidad, Panama | Mosquitoes (probably *Aedes* sp. and *Mansonia* sp.) | Probably wild and domestic mammals and birds | Central nervous system | |
| St. Louis encephalitis | Virus | United States | Mosquitoes (*Culex tarsalis, C. pipiens*) | Probably wild and domestic mammals and birds. Perhaps man as well | Central nervous system | |
| Japanese B encephalitis | Virus | Japan, Okinawa, Guam, Korea, China, Manchuria and U.S.S.R. and probably much of Far East | Mosquitoes (*Culex tritaeniorhynchus*) | Man or birds? | Central nervous system | |
| Russian spring-summer encephalitis | Virus | U.S.S.R. | Ticks (*Ixodes persulcatus*, possibly others) | Unknown | Central nervous system | Isolate virus, complement fixation, neutralizing, or hemagglutination-inhibition antibodies, pathology |
| Louping ill | Virus | England, Scotland, Czechoslovakia, "White Russia" | Tick (*Ixodes ricinus*) | ? | Blood? | |

MISCELLANEOUS

| DISEASE | ETIOLOGIC AGENT | GEOGRAPHICAL DISTRIBUTION | VECTOR | RESERVOIR | LOCATION OF ETIOLOGIC AGENT IN MAN | DIAGNOSTIC PROCEDURES |
|---|---|---|---|---|---|---|
| Enteric diseases: typhoid, bacillary and amebic dysentery, diarrheas, Asiatic cholera, certain helminth infections | | Differs in various regions | Houseflies (*Musca domestica*) et al. frequenting human excrement and food; mechanical transmission | Man | Intestines, etc. | Clinical picture, stool exam. and culture |
| Human bots (myiasis) | *Dermatobia* spp. | American tropics | Flies, mosquitoes, blood-sucking arthropods | Various mammals, birds | Superficial layers of skin | Appearance of lesion; excision |

*Table 55  Envenomization (Including Allergies)*

| COMMON NAME | SCIENTIFIC NAME (OR GROUP) | DISTRIBUTION | IMPORTANT EFFECTS ON MAN | REMARKS |
|---|---|---|---|---|
| Mites: Chiggers | *Eutrombicula alfreddugèsi* and other trombiculine larvae | Tropics and warmer temperate regions | Intense itching; dermatitis; persistent purplish ecchymoses | Avoid by use of protective clothing; dimethyl or dibutyl phthalate repellents |
| Cheese and flour mites | Several genera of ACARIDAE (TYROGLYPHIDAE) | Worldwide | Dermatitis; allergic phenomena from contact with dead bodies of mites | Infestation usually limited to handlers of dry food products |
| Rat mites | *Liponyssus bacoti* | Worldwide | Dermatitis; intense itching; hemorrhagic areas | Infests persons who work or loiter in rat-infested premises |
| Grain itch mites | *Pediculoides ventricosus* | Widespread | Dermatitis and fever | Infest threshers and persons who sleep on straw |
| Ticks: Soft ticks | *Ornithodoros* spp. | All continents | Local and systemic reactions: some species (*O. coriaceus*) extremely venomous | Avoid rest houses, rodent burrows, mountain homes |
| Hard ticks | *Dermacentor andersoni* | {Western Canada {Western U. S. A. | Tick paralysis | Early removal of ticks very important; otherwise usually fatal |
|  | *D. variabilis* | Eastern U. S. A. Pacific Coast | Tick paralysis |  |
| Black Widow Spiders | *Ixodes* spp. *Latrodectus mactans* *Latrodectus* spp. | Widespread The Americas Widespread | Tick paralysis {Local swelling; abdominal rigidity; intense pain | Morphine useful sedative; 10 cc. calcium gluconate (10%) intravenously |
| Scorpions | Order: SCORPIONIDA | Tropics and subtropics | Painful sting; neurotoxin and hemolysin injected; sometimes fatal | Ligature, incision and suction helpful; use antivenin, if available; other treatment empirical |
| Centipedes | Class: CHILOPODA | Warmer regions | Painful bite; local necrosis; generalized symptoms | Give sedatives; apply dilute ammonia, locally |
| Insects: Mayflies | Order: EPHEMERIDA | Worldwide | Asthmatic paroxysms from inhalation of insect fragments | Desensitization perhaps feasible |
| Caddis flies | Order: TRICHOPTERA | Worldwide | Asthmatic symptoms from inhalation of hairs and scales | Desensitization perhaps feasible |
| Kissing bugs (cone noses) | Fam: REDUVIIDAE | Worldwide | Painful bites, with more or less local edema and inflammation | Symptoms vary with species; may be due to Chagas' disease |
| Blister beetles (and others) | Fam: MELOIDAE Fam: STAPHYLINIDAE Fam: PAUSSIDAE | Worldwide Worldwide Worldwide | Severe blisters (from cantharidin) Delayed blistering effect Blistering from acid secretion | Symptoms result from crushing insects on skin Apply soothing lotions |
| Caterpillars (with urticating hairs and spines) | Order: LEPIDOPTERA (several families) | Worldwide | Urticaria, rash and generalized symptoms, on contact with hairs or spines | Alkaline compresses useful; supportive treatment sometimes necessary |
| Bees, wasps, certain ants | Order: HYMENOPTERA (several families) | Worldwide | Painful stings; local swelling, sometimes anaphylaxis (certain ants *bite* rather than sting) | Apply soothing lotions; administer epinephrine subcutaneously for anaphylaxis |

ever, the symptoms are extremely severe and especially if they occur in only a minority of the individuals exposed, the term is regarded as appropriate. Asthmatic symptoms, caused by the inspiration of fragments of mayfly wings, are a case in point (Table 55).

**Infestation by Insect Larvae**   Not infrequently the human body plays host to insect larvae of different types, chiefly of the order DIPTERA. This condition is termed *myiasis*, which means simply "being infested with flies." Some species, such as the Congo floor maggot, the Tumbu fly and the so-called "human bot-fly" are confirmed parasites and can live in no other way. Others, such as the flesh flies and blue-bottles, may develop either in non-living organic matter or in living tissue. A third group occasionally adapt themselves to the intestinal tract or to the genito-urinary passages, where they cause varying degrees of irritation and distress. These three types of parasitism are termed "specific," "semi-specific" and "accidental," in the order named. Very rarely the larvae of beetles (COLEOPTERA) have been recovered from man, in which case the term *canthariasis* is more appropriate. The term *scholeciasis*, is applied to the presence of lepidopterous larvae in the human intestinal tract.

**Dermatoses**   Closely related to the irritation caused by insect bites are various skin conditions due either to this cause or to the actual presence of arthropods in the skin, as in the case of infestation by *Sarcoptes scabiei* (Linn.), the well known itch mite of man.

Although a transient dermatitis may be evident in connection with the bite of one (or a few) blood-sucking insects, a persistent dermatosis is usually the result of attack by large numbers over a considerable period of time. This is particularly true in *pediculosis*, caused by prolonged harboring of the human louse, *Pediculus humanus* Linn.

Specific types of dermatosis are described in detail in connection with the discussion of particular species groups. Species and groups already listed under Envenomization (Including Allergies), Table 55, are not repeated in Table 56.

## Structure, Classification and Biology of Medically Important Arthropods

*Characterization*   The Phylum ARTHROPODA is the most highly evolved of all invertebrate groups. Its members are characterized by a chitinous exoskeleton, a more or less marked segmentation of the body both externally and internally, and the presence of several pairs of jointed appendages. In such a vast group (well over half a million described species) it is not surprising that some forms fail to manifest all the characteristics listed. Thus body segmentation is not evident in the ticks, while certain larval forms, such as the maggots of flies, have no appendages at all. Their life histories, however, furnish ample evidence for their inclusion with the rest.

The five medically important classes will be discussed in turn.

*Table 56  Dermatoses of Arthropod Origin*

| COMMON NAME OF ARTHROPOD | SCIENTIFIC NAME (OR GROUP) | DISTRIBUTION | EFFECTS ON MAN | REMARKS |
|---|---|---|---|---|
| Itch Mites (scabies) | *Sarcoptes scabiei* | Worldwide | Burrows in skin, causing chronic dermatosis (acariasis) | Transmitted by direct contact or by clothing, bedding. Eurax cream, Kwell ointment. |
| Hard Ticks | *Amblyomma* spp. *Hyalomma* spp. *Haemaphysalis leachi* | Widespread South Africa South Africa | Cause extreme annoyance | Protective clothing helpful. DDT effective against larval forms. Vectors of certain rickettsial diseases |
| Springtails | Order: COLLEMBOLA (Several species) | Worldwide | Sharp bites, followed by pruritus | Ordinarily phytophagous. Introduced into houses (and hospitals) on garden vegetables and flowers |
| Lice: | | | | |
| Head lice | *Pediculus humanus* var. *capitis* | Worldwide | Hair becomes matted, with fetid odor | Delousing spray or powders (DDT, lindane, etc.) see p. 749. Body louse vector of epidemic typhus, relapsing fever and trench fever |
| Body lice | *P. humanus* var. *corporis* | Worldwide | Reddish papules; pruritus, followed by induration and pigmentation | |
| Pubic lice | *Phthirus pubis* | Worldwide | Intense irritation; attacks not necessarily limited to pubic region | |
| Bedbugs | *Cimex lectularius* *Cimex hemipterus* *Cimex* (*Leptocimex*) *boueti* | Worldwide Tropical and subtropical South America, Africa, New Guinea | Periodic blood-suckers; some persons suffer from bites, others immune to attack | No proved role in disease transmission; (mechanical vectors under experimental conditions) |
| Fleas: | | | | |
| Human flea | *Pulex irritans* | Worldwide | Marked dermatitis frequent | Apply soothing lotions. Vectors of important disease agents. Avoid contact |
| Dog flea | *Ctenocephalides canis* | Worldwide | Marked dermatitis frequent | |
| Cat flea | *Ctenocephalides felis* | Worldwide | Marked dermatitis frequent | |
| Tropical rat flea | *Xenopsylla cheopis* | Spreading from topics | Marked dermatitis frequent | |
| Other rodent fleas | *Xenopsylla* spp. | Widespread | Marked dermatitis frequent | |
| Chigoe flea (jigger) | *Tunga penetrans* | Tropical Africa and America | Burrows in skin; introduces tetanus, gas gangrene, other organisms | Remove flea aseptically. Dilute lysol bath before and after removal recommended |
| Flies (all types): | | | | |
| Punkies | *Culicoides* spp. | Worldwide | Nodular, inflamed swelling, becoming vesicular | Attack in daytime; fierce biters. Transmit certain helminth infections |
| Black flies | *Simulium* spp. | Worldwide | Hemorrhagic punctures: pain, swelling, general discomfort | Vectors of onchocerciasis |
| Sandflies | *Phlebotomus* spp. | Widespread in warmer regions of the world | Stinging bite, followed by itching; whitish wheals | Night biters. Prefer ankles, wrists. Vectors of several diseases |
| Mosquitoes | Family: CULICIDAE | Worldwide | Swelling, itching, annoyance, according to susceptibility of individual | Over 1500 species, of various biting habits. Vectors of several diseases |
| Horse and deer flies | Family: TABANIDAE (*Tabanus, Chrysops*) | World wide | Painful bite; no poisonous after effects | Daytime biters. Vectors of loiasis, tularemia |
| Snipe flies | Family: RHAGIONIDAE | Europe, Australia, the Americas | Painful bite; no poisonous after effects | Daytime biters; few species attack man. Not vectors of disease |
| Stable flies (dog flies) | *Stomoxys calcitrans* | Worldwide | Painful bite; no poisonous after effects | Fills to capacity in 3–4 minutes. May be mechanical vector of disease |
| | *Stomoxys* spp. (3) | Africa | Painful bite; no poisonous after effects | (As above) |
| Tsetse flies | *Glossina* spp. | Africa | Painful bite; no poisonous after effects | Cyclical vectors of various trypanosomes of man and animals |

### Class Crustacea

The members of this large group of aquatic arthropods are familiarly known as crabs, crayfish, lobsters, shrimps, prawns, etc. All species breathe by true gills and are characterized by the presence of two pairs of antennae and at least five pairs of legs. The openings of their reproductive organs are usually far forward on the body (Fig. 283).

**Subclass Copepoda**   These are small, elongate, distinctly segmented forms, with paired biramous appendages, six on the head and five on the anterior trunk region.

Two important parasites of man, *Diphyllobothrium latum* (broad tapeworm and *Dracunculus medinensis* (guinea worm), pass a portion of their life cycle in copepods, notably species of *Cyclops* and *Diaptomus*, which acquire infection by swallowing microscopic stages of the parasites.

**Subclass Malacostraca**   These are the larger CRUSTACEA. The better known forms fall in the Order DECAPODA, certain species of which act as intermediate hosts for *Paragonimus westermani* (Kerbert), the lung fluke of man. Species of marine crabs which migrate up fresh-water streams, and less frequently fresh-water crayfish, are natural hosts in Korea and Japan while various fresh-water crabs serve in a similar capacity in other areas.

### Class Arachnida

This group, which includes the spiders, scorpions, ticks and mites, is of great medical importance. Because of the many diseases capable of transmission by arachnids (especially the ticks) this class will be treated separately on pp. 655–682.

### Class Pentastomida (Linguatulida)

This group is treated by some authors as an order of the Class ARACHNIDA; by others they have been included in the Order ACARINA (ticks and mites). Modern usage, however, regards them as constituting a distinct class of arthropods. They are degenerate, wormlike parasites, with neither circulatory nor respiratory organs. The adults possess two pairs of hooks near the mouth; otherwise they are without appendages. Their larvae, however, bear two pairs of very short legs (Fig. 283).

As a rule the adults live in the respiratory passages of carnivorous reptiles, birds and mammals, the eggs being discharged in the sputum or nasal mucus. The intermediate host, usually an herbivore, takes up the eggs in food or water. The larvae emerge in the intestine, migrate to the liver, spleen, lymph nodes or lungs and there become encapsulated. From the nature of the life cycle it is evident that man is more likely to function as the intermediate than as the definitive host. At least four species have been recorded from human tissue.

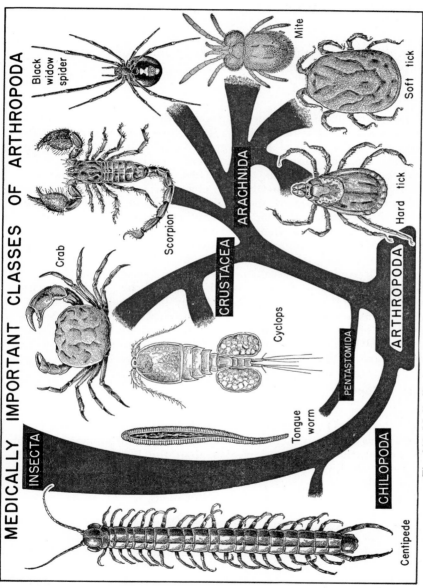

Fig. 283. Medically important classes of ARTHROPODA—selected examples.

*Armillifer* (*Porocephalus*) *armillatus* is a relatively common human parasite in Africa. *Armillifer moniliformis* has been recorded from China, Sumatra and Manila. *Linguatula serrata* Frölich has been taken from man in Africa, Panama, Germany, Switzerland, United States (Texas) and Brazil. *Pentastoma najae* has been recovered from man at least once in India. Infection with pentastomids has been termed *linguatulosis* or *porocephaliasis*, depending on the genus of parasite involved. Pulmonary infection by linguatulids may lead to symptoms suggestive of tuberculosis.

### Class Chilopoda

The centipedes are elongate arthropods with a conspicuous pair of legs on each segment of the body. They have poison glands in the claws of the first pair of leglike appendages, and by injecting this material into their prey (insects and other small animals) cause immediate paralysis or death. Only a few, however, have jaws sufficiently strong to penetrate the skin of man. Two American species, *Scolopendra heros* Girard and *S. morsitans* Linn., are large forms (4 to 6 inches in length) capable of inflicting painful bites. Certain tropical species, among them the 10 inch *Scolopendra gigantea*, are reputed to be very poisonous, but positive record of death from centipede bite is lacking. Hospitalization for a period of two to five days, however, is sometimes necessary. Persons are bitten usually in bed or when putting on clothing in which centipedes have hidden during the night. When pinched or impeded they bite in self-defense.

**Symptoms and Treatment** There are usually local, necrotic lesions at the site of the two punctures, and the patient may suffer headache, fever, vomiting and sometimes coma. Sedatives should be given to relieve the pain. Dilute ammonia, applied locally, is recommended also.

### Class Diplopoda

Millipedes, sometimes confused with centipedes, belong to a distinct class, the DIPLOPODA. They are characterized by the presence of *two* pairs of legs on each apparent segment, and in every case these legs are much smaller and weaker than the locomotor organs of centipedes. Millipedes cannot bite man and are usually regarded as of no medical importance, though some collectors report irritation of the skin from handling the living specimens.

### Class Insecta (Hexapoda)

The vast majority of arthropod-borne diseases are insect-borne. This is not strange when one considers that the Class INSECTA alone is vastly larger than all the other classes put together and that there are few places on the earth's surface where man is not in constant and intimate association with insect forms. For information concerning the medically important groups, see pp. 683–793.

# 70  The Class Arachnida

The ARACHNIDA constitute one of the more important classes of arthropods. Typical forms have the ·head and thorax fused together, forming a cephalothorax. Adults normally possess four pairs of legs. The class includes at least nine distinct orders, but only three, the SCORPIONIDA, ARANEIDA and ACARINA, are of medical importance. These will be discussed in turn.

## The Order Scorpionida (Scorpions)

Scorpions are found largely in the warmer regions of the world. They have exceedingly large *pedipalps*, furnished with stout pinching claws. The cephalothorax is compact but the abdomen is conspicuously segmented. The anterior portion of the abdomen is broad, while the posterior five segments are much narrowed, forming a conspicuous tail at the tip of which is a bulb-like enlargement, bearing the poisonous sting. It is this sting, and not the anterior claws, which is dangerous to man. Some species carry the tail over the back in a threatening attitude as they run about; in others, it merely drags along behind. Over 300 species are known, but only a limited number inject sufficient poison to make their stings a matter of concern (Fig. 283).

*Centruroides sufusus* Pocock is credited with having caused the death of some 1600 persons, mostly children, in the State of Durango, Mexico, over a period of thirty-six years. At least four other species of the same genus are regarded as capable of inflicting fatal stings. One hundred forty-five deaths are reported from 1328 stings (mostly children) in Bello Horizonte, Brazil, *Tityus serratulus* being probably the chief offender. The Egyptian species, *Buthus quinquestriatus* Hemprich and Ehrenberg, is exceedingly dangerous, the mortality rate among children under five being nearly 60 per cent. Dangerous species exist in Trinidad, North Africa, India, Palestine, Manchuria and the Malayan region. Tropical forms sometimes attain a length of seven or eight inches, but it is not always the largest species which are most poisonous.

**Habits and Life History**  Scorpions are nocturnal, feeding on spiders and larger insects which they seize with their claws (pedipalps) and sting to death. During the day they lie hidden beneath débris of all kinds such as loose stones or bits of bark, as well as under buildings and lumber piles. Those which invade houses may hide in shoes or clothing, as day approaches. The sexes are similar in appearance but the males have somewhat larger pedipalps and longer tails.

**Symptoms**  The patient is first conscious of a burning pain, after which there are excessive salivation, drowsiness, nausea and vomiting with profuse sweating. The tongue is sluggish and the muscles

**655**

of the jaw are contracted. Speech may be impossible and the giving of medicines is difficult. The temperature rises to 104° or 104.8° F., the patient is very sensitive to light, and there may be hemorrhages into the stomach, intestine or lungs. There is dyspnea, but never cyanosis. Reflexes become exaggerated and sometimes conspicuous strabismus or even convulsions may ensue. Oliguria is frequently observed. If the patient survives three hours the prognosis is good, though there is record of death as late as the fifteenth day. The poison acts on the nervous system and kills by its effect on the cardiac and respiratory centers. Pulmonary edema may be present.

**Treatment**   A tight ligature should be applied proximal to the sting and an incision made at the site, suction being applied to remove the venom. Sedatives should be given to induce sleep. A drop of strong ammonia, locally applied, is also helpful in relieving pain. Standardized antivenin may be given intravenously, subcutaneously or intraspinally. Intravenous glucose (10 per cent) followed by insulin is recommended as supportive treatment. Epinephrine is also useful. Artificial respiration may be required.

**Control**   General extermination of scorpions is impracticable, but they may be destroyed in houses by sulfur fumigation. New buildings should be so constructed as to make their ingress impossible or rare. The removal of ivy from walls has been advocated as a control measure, since the vines furnish excellent hiding places for scorpions (Brazil). Poultry are valuable allies in destroying scorpions about yards and wood piles, as they seem unaffected by the venom and relish the scorpions as food.

**Whip Scorpions**   "Whip scorpions" belong to the PEDIPALPIDA. They are distinguished by the slender, whip-like character of the first pair of legs, also (in certain species) by the presence of a slender whip-like appendage on the last abdominal segment. Whip scorpions have no sting, but depend for defense upon the secretion of a repellent fluid which has the odor of vinegar and which is responsible for the common name "vinegerone." This secretion may be irritating to sensitive skin; otherwise, they are quite harmless, in spite of widespread opinion to the contrary.

## The Order Araneida (*Spiders*)

There are more than two thousand genera of spiders distributed within some thirty families. Typical spiders bear up to eight eyes on the cephalothorax, which is joined to the abdomen by a rather slender pedicle. The abdomen is unsegmented. The *chelicerae* or jaws each contain a poison gland which opens near the tip of the second (distal) segment. Pedipalps, of six segments, precede the four pair of legs and may give the impression that five pairs of legs are present. Pedipalps of male spiders function in the transfer of spermatozoa to the female at the time of mating. A spider's "silk" is produced from three or four pairs of spinnerets, located near the tip of the abdomen on the ventral side.

Only a few species are actually dangerous to man. Medical interest centers in two groups, termed respectively *tarantulas* and *black widows,* which may be distinguished as follows.

## Tarantula Group

The term "tarantula," as employed in Europe, relates specifically to *Lycosa tarentula* (Family Lycosidae). The bites of Lycosidae, however, are not very serious. They have never been shown to cause death in man and, with the exception of a few American species, cause no great discomfort. The Russian tarantula, *Trochosa singoriensis,* is much feared, but the fear is probably without foundation.

In America the term "tarantula" is loosely used for any of the larger hairy spiders, most of which fall in the superfamily Avicularoidea. They are found in Central and South America as well as in the southern and southwestern United States. They may be distinguished from all other spiders by the fact that their *chelicerae* (jaws) are paraxial, that is, they both extend forward and operate vertically, with a downward stroke, rather than against one another from opposite sides (diaxial articulation). Members of the genus *Eurypelma* are typical. With their heavy bodies and leg spread of five or more inches they excite much apprehension, but the effect of their bite is trivial. *Sericopelma communis,* the "black tarantula" of Panama, is probably the most venomous of the group.

Sometimes confused with these American tarantulas are certain large spiders (Family Heteropodidae) found frequently in shipments of tropical fruit, particularly bananas. They may be recognized by their smoother bodies, longer legs and diaxial jaws. *Heteropoda venatoria* Koch is the species most commonly seen. Its bite is painful but not serious.

## Black Widow Group

Of much greater importance than the three foregoing families is the family Theridiidae. This group includes a number of rather small, dark spiders falling in the genus *Latrodectus,* the bites of which are extremely poisonous and sometimes fatal. Best known is the American species *Latrodectus mactans* (Fabricius), which is widely distributed from southern Canada to parts of Chile and Peru.

**Recognition Characters** (Fig. 283)  The female black widow is of a shining black color above, with certain reddish markings on the under side of the abdomen. The largest of these is usually shaped like an hour-glass and is directly ventral. The other spot (or spots) occur almost at the tip of the abdomen in the vicinity of the spinnerets. The abdomen itself is nearly spherical and has been likened to a shoebutton. The hind tarsus bears a comb of spines.

Male specimens, also the young of both sexes, usually have irregular yellowish markings on the upper surface. Females grow to about half an inch in length, not including the legs. The males are somewhat smaller.

**Habits and Life History**  Black widows are found largely in cellars, privies, manholes, culverts, or under rocks, bridges or hollow logs. Here they spin a loosely woven, irregular web in which insects and other small prey are captured. After mating, the female lays some three or four hundred eggs, enclosed in a dense ball of silk nearly three-eighths of an inch across. (The name "black widow" is derived from the fact that the males are frequently devoured by their mates after mating). The young spiders hatch in three or four weeks and scatter over the web. At first they are of a light tan color, but become darker with succeeding molts. A single female may construct as many as nine successive egg sacs, though the fertility of the latter batches may be somewhat reduced, due to exhaustion of sperm. Spiders hatching in midsummer may complete their development the same season, but hibernation in all stages is not uncommon. The males pass through five instars, the females seven or eight.

The males seldom or never bite and it would not be important if they did so, as extracts prepared from mature males have been found less than one-fortieth as poisonous as those prepared from females. Female venom, on the other hand, has been shown to be fifteen times as potent, on a dry weight basis, as that of *Crotalus albicans,* the prairie rattlesnake. It differs chemically from snake venom, however, being neither an alkaloid nor a glucoside, but a toxalbumen.

Black widow spiders ordinarily bite only legitimate prey, but when frightened or injured, strike in self-defense. A female, guarding her egg sac, is particularly vicious and since the under side of privy seats is a favorite location for egg laying, it follows that a majority of recorded bites are received in outhouses and latrines, the male genital organs being the parts most commonly attacked.

**Symptoms of Spider Poisoning (Arachnidism)**  The spider bite itself is not always felt, or if so, is no more painful than a pin prick. Two tiny red spots usually appear and there may be some local swelling, but the more serious symptoms are general in character. Within ten minutes there is usually cramping pain, the distress involving successively the abdomen, legs, chest and back. At the end of an hour the patient may be writhing in agony. All of the larger muscle groups show marked rigidity, the condition being especially marked in the muscles of the abdominal wall. In cases in which an incision has been made the intestine has been found to be extremely contracted and spastic. (This may result in paralytic ileus.) Acute symptoms persist from twelve to forty-eight hours. These include elevation of temperature and blood pressure, as well as increased spinal fluid pressure. There is a definite leukocytosis. Nausea, excessive perspiration and respiratory embarrassment are common. There may be chills, hyperactive reflexes, priapism and sometimes a macular rash. Numbness and tingling of the feet may persist for some days after recovery. It is reported that 4 per cent of the typical cases result fatally. When the bites are on the extremities, however, symptoms are usually less severe.

The Russian species, *Latrodectus lugubris*, also called "kara-kurt" or "black wolf," is quite as dangerous as the American species. Other members of the genus occur in southern Europe, Australia, New Zealand, the Philippines, Madagascar, South and West Africa and Brazil.

An altogether different spider, *Glyptocranium gasteracanthoides* Nicolet, an orb-weaver falling in the Family ARGIOPIDAE, is regarded in Peru as particularly venomous.

**Treatment** The use of opiates to relieve pain, also hydrotherapy in the form of hot baths or hot packs, are desirable procedures. Intramuscular injections of standardized antivenin is the preferred treatment, but is not always practicable, as spider antivenins are strictly specific and the preparation at hand may not be suitable for the species concerned. Intravenous administration of 10 ml. of 10 per cent calcium gluconate is the best supportive treatment. Spinal puncture and intravenous injection of 10 per cent magnesium sulfate (20 ml.) have also been recommended. Intramuscular injection of convalescent serum has not given consistent results.

In the case of bites on the extremities, a tourniquet may be applied above the site and, following incision, the venom extracted by means of a mammary pump.

**Prophylaxis** There is experimental evidence in relation to the *Latrodectus* of Russia, which indicates that repeated injections of nonfatal doses of spider venom may confer immunity to the bites.

All persons, and especially children, should be warned against the habits of these spiders, and should exercise care when visiting privies or handling old lumber.

**Control** Ordinary sprays do not kill black widow spiders. Creosote, however, is an effective repellent and may be sprayed under toilet seats and into corners of basements and outbuildings with good effect. Egg sacs and webs may be brushed down with a broom and either crushed or burned. Blow torches should be used only in situations where the fire risk is minimal. The wearing of gloves by persons working in the vicinity of spiders is desirable.

Natural enemies ordinarily keep this species from becoming extremely abundant. The blue mud-dauber wasp, *Chalybion cyaneum* (Klug), frequently provisions its nest with black widows. There are also forms which prey on the eggs, such as the larvae of *Baeus latrodecti* Dozier, a species of wasp, and also the larvae of a small fly, *Pseudogaurax signata* (Loew). The successful introduction of a California species of *Baeus* into Maui (Hawaiian Islands) to assist in the control of black widows was accomplished in 1940.

**Jointed Spiders** The "jointed spiders," also called "sun spiders" or "wind scorpions," fall into the SOLPUGIDA. They differ from true

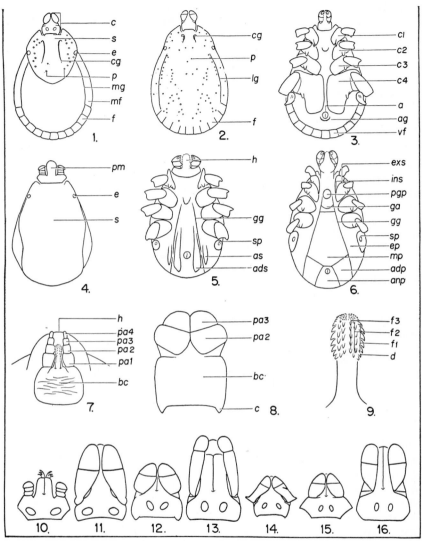

Fig. 284. Morphology of adult ticks. 1. *Dermacentor* female, dorsal view: *c*, capitulum; *cg*, cervical groove; *e*, eye; *f*, festoon; *mf*, marginal fold; *mg*, marginal groove; *p*, punctations; *s*, scutum. 2. *Dermacentor* male, dorsal view: *cg*, cervical groove; *f*, festoon; *lg*, lateral groove, *p*, punctation. 3. *Dermacentor* male, ventral view: *a*, anus, *ag*, anal groove; *c1*, coxa I (bifid); *c2*, coxa II; *c3*, coxa III; *c4*, coxa IV; *vf*, ventral festoon. 4. *Boophilus* male, dorsal view: *e*, eye; *pm*, piercing mouth parts; *s*, scutum. 5. *Boophilus* male, ventral view: *as*, accessory shield; *ads*, adanal shield; *gg*, genital groove; *h*, hypostome; *sp*, spiracular plate. 6. *Ixodes* male, ventral view: *adp*, adanal plate; *anp*, anal plate; *ep*, epimeral plate; *exs*, external spur on coxa I; *ga*, genital aperture; *gg*, genital groove; *ins*, internal spur; *mp*, median plate; *pgp*, pre-genital plate; *sp*, spiracular plate. 7. *Ornithodoros* (ARGASIDAE), ventral view: *bc*, basis capituli; *h*, hood; *pa1*, palpal article 1; *pa2*, palpal article 2; *pa3*, palpal article 3;

spiders in having the abdomen segmented and more broadly joined to the cephalothorax. Their chelicerae, which are two-segmented, are large, powerful, and capable of inflicting a painful bite, but the effect is transitory, as no poison glands are present. Because of the depth of penetration, the possibility of secondary infection, however, should not be overlooked. The group occurs largely in desert, tropical and subtropical regions. Solpugids are chiefly nocturnal.

## The Order Acarina *(Ticks and Mites)*

Members of this order can, as a rule, be readily distinguished from other ARACHNIDA as well as from insects by the general absence of body segmentation. A head is lacking and, with the exception of some adult mites, there is a strong fusion of thorax and abdomen with no external sign of demarcation. Wings or antennae are never present. As with spiders and scorpions, the adults have four pairs of legs, but the larvae have only three pairs (exceptionally less in some mites). The two major groups can be best discussed separately.

### The Superfamily Ixodoidea *(Ticks)*

The ticks are further characterized in general as follows. Eyes, when present, are simple. The mouth parts consist of a pair of dorsal cutting organs, the *chelicerae;* a ventral, characteristically toothed *hypostome* for anchoring the tick to its host; and paired *palpi* lateral to the mouth. The mouth consists of a chitinous ring lying at the base of, and between, the chelicerae and the hypostome.

The superfamily IXODOIDEA is ordinarily divided into two family groups, the ARGASIDAE and the IXODIDAE. These may be separated on the basis of a single structure, the *scutum,* which is lacking in the ARGASIDAE in all stages ("soft ticks") and present in the IXODIDAE in all stages ("hard ticks"). In the ixodid female, the scutum covers only the anterior part of the dorsal surface; in the male it covers most of the dorsal surface. The two groups are further characterized by ventral mouth parts and only slight sexual dimorphism in the argasid ticks; and by mouth parts that project in front of the body when viewed dorsally, and marked sexual dimorphism in the ixodid ticks. (Fig. 284.)

A third family, the NUTTALLIELLIDAE, is represented by the single, rare, African species *Nuttalliella namaqua* Bedford. The species is morphologically intermediate between the argasid and the ixodid ticks and is of no known medical importance.

**The Family Ixodidae *(Hard Ticks)*** Numerous species of ixodid

*pa4,* palpal article 4. 8. *Dermacentor* male, dorsal view: *bc,* basis capituli; *c,* cornu; *pa2,* palpal article 2; *pa3,* palpal article 3. 9. Hypostome of *Amblyomma: f1,* file 1; *f2,* file 2; *f3,* file 3; *d,* a single denticle. 10 to 16. Typical Capitula (IXODIDAE) females, dorsal view: 10. *Boophilus;* 11. *Ixodes;* 12. *Dermacentor;* 13. *Amblyomma;* 14. *Haemaphysalis;* 15. *Rhipicephalus;* 16. *Hyalomma.* (Courtesy Dr. R. A. Cooley, Rocky Mountain Laboratory, U.S.P.H.S.)

ticks are of the greatest medical importance as reservoirs or vectors of agents of disease which affect man and the lower animals. Among the agents transmitted to man are rickettsiae, viruses, bacteria, and others the nature of which is unknown. The rickettsial diseases of man comprise American spotted fever, fièvre boutonneuse (including Kenya typhus, South African tick-bite fever, and Indian tick typhus, which are probably identical), Siberian tick typhus, North Queensland tick typhus, and Q fever. Colorado tick fever and Russian spring-summer encephalitis are caused by viruses, and tularemia is a bacterial disease. The agents of Bullis fever, a disease which as yet is not definitely known to be tick-borne, and of tick paralysis have not been discovered but the latter disease is believed to be caused by a toxin. Methods of transmission include tick bite and contact of tick feces or crushed tick tissues with the skin. The tick-borne diseases of animals are numerous and result in vast economic losses; moreover, heavy infestation may result in severe anemia or death, even in large animals, from blood loss alone.

**Life History** All species of ixodid ticks pass through four stages, viz., egg, larva, nymph and adult. The eggs are deposited on the ground where after varying lengths of time they hatch, giving rise to hexapod (six-legged) larvae which soon seek a blood meal. Some species show marked host specificity while others use a wide variety of hosts. In multiple-host ticks the engorged larvae drop from the host after several days of feeding, and seek a cool place where they remain until molting takes place. The resulting octopod (eight-legged) nymphs then feed on a second host, again drop to the ground and await molting. The ticks emerge from this second molt as adults, males and females. An interval of a week to ten days is required for engorgement of the female, during which time mating takes place. This life cycle normally requires from a few weeks to two or more years, according to the species and host availability. The number of eggs also varies greatly. A maximum of 18,497 has been recorded for a single *Amblyomma maculatum*. After egg laying is completed the female dies.

Some ixodid ticks, e.g., the southern cattle tick, *Boophilus annulatus* (Say), does not drop from the host between feedings. Such ticks are designated as one-host ticks.

The family IXODIDAE consists of at least ten well-defined genera composed of over three hundred species. Five genera are of especial importance to man. These are *Dermacentor*, *Amblyomma*, *Rhipicephalus*, *Haemaphysalis* and *Ixodes*. Species of the genus *Amblyomma* are chiefly tropical or subtropical in their distribution. The other genera have representatives that are worldwide or nearly so in their range.

GENUS *Dermacentor*. These are usually ornate ticks with eyes, festoons, and short palpi. There are about 20 species. *Dermacentor andersoni* Stiles is widely distributed in southern British Columbia, Alberta, and southwestern Saskatchewan, throughout the Rocky Mountain States and southward into northern Arizona and northern New Mexico. The larvae and nymphs feed on small animals such as ground squirrels, pine squirrels, chipmunks, woodchucks, and various kinds of mice, while the adults feed on larger animals including man. This species transmits Rocky Mountain spotted fever, tularemia, and Colorado tick fever, and is a suspected vector of Q fever; it also causes tick paralysis. *Dermacentor variabilis* (Say) is found in the States east of the Rocky Mountains, including eastern Texas, and occurs also near the west coast of California and Oregon. This species is found frequently in wooded areas and along streams. In the eastern States, mice are the principal hosts of the larvae and nymphs; in Iowa cottontails are also reported as important hosts. The adults are frequently found on dogs. This tick is a vector of Rocky Mountain spotted fever and tularemia and it causes tick paralysis. Colorado tick fever virus has been reported in ticks of this species collected on Long Island, New York. *Dermacentor occidentalis* Neum., the Pacific coast tick, occurs chiefly in California and extends north into Oregon. It has a wide variety of hosts. Stage-to-stage and generation-to-generation transmission of spotted fever rickettsiae has been shown experimentally. It is probably a natural vector of spotted fever and tularemia.

Genus *Amblyomma*. Ticks of this genus are also usually ornate, with eyes and with festoons. The palpi are long and thin with article (segment) 2 especially long. These ticks are widely distributed in the tropics and subtropics. There are about ninety described species, twenty of which are reported from Panama. *Amblyomma americanum* (Linn.), the Lone Star tick, is found from central Texas eastward to the coast and southward to South America. It has a wide range of hosts and bites man in all stages. Its bite is painful and is often followed by suppurating sores. It is a vector of Rocky Mountain spotted fever and tularemia and it has been suspected of causing tick paralysis. Wild-caught ticks have produced Q fever in guinea pigs. In Texas this tick has been suspected as a vector of a clinical syndrome termed Bullis fever. *Amblyomma cajennense* (Fabr.) occurs in extreme southern Texas, Mexico, and in Central and South America. Its bite is severe and is frequently followed by sores that heal with difficulty. It is a proved vector of spotted fever in Colombia and Brazil and has been found spontaneously infected with the rickettsiae of this disease in Mexico where it can be considered as a probable vector.

Genus *Rhipicephalus*. Ticks of this genus are usually inornate, with eyes and festoons. In the commoner species the *basis capituli* is hexagonal dorsally. There are about forty species. *Rhipicephalus sanguineus* (Latr.), the cosmopolitan brown dog tick, has as its principal host the dog although it feeds on many other animals including man. It is widely distributed around the world in the tropics and subtropics, and in cooler climates it sometimes becomes established in kennels and in houses where dogs are kept as pets.

This tick is a vector of spotted fever in Mexico and of fièvre bouton-neuse in the Mediterranean region and in Africa. It has also been found spontaneously infected with the etiologic agents of Indian tick typhus in northern India and of Q fever in the United States.

GENUS *Haemaphysalis*. This is a genus of small, inornate and eye-less ticks. Festoons are present. The second article of the short palpi projects laterally forming an acute angle. *Haemaphysalis leporis-palustris* (Packard), commonly known as the rabbit tick, is some-times found on domestic animals and the immature forms have been reported from nearly sixty species of ground-frequenting birds. Four hundred ninety-five ticks were recovered from one brown thrasher, *Toxostoma rufum*. This suggests a possible wide dissemination by such birds. This tick very rarely bites man; however, it serves as an important vector of Rocky Mountain spotted fever and tularemia among rabbits, which in turn are hosts to *D. andersoni* and *D. variabilis*, vectors to man. The species has been found naturally in-fected with Q fever rickettsiae in Virginia. *Pasteurella tularensis* has been recovered from *Haemaphysalis chordeilis* (Packard) col-lected from the sage hen, *Centrocercus urophasianus*. *Haemaphysalis leachi* (Audouin), a dog tick of Africa, is considered a vector of South African tick-bite fever. *H. humerosa* is a vector of Q fever among bandicoots in Australia and *H. bispinosa* is reported as a po-tential vector in the Q fever cycle in that country.

GENUS *Ixodes*. Ticks of this genus are eyeless and without fes-toons. The palpi may be long or short but when closed do not form a cone as in the genus *Haemaphysalis*. There are more than fifty species. Distribution is worldwide. *Ixodes pacificus* Cooley and Kohls has been found naturally infected with *P. tularensis* in Oregon. This tick bites man freely and the mouth parts are sometimes left in the skin when the tick is removed. Severe reactions may follow. Several species cause tick paralysis; among these are: *I. holocyclus* Neum. in Australia; *I. persulcatus*, which is both a reservoir and vector of Russian spring-summer encephalitis; *I. ricinus* (Linn.), the Euro-pean castor bean tick, which is a vector of the virus disease, louping ill, in sheep in southern Scotland. This virus is infectious for man and very similar to the virus of Russian spring-summer encephalitis.

**Control**   Various methods of control have been attempted with definite gains in local areas. Repeated dipping of cattle and grazing control have been highly successful. Some of the newer insecticides such as DDT, chlordane, toxaphene, and benzene hexachloride, are effective in controlling ticks on pets and livestock, or on vegetation along trails and roadsides where ticks concentrate. Where feasible, the elimination of small animals which serve as hosts of the im-mature stages of ticks results in a temporary reduction in the tick population.

Heavily infested areas should be avoided, when possible, in the spring and early summer months. High boots or leggings afford considerable protection. At any rate the body should be carefully examined at least once and preferably twice a day. Special attention should be given to the perineal region, for some species of ticks produce no sensation while feeding and not infrequently ticks nearly engorged have been found on individuals of cleanly habits. Clothing dipped in M-1960, a 9.1 per cent water emulsion of repellent consisting of 30 parts benzyl benzoate; 30 parts *n*-butyl acetanilide; 30 parts of 2-butyl-2-ethyl-1,3-propanediol; plus 10 parts of an emulsifier protects individuals from ticks. Clothing so treated also protects against fleas and chiggers and helps prevent annoyance by mosquitoes.

**The Family Argasidae (Soft Ticks)** This family consists of four genera, viz., *Argas, Otobius, Antricola* and *Ornithodoros.*

Ticks of the genus *Argas* have the margin of the body distinctly flattened and the structure of the marginal integument differs from that of the rest of the body; a definite *sutural line* which separates the dorsal and ventral surfaces is usually present. *Argas persicus* (Oken), a widely distributed species, is a common vector of fowl spirochetosis and occasionally feeds on man. Some other species which are reported to bite man are *Argas brumpti* Neumann, *A. reflexus* (Fabr.), and *A. mianensis* Brumpt. The last species is believed to be a vector of a spirochete causing Mianeh fever, a form of relapsing fever of man in Iran. However, since *Ornithodoros tholozani* is a known vector of relapsing fever in this area, it seems possible that cases of relapsing fever ascribed to *A. mianensis* are actually attributable to *O. tholozani.*

The genus *Antricola* has recently been erected for two species associated with bats, viz., *A. coprophilus* (McIntosh), from Arizona and Mexico and *A. marginatus* (Banks) from Cuba. These ticks have a scoop-like hypostome.

The genus *Otobius* also contains two species, viz., *O. megnini* (Dugès), the widely distributed spinose ear tick of cattle and other domestic animals and certain wild ruminants, and *O. lagophilus* Cooley and Kohls, which is parasitic on rabbits in the western United States and southern Alberta. Both species are marked by a spinose integument in the developmental stages and by vestigial mouth parts in the adults. The adults do not feed but the nymphs may remain attached in the ear for several months. *Otobius megnini* is occasionally found in the ear of man.

The genus *Ornithodoros* is by far the largest and most important of the four genera. According to recent classifications it contains at least forty-six species. Few genera of arthropods contain a larger number of species parasitic on man. At least twelve species are known vectors of relapsing fever and others are under suspicion on epidemiological grounds. Some species inflict severe bites. Although members of the genus are found in many parts of both the eastern and the western hemispheres, some species are known only locally. For example, *O. parkeri* has been found only in the western United States, *O. hermsi* in western United States and southern British Columbia, and *O. gurneyi* is known only from Australia. Other species have a much more general distribution; for example *O. savignyi* is reported from many parts of Africa and from Arabia and India.

Ticks of the genus *Ornithodoros* are more or less flattened, the degree depending on the amount of feeding. In contrast with the genus *Argas*, only a very few species are marginated and the sutural line separating the dorsal and ventral surfaces is absent. Spines, characteristic of the developmental forms of *Otobius*, are never present. The hypostomes are of various shapes but never vestigial as in the adults of *Otobius* or scooplike as in *Antricola*.

Much detailed information is available concerning some species but of others almost none. *Ornithodoros eremicus* Cooley and Kohls is known only by a nymph from the deer mouse, *Peromyscus maniculatus*, taken in southern Utah, and *O. cooleyi* McIvor by a female recovered from a shipment of pelts from southern Nevada. *Ornithodoros nattereri* Warburton was described in 1927 from specimens in the Vienna Museum, collected in Brazil more than 100 years previously.

Biologically, ticks of the genus, thus far studied, are characterized by rapid feeding (exceptions in the larval stage of some species), multiple nymphal stages and longevity. They feed on both warm- and cold-blooded animals. As a rule, a complete blood meal is necessary prior to each molt but in some species both larval and first nymphal "skins" are shed after the larval feeding without an additional blood meal. This phenomenon occurs only in species the larvae of which require several days to engorge. Thus far, it has been observed in *O. talaje* (Guérin-Meneville), *O. coriaceus* Koch and in several of the species parasitic on bats. The larvae of *O. moubata* (Murray) do not feed but molt to the first nymphal stage a few hours after hatching. *Ornithodoros delanoei acinus* Whittick may require several feedings between molts.

In contrast to the *one* nymphal stage which is constant in ixodid ticks, the number of nymphal stages in the argasid ticks may vary with the several species and even within the species. In *O. hermsi* a minimum of two nymphal stages and a maximum of four have been observed while in *O. coriaceus* the number varies from three to six. There is a definite tendency for males to mature earlier than females, e.g.: in *O. turicata* (Dugès) following the third nymphal molt numerous males and a few females appear; following the fourth nymphal molt a few males and many females appear, while the few remaining ticks that require a fifth nymphal molt are all females.

Oviposition has not been observed prior to copulation. However, after one mating fertile ova may be produced over a period of many months. As a rule, a blood meal is required before each oviposition but in some species, notably *O. nicollei* Mooser, there is a tendency to oviposit a second time without further feeding. The number of eggs at a single oviposition varies with the species; as few as twenty have been observed in *O. stageri* Cooley and Kohls and more than 700 in *O. rostratus* Aragão.

The size varies widely. The adult of *O. normandi* Larrousse, a Tunisian species, is only 3 mm. long while the engorged female of *O. delanoei acinus* Whittick from British Somaliland, reaches a maximum of 27 mm. With the exception of the larvae of some of the bat ticks, host specificity is not marked, e.g., *O. capensis* Neumann, normally a parasite of certain marine birds, feeds readily on man and on laboratory animals.

The tick biotopes are as varied as the host habitats. Most species tolerate low temperatures but do not withstand high temperatures and dryness. *Ornithodoros moubata* is adversely affected by excessive moisture.

Numerous species of the genus are best known as vectors of relapsing fever spirochetes (see Relapsing Fever, p. 95). Some, notably *O. parkeri* and *O. nicollei*, are very efficient experimental vectors of the American spotted fevers.

For the identification of species it is necessary to consult original papers. Pertinent information concerning some of the better known species which bite man follows.

*Ornithodoros hermsi* Wheeler, Herms and Meyer is a vector of relapsing fever in California, Colorado, Oregon, Washington, Nevada and Idaho, and probably in southern British Columbia. This species is parasitic chiefly on tree squirrels (*Tamiasciurus*) and chipmunks (*Eutamias*) which inhabit wooded areas at relatively high elevations; the ticks have been collected in large numbers from the cracks and crevices of decaying Douglas fir, *Pseudotsuga taxifolia*. Such biotopes may act as tick reservoirs, from which ticks are transported into mountain homes either by the rodent host or possibly by means of the infested wood which is, at times, used for fuel. This is the only known species whose "coxal fluid" is not fluid; it appears as a fine white crystalline deposit.

*Ornithodoros turicata* (Dugès) is a vector of relapsing fever in Texas, Kansas, Oklahoma, New Mexico and in Aguascalientes, Mexico. It is also present in Arizona, California, Colorado, Utah and Florida. It has a wider variety of hosts and habitats than either *O. hermsi* or *O. parkeri*. Among the hosts are numerous mammals, wild and domestic, as well as snakes and terrapins. It is markedly androphilic. In Texas, it has been found in great numbers in limestone caves. In Kansas, approximately 2000 specimens were collected in an abandoned pack rat's (*Neotoma*) nest inhabited by numerous terrapins, *Terrapene ornata*. In New Mexico, this species was first reported from cattle and was subsequently collected over large areas within the mounds of kangaroo rats, especially *Dipodomys spec-*

*tabilis baileyi,* and from rodent burrows beneath calcareous mounds in "borrow pits." In Oklahoma, they appeared in vast numbers in a storm cellar to which rats and mice had access. In Mexico, these ticks are reported as commonly present in chicken yards. All (100 per cent) of the progeny of a single oviposition of an infective female have been shown to transmit relapsing fever spirochetes (transovarial transmission). The larvae may infect white mice in less than one minute of feeding.

*Ornithodoros parkeri* Cooley has a quite general distribution in Nevada, Utah and California and is also present in parts of Wyoming, Colorado, Washington, Oregon, Idaho and Montana. In contrast with *O. hermsi,* this species is found in burrows in such varied type areas as grassy slopes, sagebrush prairies, and semidesert regions, from low elevations, such as the San Joaquin Valley in California, to elevations of 7000 feet on plateaus in southern Wyoming.

It has been observed most frequently in association with prairie dogs *(Cynomys).* Other natural hosts are jack rabbits *(Lepus),* cottontail rabbits *(Sylvilagus),* mice *(Peromyscus),* ground squirrels *(Citellus),* weasels *(Mustela),* and the burrowing owl, *Speotyto cunicularia.* It is a vector of relapsing fever in California, and spirochetes which produce typical relapses in experimental animals have been recovered from ticks collected in Wyoming, Montana, Utah, California, Nevada, Oregon and Idaho. *Coxiella burnetii* and *Pasteurella tularensis* survive and retain their virulence in the tissues of the tick for many months. Infection does not take place during feeding, but tick excrement is infective. *Ornithodoros parkeri* differs biologically from the closely related species, *Ornithodoros turicata* (Dugès), in that the former transmits spotted fever readily by bite. Transovarial transmission to the fourth generation has been shown experimentally in *O. parkeri.*

*Ornithodoros talaje* (Guerin-Méneville) is cosmopolitan in the tropics and sub-tropics of the Americas. It is a vector of relapsing fever in Guatemala, Panama and Colombia; relapsing fever spirochetes have been recovered from ticks collected in Arizona, Kansas and Texas. It occurs also in California, Kansas, Nevada and Florida and as far south as Argentina in South America. The larvae are common parasites of *Rattus norvegicus* in Panama; later stages are frequently found in crude beds made of bamboo. It has been recorded from numerous mammals, birds and reptiles. The larvae require several days to engorge, after which there are two successive molts without further feeding.

*Ornithodoros rudis* Karsch (=*O. venezuelensis* Brumpt) (=*O. migonei* Brumpt) is considered the most important vector of relapsing fever in Panama, Colombia, Ecuador and Venezuela, where it is often found in large numbers in primitive dwellings. It is also reported from Paraguay. Man is the only known host. This is a small species and the larvae were formerly confused with the larvae of *O.*

*talaje*. The larvae of O. *rudis* feed rapidly and molting is regular (see O. *talaje*, above).

*Ornithodoros moubata* (Murray), the eyeless tampan, is considered the most important vector of relapsing fever in Africa, where it is widely distributed from Sierre Leone, eastward (discontinuous) to the Red Sea, and southward to Cape Colony. It is also reported from northwestern Madagascar. It is found commonly in the dust of the earth floors of native huts and rest houses and feeds on man and domestic animals.

Following hatching of the eggs, the larvae remain quiescent and within a few hours molt to the first nymphal stage without feeding; in this stage they may survive for many months without a blood meal.

Some species of *Ornithodoros* transmit relapsing fever spirochetes by *bite* but the secretions of both salivary and coxal glands are media of transmission for this species. Although O. *moubata* transmits spirochetes other than *S. duttoni*, experimentally, ticks that have acquired such foreign spirochetes (e.g., from *S. hermsi*) become dwarfed and females fail to oviposit.

*Pasteurella tularensis* is transmitted, experimentally, but the infection ultimately proves fatal to the tick. Stage-to-stage and transovarial transmission of *Coxiella burnetii* have been demonstrated.

*Ornithodoros savignyi* (Audouin), the eyed tampan, has a wider distribution in Africa than O. *moubata* and is also known in the Bombay and Madras Presidencies in India. It has also been reported from Arabia but these reports are in question. It feeds on a number of species of domestic animals and on man. This species is closely related to O. *moubata* but can readily be identified by the presence of two pairs of eyes. It has frequently been reported as a vector of relapsing fever spirochetes but authentic records of the recovery of spirochetes from ticks of this species, as collected in nature, cannot be found.

*Ornithodoros erraticus* (Lucas) (=O. *marocanus* Velu) (see comments under Relapsing Fever) is widely distributed in North Africa and is the only known vector of relapsing fever in Spain and Portugal. It is also found in Iran. It has been taken from pigsties and from the burrows of numerous species of mammals. Its presence in Senegal and the recovery of the spirochete, *Borrelia crocidurae*, from it and from the shrew, *Crocidura stampflii*, may explain the presence of relapsing fever at Dakar. The present known eastward limit for this species in Africa is Kenya.

*Ornithodoros coriaceus* Koch, the "pajaroello," is a large species found locally in California and in Oaxaca, Mexico. It is parasitic on large mammals and bites man freely. In California it is frequently found in deer beds among the scrub oaks, *Quercus dumosa*. It is the only known species in the Americas that has eyes. In freshly molted specimens the delicately sculptured mammillae give to the integument a patina of fine shagreen. The larvae are extremely active and, like the larvae of *O. talaje,* require several days to engorge, becoming enormously distended, after which there are two successive molts without further feeding.

This species is not known to transmit any disease agent but its bite is extremely venomous. In some areas the bite is more dreaded than the bite of a rattlesnake. A sharp pain is rapidly followed by extensive swelling and numbness. A crust with exuding lymph at the site of the puncture wound may persist for several months.

*Ornithodoros verrucosus* Olenev has been reported from a cave in the North Caucasus. It is a small species characterized by large, thick mammillae. This species bites man readily and is considered a vector of relapsing fever.

*Ornithodoros gurneyi* is the only species of the genus known on the mainland of Australia. It has been taken in New South Wales and from kangaroos' bedding areas in Queensland. Systemic paralysis, blindness and unconsciousness are said to follow the bite of this tick.

*Ornithodoros nicollei* Mooser is a native to the states of Guerrero, Puebla, Colima and Jalisco in Mexico. Known natural hosts are *Neotoma,* dogs, and man, and it has been found on a rattlesnake in the Zoo in St. Louis, Missouri. It is found in houses in Mexico.

Females frequently oviposit twice following a single blood meal with an interval of several months between the ovipositions. The rate of hatching of the eggs is relatively high and eggs deposited one year following the last mating have proved 98 per cent fertile.

Infectious agents have not been recovered from this species collected in nature. However, it is similar to *O. parkeri* in that, experimentally, it transmits the rickettsiae of the spotted fevers of the United States, Colombia and Brazil; transovarial transmission has also been demonstrated.

*Coxiella burnetii* and *Pasteurella tularensis* are conserved in the tissues of *O. nicollei* for more than 200 days, as shown by injection, but neither organism is transmitted during tick feeding. As in *O. moubata, P. tularensis* is harmful to this species; molting is delayed and the infected ticks become dwarfed.

*Ornithodoros rostratus* Beaurepaire-Aragão has been reported from southern Brazil, northern Argentina and from Paraguay and Bolivia. In Brazil it is found in houses and is known as Garrapato du chão. It bites man and produces extensive areas of ecchymosis. The prolonged hemorrhages seen in experimental animals following tick feeding suggest the presence of a powerful anticoagulant. The larvae are reported as requiring several hours or even days for engorgement but they have been observed to engorge and detach voluntarily in less than a half hour.

*Ornithodoros brasiliensis* Aragão is a large species from the state of Rio Grande do Sul, Brazil. It feeds on mammals and birds and produces local and systemic reactions in man. Erythema and papule formation at the site of puncture are followed by headache and fever.

*Ornithodoros tholozani* (Laboulbène and Mégnin) (=*O. papillipes* Birula) is a vector of relapsing fever in the Caucasus, Turkestan, Iran, Syria, Palestine, Northern India, and the island of Cyprus. Among its hosts are the camel, chickens, and various species of rodents. In some areas it is found commonly in caves. In Turkestan it is found in stables. (Taxonomists differ as to whether *O. crossi* Brumpt is a synonym of *O. tholozani*, a variety of the species, or a valid species. It was discovered in stables in northern Punjab, India.)

*Ornithodoros asperus* Warburton has been taken at Bileck-Steppe in eastern Iraq; spirochetes were recovered from these ticks. The host is unknown.

*Ornithodoros lahorensis* Neumann was originally described from the Punjab where it was found in old sheepfolds feeding on sheep which were dying of anemia. It is now also known from Yugoslavia, Turkey, Palestine, Iran, Russian Turkestan, and Kashmir. Like *O. savignyi*, this species has been reported as a vector of relapsing fever spirochetes but such reports cannot be confirmed.

*Ornithodoros pavimentosus* Neumann is known from Great Namaland and Namaqualand in South-West Africa. It is somewhat similar to *O. savignyi* in appearance but its behavior is nearer to that of *O. moubata* in that it is found commonly in huts and in travelers' rests where it frequently attacks man; the bite is very severe.

*Ornithodoros normandi* Larrousse, one of the smallest known species, is reported as abundant in rodent burrows near Kef, Tunisia. It bites man readily. Relapsing fever has been reported from northern Tunisia but the role of this species, if any, has not been determined.

*Ornithodoros foleyi* Parrot was described from specimens collected near the confluence of the Igharghar and Tinikert rivers, Algeria. It feeds on dromedaries and man. The local lesions caused by the bite are said to resemble a furuncle or syphilitic chancre.

*Ornithodoros tartakovskyi* Olenev is a small species found in the burrows of rodents in the desert steppe region of Central Asia and in hedgehog burrows in Turkmenistan. It is reported as a vector of relapsing fever in these areas.

### The Genera of Ticks (Ixodoidea)

The present limited knowledge of ticks of the world makes it impossible to make fully adequate keys to the genera. The following simplified keys are intended to be useful to the field worker. Some rare genera and some that have not been thoroughly studied are omitted, but their omission will not reduce the value of the keys in the very great majority of cases.

*Table 57    Keys to the Families and Genera of Ticks*

**Key to Families of the Ixodoidea**

1    (2)    \* Lacking a scutum or "shield" in all stages ("soft ticks") ............. *Argasidae*

2    (1)    With a scutum or "shield" in all stages; scutum in females small, covering anterior part of the dorsal surface, in males covering most of the dorsal surface ("hard ticks") .......... *Ixodidae*

**Key to Genera of the Argaside:† *Adults and Nymphs***

1    (2)    Nymphs (the stage usually seen) with integument beset with spines, hypostome well developed, adults with granular integument, hypostome vestigial; lacking a definite impressed sutural line separating the dorsal and ventral surfaces ............. *Otobius*

2    (1)    Adults and nymphs with integument essentially alike and lacking distinct spines; hypostome of various forms but never vestigial; sutural line separating the dorsal and ventral surfaces present or absent .......... 3

3    (4)    Hypostome broad at the base and scooplike; sutural line separating the dorsal and ventral surfaces absent. (Associated with bats) ............... *Antricola*

4    (3)    Hypostome of various forms but never scooplike; with or without a sutural line separating the dorsal and ventral surfaces .................... 5

5    (6)    No sutural line separating the dorsal and ventral surfaces; margin of the body rarely distinctly flattened and usually similar in structure to the general integument ............. *Ornithodoros*

6    (5)    Usually with a sutural line separating the dorsal and ventral surfaces; margin of the body distinctly flattened and different in structure from the general integument .............. *Argas*

\* Digits in parentheses indicate alternative (e.g., negative condition with respect to the character being considered). For example if tick in 1 (2) above *has* a scutum, proceed to 2 (1).

† Modified from Cooley, R. A. and Kohls, G. M., 1944. The Argasidae of North America, Central America, and Cuba, University Press, Notre Dame, Ind. 152 pp.

*Table 57 Continued*

**Key to Genera of the Ixodidae: *Adults‡***

| 1 | (2) | With eyes .......................... | 3 |
|---|-----|-------------------------------------|---|
| 2 | (1) | Without eyes ...................... | 15 |
| 3 | (4) | Scutum ornate (usually) ........... | 5 |
| 4 | (3) | Scutum inornate (*Rhipicephalus* is rarely ornate) ................. | 7 |

5 (6) Palpi short; denticles almost always in 6 rows (rarely 8) 3 on a side and expressed 3/3 (or 4/4) and occupying most of the length of the hypostome *Dermacentor*

6 (5) Palpi long and thin (with rare exceptions); denticles usually 3/3 or 4/4 and occupying the distal part of the hypostome ..................... *Amblyomma*

| 7 | (8) | Eyes marginal ..................... | 9 |
|---|-----|-----------------------------------|---|

8 (7) Eyes not marginal (Old World only) *Hyalomma*

| 9 | (10) | With festoons .................... | 11 |
|---|------|-----------------------------------|----|

10 (9) Without festoons ................ *Boophilus*

11 (12) Ventral shields or plates (back of the hind legs) absent in both sexes .... 13

12 (11) Ventral shields or plates (back of the hind legs) present in males, absent in females ..................... *Rhipicephalus*

13 (14) Spurs on coxa IV of male very long (Africa) ....................... *Rhipicentor*

14 (13) Spurs on coxa IV short or absent in both sexes (tropical and subtropical America) ..................... *Anocentor* (*Otocentor*)

15 (16) Usually ornate (tropical and subtropical, on reptiles almost exclusively) *Aponomma*

16 (15) Inornate (world-wide, generally on land vertebrates other than reptiles) 17

17 (18) With festoons; palpi short, usually massive and conical when closed; anal groove contouring the anus posteriorly ...................... *Haemaphysalis*

18 (17) Without festoons; palpi short or long and when closed with sides parallel, not forming a cone; anal groove contouring the anus anteriorly or, rarely, encircling it ............. *Ixodes*

‡ Furnished by Dr. R. A. Cooley and Glen M. Kohls, Rocky Mountain Laboratory, U. S. P. H. S.

**Definitions and Explanations***

**Articles**   Applicable to the legs and palpi; the divisions which make up the appendages, erroneously spoken of as "joints."

**Articulation**   The joining of two articles; they may be immovable (fused) or movable in some palpi.

**Basis capituli**   The basal portion of the capitulum to which the hypostome, chelicerae and palpi are attached, often abbreviated to "basis."

**Buttons**   In *Argas;* circular elevations on the integument, each with a central pit and often with a hair in the pit.

**Camerostome**   In *Ornithodoros;* the depression or cavity in which the capitulum lies, usually less definite in engorged specimens.

**Capitulum**   The movable anterior portion of the tick including the attached mouth parts.

**Cheeks**   In *Ornithodoros;* the paired flaps at the sides of the camerostome; they may be either movable or fixed, and they increase in size progressively in the successive stages of development.

**Chelicerae**   In all ticks in all stages; the paired dorsal members of the piercing mouth parts with movable barbs or teeth at their tips which serve for cutting; they are capable of being extended or withdrawn.

**Cornua**   Projections extending caudad from the posterolateral corners of the basis capituli.

**Coxae**   On the ventral surface of all ticks, in all stages; the paired plates to which the legs are attached.

**Denticles**   The recurved barbs or "teeth" on the hypostome in nearly all ticks, in all stages.

**Discs**   In the ARGASIDAE; limited areas or spots which are the external evidence of modification of the structure of the body wall at the points of the attachment of dorsoventral muscles. They may be superficial or depressed, faint or distinct.

**Dorsal Humps**   In *Ornithodoros;* humps or elevations on the dorsal walls of the articles of the legs and not including the subapical dorsal protuberances.

**Eyes**   Small, simple, smooth, shining organs found on many IXODIDAE and situated in or near the lateral borders of the scutum—not on the basis capituli as might be suspected. They are "marginal" if situated on the edge of the scutum, "not marginal" if placed a short distance away from the edge. Often present in nymphs and larvae. When present in the ARGASIDAE they are found on the sides of the ticks.

**Festoons**   In some genera, in both sexes; the uniform more or less rectangular areas near the posterior margins, on dorsal and ven-

* Furnished by Dr. R. A. Cooley, Rocky Mountain Laboratory, U.S.P.H.S.

tral surfaces, limited by depressed lines. In some species the limiting line is absent on the anterior side.

**Files**  The longitudinate rows of denticles on the hypostome.

**Grooves**  In nearly all ticks; in the IXODIDAE the principal ones are on the dorsal surface, in the females the marginal grooves, in males the lateral grooves, in both sexes the cervical grooves, and on the ventral surface the anal groove and the genital groove. In both sexes of the ARGASIDAE the principal grooves are ventral and are the preanal, median postanal, and the transverse postanal grooves. Some species have dorsoventral grooves at the sides.

**"Hairs"**  Hairs may be long or short, tapering or not tapering, pointed or blunt, forked or barbed.

**Hood**  In *Ornithodoros;* the anterior projection of the body wall; it may be large, small, or absent.

**Hypostome**  The ventral member of the piercing mouth parts in the adults, nymphs, and larvae of nearly all ticks. It usually has numerous recurved barbs or "teeth" (denticles) which serve to fasten the tick to the host.

**Mammillae**  In nymphs and adults of *Ornithodoros;* the characteristic small elevations of various forms on the general surface of the body in contradistinction to "granulations" (in *Otobius*), "tubercles" (in *Antricola*), and "wrinkles" (in *Argas*).

**Marginated**  Having a margin which is distinct in appearance or structure.

**Ornamentation**  The symmetrical pattern of color superimposed over a darker color, and spoken of as "white," "gray," "rose," etc.; applicable to many IXODIDAE, but generally found only on adults.

**Palpi**  In all ticks in all stages the paired structures attached to the basis capituli. They have four divisions or articles which in the ARGASIDAE are easily visible with all articles movably attached. In the IXODIDAE article 1 is not easily seen. The articulation between articles 1 and 2 may be movable or immovable. If immovable, articulations are spoken of as "fused."

**Plaques**  On the ventral surface of some males; small sclerotized spots, in symmetrical pairs, anterior to the festoons.

**Posterodorsal Elevation**  In some genera (notably *Hyalomma, Amblyomma,* and *Dermacentor*); the elevation on the dorsal surface at the base of article 2 of the palpus, rarely pronounced, as in *Dermacentor reticulatus.*

**Pulvillus**  Cushion-like structure, near the claws, at the tip of the leg; may be present or absent.

**Punctations**  In all ticks in all stages; the pits or depressions on the surface of the body or its appendages.

**Sclerotization**  The thickening or strengthening of the wall of the body or parts of the body or appendages.

**Scutum**    The sclerotized "shield" on the dorsal surface; present in "hard" ticks (Ixodidae), absent in "soft" ticks (Argasidae). In females, nymphs, and larvae it is found at the anterior end of the body; in males occupying all or nearly all the dorsal surface.

**Sexual Aperture**    In all adult ticks the opening on the median line of the venter between the coxae, covered with a flap in some males; absent in nymphs and larvae.

**Similar**    In the Argasidae; sexes are similar if separable only by size or differences in the morphology of the sex aperture; dissimilar if there are other morphologic differences of the body or appendages (as in *Antricola*). Adults and nymphs are similar if separable only by the presence of a mature sex aperture which is absent in the nymph; dissimilar if (as in *Otobius*) the adults and nymphs have other differences in body structures.

**Spines**    In nymphs of *Otobius*; the erect hair-like appendages which are thickened near their bases.

**Spiracular Plates**    The paired plates of various shapes on the sides anterior to coxa IV in the Argasidae, and posterior to coxa IV in the Ixodidae. Present in adults and nymphs, absent in larvae.

**Spurs**    In most genera, in all stages; posterior projections on the posterior side of the coxae; they may be large or small, pointed or rounded, present or absent; when the two on coxa I are long they may be spoken of as bifid.

**Subapical Dorsal Protuberances**    In *Ornithodoros*; the dorsal protuberance near the distal end of the leg; when much drawn out it results in what is called a "bifurcate" tarsus.

**Sutural Line**    A definite line of cleavage in *Argas*, separating the dorsal and ventral surfaces. In molting the integument splits along this line, permitting the escape of the tick.

**Tubercles**    In *Antricola*; the small elevations on the surface of the body, usually bearing hairs, comparable to the mammillae in *Ornithodoros*.

**Ventral Plates**    In males of *Ixodes*; the sclerotized plates which form a large part of the ventral surface and are designated as median (the anterior middle plate), anal (the posterior middle one), adanal (paired lateral plates next to the end plate), and epimeral (paired plates out side of the adanals, often not plainly visible). A small plate, the pregenital plate, is sometimes present in front of the sexual aperture.

**Ventral Scutes**    The sclerotized plates sometimes present on the ventral surface of festoons; they may extend as shelves beyond the margin of the festoons.

**Ventral Shields**    On the ventral surface in males of *Rhipicephalus*, *Boophilus*, and *Hyalomma*; the irregularly shaped shields usually attached in front and free behind, and designated as adanal, and accessory plates.

## Descriptions of Genera*

*Argas*. Body flattened, dorsal and ventral areas about equal; margins distinctly flattened (marginated), made up of radial striae or quadrangular plates. Sutural line separating dorsal and ventral surfaces usually present. Flattened margins not obliterated even when the tick is fully fed. Capitulum either distant from or near to the anterior border. Integument leathery, minutely wrinkled or in folds of many shapes, often intermingled with small, rounded buttons each with a pit on top and often bearing a hair in the pit. Discs present on both dorsal and ventral surfaces and placed in more or less radial lines. Eyes absent.

*Otobius*. Adults and nymphs dissimilar, with sexes similar. Adults with the integument granulated; nymphs striated and with spines. Without change of pattern of the integument at the sides. Capitulum distant from the anterior margin in adults; near the margin in nymphs. Hood and eyes absent. Hypostomes of nymphs well developed; vestigial in adults.

*Ornithodoros*. Body more or less flattened but rarely marginated. Sutural line separating dorsal and ventral surfaces absent. Surface usually very convex dorsally when distended with blood. Dorsal humps and subapical dorsal protuberances when present on legs become progressively more prominent in the successive nymphal stages. Capitulum either subterminal or distant from the anterior margin. Hypostome well developed and usually essentially alike in the two sexes and in nymphs and adults. Integument with discs and mammillae commingling in a variety of patterns. Hood, camerstome, and cheeks present or absent. Eyes present or absent.

*Antricola*. Dorsal wall flattened and marginated; sutural line separating dorsal and ventral surfaces absent; ventrally, the body convex and deep. Integument semitranslucent with the surface smooth, shining, and with tubercles. Discs absent on the venter. Mouth parts adapted for quick feeding and not for clinging to the host; hypostome convex ventrally, concave dorsally (internally) and lacking effective denticles; chelicerae large and effective. Anal ring large. Eyes absent. Eggs small, and the small larvae with bulbous pulvilli in place of claws.

*Amblyomma*. Usually ornate with dark spots and stripes on a pale background. Eyes and festoons present. Palpi usually long with article 2 especially long. Articulation between palpal articles 1 and 2 movable (not fused). Basis capituli of variable form, often subquadrangular or subtriangular. Males without the adanal shields found in *Rhipicephalus*, *Boophilus*, and *Hyalomma* though ventral plaques or ventral scutes may be present. Spiracular plates subtriangular or comma-shaped. Nymphs resemble adults but differ in the shape of the spiracular plate and are seldom ornate.

* Furnished by Dr. R. A. Cooley, Rocky Mountain Laboratory, U.S.P.H.S.

*Aponomma.* Characters as in *Amblyomma,* excepting that the eyes are absent.

*Dermacentor.* Ornate; with eyes, and festoons (11 in number). Basis capituli quadrangular dorsally. Hypostome with three (rarely four) rows of denticles on each side of the median line. Palpi short, broad or moderate in width and with a posterodorsal elevation present; article 1 fused with article 2. Coxae I to IV increasing in size progressively and coxa IV of male very large; coxa I bifid. Spiracles suboval or comma-shaped. Postanal groove present. Male with no ventral plates or shields.

*Anocentor (Otocentor).* Inornate, without ventral plates or shields; postanal groove present but faint. Basis capituli rectangular dorsally. Coxa I with short spurs in both sexes. Palpi short, moderate in width, and when closed not covering the chelicerae dorsally; palpal article 1 fused with article 2; denticles arranged in four rows on each side of the median line; eyes present (obsolescent). Festoons present (seven in number). Lateral grooves absent in the male; marginal grooves absent in the female.

*Ixodes.* Sexual dimorphism pronounced. Inornate, without eyes and without festoons. Palpi and basis capituli variable in form. Articulation between palpal articles 1 and 2 movable. Coxae either with or without spurs; spurs on coxa I when present are variable. Anal groove contouring the anus anteriorly or rarely encircling it. Male with ventral plates present—one median, one anal, two adanal, and two epimeral plates; a pregenital plate sometimes present.

*Hyalomma.* Ornamentation, if present, confined to the legs. Eyes present, hemispherical, not marginal. With or without festoons. Palpi usually long; articulation between articles 1 and 2 movable. Basis capituli subtriangular dorsally. Female resembles *Amblyomma.* Male with a pair of adanal shields and with or without accessory adanal shields, and usually with two posterior abdominal protrusions capped by sclerotized points. Coxa I bifid. Spiracular plates comma-shaped.

*Haemaphysalis.* Usually of small size. Inornate, without eyes but with festoons; with palpi usually short, conical and with second article projecting laterally beyond the basis capituli which is rectangular dorsally. With a dorsal process on first trochanter. Sexual dimorphism slight. Ventral plates and shields on males absent. Spiracular plates of male oval or comma-shaped; in females rounded or oval.

*Rhipicephalus.* Usually inornate, with eyes and festoons; palpi short and basis capituli usually hexagonal dorsally. Coxa I bifid. Males with a pair of adanal shields and usually a pair of accessory shields. Spiracular plates comma-shaped, short or long.

*Rhipicentor.* Inornate, with eyes and festoons. Palpi short; basis capituli hexagonal dorsally and with very prominent lateral angles; coxa I bifid in both sexes. The male resembles *Rhipicephalus* dorsally and *Dermacentor* ventrally; coxa IV much the largest. Ventral plates and shields lacking. Spiracular plate of the female subtriangular, of the male, comma-shaped.

*Boophilus.* Poorly sclerotized. Inornate, with eyes but without festoons. Palpi very short, compressed, more than usually separated, and with dorsal and lateral transverse ridges on the articles. Basis capituli hexagonal dorsally. Anal groove in male faintly indicated, obsolete in the female. Males with adanal and accessory adanal shields. Spiracular plates rounded or oval in both sexes.

### Acarina Other Than Ticks (Mites)

More than two hundred families of mites have been described. The species comprising most of these families are free-living, but those of a few are parasites of plants or animals.

The known parasitic species found on animals exhibit different degrees of parasitism. Some are parasitic in all active stages (scabies mites); some during only the larval stage (chiggers); some are fortuitous parasites ("cheese mites"); while still others, such as the rare *Holothyrus coccinella*, produce harmful effects by means of an irritant poisonous fluid.

The mites affecting man may be considered in three groups: (1) species which cause a dermatitis (DERMANYSSIDAE, PYEMOTIDAE, ACARIDAE, GLYCYPHAGIDAE); (2) the "chiggers," larval mites of the family TROMBICULIDAE, many of which may cause a dermatitis and some of which are vectors of the rickettsiae of scrub typhus (tsutsugamushi); (3) the itch mite, *Sarcoptes scabiei* (SARCOPTIDAE).

**Dermanyssidae** *Bdellonyssus bacoti* (Hirst) (the genus *Liponyssus* of authors has been synonymized under *Bdellonyssus*, and literature to these mites should be checked under both names), the tropical rat mite, is one of the species most troublesome to man throughout the world. Its bite is very painful and is followed by intense itching and the formation of small hemorrhagic areas. The mites normally feed on rats and readily attack man in restaurants, warehouses, etc., where rats are prevalent. Control of this mite depends upon rat control. The tropical rate mite has been found capable of transmitting typhus and rickettsial pox experimentally.

*Bdellonyssus sylviarum* (C. & F.), the northern fowl mite, occasionally bites man and has been found to be infected with western equine encephalitis in California, and the Newcastle disease virus of chickens in Iowa. It is to be found throughout the temperate regions, being parasitic on domestic fowls and many wild birds.

*Dermanyssus gallinae* (Degeer), the chicken mite, is primarily a pest of chickens, but also parasitizes various wild birds. This species sometimes bites man, causing mild dermatitis and itching. It has been found naturally infected with the St. Louis encephalitis virus. It is widespread throughout the world.

*Allodermanyssus sanguineus* (Hirst), the mouse mite, is generally found infecting mice. It occasionally bites man in the northeastern United States and transmits a relatively mild rickettsial disease known as rickettsialpox. The bites of the mite apparently cause no discomfiture. The known distribution is the United States and northern Africa.

**Pyemotidae (=Pediculoididae)**   *Pyemotes* (= *Pediculoides*) *ventricosus* (Newport) is a widely distributed predaceous mite which attacks the larvae of a number of insects. However, it also attacks man, producing a dermatitis known as "straw itch." The nongravid female is tiny and elongate, but in the pregnant female the abdomen becomes enormously distended and globoid. The species is ovoviviparous. The eggs hatch, the young mites develop to maturity, and the newly adult females are often fertilized within the body of the mother before escaping to the outside. Numerous epidemics of dermatitis are attributed to infestation with this mite. Farmers feeding grain through threshing machines or sleeping on straw mattresses are often affected. Mite-laden dust from harvesting machines may be carried considerable distances and result in the infestation of inhabitants of nearby dwellings. The resulting dermatitis, sometimes covering the entire body, has been confused with chickenpox, smallpox, and scabies. A relatively high fever is not uncommon.

For *control*, burning of the grain stubble is recommended to destroy the mites and the insect larvae on which they feed. Pyrethrins and piperonyl butoxide can be used on straw with good results.

**Acaridae (=Tyroglyphidae)**   This is a cosmopolitan family of tiny mites that infest a wide variety of materials such as cereals, grains, and other stored products. In one stage (hypopial) they may attach themselves to living insects which then serve as disseminators. The dermatitis resulting from infestations with these mites is similar to that produced by the "straw itch" mite, *Pyemotes ventricosus*. Several species are concerned. The rash caused by *Tyrophagus castellanii* (Hirst) is designated as "copra itch," and that caused by *Acarus siro* L., "vanillism" (in vanilla pod handlers). Some species have been reported from both the urinary and intestinal tracts. *Tyrophagus longior* (Gervais) may be ingested, especially in cheese, and may be found subsequently in the feces. It is not known, however, to produce a true intestinal infestation. The characteristic pungent flavor of Altenburger Milbenkäse is due to mites. Contact with the excrement or powdered bodies of these mites may readily result in allergic phenomena. *Glycyphagus domesticus* (Degeer) in the closely related family GLYCYPHAGIDAE causes the well known "grocers' itch."

**Trombiculidae**   Chiggers (red bugs, harvest mites, bête rouge, etc.) are the parasitic larval mites of the family TROMBICULIDAE that infest vertebrates. In some areas the term "chigger," probably a corruption of "chigoe," is also applied to the burrowing flea. The larvae are almost microscopic in size. The adults seldom exceed 1 mm. in length, and are often brilliantly colored. The nymphs and adults are predators, living upon small arthropods and their eggs. In the laboratory, mosquito eggs and springtails seem to be the preferred food of certain species. The family is cosmopolitan in distribution, ranging from Alaska and Labrador in the north to New Zealand in the south, and from sea level to over 16,000 feet in the Andes. Eggs, which are deposited on the ground in light soil, give rise to hexapod larvae which attach to their hosts, including man, by hooked mouth parts, but they do not burrow into the skin. After a prolonged period of feeding the engorged larvae fall to the ground and molt. In the

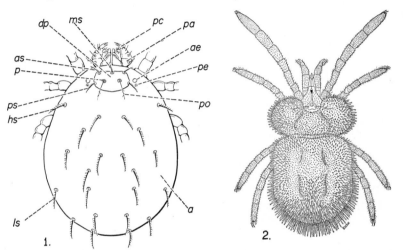

Fig. 285. *Eutrombicula alfreddugèsi* (Oudemans). 1. Larva (North American chigger), greatly enlarged. 2. Adult. *a*, abdomen; *ae*, anterior eye; *as*, anterolateral seta; *dp*, dorsal plate; *hs*, humeral seta; *ls*, lateral seta I; *ms*, median seta; *p*, pseudostigma; *pa*, palpus; *pc*, palpal claw; *pe*, posterior eye; *po*, pseudostigmatic organ; *ps*, posterolateral seta. (Modified from Ewing.)

nymphal and adult stages they are predaceous. In northern United States there is only one or possibly two generations a year, but in Florida the generations are continuous.

Chiggers usually produce intense itching and a severe dermatitis. At times there is also extravasation of blood from subcuticular capillaries, producing bluish or purplish ecchymoses visible for months. Secondary infections due to scratching, and loss of sleep, result in a reduced efficiency of troops or other organizations in the field. *Eutrombicula alfreddugèsi* (Oudemans) is the common chigger of the United States and is especially prevalent in the southern states during summer and fall (Fig. 285).

A rickettsial disease commonly known as scrub typhus, tsutsugamushi disease, flood fever, etc., occurs in Japan, Formosa, Australia, Sumatra, Malaya, India, Indo-China, Java, Philippine Islands, Burma, New Guinea, Bougainville, and adjacent areas, and is transmitted by the larval trombiculids or chiggers. The *Rickettsia tsutsuga-mushi* are found in the trombiculid mites and their normal hosts, small rodents. Man picks up the disease from the mites when an infected trombiculid accidentally gets on him and feeds. The disease is transmitted only by the parasitic larva, and the rickettsiae survive through the nonparasitic nymphal and adult states to be passed through the egg to the next generation.

Most areas where scrub typhus is a problem are characterized by abundant food for rodents like that supplied by abandoned gardens, plantations, primary jungle, and marginal agricultural lands subjected to floods or seasonal activity such as harvesting of natural products. "Fringe habitats" surrounding grassy areas are dangerous locations.

*Trombicula* (*Leptotrombidium*) *akamushi* (Brumpt), *T.* (*L.*) *deliensis* Walch, *T.* (*L.*) *pallida* Nagayo et al., *T.* (*L.*) *intermedia* Nagayo et al., and *T.* (*L.*) *scutellaris* Nagayo et al. have been reported as carriers of the scrub typhus rickettsiae.

*Control* consists in removing scrub growth, and oiling and burning areas around encampments. Chemical control of the mites can be obtained by use of sulfur, chlordane and chlorinated camphene, hydroxypentamethylflavan, DDT in calcium carbonate, benzene hexachloride, crude benzene hexachloride dust, and others. Personal protection can be had by treating clothing with dimethylphthalate, dibutylphthalate, benzene, 2-thenylsalicylate, or "M-1960."

**Sarcoptidae**    Members of this family of "itch mites" produce skin diseases in many species of birds and mammals. Members of the genus *Sarcoptes* are burrowing mites, and may infest man (*Sarcoptes scabiei* var. *scabiei* (De Geer), sheep (*Sarcoptes scabiei* var. *ovis* Mégnin), pig (*Sarcoptes scabiei* var. *suis* Gerlach), goat (*Sarcoptes scabiei* var. *caprae* Fürstenberg), and other animals.

*Sarcoptes scabiei* (De Geer) of man, the human itch mite, is a minute, oval mite with transversely striated skin, short dorsal spines, and short stubby legs, the last two pairs of legs of the female ending in long whiplike setae. Eggs are laid in the burrow the female makes in the horny layer of the skin. These eggs hatch and the six-legged larvae leave the burrows and move about on the skin looking for food and shelter. Immature forms do not make permanent burrows, and fertilization of the female probably takes place on the skin. The mature female usually stays in the burrow her entire life.

These mites cause severe itching, especially at night. A characteristic rash, due to both the mite and scratching, appears. Areas usually affected are those under the arms, around the waist, on the wrists, on the inner sides of the thighs, and on the ankles. Many of the skin symptoms are due to secondary infections. The highest incidence of scabies is in the winter when people are inclined to sleep together for warmth. Scabies is acquired through such close personal contact with an infected person, and it is not believed that casual contact is important in the dissemination of this mite.

For treatment see scabies p. 601.

# 71　The Class Insecta (Hexapoda)

## Introduction

This, the largest and most important class of arthropods, both medically and otherwise, is characterized by the division of the body into three distinct portions; a head, composed of six (possibly seven) fused segments; a thorax of three segments, usually well marked, and an abdomen of eleven segments of which only five to eight are usually visible. The head bears the mouth parts, a single pair of antennae and the eyes, when present. Adult insects display three pairs of legs, borne ventrally by the three thoracic segments. The majority of insects have wings, borne dorsally on the last two thoracic segments. Caudal appendages, called *cerci*, are often present on the last abdominal segment.

Insects are found under a wide variety of environmental conditions, but only those which live as parasites in some stage of their existence or which have intimate contact with the human body or with human food are ordinarily concerned with problems of health and disease.

Some thirty-three orders of insects are recognized at the present time. Of these only twelve may be listed as of medical interest, and some of these are important only in a very limited way. In the list which follows, the four most important orders are marked with an asterisk. These will be discussed at length; the others in less detail.

The order of presentation is, in general, from the simple to the complex, the COLLEMBOLA for instance being much more primitive both in structure and life history than the DIPTERA, HYMENOPTERA and other highly evolved groups.

### List of Medically Important Orders

1. COLLEMBOLA (Springtails)
2. ORTHOPTERA (Cockroaches and others)
3. EPHEMERIDA (Mayflies)
4. TRICHOPTERA (Caddis flies)
5. MALLOPHAGA (Bird lice)
*6. ANOPLURA (Sucking lice)
*7. HEMIPTERA (Bugs)
8. COLEOPTERA (Beetles)
9. LEPIDOPTERA (Butterflies, Moths)
*10. DIPTERA (Flies)
*11. SIPHONAPTERA (Fleas)
12. HYMENOPTERA (Ants, Bees, Wasps)

## Order Collembola

The Collembola are primarily phytophagous and are not usually thought of as medically important insects. Two Australian species, however, *Entomobrya multifasciata* Tullb. and *E. tenuicauda* Schött, have recently been recorded as attacking man, the patients complaining of a sharp, biting sensation followed by irritation and papules

* These orders are of outstanding medical importance.

**683**

similar to mosquito bites, with pruritus. These forms derive their common name from the fact that they possess a forked muscular appendage at the posterior end of the abdomen, which is used in springing into the air (Fig. 286). They are entirely wingless, and their

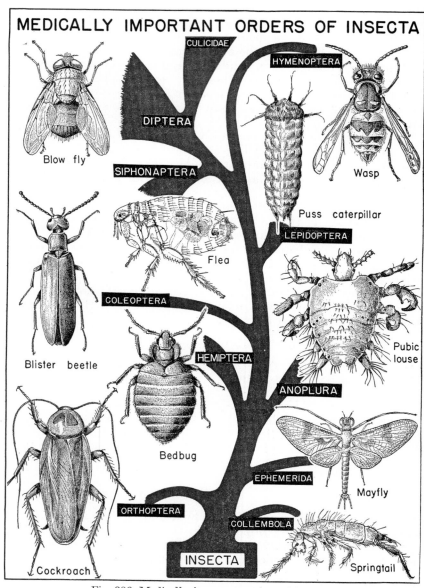

**MEDICALLY IMPORTANT ORDERS OF INSECTA**

CULICIDAE

HYMENOPTERA

DIPTERA

Blow fly

SIPHONAPTERA

Wasp

Puss caterpillar

Flea

LEPIDOPTERA

COLEOPTERA

Blister beetle

Pubic louse

HEMIPTERA

ANOPLURA

Bedbug

EPHEMERIDA

Mayfly

ORTHOPTERA

COLLEMBOLA

INSECTA

Cockroach

Springtail

Fig. 286. Medically important orders of insects.

mouth parts are of the chewing type. Most species are less than an eighth of an inch in length.

## Order Orthoptera

Of the ORTHOPTERA, only the roaches (Family BLATTIDAE) are believed to be concerned in the transmission of disease. They are cosmopolitan in distribution. These insects frequent filthy situations and are known to feed on both excrement and sputum, if opportunity affords. Soon after, they may be found on human food, where,

*Table 58   Key to Domestic Cockroaches in U.S.A.*

1   (6)   Larger species (1¼–2 inches in length) ............ 2
2   (5)   Wings well developed, extending to or beyond the last abdominal segment; general color reddish brown .... 3
3   (4)   Wings with a bright yellow heavy line on the outer edge of the basal half of the wing—*Periplaneta australasiae* F. (Australian cockroach).
4   (3)   Wings uniformly reddish brown—*Periplaneta americana* L. (American cockroach).
5   (2)   Wings vestigial in female; in male usually reaching within four segments of tip of abdomen; general color black or very dark brown. Sluggish species, prefers very damp environment—*Blatta orientalis* L. (Oriental cockroach).
6   (1)   Smaller species (less than ¾ inch in length) ......... 7
7   (8)   Thorax bearing two dark, longitudinal dorsal stripes. Wings uniform in color—*Blattella germanica* L. (German cockroach).
8   (7)   Thorax without longitudinal dorsal stripes. Wings with two cross bands of light yellow, one at the base, the other a little farther back—*Supella supellectilium* Serv. (Tropical cockroach).

both by their feces and by regurgitation, they unburden themselves of their bacterial flora. Cholera vibrios have been found alive in cockroach feces as long as 79 hours after ingestion. Organisms cling, likewise, to their antennae, legs and body hairs, only to drop off at some later time and thus spread contamination.

There is evidence to indicate that roaches may serve as intermediate hosts of certain helminths.

Roaches are fast-running flattened insects with long slender antennae and semitransparent brownish wings (in the wing-bearing species) (Fig. 286). The head is turned so far under that the mouth parts are actually directed backward. Mouth parts are of the chewing type. Not all species enter buildings. The adults of the five types most commonly encountered in houses in the United States may be differentiated as shown in Table 58.

**Habits and Life History** Cockroach eggs are deposited in a leathery capsule which may often be seen protruding from the body of the female, who sometimes carries it for days. Eventually she either glues the capsule to some object or merely drops it. The twenty or thirty eggs (*Blattella*) hatch into tiny nymphs which closely resemble the adults except that they have no wings. A gradual metamorphosis ensues. Roaches are nocturnal in habit, hiding during the day in sheltered, darkened places. They have scent glands which secrete an oily liquid responsible for the characteristic "roachy" odor.

**Control of Roaches** 1. Fumigation by professionals with hydrogen cyanide is the most effective procedure; however it is necessary to evacuate the premises during the fumigation and the rooms must be constructed well enough to permit them to be made "gas-tight" without too much labor or expense.

2. An alternative method is the heating of rooms to 130° or 135° F. for a period of not less than three hours.

3. Under ordinary circumstances the use of various powders and pastes is probably to be preferred:

(*a*) Sodium fluoride may be sprinkled or blown into crevices where it is allowed to remain for two or three days. The roaches run through the powder, which kills either by contact or as a stomach poison. (These insects usually clean their legs and antennae by means of their mouth parts, thereby taking considerable of the powder into the alimentary tract.) Sodium fluoride may also be combined with food materials and made to function as a poison bait. Children and pets should of course be kept from contact with the poison, and special care should be exercised in and about kitchens and food establishments where sodium fluoride may perhaps be mistaken for flour, baking powder, or borax. Certain manufacturers have recently taken to coloring their product a bluish-green, in order to make it readily distinguishable from edible or harmless substances.

(*b*) Pyrethrum powders, dusted about the rooms, are reasonably effective; however, the pyrethrum must be fresh and the apparently dead roaches should be swept up and destroyed, since many will be merely stupefied by the pyrethrins, and will revive if left about.

(*c*) Borax, as a roach powder, is none too effective and is recommended only in case other materials are not available.

(*d*) Phosphorus paste (purchasable at drug stores) may be smeared inside of cardboard rolls which are then left or fastened where roaches are known to run. This method is highly recommended for use in very damp climates.

4. Sprays of various types are also used:

(*a*) Ordinary sprays, applied either by hand or with power sprayers, kill by contact only; hence the roaches must be hit and made wet by the spray, a fact which necessitates driving the spray deep into cracks and corners of the room. Five per cent DDT and 2 per cent chlordane in kerosene is probably the best residual spray.

(*b*) Vapor sprays, produced by electrically operated vaporizers, are markedly superior to the above, since the oil-pyrethrum preparations are broken up into fine mist which penetrates all crevices and hiding places by diffusion. Cracks about doors and windows should be stopped tight, as the roaches are irritated by the mist and if not confined will migrate from the room before being killed.

After eradicating cockroaches by any of the above methods it is desirable to fill all cracks which might serve as hiding places with plastic wood, putty, or plaster of Paris, as prophylaxis against their return.

5. Five per cent DDT (dichloro-diphenyl-trichlorethane) may be used either as an oil emulsion (spray) or as a dust. In and about kitchens the latter is preferable as it is not then necessary to extinguish fires during the work. As high a concentration as 20 per cent may be used for quick effects. The dust should be placed in cracks and runways; meter boxes, space behind meter boards and cracks in tables should not be overlooked. Because of its residual effect, treatment with DDT usually controls the roaches for at least ten weeks. DDT is not used directly upon the floor except in empty buildings. *Dishes and utensils used in preparation of food should be kept from contact with the insecticide.*

Orthoptera of the family PHASMIDAE (walking sticks) have been known to discharge an irritating fluid, which in the case of *Anisomorpha buprestoides* (Stoll) is capable of being squirted a distance of some two feet. If introduced into the eye, it causes excruciating pain.

## Order Ephemerida

The EPHEMERIDA, commonly known as lake flies, shad flies, or Mayflies, are of medical interest only because of their relation to certain allergic conditions. For example, *Hexagenia bilineata*, a common species along the shores of Lake Erie, occurs in such numbers in midsummer that cast skins (exuviae) are everywhere present on buildings, trees, and shrubbery. Persons breathing fragments of these exuviae may become highly sensitized and severe asthmatic paroxysms have been recorded (Table 55). There is some evidence that an extract made from the dried insects may be useful in desensitization.

## Order Trichoptera

TRICHOPTERA, or caddis flies, are likewise causative agents of allergic symptoms at times. These are mothlike creatures, and it is the hairs and scales from their bodies which cause disturbances.

## Order Mallophaga

MALLOPHAGA, or biting lice, are mentioned here merely to distinguish them from the sucking lice, discussed below. MALLOPHAGA abound chiefly on birds though many species are adapted to mammalian hosts. They have chewing mouth parts and feed chiefly on dandruff, scurf, or dried blood. They are exceedingly irritating when abundant and constitute a considerable problem for the veterinarian. Poultry handlers are frequently annoyed by them, but the irritation is of short duration since these species will not remain on human hosts.

The biting dog louse, *Trichodectes canis,* is an intermediate host of the dog tapeworm, *Dipylidium caninum,* a species occasionally found in man.

## Order Anoplura

Some authorities place the biting and sucking lice in the order ANOPLURA as the suborders MALLOPHAGA and SIPHUNCULATA, respectively. In this text the ANOPLURA are limited to the sucking lice; these are unquestionably of great medical importance. Apart from their significance as vectors of typhus fever, trench fever, and relapsing fever, their continued presence causes the condition known as *pediculosis,* which, in sensitized individuals may be very severe.

The group numbers approximately 200 species, distributed over four families. Only the Family PEDICULIDAE, however, contains parasites of man. All human lice are small, flattened ectoparasites, characterized by a toughened skin and the complete absence of wings. The mouth parts, which are retractile, are for piercing and sucking. The head is narrow and pointed in front. The eyes are either degenerate or wanting. The thoracic segments are fused, but the thoracic regions are well marked by the three pairs of jointed legs. The tarsi are of one segment with a single, terminal claw, which, together with a process of the tibia (tibial thumb) makes an effective grasping organ, enabling the insect to cling to hairs or fabric. Females are notched, the males rounded, at the posterior extremity. Metamorphosis is of the "gradual" type (Fig. 286).

Human lice are of two species, the pubic louse *Phthirus pubis* (Linn.), and the head and body louse *Pediculus humanus* Linn. The latter exists in two doubtfully distinct varieties, *P. humanus* var. *capitis* De Geer, found chiefly on the scalp, and *P. humanus* var. *corporis* Retzius, which occurs on all parts of the body and is usually abundant in the seams of clothing. Human lice occur from the arctic to the tropics, wherever the habits of man are such as to encourage their existence. The species and varieties may be separated as follows (Table 59).

**Life History of the Body Louse (and Other Lice)**    The body louse, *Pediculus humanus* var. *corporis,* is a small flattened insect, living permanently on the person or in the clothing of man. As with all PEDICULIDAE, its mouthparts consist of an extrusible proboscis capable of piercing the skin. The piercing structures consist of a ventrally situated labium, chiefly for support, a median hypopharynx which contains the salivary canal and a pair of bristle-like maxillae, dorsal in position. When not in use these parts are housed in a stylet sac, ventral to the food canal. Both stylet sac and buccal cavity open by way of a short, tubelike structure, the haustellum, which bears six pairs of very small teeth. These teeth are usually concealed but become everted at the time of feeding and thus serve to anchor the mouth parts to the skin. The piercing structures are then thrust forward from the stylet sac and perforate the integument. The saliva contains an anticoagulant and a pharyngeal pumping apparatus

### Table 59   Key to Human Lice

1  (2)  Abdomen very short and broad, segments 1 to 5 being closely crowded, so that the spiracles of segments 3, 4, 5 appear to lie in a transverse row; segments 5 to 8 with lateral processes; fore legs slender, with elongate claws; other legs stout, with claws short and strong; tibial "thumbs" short . .*Phthirus pubis* (crab louse of man)

2  (1)  Abdomen elongate, none of the segments bearing lateral processes. All legs stout, the fore-legs stouter than the others. Tibial "thumbs" long slender, and beset with strong spines . . . . . . . . . .*Pediculus humanus* Linn.   3

3  (4)  Smaller forms. Females 2.8–3 mm.; males 2 mm. Eggs usually glued to hair of scalp
*P. humanus* var. *capitis* De Geer

4  (3)  Somewhat larger forms. Females, 2.74–4.4 mm.; males 2.74–3.6 mm. Eggs, by preference, deposited on threads of clothing. "Cooties," "graybacks," or "seam squirrels'
*P. humanus* var. *corporis* Retzius

causes blood to flow rapidly into the louse's distensible alimentary tract. Body lice feed frequently at all stages of their existence and die within relatively few days when removed from their hosts. Lice which are very hungry, especially the nymphs, sometimes feed so voraciously as to rupture the alimentary tract. Such lice appear red throughout, and will die in a few hours. The optimum temperature for the body louse is around 87° F. They will leave a dead body, a fevered patient or an individual heated by exercise.

In their development, lice show gradual metamorphosis. Eggs ("nits") are glued to hairs or fibers by the ovipositing females, and when the young push aside the opercula seven to ten days later, they emerge as miniature replicas of their parents. They must feed within 24 hours in order to survive. Growth is rapid; a succession of three molts brings them to maturity in about two weeks under favorable conditions. Following fertilization, the females lay several eggs daily for most of the remainder of their short lives. The entire cycle from egg to egg thus requires only a month or slightly less. The female lives an additional twenty or thirty days, during which time she may deposit from 275 to 300 eggs.

Body lice hide themselves in the seams of clothing, especially those of underwear and of heavier outer garments at points of pressure. Usually they cling to the clothing even while feeding; thus they may sometimes be entirely absent from the body of even a heavily infested person. Nits as well as lice are found in the seams. Therefore it is much more important to inspect the clothing of a suspected carrier than to examine the individual himself.

The increase of body lice is facilitated by infrequent laundering of clothing, while their spread is favored by close crowding of individuals, especially in sleeping quarters. Lice may be transferred indirectly from one person to another at night when clothes are placed not in separate lockers but on hooks in open rows.

The head louse, *P. humanus* var. *capitis,* is very similar to the body louse, differing more in habits than in structure from its close relative. Head lice may be induced to live in clothing and to interbreed with body lice, but when undisturbed they confine themselves to hairs of the scalp. They are probably of minor importance in the transmission of louse-borne diseases and should be regarded principally as nuisances indicative of poor hygienic standards.

Pubic lice, *Phthirus pubis,* inhabit hairs of the genital region, less often the eyelashes, moustache, axillae and body surface (hairy individuals). They are usually acquired by sexual contact or from toilet seats. They differ markedly from body and head lice, being smaller and much less slender. Their short stocky bodies and powerful grasping legs give them their vernacular name, crab lice. The life cycle of *P. pubis* is essentially similar to that of other lice, but they are less prolific, a normal female laying not more than 30 eggs. In addition to its predilection for the genital hairs, this species is distinguished by its tendency to remain immobile for days at a time, its proboscis inserted constantly in the skin. It apparently prefers white to colored skin. Pubic lice do not transmit louse-borne diseases.

**Pediculosis**   The bites of lice often cause intense discomfort, not only when the insect is feeding but also during the hours which follow. In the case of sensitized persons, symptoms may persist for many days. Typically, a small reddish papule appears at the site of each feeding puncture. Intense pruritus follows and scratching frequently results in a "weeping" dermatitis, predisposing to secondary infection. Diffuse swelling and erythema may both occur, especially if many lice have fed in a restricted area. Healing is usually accompanied by induration and mild fissuring of the skin with the deposition of a bronze pigment which persists indefinitely.

It has been shown that repeated exposures are necessary for the development of dermal hypersensitivity, and that the feces of the louse are involved in this reaction. The pruritus is part of the syndrome of hypersensitivity. As for the bite itself, the reaction appears to involve two components, a purpuric reaction, which depends on the act of feeding, and an inflammatory reaction, dependent on sensitization. If one remains lousy over an extended period of time the deeply pigmented condition of the skin known as "vagabond's disease" results. Systemic symptoms have been recorded, including general malaise and mental depression as well as a rash somewhat resembling that of German measles.

Untreated pediculosis of the scalp results in a condition in which the hair becomes matted together by exudate from the pustular lesions and the entire mass develops a fetid odor. The severity of the condition is often aggravated by the presence of mycotic infections, certain of which may be transmitted by the louse.

**Lice as Vectors of Disease** Epidemic typhus, trench fever and louse-borne relapsing fever have each been treated at length in earlier pages of this work. In the case of typhus, infection is transmitted chiefly by the feces of the louse upon the skin or by air-borne rickettsiae of fecal origin. The bite of the louse is of doubtful importance, but crushing of the louse upon the body, particularly if the skin be broken (as by scratching), is a common means of transmission.

With trench fever (Wolhynia fever) transmission takes places through contamination with louse feces and probably also by the bite. It is of interest to note that trench fever, in World War I, was second only to scabies as a cause of absence from duty.

The spirochetes of relapsing fever normally leave the alimentary tract of the louse and multiply in its body cavity. They are transmitted to man only when the louse is crushed and rubbed into the skin.

**Treatment of Pediculosis** Treatment of pediculosis is of scant value unless combined with measures designed to rid the individual of his parasites. However, temporary relief from skin irritation may be secured by use of spirits of thymol, 1 per cent. Ten per cent thymol in olive oil is also recommended.

When a considerable portion of the body surface is involved, the following procedure has been found very effective:

1. Wash the skin with acetone.

2. Apply an anti-itch mixture containing 5 per cent benzocaine (local anesthetic), 2 per cent methyl salicylate, 0.5 per cent salicylic acid. The preparation is made up to volume with 70 per cent alcohol. Such treatment is desirable in the case of laboratory workers who intentionally permit lice to feed upon their person as part of their routine duties.

**Prophylaxis and Control** Under normal circumstances, ordinary cleanliness, with frequent changing and laundering of garments, provides insurance against lousiness. On the other hand, crowded conditions and lack of sanitary facilities, together with circumstances which prevent a change of clothing, always make the louse problem more severe. For these reasons populations living in colder climates frequently suffer most, though lousiness in warmer regions is by no means rare.

Control procedures fall into two categories: (1) those concerned with the individuals directly; (2) those concerned with mass treatment of populations or troops.

1. Treatment of Individual

   a. Head Lice

      (1) *Insecticide, Spray, Delousing,* containing 6 per cent DDT, 68 per cent benzyl benzoate, 12 per cent benzocaine (ethyl para-amino-benzoate) and 14 per cent non-ionic emulsifiers, is the preparation of choice. The stock solution must be diluted just prior to use as follows: 1 part concentrate to 5 parts of water. The hair should be thoroughly wetted by spraying or sponging the mixture onto the head. Approximately 50 ml. are required for one treatment. For best results, the hair should not be washed for from 10 to 14 days following the treatment. Normally, one application will give complete control, but occasionally a second treatment will be needed after about one week. Care should be taken not to get any of the material in the eyes or open cuts.

      (2) *Insecticide, Powder, 10 per cent DDT,* in pyrophyllite, or talc also gives excellent control. Dust the head thoroughly and work down to the base of hair with finger tips. Repeat at end of one and two weeks to kill lice hatched from eggs. The hair should not be washed while treatment is in progress as DDT is not an ovicide.

      (3) *Insecticide, Powder, Pyrethrins (or Allethrin) and Synthetics,* containing pyrophyllite, various synergists, conditioners and antioxidants, is another excellent material. It is used in the same manner as *Insecticide, Powder, 10 per cent DDT.*

      (4) *Insecticide, Powder, Dusting, 1 per cent Lindane* is also satisfactory. It is used in the same manner as *Insecticide, Powder, 10 per cent DDT.* When this material is used the following precautions should be taken: Do not use more than 60 gm. on one individual, redusting will not be performed until after the lapse of seven (7) full days from the time of completion of a previous dusting, do not use in conjunction with insect repellents or other oily liquids applied to the skin.

   *NOTE:* With the above treatments it is not necessary to clip the hair.

   b. Body Lice

      (1) *Insecticide, Powder, 10 per cent DDT,* is the material of choice for the control of body lice, except in areas where lice are resistant to DDT, when *Insecticide, Powder,*

*Dusting, 1 per cent Lindane,* or *Insecticide, Powder, Pyrethrins (or Allethrin) and Synthetics* should be used. Remove clothing, turn inside out and dust lightly over entire inner surface, rubbing powder well into all seams. The powder remains effective for one month or longer if not washed off.

(2) *Insecticide, Powder, Pyrethrins (or Allethrin) and Synthetics* also gives excellent control. It is used in the same manner as *Insecticide, Powder, 10 per cent DDT,* except that retreatments will be necessary after 1 and 2 weeks.

(3) *Insecticide, Powder, Dusting, 1 per cent Lindane,* is another excellent insecticide. It is used in the same manner as *Insecticide, Powder, 10 per cent DDT,* except that retreatments will be necessary after one and two weeks. The same precautions should be observed that were pointed out in the section on the control of head lice.

c. Pubic Lice

(1) *Insecticide, Spray, Delousing,* is the preparation of choice in the control of pubic lice. It should be diluted and applied to all the regions of the body where coarse hair is present in the same manner as described under the section on head lice. Repeat every few days for two weeks.

(2) *Insecticide, Powder, 10 per cent DDT,* is an excellent material for the control of pubic lice. The powder should be thoroughly applied to all regions of the body where coarse hair is present. Repeat every few days for two weeks.

(3) *Insecticide, Powder, Pyrethrins (or Allethrin) and Synthetics* also gives excellent control. It is used in the same manner as *Insecticide, Powder, 10 per cent DDT.*

(4) *Insecticide, Aerosol, DDT and Pyrethrins (or Allethrin)* is another formulation that may be used. The aerosol should be applied to all the regions of the body where coarse hair is present. Repeat every few days for two weeks. Care should be taken not to get any of the aerosol in the eyes.

2. Mass Delousing of Populations or Troops

a. Mass delousing of large numbers of people by use of louse powders applied with a dust gun or power blower has proved entirely practicable in many areas throughout the world. *Insecticide, Powder, 10 per cent DDT,* is the material of choice, but in some areas of the world, where body lice are resistant to DDT, *Insecticide, Powder, Dusting, 1 per cent Lindane,* must be used. In mass delousing each person should be treated in the following manner:

(1) Dust inside of hat and replace on head.

(2) Extend arms at side, shoulder height. Insert delivery tube

slowly up each sleeve between skin and inner garment. Blow powder into armpit and about shoulder.

(3) Insert tube at back of neck and dust back and neckband.

(4) Insert tube in front at neck and dust toward armpits, both sides of body, chest and abdomen.

(5) Loosen trousers, insert tube between skin and innermost garment, and powder generously crotch and pubic area, also underwear, especially waist and side seams.

(6) Insert tube down rear of trousers next to skin and powder buttocks and rear of crotch.

(7) Dust socks thoroughly.

(8) Dust should be applied to each layer of clothing in each of the above steps.

(9) Dust any blankets or bed rolls that individuals may possess.

Normally, one application of 10 per cent DDT is sufficient to control an infestation, but occasionally a second application may be needed after one week. When *Insecticide, Powder, Dusting, 1 per cent Lindane,* is used, repeat treatment at one and two weeks, observing the same precautions that were pointed out in the section on head lice.

*b.* Whenever it is practicable mass delousing should also be accompanied by cleansing of the people and disinfestation of clothing, towels, bedding and equipment.

*c.* Disinfestation of clothing, towels, bedding and equipment.

(1) In areas where lice are not resistant to DDT this can readily be done by thoroughly spraying the articles with 5 per cent DDT in kerosene or a 2 per cent DDT emulsion. The residual effect of DDT is such that any lice that emerge from eggs will be killed and the articles will contain a dosage of DDT that will be toxic to lice for about one month if the DDT is not removed sooner by laundering. *Insecticide, Powder, 10 per cent DDT,* may also be used for this purpose. In areas where DDT resistance is encountered, *Insecticide, Powder, Dusting, 1 per cent Lindane* or a 1 per cent lindane emulsion may be used. The articles should be retreated at one and two weeks.

(2) Dry heat at 140° F. for 20 minutes kills all lice and nits. Exposure for 1 minute at 159° F. is equally effective. This method is not harmful to any materials but woolens. A hot iron is very adequate in disposing of the lice where only a few garments are involved.

(3) Hot water at 150° F. for five minutes will kill all stages of lice. Such treatment, however, may not be used for webbing, rubber, felt or leather goods. Woolens are liable to undue shrinkage, unless especially handled.

(4) Live steam at 259° F. for 10 minutes kills both eggs and

lice, but steam under pressure at 267° F. is preferable since it has better penetrating power. Equipment may range from elaborate steam chambers mounted on railway cars to the primitive but very effective "Serbian barrel." Again, woolens, leather, rubber, felt and webbing are subject to damage by such procedure.

(5) Chemical treatment is usually reserved for materials which might be damaged by other methods. Immersion in a 2 per cent solution of cresol for 30 minutes at 100° F. is an effective procedure. Washing in a 5 per cent solution may be substituted if time is limited.

The impregnation of garments by immersing them in a 2 per cent emulsion of DDT gives excellent results for almost all types of clothing and equipment. Fabrics so treated may be laundered repeatedly and still remain immune from infestation for several weeks.

(6) Fumigation of clothing may be accomplished by use of methyl bromide, carbon bisulfide or hydrocyanic acid gas. Methyl bromide is the fumigant of choice. Carbon bisulfide is highly inflammable and hydrocyanic acid gas is very poisonous to man, so for these reasons fumigation with these materials should be handled only by expert and experienced personnel. Methyl bromide may be employed either in a gas-tight fumigation vault for disinfesting large quantities of clothing or in small, sealed units for disinfesting a limited quantity of clothing. In the latter case a gas-proof bag is loosely filled with clothing and a glass capsule, about five inches long, containing the fumigant, is placed in a pocket inside the bag. The mouth of the bag is tightly closed and the capsule is broken by pressure from the outside. After an interval of 20 to 45 minutes (depending on the temperature) the bag is opened and the clothing is removed. The clothing should be aired for at least 10 minutes before it is worn.

(7) Storage alone will free clothing of lice, as the active parasites all die if deprived of food for 10 days. A total of 30 days will take care of any that may have hatched during the period of storage. Exposure of clothing to the hot sun or to zero temperatures is also practiced, when climatic conditions permit.

*NOTE:* Disinfestation by heat as covered in (2), (3) and (4) above will also kill rickettsiae.

d. Barracks or other quarters may be fumigated, or sprayed (4 per cent cresol) while bedding and hangings should be treated in the same manner as clothing. For further discussion of control of insects in quarters, see Order HEMIPTERA, page 698.

## Order Hemiptera* *(True Bugs)*

The members of this order may be winged or wingless. The former species possess four wings, the first pair being thickened at the base, with membranous extremities, overlapping at the tip. The mouth parts are for piercing and sucking; the rather conspicuous beak which arises from the front of the head, lies against the ventral surface of the thorax when not in use. (In the closely related HOMOPTERA the beak arises from the posteroventral portion of the head.) The metamorphosis is of the gradual type.

This is a large order, containing some 30,000 described species. The great majority are feeders on plant juices but at least two families are of considerable medical importance: The CIMICIDAE or bedbugs are a great nuisance, and constitute a control problem in hotels, dormitories, barracks and many private homes; the family REDUVIIDAE (giant bedbugs, kissing bugs) include several species capable of transmitting South American trypanosomiasis (Chagas' disease). Members of at least seven other families occasionally inflict painful bites. These nine groups may be separated according to the key on page 697.

### Family Cimicidae *(Bedbugs)*

**Life History and Feeding Habits, Including Effect of Bites**    Bedbugs are intimate associates of man wherever unhygienic conditions prevail. They inhabit his houses, barracks and other abodes, secreting themselves in crevices of walls, floors and furniture. They are flattened insects with an oval contour and a reddish color. Despite their ungainly appearance they can run at fair speed.

Adult bedbugs are about a quarter of an inch in length. They are wingless in all stages. Their piercing and sucking proboscis, when not in use, is carried flexed upon the ventral surface of the head and thorax.

Bedbugs feed on man only periodically, usually at night. Engorgement seldom requires more than ten to fifteen minutes. After their meal the insects return to their hiding places. The bites may become erythematous and swollen and are sometimes characterized by severe and prolonged itching. Scratching may result in secondary infection. These insects have been experimentally incriminated as carriers of human disease, but there is no direct evidence that either their biting or their feces transmits infection from man to man under natural conditions. It may be pointed out that bedbugs rarely pass feces while feeding.

Fertilized female bedbugs deposit their operculated eggs singly, gluing them to solid supports in the crannies which harbor the insects by day. A single female may deposit over 500 eggs in batches of ten

* The Order HEMIPTERA is sometimes used to include also the HOMOPTERA (plant lice, cicadas, and other plant feeders). When such a classification is adopted the *true bugs* are referred to the Suborder HETEROPTERA.

to sixty over a period of several months. The average is probably near 200. The eggs require about a week for development, longer if the temperature is low. Newly hatched bedbugs resemble adults in miniature and are therefore known as nymphs. In case human hosts

*Table 60   Key to Families of* Hemiptera *Biting Man*

| 1 | (4) | Antennae shorter than the head, usually hidden in a cavity beneath the eyes. All species aquatic . . . . . . 2 |
|---|---|---|
| 2 | (3) | Hind tarsi bearing distinct claws. Membranous portion of fore wing with distinct veins. Ocelli never present <br> Belostomatidae (giant water bugs) |
| 3 | (2) | Hind tarsi with bristle-like claws. Head inserted deeply into prothorax . . . Notonectidae (back swimmers) |
| 4 | (1) | Antennae as long as the head, usually free and composed of four segments . . . . . . . . . . . . . . . . . . . . . . . 5 |
| 5 | (10) | Beak composed of three segments . . . . . . . . . . . . . . . 6 |
| 6 | (7) | Fore wing without an embolium (elongate costal area). If fore wing is vestigial, ocelli are present <br> Reduviidae (kissing bug family) |
| 7 | (6) | Fore wing usually with a well developed embolium, in which case ocelli are present. (If embolium is vestigial, ocelli are absent.) . . . . . . . . . . . . . . . . . . . . . . 8 |
| 8 | (9) | Fore wings lacking or vestigial; confirmed blood suckers— . . . . . . . . . . . . . . . . . . . . Cimicidae  (bedbugs) |
| 9 | (8) | Fore wings usually well developed; normally plant feeders . . . . . . . . . . . Anthocoridae (flower bugs) |
| 10 | (5) | Beak composed of four segments . . . . . . . . . . . . . . . . .11 |
| 11 | (16) | Front legs normal, fitted for walking . . . . . . . . . . . . .12 |
| 12 | (13) | Ocelli usually present; no transverse incision anterior to ocelli; membrane of fore wing with 4 or 5 simple veins . . . . . . . . . . . Lygaeidae (chinch bugs, etc.) |
| 13 | (12) | Ocelli invariably absent. Wing pattern variable . . . . .14 |
| 14 | (15) | Body exceedingly flat . . . . . . Aradidae (fungus bugs) |
| 15 | (14) | Body contour not especially flattened <br> Pyrochorridae (cotton stainer bugs) |
| 16 | (11) | Front legs fitted for grasping prey, the foretibiae being armed with strong spines . . Nabidae (damsel bugs) |

are not available, bedbugs will readily feed on other mammals. The normal life span is from six to eight months.

Two common species of bedbug infest man: *Cimex lectularius* Linn. in most temperate regions and *C. hemipterus* (Fabr.) in the tropics, especially Asia. These species are almost identical in appearance. Closely related forms attend other warm-blooded vertebrates such as bats, but these very rarely attack man. Bat bedbugs *(Cimex pilosellus* [Horvath]) are easy to recognize by reason of the abundant hair on the body. In New Guinea man is attacked by still another species, *Leptocimex boueti* (Brumpt), whose long antennae and long legs (especially the last pair) distinguish it from related forms (Fig. 287).

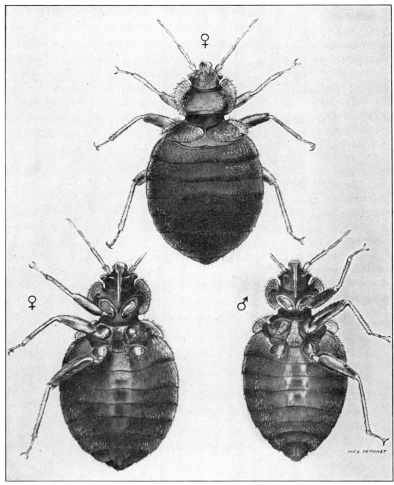

Fig. 287. Bedbug, *Cimex lectularius.* (Courtesy National Institutes of Health, U. S. Public Health Service.)

**Control**   DDT (dichloro-diphenyl-trichloroethane) is by far the most desirable of all insecticides recommended for the control of bedbugs. Mattresses treated with this substance remain free from bedbugs for sixty days or more. (See Table 69, p. 748.)

The most practicable procedure for army barracks is the spraying of beds and mattresses with a 5 to 10 per cent preparation of DDT in kerosene. Fourteen pounds in thirty-five gallons serve very well. A paint pressure outfit, operated by gas engine (or hand pump) is preferable to small equipment, as the latter wastes and spills. Best results are obtained if windows are closed during the work, operators being provided with respirator masks. One quart of spray should treat five units, a unit consisting of one bed and one mattress. The men may return to quarters as soon as treatment is completed. Rubber hose, used for dispensing the spray, should be thoroughly cleansed with soap and hot water to prevent deterioration.

Fumigation with hydrocyanic acid gas still remains an effective control procedure. It should not be undertaken save by experienced personnel. One pound of sodium cyanide is usually sufficient for 1000 cubic feet of air space.

A less dangerous fumigation may be carried out by burning sulfur, 2 pounds to 1000 cubic feet of air space. Metal objects likely to tarnish from sulfur fumes should be removed.

Where fumigation is impracticable, superheating of the room to 125° F. will be found effective. The high temperature should be maintained for ten to twelve hours, or until the heat has had opportunity to penetrate into all likely hiding places of the insects.

The use of ordinary sprays is effective only where the insecticide may be brought into direct contact with all stages of the pest. Light oil sprays containing pyrethrum are preferred. Repeated applications are usually necessary.

### Family Reduviidae (Kissing Bugs)

*Life History and Feeding Habits—Relation to Chagas' Disease* This family includes well over three thousand species, rather widely distributed. The majority feed on the blood of insects, a habit which has given them the name "assassin bugs." At least 75, however, feed on the blood of mammals, including man. Certain of these are responsible for the transmission in South and Central America of *Trypanosoma cruzi*, the causative agent of Chagas' disease. Several species of bugs may serve as vectors, notably *Panstrongylus megistus* Pinto. The opossum and armadillo are favorite hosts of this species. The bloodsucking reduviids are sometimes treated as a separate family, the "Triatomidae" (Fig. 288).

*Panstrongylus megistus.* This species is large, averaging 30 mm. in length, and may be recognized by the bright red spots on the thorax, at the base of the wings and on the lateral margins of the abdominal segments.

Both adults and nymphs hide during the day, emerging at night to seek their blood meal. In attacking human hosts they bite the cheeks by preference, near the eye, hence the common name, "barbeiros." Less commonly the angle of the mouth is the site of attack. The trypanosomes which are passed in the bug's feces may enter the puncture wound after the bug has fed, but the bite itself is probably not infective.

The females deposit their eggs, which are about 2 mm. in length, in various hiding places where they undergo incubation for approximately 20 days. Each female lays close to 200 eggs. The nymphs, which molt 5 times, develop over a period of nearly a year, and the adults live for a year or more after attaining maturity.

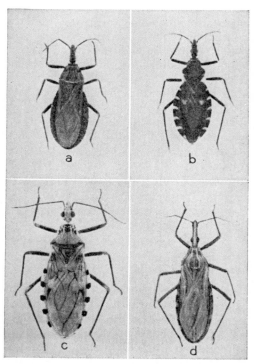

Fig. 288. Four species of REDUVIIDAE. (a) *Triatoma protracta.* (b) *Triatoma sanguisuga.* (c) *Panstrongylus geniculatus.* (d) *Mestor pallescens.* (Herms: Medical Entomology, by permission of The Macmillan Company.)

**Symptoms of the Bite**    In the case of *P. megistus* the symptoms are negligible, unless secondary infection occurs. Considerable edema about the eye (Romana's sign) is usually associated with the early stages of Chagas' disease, but this is due to the presence of the trypanosomes and not to the bite of the insect. Certain other reduviids, however, especially *Reduvius personatus* Linn, have been known to cause nausea, palpitation and generalized urticaria by their bites.

**Control**    Fumigation is feasible if the room or house may be sealed so as to prevent the strong flying adults from leaving. The reduction or elimination of the hiding places of the bug is also important. The use of bed nets is relatively ineffective, since the younger nymphal stages pass through the mesh at will. However, tests with Gammexane indicate that it is highly effective in controlling the reduviid population when used as a residual spray.

**Other Vectors and Potential Vectors** The first of the accompanying tables (Table 61) lists various species believed to be capable of

*Table 61 Reduviid Bugs Reported as Vectors of* Trypanosoma cruzi *Mexico, Central and South America*

| LOCATION | SPECIES OF BUG |
|---|---|
| Mexico | *Triatoma sanguisuga* (LeConte), *Rhodnius prolixus* Stal |
| Guatamala | *Triatoma dimidiata* (Latr.) |
| Panama | *Eratyrus cuspidatus* Stal, *Rhodnius pallescens* Barber, *R. prolixus* Stal, *Panstrongylus geniculatus* (Latr.), *Triatoma dimidiata* (Latr.) |
| Argentina | *Eutriatoma sordida* Pinto, *Psammolestes coreodes* Berg., *Triatoma infestans* (Klug) |
| Bolivia | *Eutriatoma sordida* Pinto, *Triatoma infestans* (Klug) |
| Brazil | *Panstrongylus megistus* Pinto, *Triatoma brasiliensis* Neiva, *Eutriatoma sordida* Pinto, *Triatoma chagasi* Brumpt and Gomez, *Triatoma vitticeps* (Stal) |
| Chili | *Mepraia spinalai* Porter, *Triatoma infestans* (Klug) |
| Colombia | *Rhodnius prolixus* Stal, *R. pictipes* Stal |
| Paraguay | *Eutriatoma sordida* Pinto |
| Uruguay | *Eutriatoma sordida* Pinto, *Triatoma infestans* (Klug) |
| Venezuela | *Eratyrus cuspidatus* Stal, *Eutriatoma nigromaculatus* (Stal), *Panstrongylus rufotuberculatus* (Champ.), *Psammolestes arthuri* (Pinto), *Psammolestes geniculatus* (Latr.), *Rhodnius prolixus* Stal |

*Table 62 Reduviid Bugs Naturally Infected with* Trypanosoma cruzi *(U.S.A.)*

| SPECIES | GEOGRAPHIC LOCATION | HOST ANIMALS OR HIDING PLACES |
|---|---|---|
| *Triatoma protracta* (Uhler) | New Mexico California | *Neotoma* (wood rats) |
| *Triatoma uhleri* Neiva | Arizona California | *Neotoma* |
| *Triatoma gerstakeri* (Stal) | Texas | *Neotoma* |
| *Triatoma heidmanni* Neiva | Texas | Dwellings—bedding |
| *Triatoma longipes* Barber | Arizona | Sleeping bags |
| *Triatoma protracta woodi* Usinger | New Mexico | *Neotoma* |
| *Triatoma ambigua* Neiva | Texas | *Neotoma* |
| *Triatoma sanguisuga* (LeConte) | Texas | *Neotoma* |

transmitting Chagas' disease in the areas where that disease exists (Mexico, Central and South America). It should be mentioned that *Triatoma infestans* (Klug) has recently gained considerable prominence as a vector in those countries where it occurs. The second (Table 62) tabulates those species which have been found naturally infected with *Trypanosoma cruzi* within the boundaries of the United States, where as yet no naturally infected cases of human trypanosomiasis have been found, though cases have been produced experimentally.

## Order Coleoptera (Beetles)

Typical beetles have two pairs of wings, the first of which are modified to function as wing covers and are called *elytra*. In most species the elytra are hard and horny and meet in a straight line down the back, but certain medically important species are exceptional in this respect. The second pair of wings, which are folded beneath the elytra when not in use, are usually membranous in character and when expanded constitute effective organs of flight. The mouth parts are adapted for chewing. The metamorphosis is complete (egg, larva, pupa, adult).

This is the largest order of insects (250,000 species) and its species are very widely distributed in all continents. Although much less important from a medical point of view than certain other orders (DIPTERA, ANOPLURA), COLEOPTERA affect the health of man in at least four different ways: (1) by vesicating and poisonous effects; (2) as parasitic larvae (canthariasis); (3) as hosts of helminth parasites; (4) by mechanical transmission of infective organisms.

### Vesicating and Poisonous Effects

Beetles of the Family MELOIDAE contain in their body fluids a cryptotoxic principle which, if rubbed upon the skin, has marked blistering effects. Accidental crushing of the beetles in the field may thus lead to a vesicular dermatitis with perhaps no knowledge on the part of the victim as to how or when the condition was acquired. The absence of a central puncture wound, however, will usually enable the physician to differentiate between this condition and an ordinary insect bite. The urticating principle, cantharidin, has long been used in medicine, either as a blistering agent or as a stimulant to the genital and urinary organs, under the name of "Spanish fly."

Another family, the STAPHYLINIDAE (rove beetles), also contains forms with vesicating properties. Medically important forms occur in the Orient in Java, in tropical South and East Africa and South America. The irritating substance which they produce is *not* cantharidin, though somewhat similar in its pharmacologic effect. A peculiarity of staphylinid poison is that the blistering does not occur until a day or two after contact.

A blistering effect has been reported from Southeast Africa as a result of contact with a night flying beetle of the family PAUSSIDAE, which secretes a highly acid liquid substance. Also in certain islands of the Pacific, at least two species of *Sessinia* (coconut beetles) of the Family OEDEMERIDAE are reputed to cause burning pain at the point of contact, followed by a large but relatively harmless blister.

Recent work indicates that various species of *Eobia* (OEDEMERIDAE) may cause inflammation of the skin.

A quite different example of urtication is found in the small flour beetle, *Tribolium confusum*, which gives off a gaseous substance irritating to the eyes and nasal membranes.

### Canthariasis

Infection of man by beetles at any stage of their life cycle is known as canthariasis. Intestinal, urinary, ocular, nasal and cutaneous varieties have been recorded. The condition is rare, as it follows the accidental entrance of eggs, larvae or adults into the human body. An intense diarrhea among children in Ceylon is believed to be due to intestinal canthariasis.

### Beetles as Hosts to Helminth Parasites

Various species belonging to different families are known to harbor cysticercoids of the rat tapeworm, *Hymenolepis diminuta*. Other species serve as intermediate hosts of various ACANTHOCEPHALA and nematodes.

### Mechanical Transmission of Micro-organisms by Scavenger Beetles

*Adults* of STAPHYLINIDAE (rove beetles), SILPHIDAE (carrion beetles) and HISTERIDAE all feed upon dead animal matter of one form or another. They may thus convey infection (1) upon their bodies, legs or mouthparts or (2) by way of the alimentary tract. Species of DERMESTIDAE feed on such material chiefly in the larval stage. Anthrax bacilli have been found in the feces of *Dermestes vulpinus* F. which had developed to maturity on skins of animals known to have had the disease.

***Treatment of Injury from Blister Beetles*** There is no drug known which acts as a specific in counteracting this effect. Soothing antiseptic lotions of a mild alkaline nature, with a dry dressing, are usually recommended. A saturated solution of magnesium sulfate applied as a cold compress has been found effective in treating the condition known as "Nairobi eye," an East African conjunctivitis caused by juices of crushed beetles being accidentally rubbed into the eye.

***Prophylaxis*** Prophylactic measures fall under three heads:

1. Avoid handling the beetles and especially avoid crushing them against the skin.

2. Apply a stomach poison to the vegetation on which the beetles are feeding. Calcium arsenate or arsenate of lead (one ounce to a gallon of water) is recommended (should not be used on delicate plants).

3. If the beetles are very numerous on a valuable forage crop, such as clover or alfalfa, the best control is to go over the field with a hopperdozer, as used for catching grasshoppers. U. S. Department of Agriculture pamphlets (such as Farmers Bulletin 747) give adequate instructions for such procedure.

## Order Lepidoptera *(Butterflies and Moths)*

Species in this order are characterized by the presence of numerous scales (modified hairs) on the body and wings and by the nature of their mouth parts, which are in the form of a sucking tube, coiled beneath the head when not in use. Except for a few wingless forms, two pairs of wings are present. The metamorphosis is complete. Their larvae, which are called caterpillars, may be either smooth and wormlike, or thickly covered with hairs, according to the species concerned. Most moths pupate inside of a silken covering, termed the cocoon, spun by the larva just prior to transformation.

The order is of minor significance from a medical point of view; nevertheless, as with the beetles, certain important medical relationships exist.

### Urticating Hairs

There are several groups of caterpillars which bear hairs capable of irritating the skin and mucous membranes. These may be rather simple bristles or heavy hollowed spines but all are associated with poison-secreting cells or glands. Persons coming into direct contact with such caterpillars are pierced by the hairs or fragments thereof with resultant urticating effects. The more slender types of hair may occasionally become detached and be of annoyance following their transport by the wind.

**Symptoms of Poisoning by Caterpillar Hairs**   The exact nature of caterpillar poison is unknown. Browntail caterpillar venom causes crenation of red blood cells, is soluble in alkalies and may be inactivated by exposure to a temperature of 115° C. Increased susceptibility rather than immunity appears to result from repeated exposure.

In the United States the "puss caterpillar" (*Megalopyge opercularis* S.&A.) is by far the most important species. In certain parts of Texas thousands of cases of dermatitis have been known to occur in a single season, and public schools have been closed because of its abundance on playgrounds.

There is at first an intense, burning pain, followed by an itching which may last as long as twelve hours. The affected area develops whitish papules which soon become red. There may be nausea and fever, with numbness and swelling of the part affected. In rare cases symptoms may be alarming. Paralysis may ensue, particularly if the stings are received in the region of the neck. Severe symptoms may persist for as long as six days.

The hairs of the browntail moth caterpillar, *Euproctis phaeorrhoea* (Don) produce a severe dermatitis but do not, as a rule, cause systemic symptoms. Necrosis of epidermal cells, the formation of vesicles and perivascular inflammation in the corium constitute the characteristic pathology of "browntail rash."

Windblown hairs of various species have been known to cause a painful, nodular conjunctivitis (*ophthalmia nodosa*). As many as twenty-seven nodules have been excised from the eye of a child, most of which proved on microscopic examination to contain urticating hairs.

**Treatment**    Alkaline compresses may be used to give a measure of relief. Local applications of warm ammonia water or baking soda are recommended. Camphophenique, a proprietary mixture, seems to be reasonably satisfactory. A special formula composed of carbolic acid, 2 ml., zinc oxide, 15 gm., and limewater, 240 ml. is probably the best available. The mixture should be shaken thoroughly and rubbed into the affected parts. A natural remedy, consisting of the freshly crushed leaves of the garden purslane (*Portulaca oleracea* L.) is definitely useful for the relief of pain.

Supportive treatment is sometimes necessary. If secondary infection occurs appropriate treatment should be instituted.

**Prophylaxis and Control**    All bedding and clothing contaminated with the hairs should be washed. Caterpillars may be destroyed by spraying trees and shrubs with a mixture of arsenate of lead, 7 lbs. to 150 gallons, and dehydrated lime (4 lbs). This concentration is needed to kill the caterpillars quickly, otherwise they crawl about a great deal before death, shedding hairs wherever they may go. Workmen engaged in control work should wear protective goggles.

### Scholeciasis

This is the term applied to the very rare condition in which lepidopterous larvae sometimes manage to survive in the alimentary canal. The most authentic record relates to a case of poisoning from ingesting the larva of *Pieris brassicae* (cabbage worm) with raw cabbage.

### Lepidoptera as Hosts of Helminth Parasites

The rat tapeworm *Hymenolepis diminuta* (Rudolphi) may pass its cystericercus stage in several species of Microlepidoptera.

## Order Diptera

This is the most important order of insects from a medical point of view. Malaria, yellow fever, dengue, kala-azar, oriental sore, espundia. African sleeping sickness, several types of filariasis, Carrión's disease, pappataci fever and certain of the encephalitides are transmitted by dipterous vectors. In addition, cholera, typhoid, amebiasis, bacillary dysentery and various diarrheas, also conjunctivitis and occasionally trachoma are distributed by the activities of flies.

For an account of the medically important Diptera by families see Chapter 72, p. 714.

## Order Siphonaptera (Fleas)

Fleas are laterally compressed, highly chitinized and sclerotized, small, wingless, bloodsucking ectoparasites of mammals and birds. The common species vary from 1.5 to 4 mm. in length.

The mouth parts are adapted for piercing and sucking and the powerful long legs for jumping. The impregnated chigoe flea is exceptional in that it burrows into the skin and is largely sessile.

The head bears, in addition to mouth parts, inconspicuous annulated antennae which normally lie in grooves. The eyes are simple, when present.

The thorax is divided into three segments and the abdomen is variously stated to consist of ten to twelve. Both present a series of chitinized plates, the *sclerites*. The dorsal plates are known as *tergites*, the lateral as *pleurites* and the ventral as *sternites*.

The *ctenidia*, or combs, bold backward-pointing rows of spines, are characteristic structures, the genal comb being just above the mouth parts and the pronotal comb dorsally on the first thoracic segment. Their presence or absence in either location or both locations is important in classification.

Other taxonomic characters are the shape of the head, the cranial grooves, the male terminalia, the receptaculum seminis in the female, and the location and arrangement of certain bristles, spinelets and spurs (Fig. 289).

**Life History** Flea eggs are glistening white and are deposited *dry* among the hairs of the host or in the nest. The developing embryo is provided with a sharp spine on the head by means of which the eggshell is shredded and the embryo liberated. The larvae are thirteen-segmented maggots with biting mouth parts. They feed chiefly on feces of adult fleas and of rodents. There are three larval instars. At the end of the feeding period the larva spins a cocoon and pupates. The length of the pupal stage is, to a considerable extent, determined by the existing temperature. The time required for completion of the entire life cycle varies from about three weeks to several months.

Some species may live for several months without feeding, thus enabling them to act as "preservers" of *Pasteurella pestis* in the prolonged intervals between blood meals.

There are more than 800 described species of fleas. These are grouped in six or more families of which the Pulicidae, Dolicho-

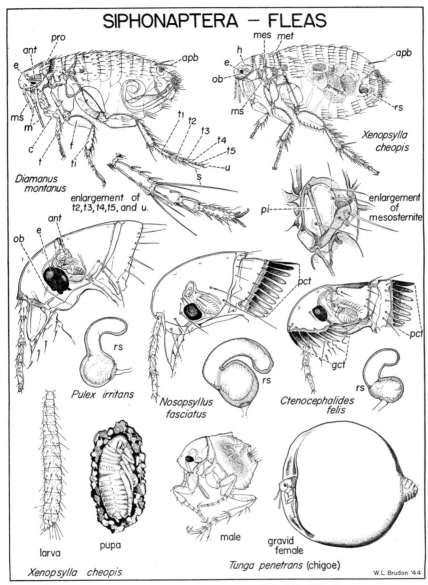

## SIPHONAPTERA – FLEAS

*Diamanus montanus*

enlargement of *t2, t3, t4, t5,* and *u.*

*Xenopsylla cheopis*

enlargement of mesosternite

*Pulex irritans*

*Nosopsyllus fasciatus*

*Ctenocephalides felis*

larva

pupa

*Xenopsylla cheopis*

male

gravid female

*Tunga penetrans* (chigoe)

W.L.Brudon '44

Fig. 289. SIPHONAPTERA: certain characters used in identification. *ant*, antenna; *apb*, antepygidial bristle; *c*, coxa; *e*, eye; *f*, femur; *gct*, genal ctenidium; *h*, head; *m*, mouth parts; *ms*, maxillary palpus; *mes*, mesothorax; *met*, methathorax; *ms*, mesosternite; *ob*, ocular bristle; *pct*, pronotal ctenidium; *pi*, perpendicular incrassation of mesosternite; *pro*, pronotum; *rs*, receptaculum seminis; *s*, spine at tip of second tarsus; *t*, trochanter; *ti*, tibia; *t1* to *t5*, tarsus 1, 2, 3, 4, 5; *u*, ungues.

PSYLLIDAE and HECTOPSYLLIDAE are of special medical importance (Table 63).

The family PULICIDAE contains *Ctenocephalides felis* (Bouché) and *C. canis* (Curtis), the cat and dog fleas respectively; *Pulex irritans* (Linn.), the human flea; several species of *Xenopsylla;* and a ground squirrel flea, *Hoplopsyllus anomalus* (Baker).

*Table 63   Key to the Families of* SIPHONAPTERA*

| | | | |
|---|---|---|---|
| 1 | (2) | The three thoracic tergites together longer than the first abdominal tergite | 3 |
| 2 | (1) | The three thoracic tergites together shorter than the first abdominal tergite | HECTOPSYLLIDAE |
| 3 | (4) | No vertical suture from dorsal margin of head to bases of antennae; frontal region almost evenly rounded along margin | 5 |
| 4 | (3) | A vertical suture passing upward from the bases of the antennae to the dorsal margin of head; margin of frontal region usually most strongly curved at vertex | 7 |
| 5 | (6) | Abdominal tergites with but a single row of setae | PULICIDAE |
| 6 | (5) | Abdominal tergites with at least two rows of setae | DOLICHOPSYLLIDAE |
| 7 | (8) | Head without a pair of dark anteroventral flaps on each side | 9 |
| 8 | (7) | Head with a pair of dark anteroventral flaps on each side | ISCHNOPSYLLIDAE |
| 9 | (10) | Occipital region without dorsal incrassation; frontal region entire | HYSTRICHOPSYLLIDAE |
| 10 | (9) | Occipital region with dorsal incrassation; frontal region divided, the anterior part bearing a border of spines | MACROPSYLLIDAE |

* From Herms, Medical Entomology, 3rd ed. Macmillan, 1943. (Modified by Stewart after Ewing.)

*Ctenocephalides felis* and *C. canis* are almost cosmopolitan. In both species, genal and pronotal combs are present. The genal comb consists of eight spines and the pronotal of sixteen. *Pulex irritans* has been reported from all of the major zoographical regions but is absent from some large cities and present in some sparsely populated areas. *Xenopsylla cheopis* is widely disseminated in many countries. It has been recorded from nineteen of the United States and has become established as far north as Michigan and Minnesota. *Pulex irritans* and *X. cheopis* are similar in that they both lack genal and pronotal combs. However, in *X. cheopis* there is one rod-like thickening of the mesosternite extending anterodorsally and another extending nearly perpendicularly. In *P. irritans* the perpendicular rod is absent. In addition, the ocular bristle of *X. cheopis* arises in front of and just above the middle of the eye, while in *P. irritans* it arises near the lower anterior margin. Other important species of *Xenopsylla* are *X. brasiliensis, X. eridos, X. nubicus, X. piriei* and *X. astia*, all of which are implicated in plague transmission.

The family DOLICHOPSYLLIDAE contains medically important species of several genera. Among these are a ground squirrel flea, *Diamanus montanus* (Baker); the temperate zone rat flea, *Nosopsyllus fasciatus* (Bosc); the South American cavy flea, *Rhopalopsyllus cavicola* (Weyenb.); and two rodent fleas from the Russian steppes and Manchuria, *Ceratophyllus tesquorum* (Wagner) and *Oropsylla silantiewi* (Wagner) respectively. All are vectors of *P. pestis* among rodents and *N. fasciatus* is also a vector of murine typhus among rats.

The family HECTOPSYLLIDAE is represented by two important genera, *Echidnophaga* Olliff and *Tunga* Jarocki.

*Echidnophaga gallinacea* (Westwood) the stick-tight flea, is widely distributed in tropical and subtropical regions, including Australia. In the United States it has been listed from twenty-two states and is reported as permanently established as far north as Virginia and Kansas. It is a serious pest of poultry in the south and attacks many species of vertebrates including dogs, cats, rats and man. When feeding, the female attaches firmly to its host. Thus rats and wild birds may function in its dispersal far beyond its normal range. Although it is reported as relatively rare on rats in the United States it is said to occur in large numbers on rats in Madagascar. *Pasteurella pestis* has been recovered from these fleas taken from the burrowing owl, *Speotyto cunicularia*, in the western states.

*Tunga penetrans* (Linn.), the burrowing flea, is widely distributed in the tropical regions of America and Africa. It is commonly known as the jigger, sand flea, or chigoe. In Latin America it is also known as *nigua* and *bicho do pê*.

The fertilized female burrows into the skin of the feet, often beneath the nail, or in other parts of the body, where its abdomen becomes greatly distended by blood and developing eggs. There is intense itching and inflammation, and not uncommonly secondary infection. In Central America tetanus and gas gangrene frequently occur. Over a four-year period 250 deaths from tetanus were reported in Costa Rica. Auto-amputation of the toes has been attributed to infestation with this flea in Angola (Fig. 290).

Surgical removal of the intact flea is recommended. This consists of slightly enlarging the entrance hole of the flea by the use of a sterile needle, followed by gentle pressure on the sides of the aperture. The entire flea is thus forced out. The wound is then cleansed and an antiseptic dressing applied. On the other hand, excellent results are reported from the use of an initial Lysol bath, followed by puncturing each flea with a needle. A second Lysol bath kills the liberated eggs and sterilizes the wound. Five other species of *Tunga* are known, one of which appears in Brazil and one in China.

**Relation to Disease**   Fleas serve as vectors of the rickettsiae of murine typhus from rat to rat and from rat to man. They are reservoirs, "preservers," of *Pasteurella pestis* and transmit this organism from rat to rat, rat to man, and man to man; and in sylvatic plague from wild rodent to wild rodent, from wild rodent to rat, and from both to man. They are also intermediate hosts of several tapeworms.

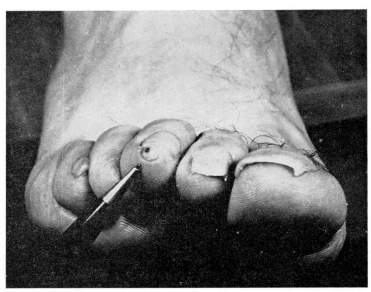

Fig. 290. Chigoe flea, *Tunga penetrans*, embedded in characteristic position below nail. (Courtesy Dr. T. H. G. Aitken.)

The bites of some fleas are extremely annoying and result in a dermatitis. The burrowing chigoe flea frequently affords entrance to pathogenic bacteria, as already pointed out.

Although the flea fauna is, to some extent, characteristic for certain hosts, host-specificity is not marked. The fleas that most frequently bite man are said to be *Ctenocephalides canis* (Curt.), *Ctenocephalides felis* (Bouché), the dog and cat fleas respectively, and *Pulex irritans* Linn., which is a common parasite also of swine and prairie dogs (*Cynomys*). *Xenopsylla cheopis* (Roth) and *Nosopsyllus fasciatus* (Bosc) are typically parasites of rats. Both are widespread and the former bites man readily. On the other hand, *Diamanus montanus* (Baker) and *Hoplopsyllus anomalus* (Baker) are parasites of certain ground squirrels. Neither is reported as a frequent parasite of man, but an interchange of parasites between rats and ground squirrels is not uncommon.

Intensive studies in widely separated endemic areas have served to amplify rather than simplify the already complex ecology of sylvatic plague. In the western United States thirty species of rodents and two species of lagomorphs have been found plague-infected, and more than thirty species of fleas are capable of harboring *Pasteurella pestis*. Of the two species of fleas most frequently found on the ground squirrel, *Citellus beecheyi beecheyi*, *Diamanus montanus* is by far the more efficient vector. This flea has also been recovered from pack rats (*Neotoma*), prairie dogs (*Cynomys*), tree squirrels (*Tamiasciurus*), rock squirrels (*Citellus*), ground hogs (*Marmota*), and from *Rattus norvegicus* and *Rattus rattus alexandrinus*. *Xenopsylla cheopis* (Roth.), the common vector in classic plague, has also been recovered from Beechey ground squirrels. The stick-tight flea, *Echidnophaga gallinacea* (West.), with a wide variety of hosts including the burrowing owl, *Speotyto cunicularia*, has been found naturally infected.

*Opisocrostis bruneri* (Baker) and *Thrassis bacchi* (Roth.), recorded from several species of squirrels, have been recently demonstrated as efficient vectors. In South Africa *Xenopsylla eridos* Roth. is considered the chief vector. Although *X. cheopis* is present in Kenya, Uganda and Nigeria, *X. brasiliensis* (Baker), often designated as "the flea of the hut," is the most important vector to man in these areas. In central Asia, *Oropsylla silantiewi* (Wagner), the tarbagan (*Arctomys bobac*) flea, and in the Russian steppes *Ceratophyllus tesquorum* (Wagner), the suslik (*Citellus*) flea, and *Neopsylla setosa* Wagner have been incriminated. In Argentina and Ecuador *Rhopalopsyllus cavicola* (Weyenb.) is reported as a vector among cavies. During epidemics *Pulex irritans* Linn., *Ctenocephalides canis* (Curt) and *C. felis* (Bouché) may function as vectors from man to man.

On epidemiologic grounds, *P. irritans* was under suspicion as the vector in the Paris epidemic (1921). On similar grounds it has been indicated as a vector in the mountainous regions of Ecuador where *X. cheopis* does not occur. In some areas in the western United States, the prairie dog (*Cynomys* spp.), a natural host of this flea, constitutes an important rodent reservoir.

*Xenopsylla cheopis* is considered the most common flea vector of murine typhus.

## Order Hymenoptera

This order includes the bees, wasps, and ants. Except for certain wingless forms, these insects are characterized by the presence of four membranous wings, the anterior and posterior wings of the same side being held together by a row of fine hooks termed hamuli. The mouth parts are formed for chewing or for both chewing and sucking, but never for sucking blood. The abdomen in the female is usually provided with a sting, piercer or saw. The metamorphosis is complete (egg, larva, pupa, adult).

Hymenoptera are of medical interest for two reasons: (1) the poisonous effects of their stings; (2) as mechanical vectors of parasites (of very slight importance).

### The Poisonous Effects of Stings

The sting of the female hymenopteron is really a modified ovipositor, composed (in the honeybee) of a central *shaft*, two lateral lancets or *darts* and two finger-like *sting-palpi*. The darts are provided with sharp, recurved teeth.

In most species the poison glands are of two types. The acid-secreting gland, a paired structure, produces a toxin which is capable of paralyzing other insects but which cannot, alone, cause their death. Formic acid is known to constitute at least a portion of the material secreted. Those species which provision their nests with living prey have only this gland present.

The second gland, usually single, produces an altogether different substance, alkaline in nature. Like the acid secretion, this substance is only mildly irritating in itself but when the two are combined, as occurs at the time of the sting, typical and painful symptoms ensue. In cases when the stinger remains in the wound the muscles continue to contract for some minutes, thereby forcing the shaft deeper into the subcutaneous tissue and causing a greater amount of poison to be discharged.

Local swelling is always characteristic and especially so if the sting should be in the vicinity of the eye or mouth. A sting on the tongue has been known to endanger life by reason of the great amount of collateral edema produced. Bee stings are rarely fatal to man; it is estimated that some 500 stings at or about the same time are necessary for a lethal dose of poison. In certain instances, however, individuals become sensitized, after which a single sting may produce alarming and occasionally fatal results, particularly if the venom is introduced directly into the blood stream.

The whole question of allergy in relation to bee venom is somewhat confused, since bees frequently carry various pollens and other substances, picked up while visiting flowers and other sources of food. These, rather than bee venom, may be responsible for the hay fever and asthmatic symptoms reported by persons handling hives, bee frames, honey or in other ways having contact with bees. Such facts argue for the utilization of whole bee extract rather than venom alone in desensitizing procedures.

There are nearly 5000 species of stinging bees.

The honeybee *Apis mellifica* falls in the Family APIDAE while bumble-bees (various species of *Bombus*) belong in the BOMBIDAE. Both, however, are included in the Superfamily APOIDEA. Unlike the honeybee, representatives of *Bombus* do not leave the stinging apparatus in the wound, but may withdraw and insert the stinger repeatedly. Certain South American bees are stingless but nevertheless cause great discomfort by biting and twisting with their mandibles. When aroused they tend to attack the scalp in large numbers. Some inject an irritating saliva at the point of the bite.

Besides the APOIDEA, the following five superfamilies of HYMENOPTERA contain stinging forms:

Certain of the FORMICOIDEA or true ants may possess dangerous stings; fire ants, harvester ants and numerous tropical species are to be avoided for this reason. The VESPOIDEA include wasps, hornets, yellow jackets, velvet ants, mud daubers and mason wasps; all are capable of stinging. Less often encountered are thread-waisted wasps of the insect-destroying SPHECOIDEA. The BETHYLOIDEA and ICHNEUMONOIDEA include various wasplike insects, most of them of little medical concern.

Due to the fact that the families and superfamies of HYMENOPTERA are separated only with considerable difficulty, it has not been deemed advisable to attempt a simplified key to the medically important groups.

**Treatment of Hymenopterous Stings**   1. If the sting remains in the tissue, as is usually the case with the worker honey-bee, it should be removed. This may be accomplished by gentle pressure and manipulation rather than by a direct grasping of the shaft, as the latter procedure will aways force more poison into the wound.

2. Apply a paste of water and bicarbonate of soda. The dressing should be replaced from time to time and treatment may be necessary for several hours. Eau de Javelle, 1 to 100, also calcium chloride in water, 1 to 60, have likewise been recommended. Ammonia is preferred by some to bicarbonate of soda. Carbolated petroleum jelly, a 2 per cent alcoholic solution of carbolic acid, ethereal menthol and iodine salve each has its advocates. Hot fomentations alone give genuine relief in many cases.

3. If the patient shows a marked degree of allergy (*anaphylaxis*), epinephrine should be administered immediately. In serious cases stimulants may be necessary.

4. A large fluid intake and catharsis are useful in hastening the elimination of the venom.

**Prophylaxis and Control**   Persons who have shown marked sensitivity to bee venom may be desensitized by use of whole bee extract (in Coca's solution) in small doses over an extended period of time. Fortunately, whole bee extract is more or less group specific, so that desensitization to many species of stinging HYMENOPTERA may be accomplished by a single course of treatment. Certain workers maintain that this is not a true desensitization, but an elevation of the threshold of immunity.

The wearing of white or light clothing when working around bees is very desirable. It is well known that black chickens, dogs and horses are stung much oftener on farms than animals of other colors.

The Mexican fire ant may be destroyed in nature by injecting a mixture of one part carbon bisulfide and three parts carbon tetrachloride into the opening of the nest and covering the aperture. An oil can with a long spout is a convenient tool. Kerosene is somewhat less effective. Similar measures may be employed in the case of ground-nesting wasps. Aerial (paper) nests, if large, may be enclosed in a bag at night and the bag and contents destroyed. Smaller paper nests and mud nests may be encompassed by use of a tin can with tight fitting lid. The site should then be daubed with creosote to repel future nest-makers.

### Mechanical Vectors of Parasites

It has been shown that at least one species of wasp, *Polistes gallicus* (Family VESPIDAE), may carry about on its wings, legs, body and mouthparts eggs of *Ascaris, Trichurus* and hookworms, also rhabditiform larvae. Undoubtedly any species which seeks food or moisture from situations in which parasite ova are found, may transport them to fruit and other human food.

# 72  The Order Diptera

The DIPTERA or true flies constitute the most important single order of insects from a medical standpoint. Almost every possible relationship to human disease is represented within the group. Some are external blood sucking parasites. Others develop as larvae within the human host. Dipterous species serve as vectors of protozoal, viral, bacterial and helminth diseases. Their vectorship is sometimes mechanical, sometimes cyclical, sometimes cyclico-propagative. The distribution of the group is world-wide, the larger number being found in warmer geographic regions.

*Characterization*  The winged members of the order have only two wings, borne by the mesothorax. The second pair of wings is represented merely by a pair of knobbed hairs, the *halteres* (see Fig. 292) which are believed to function in the maintenance of equilibrium. The mouthparts are always formed for sucking, but in comparatively few groups is there adaptation for piercing animal or human skin. The metamorphosis is complete. Of the 80,000 species of described DIPTERA a relatively small number are of medical interest. These few, however, are of tremendous importance in relation to human health.

*Classification*  It is convenient to consider the DIPTERA as falling into three suborders, the NEMATOCERA, BRACHYCERA and ATHERICERA (or CYCLORRHAPHA). The first two are frequently grouped together by classifiers as the ORTHORRHAPHA, or "straight seamed flies," the name referring to the manner in which the majority of the species emerge from the pupal skin. The name CYLORRHAPHA ("circular seamed flies") is equally significant. The three suborders may be easily differentiated (Table 64).

## Suborder Nematocera

These are the most primitive of the three groups. They include the mosquitoes, midges and many similar forms. Five families of NE-

*Table 64   Differentiation of Suborders of* DIPTERA

| SUBORDER | LARVA | PUPA | ADULT FLY |
|---|---|---|---|
| NEMATOCERA (ORTHORRHAPHA, in part) | With well developed, exserted head, and biting mandibles horizontally disposed. (In some species, mouthparts are vestigial) | Free (i.e., not enclosed in last larval skin). Adults escape by a straight or T-shaped longitudinal slit, or by a transverse slit between 7th and 8th abdominal segments | Antennae frequently longer than head and thorax; segments numerous and largely similar; arista wanting. No frontal lunule. Palpi pendulous, 4 or 5 segmented. Wing venation simple; discal cell generally absent; cubital cell (really first anal) when present, widely open |
| BRACHYCERA (ORTHORRHAPHA, concluded) | With head more or less incomplete and retractile, and with vertically biting mandibles, sometimes rudimentary | As above | Antennae variable, usually shorter than thorax; commonly of three segments, the last frequently subdivided into a number of small ringlike units. Palpi prorect, 1 or 2 segmented. Discal cell of wing usually present; cubital (1st anal) cell contracted or closed |
| ATHERICERA (CYCLORRHAPHA) | With head vestigial, mouth-parts usually reduced to simple hooks | Coarctate (i.e., enclosed within hardened larval skin). Adults escape through a circular split which releases an operculum at the anterior end | Antennae 3 segmented with an arista (usually dorsal) on segment 3. Frontal lunule present. Palpi one-segmented. Wing with discal cell usually present; cubital (1st anal) cell contracted or closed |

MATOCERA are concerned and in all five females suck blood. They may be separated as follows (Table 65):

### Table 65   Key to Important Families of NEMATOCERA

1  (8)   Wing with no indication of a fine network in addition to the veins ..................................... 2

2  (5)   Marginal vein not continued beyond the tip of the wing 3

3  (4)   Antennae longer than the thorax, of 14 segments, more or less bushy. Wings rather narrow, with setae but no scales .... CHIRONOMIDAE (including CERATOPOGONIDAE, formerly considered a subfamily of Chironomids)

4  (3)   Antennae shorter than the thorax, of 11 segments, not plumose. Wings broad, without scales or hairs
SIMULIIDAE (Black flies)

5  (2)   Marginal vein extending entirely around the wing. Second and fourth longitudinal veins forked .......... 6

6  (7)   Wings and body thickly covered with coarse hairs. Wings more or less spear-shaped with approximately parallel veins .. PSYCHODIDAE (Moth flies and sandflies)

7  (6)   Veins of the wing fringed with conspicuous scales. Wing tip rounded ............... CULICIDAE (Mosquitoes)

8  (1)   Wings marked by a net-work of fine lines in addition to the veins ..... BLEPHAROCERIDAE (Net-winged midges)

### Family Ceratopogonidae (Heleidae)

This group contains many genera but only four, *Lasiohelea, Haemophoructus, Leptoconops,* and *Culicoides* include species which suck the blood of man. The genus *Culicoides* is outstanding in this group, being represented in many parts of the world, with forty-eight authentic species listed from North America alone.

**Medical Importance**   Members of the genus Culicoides may be real pests in their own right. All are exceedingly minute, and have long been called "no-see-ums" by certain tribes of American Indians. In some areas they are termed "punkies," and in others "sandflies." They attack in the daytime, bite fiercely and their bites continue to be irritating for many days. They attack principally at the neckline, the belt line, shoe tops, or where sleeves are rolled up on the arm. A nodular, inflamed swelling is produced, which in susceptible individuals may become vesicular. The vesicle, if ruptured, yields a serous exudate, and the "weeping" continues for several days. Conspicuous red scars sometimes persist for weeks (Fig. 291).

**As Vectors**   Members of this genus serve as intermediate hosts for two species of roundworms. In Africa, British Guiana and New Guinea *Acanthocheilonema perstans* passes seven to nine days as a developing larva in the body of the fly. *Culicoides austeni* and *C. grahami* are important vectors of this species. In the British West

Indies *Culicoides furens* Poey functions similarly as the vector of *Mansonella ozzardi.*

**Diagnostic Characters** The adult flies may be recognized by their small size (up to 2¼ mm.), and their somewhat pubescent (finely hairy) wings, which in most species display a characteristic, iridescent spotting (Fig. 291). The antennae possess fourteen segments, the palpi five.

Breeding takes place in pools, ponds, slow streams, water in hollow stumps or even in moist soil, depending on the species concerned. Fresh water is usually preferred by the aquatic forms, but brackish waters are sometimes used. The larvae are small, slender, legless

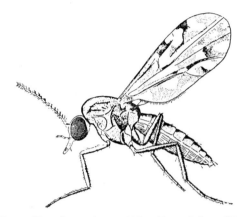

Fig. 291. *Culicoides* sp. Female specimen. (After Dampf, from Herms, Medical Entomology, by permission of The Macmillan Co.)

wormlike creatures with a distinct brownish head and twelve body segments. The pupae, if aquatic, are usually found floating vertically, their respiratory trumpets just breaking the surface.

**Control** Because of the great variety of breeding places, intelligent control depends chiefly upon a knowledge of the habits of the local species. For salt marsh types, flood gates may be effective. Channelization and removal of vegetation will help in eliminating those which breed in streams. Creosote may be used to kill larvae in tree holes. Pyrethrum sprays are effective against the adults in houses, and in the field the newer mosquito repellents give promise of good results.

### Family Simuliidae

This family contains approximately 600 species known variously as black flies, buffalo gnats, or turkey gnats, and is found throughout the world. The females of many species are vicious biters. Besides causing discomfort by their bites, certain forms (*Simulium damnosum* Theob. and *S. neavei* Roubaud in Africa; *Eusimulium avidum*

Hoffman, *Eusimulium ochraceum* Walker and *E. mooseri* Dampf in Mexico and Central America) are essential hosts of *Onchocerca volvulus*, roundworm parasite of man. At least one species, *Simulium decorum katmai*, has been incriminated as a mechanical vector of tularemia.

SIMULIIDAE are small (1 to 5 mm.), hump-backed flies with short, stubbed antennae of ten or eleven segments. The wings are characterized by two or three very heavy veins in the costal region, the remainder of the wing being supported by more delicate veins. The palpi have four segments. There are no ocelli (Fig. 292).

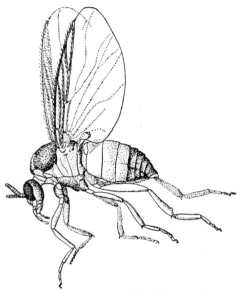

Fig. 292. *Eusimulium pecuarum*, a species of black fly. (Redrawn after Garman from Herms, Medical Entomology, by permission of The Macmillan Co.)

**Habits and Life History**    Black flies breed by preference in rapidly flowing streams, the females attaching their eggs to rocks at or beneath the surface of the water. Logs and aquatic plants may also be used and a few species are known to breed in quiet streams and ditches, attaching their eggs to the submerged tips of grasses rooted along the margin. The eggs, at first light in color, soon change to a dark brown or black. Each female deposits between three and four hundred eggs. In water at about 20° C. the eggs require five days incubation. Colder water may retard hatching for as long as thirty days.

The larvae are twelve-segmented and are provided with a disk-like, hooklet-bearing sucker at the posterior end, by which they remain attached. Silken strands, spun by cephalic silk glands, also aid in this attachment. There is, in addition, a disklike proleg near the anterior end, locomotor in function. Fan-shaped mouth brushes create a current by which microscopic food particles are drawn into the mouth. Respiration is accomplished by gills on the dorsal surface of the last abdominal segment. Larval development requires from three to ten weeks, depending on the species and environmental conditions. In some species the larvae are black in color and when present in large numbers form a conspicuous blanket on rock surfaces beneath the water.

The pupae are likewise aquatic and breathe by respiratory filaments attached to the dorsal surface of the thorax just behind the head. They are enclosed in pocket-like cocoons. The pupal stage requires three to six days. Some species produce as many as five or six generations in a single season.

In latitudes where there is a winter season, both eggs and larvae hibernate.

Adult *S. damnosum* usually remain close to the breeding area except immediately after a rain, when they may be found as much as a thousand yards away. This species bites chiefly from six to eight in the morning and again at dusk, though if there is sufficient shade it will attack at any time during the day. Curiously enough, *S. damnosum* rarely bites more than three feet above the ground, hence children placed on tables are seldom if ever bitten. A knowledge of these facts is of some importance in the avoidance of infection with onchocerciasis in *S. damnosum* territory.

**Black Fly Bites**   Only the females suck blood. The mouth parts consist of six bladelike lancets and with these they make a conspicuous puncture which remains hemorrhagic in character long after the fly has gone. Flies of this family attack usually in daylight or full moonlight. They may be a terrific pest to fishermen, campers, and troops operating near their breeding areas. Many species eagerly attack by preference the eyes, ears, and nostrils, though any exposed portion of the body is certain to be bitten. This bite itself may be painless but, soon after, much pain, swelling and general discomfort occur. The eyes may be completely closed and the face so distorted as to render the individual unrecognizable. Some persons, if severely bitten, may show a rise in temperature and intestinal disturbances. Itching sores, becoming ulcer-like, may develop and usually persist for days. Black flies are most annoying in north temperate and subarctic zones, appearing in enormous numbers when conditions favor their development. Domestic animals are frequently killed by them in the Mississippi Valley, following the recession of the spring floods. In Alaska a white-footed form, *Simulium arcticum*, is a very serious menace during certain seasons of the year. In the early part of the summer *Simulium venustum* Say is a pest in Canada and certain portions of the United States. *Simulium columbaczense* (Schiner) is a most important species in Europe, at times causing the death of large numbers of domestic animals as well as wild game.

**Treatment of the Bites**   The application of dilute alkaline solutions will usually soothe the pain and reduce the swelling. In very young children, badly bitten, supportive treatment may be required.

**Prophylaxis and Control**   The wearing of complete clothing is very desirable, thereby limiting the attacks to the hands and face. Head nets are impracticable, as a mesh sufficiently small to exclude black flies constitutes a great obstruction to vision. Smearing the face with oil of tar, or a mixture of kerosene and mutton tallow, has long been practiced by woodsmen in the north. Mixtures of kerosene and pennyroyal have also been recommended. The newer mosquito repellents (Indalone, 612, dimethyl phthalate) give promise of being helpful. Sensitive persons may find it necessary to keep out of the woods during the black fly season. Native populations appear to develop a certain amount of immunity, through exposure over an extended period of time.

The control of black flies in nature is rather impracticable. However, if labor is available, reasonably satisfactory control may be accomplished by cleaning the streams of rocks, logs, débris and concrete slabs. Another possible procedure is the removal of larvae from rock surfaces by scrubbing with wire brooms. The dislodged larvae, as they float downstream, may then be caught in a fine-mesh baffle and destroyed. Control of black fly larvae may be secured with DDT oil sprays. Effective control was obtained in Alaska, for a distance of two miles downstream from the point of application, when DDT was applied at the rate of 0.1 pounds per acre in 800 ft. swaths across streams.

The use of smudges has been found effective in repelling the adult flies.

In many localities the flies are held in check by natural enemies, which include dragonflies, robber flies, various aquatic insects and certain protozoal parasites.

### Family Psychodidae

This important family, the species of which are known variously as moth flies, owl flies, or sandflies, is characterized by small size, long legs, and the presence of abundant hair both on wings and body. The wing venation is distinctive, the longitudinal veins all arising near the base of the wing and lying practically parallel through their course. Scarcity of cross-veins and a lanceolate outline are also characteristic of psychodid wings. The antennae are long and have twelve to sixteen segments.

The medical importance may be better understood if one discriminates between the two subfamilies of which the PSYCHODIDAE are composed (Table 66).

**Psychodinae**   A single species of the genus *Pericoma* has been reported as biting man in Australia. There is also record of urinary myiasis caused by larvae of the genus *Psychoda*. In this instance it is believed that the parasites migrated from the rectum, after ingestion with garden soil.

**Phlebotominae** This subfamily is of far greater importance than the first. More than fifty species are known and in all cases the females suck blood. The group includes but one genus, *Phlebotomus*. Particular species serve as vectors of sandfly fever, kala-azar, cutaneous leishmaniasis, espundia, oriental sore, Carrión disease and possibly tropical ulcer, besides causing considerable annoyance and discomfort by their bites. The group is represented in all warmer regions of the world. Fortunately the best known species in the United States (*Phlebotomus vexator*) does not function as a vector of disease.

**Habits and Life History** (with special reference to the genus *Phlebotomus*) Most species breed in rock piles, cracks in walls, and beneath débris of various kinds. In eastern India there is some

*Table 66    Key to Subfamilies of the Sandflies* (PSYCHODINAE)

1  (2)  Second longitudinal vein branching near the base of the wings; wings usually held rooflike when at rest
                                                            PSYCHODINAE
2  (1)  Second longitudinal vein branching at a considerable distance from the base of the wing; wings usually held at an angle of 45 degrees when not in use  ..PHLEBOTOMINAE

breeding of *Phlebotomus argentipes* in grass along the margin of streams, but this is relatively uncommon. The habits of *P. papatasi* as found in Africa, Asia and southern Europe may be cited as typical of the group (see Fig. 149, p. 336).

The small (3 to 5 mm.), humpbacked, hairy flies deposit their tiny eggs in batches of fifty or more in various dark, humid places. The larvae hatch in approximately one week and proceed to feed on a variety of organic materials including the feces of lizards and the bodies of their own parents, which do not long survive oviposition. The larvae are small, whitish in color and possess twelve body segments. The ninth and tenth abdominal segments are equipped with conspicuous dorsal bristles. The three larval stages require a total of approximately thirty days for development, and the pupa about ten days more. A temperature of 70° to 80° F. is most favorable for their growth. The adults are poor fliers and do not migrate far from the breeding areas. Biting occurs at night and it is believed that the females must have a blood meal before they can develop their eggs. They do not fly if the slightest wind is stirring; hence bites may be expected only on quiet nights.

**Nature of the Bites** Attacking silently, the female *Phlebotomus* seeks out the ankles, wrists, knees and elbows, showing a preference for areas where the skin is particularly delicate or tightly drawn. A painful, stinging sensation is followed by itching which persists for some time. Firm whitish wheals which may become pustular and edematous if scratched are characteristic of attacks by *Phlebotomus*. If no secondary infection ensues, the irritation subsides in a few days, though toxemia, nausea and rise in temperature have been reported in some cases after numerous bites.

**Prophylaxis and Control**   Repellents are none too effective though some of the newer mosquito lotions are of value. Screening is impracticable, since a mesh of 25 to 30 to the inch is required to prevent their penetration. The avoidance of exposure at night is of great importance, as proved by the practice of evacuating workmen from verruga-ridden valleys (South America) at close of day. The painting of door posts and exteriors of huts with fuel oil has been found very effective in discouraging the flies from entering buildings. The keeping of animals near human sleeping quarters is believed to attract *Phlebotomus* away from human hosts.

It has been shown recently that the sprays used for the control of mosquitoes are effective in controlling *Phlebotomus*. Virtual eradication has been reported when DDT residual sprays were applied to breeding places within 200 yards of the perimeter of the community.

Indoors the use of mosquito sprays is desirable; electric fans may be useful in keeping the flies away. Peculiarly enough, *Formalin*, not useful against most insects, seems to be reasonably effective as a spray material in the case of sandflies. A crude method of reducing the numbers by the use of sticky "racquets," held for a few minutes in the corners of huts where adult flies are hiding has been advocated in Russia. The edges of the "paddle" are thickened to guard against the sticky surface coming into contact with the wall. Even soapsuds will suffice as an entangling substance. The specimens may be removed later, with alcohol, for identification.

The abolition of the breeding places is in all cases to be preferred over any other method of control. Removal of rubble, also the cementing of cracks and filling of holes, should be undertaken wherever practicable. The planting of thyme, pennyroyal and other aromatic plants is believed to have a repellent effect. Benzene polychlorines, applied to the breeding places, is believed to be effective in destroying the larvae.

## Family Culicidae (Mosquitoes)

The CULICIDAE constitute the most important single family of insects from the standpoint of human health. Distributed throughout the world from the arctic to the tropics, mosquitoes, from time immemorial, have been known as intolerable pests. More important than this, however, is their role in the transmission of human disease. CULICIDAE have been found to act as vectors of filariasis, dengue, yellow fever, the malarias and several of the encephalitides.

There are well over 1500 species of mosquitoes known. The family may be distinguished from similar nematocerous DIPTERA (midges, crane flies, fungus gnats) by two obvious characters: 1. The veins of the wings as well as the wing margin are covered by conspicuous scales. 2. The head bears a conspicuous proboscis, which extends either forward or downward when the insect is at rest.

Other family characters are as follows: Antennae long, slender, of fifteen segments, the first usually obscured by the globular second segment (pedicel). Male antennae strongly plumose; those of the female sparsely hairy. Ocelli absent. Wings narrow. Thorax without a transverse V-shaped suture on the dorsal surface. Abdomen long and slender, bearing two small caudal cerci in the female and a rather elaborate *hypopygium* (sexual apparatus) in the male.

**Classification**   The Family CULICIDAE was formerly defined to include the Subfamily CORETHRINAE, a non–blood-sucking group, dis-

## Table 67   Key to Tribes of CULICIDAE

1  (2)   Female palpi as long as proboscis or nearly so; scutellum almost always evenly rounded; wings usually spotted; male palpi long, clubbed at the tip; abdomen not covered with flat scales. Proboscis, head, thorax and abdomen forming a straight line . . . . . . . . . . . . . *Anophelini*

2  (1)   Female palpi very short; scutellum variable; wings usually without spotting; male palpi long but not clubbed at tip. Profile distinctly hump-backed . . . . . . . . . . . 3

3  (4)   Proboscis straight or very slightly curved, never tapered from base to apex; scutellum trilobed, each lobe bearing a tuft of setae . . . . . . . . . . . . . . . . . . . . . . . *Culicini*

4  (3)   Proboscis rigid, the outer portion tapered and curving downward to a conspicuous degree; scutellum evenly rounded and scaled . . . . . . . . . . . . . . . . . . . *Megarhinini*

tinguished from true mosquitoes by the fact that the proboscis is much shorter (being little longer than the head), and quite unsuited for sucking blood. At present it is the accepted practice to regard this group as constituting a separate Family, the CHAOBORIDAE.

True mosquitoes (exclusive of the CHAOBORIDAE) fall into three natural groups or tribes, the ANOPHELINI, CULICINI, and MEGARHININI. These may be separated according to the following adult characters.

**Tribe Megharinini**   This small group includes the single genus, *Megarhinus*, in which all the species are large, iridescent forms, very striking in appearance. None of them sucks blood. The larvae are found chiefly in tree holes, where they feed frequently on other mosquito larvae. The group as a whole might therefore be considered beneficial.

**Tribe Anophelini**   This important series includes approximately 200 species and is well represented throughout the world, particularly in the tropics. It is the consensus that all or practically all species should be included in the one genus *Anopheles*, though various workers recognize certain natural groups to which have been given appropriate subgeneric names, e.g., *Stethomyia, Nyssorhynchus, Lophopodomyia, Arthuromyia, Myzomyia, Kerteszia.* The genus *Chagasia,* however, is regarded as sufficiently distinct to stand alone, the scutellum in these forms being trilobed, after the manner of the CULICINI.

Most anophelines should be regarded as potential vectors of malaria, though only some fifty species actually transmit the disease in nature and less than thirty are considered really "good" vectors under ordinary circumstances.

**Habits and Life History of Anophelines** (Fig. 293)   The female *Anopheles* deposits her eggs singly or in small groups on the surface of the water. The anopheline egg is boat-shaped and is supported by a pair of rather ornate structures, termed *floats*. The margin is further ornamented in many species by a beaded "gunwale" termed the *frill*. Species may be differentiated in the egg stage without difficulty and in the case of the *Anopheles maculipennis* complex of Europe, seven biological races (species ?), quite indistinguishable in the adult form, may nevertheless be separated on the basis of the shape and ornamentation of their eggs.

Anopheline eggs tend to group together on the surface of water in triangular or stellate patterns, the tips remaining in contact as though influenced by some surface tension phenomenon.

LARVAL CHARACTERS. The eggs hatch in one to two days and the larvae, or "wigglers," proceed to feed upon various microscopic organisms (bacteria, algae and protozoa). All mosquito larvae possess a broad, flattened head which bears the eyes, the antennae and a pair of conspicuous mouth brushes used for sweeping micro-organisms into the mouth. The head of an anopheline larva is capable of a rotation of 180° in either direction from the normal, an arrangement which provides for the taking in of surface organisms wherever they may be found. For nomenclature of the hairs arising from the head see legend, Fig. 293. The distance between the inner clypeal hairs is of value in classification.

The thorax, like the head, is a flattened structure, with little or no evidence of segmentation. Legs are absent, but their future locations are indicated by segmental grouping of the thoracic hairs. For taxonomic purposes the hairs at each segmental level are numbered, beginning at the median dorsal line and continuing around to the mid-ventral region. Of especial interest are the *pleural* groups, so-called, consisting of hairs 9–12 inclusive, these four being borne together on a relatively large basal tubercle with a conspicuous lateral tooth.

The abdomen, which tapers perceptibly, consists of nine visible segments, the anterior somewhat flattened, the posterior progressively more cylindrical. Near the anterior margin of each segment, and crossing the median dorsal line, is a small, transverse bar of chitin, the *anterior tergal* plate. A minute *posterior tergal* plate is

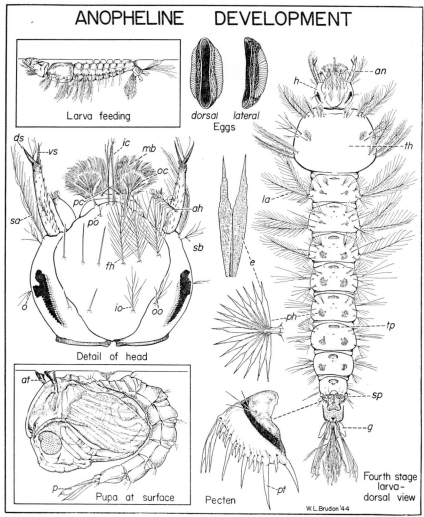

## ANOPHELINE    DEVELOPMENT

Larva feeding

*dorsal    lateral*
Eggs

Detail of head

Pupa at surface

Pecten

Fourth stage
larva-
dorsal view

W.L.Brudon '44

Fig. 293. All figures except ova pertain to *Anopheles maculipennis* Meigen. Ova (dorsal and lateral) are from *A. gambiae* Giles. *ah*, antennal hair; *an*, antenna; *at*, air trumpet; *ds*, dorsal saber; *e*, element of palmate hair; *fh*, frontal hairs; *g*, gill; *h*, head; *ic*, inner clypeal hair; *io*, inner occipital hair; *la*, lateral hair; *mb*, mouth brush; *o*, orbital hair; *oc*, outer clypeal hair; *oo*, outer occipital hair; *p*, paddle; *pc*, preclypeal hair; *ph*, palmate hair; *po*, posterior clypeal hair; *pt*, pecten tooth; *sa*, subantennal hair; *sb*, sub-basal hair; *sp*, spiracle; *th*, thorax; *tp*, tergal plate; *vs*, ventral saber.

also present on certain segments. As on the thorax the abdominal hairs are numbered outward from the median dorsal line, the most conspicuous hair (number six) being lateral in position. In anopheline species hair number one is frequently modified so as to present a palmate appearance, the elements or leaflets radiating outward from a common pedicle or stalk. Since anopheline larvae lie parallel to the water surface, these palmate hairs normally protrude through the surface film and function as "float" hairs, the tiny leaflets or subdivisions radiating in all directions. The number of pairs of "float" hairs, their location on the segment and the microscopic appearance of their elements are much used in classification.

On both thoracic and abdominal segments there is occasionally present a minute hair often near the anterior margin, not included in the conventional system of numbering. This is designated as hair number 0.

The eighth and ninth abdominal segments differ from the first seven in that they are especially modified for respiratory purposes. The two large spiracles, located well back on the dorsal surface of segment eight, are surrounded by five flaps, one anterior (called the anterior plate), two lateral (small, unsupported) and two posterior lobes which represent the posterolateral angles of the so-called posterior plate. The entire structure overhangs the ninth segment to some extent. Just beneath each lateral flap is a crescent-shaped structure, the pecten, bearing a variable number (5, 6) of rather conspicuous, backwardly directed pecten teeth. When the larva rests or feeds at the surface its entire spiracular structure perforates the surface film, a condition which requires the larva to lie horizontally and favors feeding on surface organisms. In a very few species of *Anopheles* (e.g., *A. turkhudi* List) the spiracular structure is joined to the body at an angle, resulting in an attitude more resembling that of the culicines.

The ninth abdominal segment is more or less enclosed in a tight-fitting chitinous sleeve, the dorsal plate, which fits the segment like a saddle. At least one hair, arising from the posterolateral surface on either side, is appropriately termed the "saddle hair." Arising from the posterior extremity of the ninth segment are four finger-like tracheal (anal) gills, useful in the regulation of osmotic pressure (chlorides) but not sufficient without the air-breathing spiracles, previously described. Above and below the anal gills arise strong, branching hairs which combine to form a rather elaborate caudal ornamentation (Fig. 293).

Mosquito larvae pass through four instars, the duration of larval life ranging from a few days to the entire winter, depending on the species and climatic conditions. As a rule characters sufficiently constant for classification of species are found only in the fourth stage larvae, though recent work has shown that in the case of Puerto Rican anophelines, at least, the first stage larvae may be readily distinguished. Usually, however, one had best make certain that he is dealing with the last larval stage before proceeding to make identification. The following characters will distinguish fourth stage larvae from less mature specimens:

1. Large size
2. Narrow collar (between head and thorax)
3. Leg and wing rudiments visible beneath the skin (just prior to pupation)
4. A maximum development of body hairs
5. The appearance of the imaginal eye (much larger than the larval eye)
6. The head fully as broad as long.

IMPORTANCE OF THE STUDY OF LARVAL FORMS. There are several good reasons for studying and classifying mosquito larvae:

1. In survey work, where the adult may not have been seen or collected, the identification of the larva provides a positive record of the existence of the species in the fauna.

2. Identification of the larva provides a check on the determination of the adult, especially when adult characters are obscure. (In certain species the larval characters appear to be more reliable.)

3. By collecting and rearing the larvae, perfect adult specimens of both sexes may be secured.

4. By the same procedure, the investigator may secure infection-free stock for experimental work.

THE PUPA. After completing its development, the fourth stage larva sheds its skin and becomes a pupa or "tumbler" (Fig. 293). In this stage the insect takes no food and for the most part rests quietly at the surface of the water, its two respiratory trumpets, which arise from the dorsal surface of the thorax, penetrating the surface film. Pupae nevertheless have considerable capacity for motility, being possessed of a pair of swim paddles which are situated at the posterior extremity of the abdomen. When disturbed, they go tumbling to the bottom of the pool, but return in a few moments, since they cannot long remain away from the surface for want of air. Pupae have a number of scattered hairs on the surface of the body, largely dorsal in position; the most anterior serve for purposes of flotation. In most species but two or three days are required for the complete development of the adult characters. The integument of the pupa is relatively transparent and the developing legs, wings and antennae may be easily observed.

Pupae are not readily classified; hence it is the usual practice to await the emergence of the adult before attempting to determine the genus or species.

THE ADULT ANOPHELINE. The pupal skin serves as a float or raft on which the adult may dry its wings and from which it may take off on its initial flight. Males are distinguishable from females by their bushier antennae and by the peculiarly elaborate hypopygium at the posterior extremity of the abdomen (Fig. 294). The palpi of both

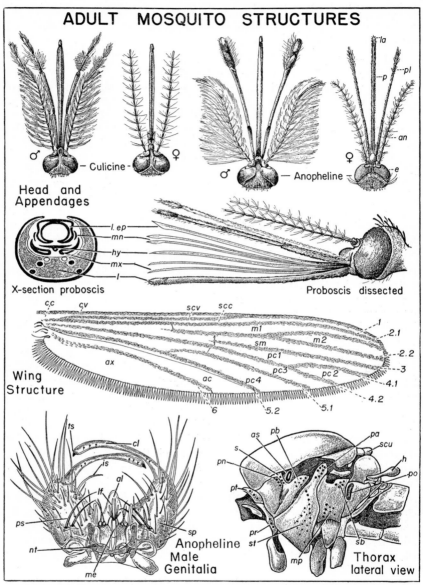

## ADULT MOSQUITO STRUCTURES

Head and Appendages

X-section proboscis

Proboscis dissected

Wing Structure

Anopheline Male Genitalia

Thorax lateral view

Fig. 294. Adult mosquito structures: *ac,* anal cell; *al,* anal lobe; *an,* antenna; *as,* anterior thoracic spiracle; *ax,* axillary cell; *bl,* blood canal; *cc,* costal cell; *cl,* clasper; *cv,* costal vein; *e,* eye; *h,* halter; *hy,* hypopharynx *ilc,* inner lobe of claspette; *is,* internal spine; *l,* labium; *la,* labellum; *lep,* labrum-epipharynx; *lf,* leaflets of meso-some; *m1, 2,* marginal cells by number; *me,* mesosome; *mn,* mandible; *mp,* mese-pimeral bristles (lower); *mx,* maxilla; *nt,* ninth tergite; *olc,* outer lobe of claspette; *p,* proboscis; *pa,* pre-alar bristles; *pb,* post-spiracular bristles; *pc1, 2,* posterior cells by number; *pl,* palpus; *pn,* pronotal bristles; *po,* posterior thoracic spiracle; *pr,* prosternal bristles; *ps,* parabasal spines; *pt,* prothoracic bristles; *s,* spiracular bristles;

sexes of anophelines are long, but in the male they are conspicuously clubbed at the tip. The sexes mate almost immediately. In some species (*Anopheles punctipennis*) the males swarm together in enormous numbers, at which time the individual females invade the swarm in search of mates. The swarming habit, however, is not universal in the group.

Male mosquitoes live a relatively short time after copulation, usually a few weeks at the most. The females set out immediately after fertilization on their quest for a blood meal. The majority of anophelines feed by preference during the twilight hours of morning and evening, although some (*Anopheles atropos*) will attack in direct sunlight as well. In most species studied it appears necessary for the female to feed on blood before she can develop her eggs. Mosquitoes deposit their eggs in batches throughout the season, the total number ranging from 100 to 500 or more. The females continue to feed throughout their life, which in non-hibernating individuals may be as long as five months. A great many species, however, hibernate as adult females, a fact which makes possible one practical means of control: to seek out their hiding places and destroy them during the dormant period. They may be found in tree holes, caves, stables, culverts, cellars and outhouses. A certain amount of moisture, combined with semidarkness, characterizes the ideal situation. Mosquitoes hibernating in houses occasionally become active during the winter and seek the warmer rooms for a blood meal.

In the spring there is a general exodus in search of breeding grounds. Specific observations have been made on the distribution flights of *Anopheles freeborni* in California. Once a breeding area has been selected the adults rarely wander more than a mile or two from that locality. Other factors also enter into mosquito distribution, such as prevailing winds, automobiles and airplanes. The last, especially, constitutes a real problem relative to the dissemination both of the insect and of mosquito-borne diseases.

**Control**  For a discussion of the control or elimination of ANOPHELINI see "Environmental Mosquito Control" (p. 738).

**Tribe Culicini**  This, the largest natural group of mosquitoes, includes over 1300 species distributed among a large number of genera. Best known are *Culex, Aedes, Psorophora, Culiseta, Mansonia* (*Taeniorhynchus*) and *Wyeomyia*. There is a wide variation in structure, biology and relation to disease. None, however, are vectors of human malaria, though certain species of *Culex* are well known vectors of malaria in birds. Species of *Culex, Aedes, Mansonia,* and *Anopheles* serve as vectors of human filariasis. *Aedes aegypti, A. albopictus* and *A. scutellaris* Walker transmit dengue fever. Yellow fever, shown in 1900 to be conveyed by *Aedes aegypti,* is now known

---

*sa,* salivary canal; *sb,* subalar bristles (upper mesepimerals); *scc,* subcostal cell; *scu,* scutellum; *scv,* subcostal vein; *sm,* submarginal cell; *sp,* side piece; *st,* sternopleural bristles, *ts,* terminal spine of clasper; 1, 2.1, 2.2, 3, 4.1, 4.2, 5.1, 5.2, 6, longitudinal veins by number.

to be transmitted by a number of species, of which *Haemagogus spegazzinii* and its subspecies *falco* are well known in connection with the problem of "jungle yellow fever" in tropical South America. *Culex tritaeniorhynchus* is a natural vector of Japanese B encephalitis, while *C. tarsalis* holds the same relation to St. Louis and western equine encephalitis in the United States. *Culex pipiens* is a suspected vector of St. Louis encephalitis. A large number of species belonging to *Culex, Aedes* and *Culiseta* have been shown to be vectors of various encephalitides under experimental conditions.

Besides this, the world's most famous "pest" mosquitoes fall in the culicine group. The northern house mosquito, *Culex pipiens*, and its counterpart in the South, *C. quinquefasciatus*, are well known examples. *Aedes taeniorhynchus* breeds in salt marshes from New York to the Guianas as well as from southern California to Peru and the Galapagos Islands. *Aedes vexans* is a very troublesome species in the Northeastern States and elsewhere. Many others of the same genus (*A. spencerii, A. punctor, A. stimulans, A. excrucians, A. communis*) play a part in rendering certain otherwise attractive regions quite unsuitable for recreational purposes. *Aedes aldrichi* is a particularly serious pest in Washington, British Columbia and Oregon. Most members of the genera *Psorophora* and *Mansonia* are fierce biters and cause extreme annoyance when present in significant numbers.

**Habits and Life History**  The biology of culicine mosquitoes is similar in many respects to that of the ANOPHELINI. We shall therefore confine this discussion largely to those features in which the CULICINI are more or less unique.

THE EGGS (Fig. 295). Culicine eggs are laid singly (*Aedes*) or in masses that float on the water (*Culex, Mansonia, Urotaenia, Culiseta*). None, however, are provided with specialized floats as in the case of anopheline eggs.

THE LARVA (Fig. 295). Culicine larvae, like anophelines, pass through four stages or instars, feed on micro-organisms by means of mouth brushes and breathe by means of spiracles at the posterior end of the body. There are certain differences, however, of a structural character, some of which have a bearing on behavior and manner of feeding, and which therefore serve as aids in the recognition of culicine larvae in the field. Other structures characterize genera and species and make possible exact classification of the several groups. We shall consider these structures briefly, beginning with the head.

Mouth brushes, eyes and antennae do not differ essentially from the same structures in anophelines. Clypeal hairs, however, are absent. The upper and lower head hairs, which correspond more or less closely to the occipital and frontal hairs of anophelines, are fewer in number and in most cases simpler in structure. The hair tuft near the base of the antennae is posterior to that organ.

Thoracic and abdominal hairs are located much as in the anophelines, but they are less frequently branched and none are of the palmate type.

The most distinctive feature of culicine larvae, however, is found on segment eight (of the abdomen), the dorsal surface of which bears a more or less elongate "siphon" or air tube. In certain species (*Culex salinarius*) this structure is almost nine times as long as

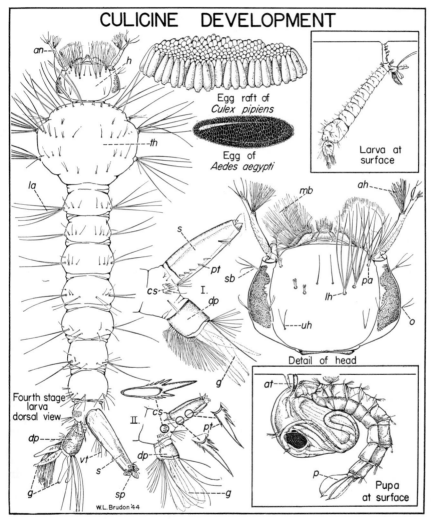

Fig. 295. All figures except as noted pertain to *Culex pipiens* Linn. Anal segments: I, *Psorophora confinnis* (L.-Arr.); II, *Aedes aegypti* (Linn.); *ah*, antennal hair; *an*, antenna; *at*, air trumpet; *cs*, comb scales; *dp*, dorsal plate; *g*, gill; *h*, head; *la*, lateral hairs; *lh*, upper head hairs; *mb*, mouth brush; *o*, orbital hair; *p*, paddle; *pa*, preantennal hairs; *pt*, pecten tooth; *s*, siphon; *sb*, sub-basal hair; *sp*, spiracular apparatus; *th*, thorax; *uh*, sutural hairs; *vt*, ventral tufts; unlabelled tuft between *lh* and *pa*, lower head hair.

broad. At its extremity are located the two spiracles, surrounded by five outwardly directed flaps. As in the anophelines the spiracles are thrust above the surface film, but because of the length of the siphon the larva itself rests well below the surface, the typical feeding angle approximating 45 degrees. Culicine larvae are not, therefore, surface feeders, a fact which makes it relatively difficult to control them by the spreading of poison dusts.

An exception to the usual behavior is found in the genus *Mansonia*, (e.g., *M. perturbans*) in which the larvae, after hatching from the egg rafts, attach themselves by their siphons to the stems of aquatic plants. They thus remain below the surface, obtaining oxygen from air spaces in the plant tissue.

Extending along the ventral surface of the siphon from the base are two rows of obliquely directed "pecten teeth," homologues of the "pecten" described in connection with the spiracular structure of anophelines. One or more pairs of hair tufts are usually found on the ventral surface of the siphon, the number and position depending on the species involved. In certain forms (*Culex restuans*) scattered single hairs are present in addition to the ventral tufts. The shape and spacing of the pecten teeth are used in separating species.

The eighth segment bears likewise, on either side, a number of backwardly directed "comb-scales," the arrangement and number of which furnish a basis for classification. The individual scales are also used in classification, being simple in *Aedes albopictus* but furnished with bars in the larva of *A. aegypti*.

The ninth segment resembles that of the anophelines, but is subject to a greater degree of variation. The dorsal plate may be a simple saddle, as in *A. stimulans*, or it may actually ring the segment. It may be that only the anterior portion of the ring encircles the segment, in which case the ventral hair tuft, being posterior, still has no contact with the ring itself (*A. sollicitans*). On the other hand if the encirclement is complete, as in *Psorophora cyanescens* or *P. confinnis*, the ventral hair tuft actually pierces the ring.

THE PUPA. Culicine pupae have no very distinctive features, save that the cephalothorax tends to be somewhat less massive than in the anophelines, a feature which has a slight effect on the position at the surface. *Mansonia*, however, is again exceptional, pupation in this genus taking place below the surface of the water. Such pupae obtain oxygen through attachment to plants by their air tubes, as do their larvae, previously described.

HABITS OF ADULT CULICINES. In such an extensive group some diversity of habit is to be expected. *Aedes aegypti* mates in the daytime, the males seeking out the females while in flight. In most species, however, the males assemble in great swarms, the females selecting their mates by darting into the swarming column. In most cases these swarms are found in the early evening hovering over some conspicuous object such as a tree, shrub or rock. For additional information on behavior see section on culicine control (p. 746).

**Considerations Relating to both Anophelines and Culicines** STRUC-
TURAL CHARACTERISTICS OF ADULT MOSQUITOES. There are a number
of structural features found in both anophelines and culicines with
which the physician should be familiar if he is to attempt identification of the medically important forms, or to understand adequately
their function in disease transmission.

1. BODY. As in all insects the body is divided into three essential
parts, a head, a thorax composed of three segments, more or less
united, and a flexible abdomen, in which eight segments are normally visible.

2. HEAD. The head, which is nearly spherical, bears the antennae,
the compound eyes and the mouth parts, the latter arranged in such
a manner as to form a piercing *proboscis*. The antennae arise high up
on the face, between the eyes. Each consists of fifteen segments, the
thirteen terminal segments being rather slender, elongate and beset
with hairs. The antennal hairs are longer and more numerous in
males.

The proboscis arises from the lower portion of the face and extends
forward and downward from the head (more forward in the case of
anophelines). The proboscis is flanked on either side by a *palpus*
which is approximately as long as the proboscis save in culicine females, where the palpi are exceedingly short. Four palpal segments
are visible in anophelines, three in culicines. Certain species have the
palpi ringed and/or tipped with white. The proboscis itself consists
of six slender stylets (labrum-epipharynx, hypopharynx, two mandibles, two maxillae) enclosed in a *labial sheath* which terminates distally in a pair of olive-shaped *labella* This labial sheath, which is
open on the dorsal surface, is drawn backward at the time of feeding,
thus permitting the other elements to enter the skin. The *mandibles*
(which terminate simply) and the *maxillae* (which bear saw teeth
near the tip), are especially concerned with the initial penetration.
The labrum-epipharynx and hypopharynx are then inserted, at
which time the saliva is forced down the slender channel of the hypopharynx by action of the salivary pump. It is at this time that the
sporozoites of malarial organisms may pass from the salivary gland
cells of the female anopheline into the blood stream of the human
host. The blood, rendered less coagulable by the mosquito's saliva, is
then withdrawn by way of a canal whose floor is the hypopharynx but whose walls and roof are formed by the labrum-epipharynx.

3. THORAX. The dorsal surface of the thorax is modified in that the
first (prothoracic) and third (metathoracic) segments are obscured
by the enormous development of the second (mesothoracic), or
wing-bearing segment. The major portion of the dorsum is designated as the *mesonotum*, behind which a more or less semicircular
unit, the *scutellum*, is appended as a backwardly directed shelf.
The metathorax is represented dorsally by a very narrow region
(metanotum) which bears the balancers or halteres. The presence

or absence of setae on the postnotum are of value in making an identification.

The wings show a fairly primitive pattern in which eight longitudinal veins are recognized. The anterior margin is formed by the *costa*, after which follow *subcosta, first longitudinal vein, second l. v.* (branched), *third l. v., fourth l. v.* (branched), *fifth l. v.* (branched), and *sixth longitudinal vein.* Vestiges of obsolete veins are sometimes visible posterior to veins *five* and *six.* Cross-veins are typical between *costa* and *subcosta*, between *subcosta* and vein *one*, between *one* and *two* and between *two* and *three;* variable between *three* and *four*, also between *four* and *five*. The marginal cells of the wing are designated, from front to rear, as: *costal cell, subcostal, first marginal, second marginal, submarginal, first posterior, second posterior, third posterior, fourth posterior, anal* and *axillary.*

The scales, which adorn all veins as well as the wing margin, may be of three colors: culicines possess only translucent gray scales, the even distribution of which gives to culicine wings a uniform (unspotted) appearance. Anophelines likewise may display only grayish scales, but they are usually grouped in such a manner as to give the effect of definite spots. The more striking spots of forms like *Anopheles albimanus* or *A. gambiae*, are due, however, to the presence of two other types of scales, some black (really dark brown), others white (more often ivory yellow). These are usually sharply segregated, resulting in a definite number of light and dark spots, exceedingly useful in classification. The scales forming the fringe along the posterior margin of the wing may likewise form spots of taxonomic value.

The three pairs of legs are borne ventrally by the three thoracic segments. The small basal segment of the leg (*coxa*) is joined by means of a still more obscure segment, the *trochanter*, to the conspicuous *femur*, (the first segment visible in dorsal view). This is followed by the *tibia* and the five segments of the *tarsus*. Light bands and spots occurring on the various segments of the legs are described as basal (toward the body), apical (toward the extremity) or subapical, according to their position on the segment concerned.

The lateral wall or pleural surface of the thorax is made up of a number of chitinous areas or *sclerites*, the largest of which pertain to the mesothorax. These sclerites bear definite groups of bristles varying in size, position and number, according to the species. These bristle groups are shown and named in Fig. 294. The thorax also bears two pairs of lateral spiracles.

4. The *abdomen* is cylindrical and slightly tapering. The dorsal and ventral sclerites of each segment meet in a lateral, horizontal line. Each visible segment bears a pair of spiracles. The last (tenth) segment of the female bears a pair of short, backwardly directed, dorsal finger-like structures (cerci). The males have a very elaborate terminal structure, the *hypopygium*, formed of the ninth and tenth segments, which, together with segment eight, undergo a rotation

of 180° at the time of emergence from the pupal skin. This peculiar happening causes the morphologically dorsal structures to appear ventral and vice versa, a situation which causes no little confusion to the student of morphology. When once the relationships are understood, however, the hypopygium furnishes excellent characters for the separation of species. The hypopygium of *Anopheles quadrimaculatus*, with all parts labelled, is shown in Fig. 294.

Bands and spots on the abdominal segments are due to the distribution of variously colored scales. These are referred to as *basal*, if found on that margin which is nearer the thorax, *apical*, if on the caudal margin.

INTERNAL ANATOMY. An understanding of the internal organization of the mosquito is very necessary in connection with malaria survey work. When the stomach of an anopheline female is found to bear one or more oocysts on its external surface, it means that there must be a human reservoir in the area. When sporozoites are found in the salivary glands it means that the species is able to transmit malaria. The following description is intended to furnish a suitable background for mosquito dissection, the techniques of which are set forth on p. 849.

The body plan of a mosquito may be described as consisting of two concentric cylinders, the outer cylinder being the body wall, the inner, the alimentary tract. The space between them is termed a hemocoel and is filled with the mosquito's "blood." Above the alimentary canal is a tubular blood vessel termed the "heart," delicate in structure and difficult to demonstrate.

The food canal may be divided into the foregut, midgut and hindgut. The foregut is subdivided into the pharynx (with pharyngeal pump), the esophagus, which bears two dorsal and one ventral diverticula (food reservoirs) and the proventriculus. The midgut consists merely of the stomach, or ventriculus, an elongate sac at whose posterior extremity are attached the five excretory (malpighian) tubules.

The hindgut consists of a relatively slender, somewhat folded intestine, followed by an expanded rectum. The walls of the latter structure are characterized by the presence of a number of peculiar elevations, termed rectal papillae.

The malariologist will be concerned only with the dissection of females, since this sex alone is adapted, by its blood-sucking habits, to serve as a vector of disease. In gravid females the ovaries become relatively enormous, a condition which interferes considerably with successful dissection of the alimentary tract.

Between the food canal and body wall is a variable amount of whitish adipose tissue which presents a rather loose-knit appearance. When abundant it may complicate the observation of dissected structures. Traversing the adipose tissue and uniting the alimentary canal to the body wall will be found numerous tracheal threads. These are a part of the insect's respiratory system.

Of particular interest are the salivary glands, a pair of tiny, three-lobed structures situated in the anterior portion of the thorax on the ventral side. Each gland is served by a slender duct, the two ducts uniting anteriorly before opening into the pharynx from below. At this point (juncture with pharynx) is a specialized structure, the salivary pump, which forces the saliva into the hypopharyngeal canal.

The salivary glands are relatively minute and should not be confused with the dorsal and ventral diverticula of the esophagus. (See instructions on dissection for further details, p. 849.)

**Practical Determination of Genera and Species**   Since there are available a number of excellent publications treating of the bionomics and classification of CULICIDAE, it has not been deemed advisable to furnish keys to the various genera and species in this volume. Students who desire to do serious work of this nature will find it necessary to consult the technical literature in any case, while others whose interest in identification is concerned solely with mosquitoes as vectors of disease will ordinarily make use of the services of specialists in determining the species concerned. The following works of reference are recommended:

1. Barraud, P. J.: A Revision of the Culicine Mosquitoes of India. Pt. 22, Ind. J. Med. Res. *14*(3):555–563, 1927.

2. Bates, Marston K.: The Natural History of Mosquitoes. New York, The Macmillan Company, 1949.

3. Dyar, Harrison G.: The Mosquitoes of the Americas. Washington, Carnegie Institution, 1928.

4. Edwards, F. W.: Diptera. Fam. Culicidae. (Wytsman, P.) Genera Insectorum, 194. Fasc. 1932.

5. Edwards, F. W.: Mosquitoes of the Ethiopian Region. III, Culicine Adults and Pupae. Brit. Mus. (Nat. Hist.) London, 1941.

6. Freeborn, S. B., and Brookman, B.: Identification Guide to the Mosquitoes of the Pacific Coast States. U.S. Public Health Service Mal. Contr. in War Areas, Atlanta, Georgia, 1943.

7. Howard, L. O., Dyar, H. G., and Knab, F.: The Mosquitoes of North and Central America and the West Indies. Washington, Carnegie Institution, Publ. No. 159, Vols. I–IV, 1913–1917.

8. King, W. V., Bradley, G. H., and McNeel, T. E.: The Mosquitoes of the Southeastern States. (U.S.D.A. Misc. Publication 336. Rev.) Washington, 1942.

9. Komp, W. H. W.: The Anopheline Mosquitoes of the Carribbean Region. U. S. Public Health Service. National Institute of Health Bulletin 179. Washington, Government Printing Office. 1942.

10. Matheson, Robert: The Mosquitoes of North America. Ithaca, N. Y., Comstock Publishing Co., 1944.

*11. Ross, E. S., and Roberts, H. R.: Mosquito Atlas. Part I. The Nearctic Anopheles. Important Malaria Vectors of the Americas and Aëdes aegypti, Culex quinquefasciatus. Part II. Eighteen Old World Anophelines Important to Malaria. Published by the American Entomological Society and the Academy of Natural Sciences. Philadelphia, 1943.

*12. Russell, P. F., Rozeboom, L. E., and Stone, Alan: Keys to the Anopheline Mosquitoes of the World. Published by the American Entomological Society and the Academy of Natural Sciences, Philadelphia, 1943.

*13. Simmons, J. S., and Aitken, T. H. G.: The Anopheline Mosquitoes of the Northern Half of the Western Hemisphere and of the Philippine Islands. Army

Medical Bulletin No. 59 (special issue). Published at Medical Field Service School, Carlisle Barracks, Pennsylvania, 1942.

*14. Yamaguti, S., and LaCasse, W. J.: Mosquito Fauna of Guam. Office of the Surgeon, Hq. 8th Army, APO 343, 1950.

*15. Yamaguti, S., and La Casse, W. J.: Mosquito Fauna of Japan and Korea. Office of the Surgeon, Hq. 8th Army, APO 343, 1950.

*16. Yamaguti, S., and LaCasse, W. J.: Mosquito Fauna of North America. Part I, Genus *Anopheles*. Office of the Surgeon, Hq. Japan Logistical Command, APO 343, 1951.

*17. *Ibid.:* Part II, Genera *Megarhinus, Wyeomyia, Uranotaenia* and *Culiseta*.

*18. *Ibid.:* Part III, Genera *Orthopodomyia, Mansonia* and *Psorophora*.

*19. *Ibid.:* Part IV, Genera *Culex* and *Deinocerites*.

*20. *Ibid.:* Part V, Genus *Aedes*.

**Mosquito Bites**   The nature and appearance of mosquito bites are too well known to require discussion here. However, since they cause a tremendous amount of discomfort which often leads to scratching and secondary infection, it seems desirable to list briefly a few of the preparations which have been recommended for relief of the swelling and itching associated with the bites. The following are perhaps the most effective:

1. Weak ammonia water.

2. Hydrogen peroxide.

3. 1 per cent solution of menthol in 95 per cent alcohol.

4. Saponated petroleum (30 ml.) containing iodine (5.0 gm.); also recommended for wasp stings.

5. Carbolic solution (1:40) followed by a dressing of boracic ointment.

6. "Circa 42," a compound developed by the Bureau of Entomology, U. S. Dept. of Agriculture, and prepared according to the following formula:

| | |
|---|---|
| n-butyl-p-aminobenzoate | |
| (May be purchased commercially under the name of Butesin) | 100 gm. |
| benzyl alcohol | 170 ml. |
| anhydrous lanolin (melted) | 20 ml. |
| cornstarch | 640 gm. |
| sodium lauryl sulfonate | 64 gm. |

Plus sufficient additional benzyl alcohol to produce a paste of desirable consistency.

The skin should be made wet before applying the preparation. "Circa 42" has been found effective for the bites of all types of arthropods, likewise in the treatment of poison ivy and of certain mycotic infections. Sweating, bathing and friction from clothing all tend to nullify its effect; nevertheless it is probably superior to most of the preparations listed above. In general it may be said that under tropical conditions it is better to avoid the use of salves and greases in the treatment of bites, scratches and other small lesions. The aim should be to get and keep the lesion *clean* and *dry*.

7. Tincture of iodine covered with collodion solution allays itching and prevents injury from scratching.

* Available to the Armed Forces through channels.

## Environmental Mosquito Control

The control of mosquitoes is an essential public health measure in most subtropical and tropical areas of the world. Breeding grounds must be rigidly controlled if the mosquitoes serving as vectors for such diseases as malaria, dengue, the encephalitides, filariasis and yellow fever are to be curbed. Emphasis is placed upon control measures for both adults and larvae; individual methods of protection such as repellents, protective clothing and bed nets as well as chemotherapy (suppressive treatment) are discussed under the pertinent diseases (see p. 323 for antimalarial measures).

### Anopheline Control.   *Measures to Control Adult Anophelines*

Camp sites and other installations should be carefully selected and situated at least one mile distant on the windward side, if possible, from actual or potential breeding areas, native villages or dwellings.

SCREENING. All buildings should be properly screened with good quality electrogalvanized 18-to-the-inch mesh wire. In tropical areas near the sea it is necessary to use wire of a noncorrosive material such as bronze, aluminum or plastic. A hard drawn wire, 99.8 per cent copper and of heavy grade, is suitable. Screen doors should open outwards, should be sturdily constructed and should be located on the windward side of buildings. In highly malarious areas two such doors, separated by a six foot vestibule, are recommended.

Particular attention should be paid to the closing of cracks in floors and walls. Knot-holes, openings under the eaves, and spaces created by outlets for pipes and wires should also be sealed. A satisfactory substance for this purpose is provided by a mixture of water and shredded toilet tissue or newspaper which has been boiled with flour until fairly homogeneous. The addition of sand and cement forms a plastic which may be molded to fill holes, cracks and crevices and which hardens without undue shrinkage.

INSECTICIDES. Spray-killing of adult mosquitoes in buildings or shacks is carried on in various ways. In closed or mosquito-proofed structures, the interior should be sprayed twice daily, preferably in the early evening and again before sunrise. On the other hand, efficient results in malaria control have been obtained in native villages in India by spraying openly constructed huts inside and out once a week with a pyrethrum insecticide; in this case the mosquitoes which normally roost in the thatch after feeding and remain there until ready for the next blood meal are killed before becoming infective. The newer residual sprays containing DDT or some other new insecticide give good control in most areas and require less frequent applications.

Insecticides may be applied by hand-operated sprayers of the ordinary Flit type or dispersed from a pressure sprayer with a fine nozzle. Two types of chemicals are used, pyrethrins and one of several newer synthetic insecticides such as allethrin, DDT, lindane, dieldrin, etc. Pyrethrum is extracted from the dried flowers of *Chrys-*

*anthemum cinerariaefolium,* while the second group is synthesized chemically.

PYRETHRINS. These are usually available in one of three forms, as follows:

1. Concentrate. This is a 20 to 1 concentrate, each gallon containing the oleoresins of approximately twenty pounds of pyrethrum flowers and containing not less than 75 to 100 gm. of total pyrethrins per gallon. Prior to use this concentrate is diluted with fourteen parts of white odorless kerosene. About one-half ounce of this diluted concentrate is required for the effective spraying of 1000 cubic feet.

2. Ready-to-Use Sprays. In areas where kerosene is not available a ready-to-use pyrethrum spray should be obtained.

3. The pyrethrum aerosol dispenser used during the past several years is a small metal pressure cylinder containing one pound of a mixture of 0.4 per cent pyrethrum and 8 per cent oil of sesame (a synergist or activator) in freon. Each cylinder is sufficient for adequate spraying of 150,000 cubic feet or for 12 to 14 minutes of constant spraying. Recently the Army has standardized an aerosol 12 oz. dispenser containing 0.4 per cent pyrethrins, 2 per cent DDT, 1 per cent piperonyl butoxide and 5 per cent alkylated naphthalene.

ALLETHRIN. One of the newer synthetic organic insecticides, allethrin, having insecticidal properties similar to pyrethrum, is now being used in a formula recently standardized by the U.S. Army to replace pyrethrum in a 12 oz. aerosol dispenser having the following formula: 0.8 per cent allethrin and related products, 2 per cent DDT, and 5 per cent alkylated naphthalene.

DDT. DDT gains entrance into the insect's body through the chemotactic sensory organs located in the tips of the tarsi or through the gut. Lethal action is obtained through irritation and paralysis of the nervous system. DDT may be sprayed on walls, screening or tents, where it has a marked residual effect on adult mosquitoes, flies, sandflies, bedbugs, etc., which persists for several weeks. Dosages which have been found to be effective against insects are not harmful to humans. Dishes, cutlery and food should be covered or removed during spraying. Oil emulsions and solutions containing DDT are absorbed through the skin and are toxic following repeated exposures. DDT used as a dust in various inert diluents may be safely applied to the human skin. Some of the more commonly encountered forms of DDT insecticides used for control of medically important arthropods are sprays containing 1 to 5 per cent DDT dissolved in kerosene or other petroleum oils, 20 per cent DDT in solvent for airplane spraying, 25 per cent DDT emulsion concentrate for making aqueous emulsions, 5 per cent DDT with 2 per cent chlordane in oils for roach and ant control, and aerosol bombs containing 2 per cent DDT together with pyrethrum or allethrin. Some DDT dust preparations commonly encountered are 75 per cent DDT water-dispersable powder, and 10 per cent DDT in pyrophyllite or talc as a dusting powder.

LINDANE. Lindane is the common name for an insecticide containing 99.0 per cent of the gamma isomer of benzene hexachloride. It is a central nervous system stimulant which is approximately twice as toxic as DDT. Lindane is effective against lice, flies, fleas, ticks, mites, mosquitoes, sandflies, roaches and other household and agricultural insect pests. It is slightly volatile and has a residual effectiveness of 2 to 4 weeks, and is available in formulations of wettable powder, emulsifiable concentrate, solutions, and dusts.

DIELDRIN. Dieldrin is one of the synthetic chlorinated hydrocarbon insecticides, also sometimes known as compound 497 or Octalox. It is absorbed readily from the skin as well as through other portals, acting as a central nervous system stimulant which is about 5 times as toxic as DDT. Dieldrin is effective against mosquitoes, flies, fleas, roaches, ticks, mites, ants and other pests. It is slightly volatile but exhibits good residual properties. Dieldrin is available in formulations of wettable powder, emulsifiable concentrates, solutions, and dusts.

**Measures to Control Larval Anophelines**   The females appear to be quite selective in their egg laying habits, utilizing only those waters best adapted for the development of the species concerned. Thus *A. quadrimaculatus* Say seldom breeds in dense shade, or in wholly unshaded waters. A certain amount of aquatic vegetation also seems necessary for the proper development of *A. quadrimaculatus*. This depends not so much upon the amount of foliage present as upon the "intersection line" where air, water and plant surface meet each other. *Anopheles freeborni* Aitken, common in Southern California, tends to avoid impounded waters. *A. albimanus* Wiedemann is a hardy species breeding in the fresh, sunlit pools of streams, swamps and marshes in humid regions. *Anopheles bellator* Dyar & Knab is a forest mosquito, breeding in rain water at the base of bromeliad plants, high up in the branches of trees. *Anopheles aquasalis* Curry favors brackish water but will tolerate either sunlight or shade. *Anopheles superpictus* Grassi favors seepages, small trickles and occasional small pools. *Anopheles gambiae* Giles seeks sunlit pools, usually of rain water that has settled in borrow pits, hoofprints and natural depressions, and avoids all moving water. *Anopheles funestus* Giles, however, prefers pools of permanent character. *Anopheles minimus* Theobald is found in slowly running water, in streams, springs, ditches and rice fields. Recent work on this species has shown that the larvae will develop in water far more heavily polluted than the female will use for oviposition.

One of the most important aspects in the field control of malaria is the elimination of man-made anopheline breeding areas. In endemic regions much acute malaria may be traced directly to such artificial breeding areas as wheel ruts, borrow pits, the obstruction of streams and irrigation ditches, improper management of irrigation water and similar artificial collections of standing or impounded water. The measures which are included within this category have as their objectives either the elimination of collections of water suitable for larval development or alteration of the conditions in such a way as to render the water unsuitable. These procedures include filling, drainage, flow regulation, alteration of the salt content, oiling or dusting, edging, control of sun or shade and the use of fish predatory upon the larvae.

FILLING. This method of eliminating breeding areas is permanent but expensive; wheel ruts, borrow pits and small swamps should be filled whenever possible.

DRAINAGE. If permanent fills are not feasible, drainage to eliminate mosquito breeding areas should be undertaken. Open drainage ditches or subsoil drains may be utilized to remove residual surplus surface water or underground water which may cause surface seepage. In some cases it is possible to remove surface water by vertical

*Table 68   Recommended Mixes for Concrete**

|  | CEMENT | DRY SAND | GRAVEL |  | WATER |  |
|---|---|---|---|---|---|---|
| Inverts (Panama) ..... | 1† | 2¼† | 3† | 6 | gal. | Wet |
| Sidewalls ............. | 1 | 2¼ | 3 | 6 | gal. | mix |
| 18″ × 24″ Tile ........ | 1 | 3 | 2 | 1½ | gal. | Dry |
| 4″ × 6″ Tile .......... | 1 | 3 | 0 | 2 | gal. | mix |

\* After Elmendorf, Lee and Mulrennan.
† Volumetric units based on standard sack of cement (1 barrel = 4 sacks).

drainage. This may consist simply of boring holes into the ground to a sufficient depth to penetrate an impervious stratum which prevents seepage of ground water to lower levels. Malaria engineers should be consulted, as it is sometimes necessary to install pumps or tide gates.

Open drains are maintained more satisfactorily if they are lined with rocks or concrete. The Panama invert, a concrete gutter pre-cast in sections, is an excellent type (Table 68).

Subsoil drainage is effected by lining ditches with baked unglazed or concrete tiles. Under emergency conditions bamboo or saplings may be substituted by laying them lengthwise in the ditch and covering them with stones and soil.

Ditching by dynamite is an efficient, rapid and cheap method. The distance between borings and the amount of dynamite necessary will vary with the type of soil and quantity of moisture present.

SALINITY. Lagoons and marshes of brackish water along the sea coast are often important breeding areas. Some anopheline larvae require water with moderate salt content; others cannot breed in brackish collections. Such breeding areas frequently may be controlled completely by the introduction of tide gates eliminating the salt water or by the construction of channels permitting a freer flow of sea water, thus increasing the salinity of the area.

LARVICIDES. Breeding areas that cannot be eliminated by filling or draining may be controlled by the judicious use of larvicides. A number of preparations such as DDT, lindane, dieldrin, Paris green, or volatile oils are useful in controlling anopheline larvae. These will be considered separately.

1. DDT. Mosquito larviciding with DDT is done largely with ground-operated equipment. In general, oil solutions of DDT are sprayed at the rate of 0.1 to 0.2 pounds of DDT for each acre of water surface. Usually 1 to 5 per cent solutions in petroleum oils are used. If a 5 per cent solution is used only 1 to 2 quarts are required to apply 0.1 or 0.2 pounds, respectively, however it is difficult to get an even distribution with such small quantities of solution to an acre, and for this reason it is frequently desirable to use a larger quantity of spray having a lower concentration. The spray nozzle should liberate as fine a spray as possible in such a manner as to obtain the maximum drift over the water. Larvicide should be applied every 1 to 3 weeks during the mosquito-breeding season, depending on temperature, degree of infestation and other factors. A prolonged residual effect can be obtained in static pools with heavy applications of DDT applied to give 1 pound of DDT to an acre.

Aircraft dispersal of DDT in mosquitocidal operation is advisable and practical under certain situations, but should only be attempted on the advice of qualified officials who have carefully weighed the numerous factors involved. The DDT formulation normally used by the Armed Services for aircraft spraying contains 20 per cent DDT in 80 per cent solvent.

Dusts containing DDT may also be used effectively for mosquito larviciding. The Army QM standard-issue dust mixture (10 per cent DDT in talc or pyrophyllite) is ordinarily diluted to a 1 or more per cent DDT mixture by adding an inert carrier as follows: for a 1 per cent mixture, add 1 part of the 10 per cent dust to 9 parts of carrier, etc. A hand-operated rotary type duster is the most satisfactory duster for drifting the dust over the area being treated. The amount of DDT needed per acre usually ranges from 0.1 to 1.0 pound per acre, depending on degree of infestation, amount of vegetation, whether residual effect is desired, etc.

2. LINDANE. If DDT-resistant mosquitoes are encountered, a 0.4 per cent lindane spray applied as a fine mist at the rate of 3 gallons per acre of water surface is recommended as a larvicide. This spray may be prepared by adding one part of 20 per cent emulsifiable concentrate to 49 parts of water and mix thoroughly.

3. DIELDRIN. A spray preparation containing 0.3 per cent dieldrin, applied as a fine mist to breeding areas at the rate of 2 to 4 gallons per acre, depending on amount of vegetation and type of equipment available, will give control of mosquito larvae. This spray may be prepared by addition of 1 part of 18 per cent emulsifiable concentrate to 59 parts of water.

4. PARIS GREEN. This emerald green, micro-crystalline powder (an aceto-arsenite of copper) is a potent gastro-intestinal poison for surface-feeding mosquito larvae. Since *Anopheles* larvae are surface

feeders, Paris green is particularly effective against them although if it floats long enough in still water, or if the water is shallow, some *Aedes* and *Culex* larvae will also ingest the poison. When carried to the bottom with wet pebbles Paris green is more effective against culicines.

The solubility of Paris green in water should not exceed 3 per cent. It should contain at least 50 per cent arsenious oxide and should also pass a 300 to 325 mesh sieve. As mixed for field use, Paris green should kill all second, third and fourth instar anopheline larvae within two hours.

For application as a dust, Paris green is mixed with finely powdered road dust, charcoal, slaked lime, powdered soapstone, or other dust which has been sifted through a 30 mesh screen. Paris green is mixed with such diluents in a proportion varying from 1 to 5 per cent by volume for hand operated blowers and up to 25 per cent or more for dusting from airplanes. When lime is used as the diluent it is recommended that Paris green be added in the proportion of 10 per cent by weight, the equivalent of 5 per cent by volume. The efficacy of this dust should be checked in the field from time to time by dipping for larvae twelve to twenty-four hours after application, or checking the kill of larvae in "planted" petri dishes.

Mixtures containing Paris green can be applied to large streams, ponds or lakes by blowing the dust into the air on the windward side so that it forms a cloud and is carried over the water. Portable or motor-driven blowers are most satisfactory, the latter being mounted on trucks or boats.

Hoppers and "venturis" attached to airplanes facilitate the dusting of large areas by air. Such operations are most effective when there is relatively little motion of the air. In warm weather under average conditions Paris green should be applied every five to seven days, or as soon as fourth stage larvae are encountered.

Paris green may likewise be used efficiently by dustless methods, using the following stock suspension:

| | |
|---|---|
| Kerosene oil | 1 pint |
| Paris green | ½ pint |
| Egg albumen (dry powdered) | ¼ teaspoonful |

Twenty-five to 27 ml. of this stock suspension is mixed with 5 quarts of water and distributed by a standard knapsack sprayer. The addition of two teaspoonfuls of castor oil increases the effectiveness. If powdered egg albumen is not available the mixture may be used with reasonable efficiency in its absence provided the sprayer is constantly agitated while in use. A 5 quart mixture is sufficient for approximately 500 square feet of water surface.

The Paris green suspension may likewise be prepared for distribution by hand casting. Egg albumen is omitted. Approximately 30 ml. of the mixture is thoroughly churned with about 3 liters of damp sand or gravel. The optimal degree of moisture of the diluent must be determined by trial and error. If too wet it does not spread well and if too dry the Paris green kerosene mixture adheres to dry particles of sand and is carried to the bottom. Dry and wet sand at a streamside may be blended to give the correct mixture. This method of use may be quite efficient.

5. OILS. Oils and oil mixtures are toxic on ingestion and also on contact with the tracheal cells of the larvae and pupae. Oils are effective against all surface-breathing species. The *Mansonia* group secures its oxygen from aquatic plants and consequently is not affected by oil. The specifications for an ideal larvicidal oil are as follows:

| | |
|---|---|
| Specific gravity 20/4 | 0.83–0.86 |
| Viscosity (Saybolt Universal at 100° F.) | 21–43 |
| Initial boiling point | 297°–414° F. (165°–230° C.) |
| Final boiling point | Max. 800° F. (426.7° C.) |
| Spreading coefficient | Min. 17.0 |

Diesel Oil No. 2 is highly satisfactory. About nine gallons per acre are required to produce a stable and uniform film. In practice, however, the actual amount required may vary from 9 to 20 gallons per acre depending upon the amount of flotage and vegetation. It is usually necessary to apply oil every five to seven days depending upon the rate of development of larvae.

Undiluted waste motor oils alone are of little value. They spread poorly and contain none of the toxic volatile substances. When mixed with kerosene in the proportion of approximately 1 to 3 they are effective and useful. The exact amount of kerosene required must be determined by observing the spreading quality of the mixture. The addition of approximately 2 per cent castor oil or 0.5 per cent cresol improves the spreading quality of the film.

Mosquito breeding in water stored for human use in tanks, cisterns and wells may be controlled by the use of screens, covers, kerosene or gasoline alone. These rapidly volatilize without impairing the water. If gasoline is to be used it must be lead-free. DDT in alcohol has been used to control *Aedes aegypti* breeding in containers; pyrethrum powder can also be used without impairing the potability of the water. In many places in South America native fish introduced into water barrels and tanks controlled the breeding of *Aedes*.

Oils may be applied effectively by spraying or by the use of continuous oiling devices. The knapsack sprayer consists of a container, hand pressure pump and spray nozzle and is carried and operated by one person. Most sprayers of this type have a capacity of 4 to 5 gallons and a spraying range of 25 feet. Such apparatus is both practical and economical for treating ditches, small ponds or puddles. Small collections of water may be treated by means of oily mops, oil soaked waste tied to a stick or other similar improvisations.

Large bodies of water are usually reached by motor driven power sprayers mounted on a vehicle or boat. Airplanes may be equipped to oil extensive breeding areas.

Oil may be distributed on small streams or in ditches by the use of continuous oilers. Such devices are not entirely reliable and require supervision. Drip oilers may be made from discarded oil drums or barrels punctured at the base to yield a flow of 10 to 20 drops per minute for each foot of width of the water surface. In home-made containers a nail hole may be used, with a nail left loosely in the hole. Sometimes string may be tied around the nail head to form a washer. The cans should be elevated several feet above the stream.

Submerged oilers may consist of oil balls or cans. The former is made by wrapping oil-soaked sawdust, cork dust, or finely pulverized coconut husks in burlap and submerging it. The latter usually consists of a discarded gasoline tin with two holes arranged so that water enters one as oil leaves the other; the openings frequently become clogged.

Oil booms used to combat larval drift in a stream are constructed of materials obtained locally and are placed across the channel. The booms should permit the water to flow freely under them while the larvae are held back in the surface scum and killed by oil-soaked sawdust or chaff that has been thrown on the water above the boom.

There are certain situations, however, in which oil may not be used. For example, large wooden tanks built for the storage of water for fighting fire or other purposes are usually lined with a bituminous material which is likely to be injured by contact with larvicidal oils. In such a case creosol larvicides are recommended.

CHANNELING AND FLUCTUATION. In regions with marked rainy and dry seasons there is considerable fluctuation of water levels in streams. This is an important factor in areas where malaria vectors develop in nearly dry stream beds. Such localities can be controlled by ditching to concentrate the flow into a single channel or by constructing dams equipped with automatic siphons or hand operated sluices to flush out the breeding areas periodically.

Fluctuation of the water level in a series of reservoirs also has been used successfully to control the development of mosquitoes. Lowering of the level may strand larvae and eggs and destroy them by desiccation or force larvae to open water where they are accessible to carnivorous enemies. Subsequent raising of the water level drives larvae out of pockets where they were temporarily free from attack.

EDGING. The removal of vegetation from the margin of a stream, lake or reservoir is an important control measure. Such a procedure tends to clear and straighten the channel of small streams or irrigation ditches and so destroy potential breeding areas. Similar clearing of the shore line about lakes or ponds removes littoral protection for larvae even though the water level may fluctuate.

SHADE. Certain anopheline larvae flourish in sunlit water while others must have shade. The elimination of trees and brush along the banks of streams and other small pools of water to provide free entry of sunlight will eliminate the larvae requiring shade. Conversely, planting along the banks of streams and ditches will eliminate those which need sunlight. These measures, however, should not be undertaken until a complete survey of the anophelines of the area has been made, since alteration of the sun and shade factors, while eliminating one species, may lead to the establishment of others which thrive under the altered conditions.

BIOLOGICAL MEASURES. The introduction of top minnows such as *Gambusia*, which feed upon mosquito larvae and pupae, is a very efficient method of control for use in lakes, ponds and circumscribed collections of water, especially where aquatic vegetation is not abundant.

"Biological" control of this nature represents merely an extension of the "natural" control factors which are in operation at all times. Not only fishes, but also water bugs (NOTONECTIDAE) and other aquatic predators (e.g., dragonfly nymphs) play an important, though sometimes unappreciated, role in keeping the numbers of mosquito larvae within normal averages.

**Species Elimination**   In some areas it may be found less expensive in the long run to attempt the complete elimination of a malaria-carrying species rather than continue indefinitely the application of measures which rarely succeed in accomplishing more than a general reduction of the mosquito fauna for a given season. The extermination of *Anopheles gambiae* in Brazil is an excellent example of a species-elimination program, carried out on a relatively large scale. No such plan should be undertaken, however, without complete knowledge of the habits and ecologic relationships of the species concerned, lest time, money and manpower be wasted in what may later prove to have been a hopeless effort. Until data have been accumulated showing the feasibility of the undertaking, it is always best to gauge the mosquito-reduction program for maintaining merely a "safe index," in other words, that degree of control under which the chances of a non-immune being bitten by an infected anopheline are of negligible significance.

**Culicine Control.**   *Measures to Control Adult Culicines*   Most of the environmental control measures described for both adult and larval anopheline mosquitoes are applicable to the culicine group or may be modified to meet the particular situation (see pp. 738 to 745). The following information is offered as a guide to some of the problems of control.

As with anophelines, some forms (including most species of *Aedes*) live only through the summer season. Others (*Culex*) usually hibernate as adults. Domesticated species, as might be expected, feed eagerly on human blood and seem to prefer it. Semi-domesticated and wild species vary in their feeding preferences. *Culiseta* attacks man rather rarely. *Culex apicalis* is believed to feed exclusively on the blood of frogs and other poikilothermic vertebrates. There is a long list of forest and open country species which subsist normally on the blood of wild mammals and birds, but which transfer to man as soon as he becomes available.

Feeding hours tend to be rather constant for the various groups. *Aedes aegypti* and *A. albopictus* are daylight biters. *Culex pipiens* and *C. quinquefasciatus* feed either at night or in darkened rooms. *Aedes stimulans*, *A. excrucians* and several others prefer late afternoon for feeding but *Aedes spencerii* attacks in bright sunshine.

Culicines in general show a greater flight range than anophelines. *Aedes sollicitans* has been known to migrate as much as forty miles, *Aedes vexans*, at least ten. *Aedes cantator* and *A. taeniorhynchus* are also known for their migrations. Some (*A. aldrichi*) restrict their migrations to wooded areas. Domesticated and semi-domesticated species, however, remain fairly close to their breeding grounds.

**Measures to Control Larval Culicines** All members of the four genera, *Culex*, *Mansonia*, *Uranotaenia* and *Culiseta*, deposit their eggs in rafts on the surface of the water (Fig. 295). In the case of *Culex pipiens* each female, fresh from hibernation, lays 100 to 400 eggs in a single mass. Each egg floats "on end," with the more slender extremity uppermost, an arrangement which gives to the "raft" a more or less concave appearance (as viewed from above).

In most other genera of culicines the eggs are laid singly in water, near water, or where water is likely to be. Species of *Psorophora* deposit eggs directly upon the ground. Protected by heavy, spiny coats they may remain dormant for months or even years, but hatch quickly when water finally becomes available. Larval development is then very rapid, requiring, as a rule, only a few days.

Most species of *Aedes* leave their eggs during the summer in the bottoms of dried-out pools, swamps and marshes. Such eggs remain dormant throughout the fall and winter (even if submerged), not hatching until the following spring. A few species of *Aedes*, however, produce at least two broods a year. *Aedes varipalpus* and *A. triseriatus* usually seek tree holes in which to deposit their eggs. *Aedes aegypti*, being a domesticated species, oviposits on or just above the surface of water in various small containers near the habitation of man. These eggs, unlike certain species mentioned above, hatch very quickly. Where temperature permits, breeding of *A. aegypti* goes on throughout the year. This species cannot survive outside of tropical and subtropical latitudes, though it may migrate into temperate regions and reproduce successfully during the summer months.

It is convenient to classify culicines into three general groups on the basis of the type of habitat selected for breeding purposes:

1. Domesticated species, which, like *Aedes aegypti*, *Culex pipiens* and *C. quinquefasciatus*, breed in and about human dwellings.

2. Semi-domesticated species, which may breed either close to human habitations or in other situations, as opportunity affords.

3. Wild species, which avoid the habitations of man, being found in salt, brackish or fresh-water marshes, in swamps, woodlands, prairies or other natural situations. The greater number of culicine

## Table 69   The Chemical Control of Arthropods of Medical Importance*

| ARTHROPOD | PLACE OF TREATMENT | CHEMICAL | AMOUNT AND METHOD USED | TOXICITY TO HUMANS |
|---|---|---|---|---|
| Mosquito and fly adults. | 1. Inclosed spaces as barracks, rooms, barns, airplanes, etc. | 1. Aerosols† Pyrethrum–DDT Aerosol. 1% pyrethrins + 2 to 3% DDT + 2% sesame oil in freon. | Aerosol bomb—spray 4 sec. per 1000 cu. ft. Spray into air. Spray 2 or 3 times this amount for aircraft disinsectization. | None. |
| | | 2. DDT‡ Spray Residue Deposit. a. DDT in kerosene (5% DDT in crude kerosene). Use technical DDT at rate of 7 oz. per gallon of kerosene to make 5% spray. | Heavy spray on interior of buildings (1 qt. per 250 sq. ft.). Particular attention to where flies and mosquitoes rest. One application will usually control flies and mosquitoes in treated buildings for 2–3 mo. When DDT-resistant strains of flies or mosquitoes are encountered, sprays containing 0.5 to 1% of dieldrin or lindane may be used effectively. | No appreciable toxicity when used properly at recommended dosages. Protect foods, dishes, and cutlery. |
| | | b. DDT-water emulsion concentrate. | 1 part of 25% concentrate to 4 parts of water and use same as in (2) above. (Note: emulsion conc. should only be used when specifically authorized.) | Relatively non-toxic when properly used at recommended dosages. |
| | | 3. Pyrethrum Extracts (1 lb. pyrethrum, containing 1% pyrethrins per gallon of kerosene). | 100 ml. per 1000 cu. ft., sprayed into the air as space spray. | None. |
| | | 4. Pyrethrum plus synthetic organic compounds such as Thanite. | 100 ml. per 1000 cu.ft., spray into the air. | None. Irritating to some. |
| | 2. Outdoors, by spraying from airplanes. | 1. Insecticide, Airplane Spray, 20% DDT (DDT in fuel oil and auxiliary solvent) or 5 to 10% DDT in fuel oil. | One-tenth to 0.25 lb. of DDT per acre will greatly reduce adult mosquito and fly populations and control mosquito larvae for one to two weeks. | Non-toxic when used properly at recommended dosages. |
| | 3. In jungle or other vegetated areas. | 1. Mists, fogs, aerosols etc. made from 5 to 10% DDT in kerosene or fuel oil, lub. oil, or a mixture of these; or 20% airplane spray as above. | One to two quarts per acre will usually give temporary control. Around a clearing, apply spray on vegetation in a 50-foot or wider band encircling area to form a barrier, with mist blowers, fog generators or aerosol generators. | Non-toxic when used properly at recommended dosages. Avoid prolonged contact. |
| Mosquito larvae | 1. Streams, lakes, swamps, pools, ruts and water-containing receptacles around houses. | 1. DDT Oil Solutions (1-5% DDT in kerosene, diesel, or fuel oil). | Prepare by adding 2 lbs. DDT per 25 gallons of oil. Use 5 qts. of 1% DDT or 1 qt. of 5% DDT per acre of water. Apply with a fine spray nozzle with main emphasis where aquatic vegetation is thick, particularly along water margins. | Avoid prolonged contact. |
| | | 2. DDT-water Emulsion Concentrate (25% DDT). | Dilute 1 part concentrate with 24 parts water. Use 10 qts. of dilute spray per acre. Emphasis on water margin as above. This preparation can be used safely on agricultural crops or other vegetation where oil preparations may cause injury. Lasts 7 to 10 days. | Non-toxic when used at recommended dosage. Avoid prolonged contact. |
| | | 3. Insecticide, Airplane Spray, 20% DDT (DDT in fuel oil and auxiliary solvents). | Spray from airplanes. Amount and method as listed above for adults (2). | Same as above. |
| | | 4. Petroleum Oil. Light fuel oil of No. 2 grade or Bunker "C" diluted ⅓ with kerosene. | 15–25 gallons per acre depending on density of aquatic vegetation. Apply as a spray every 7-10 days. | Essentially non-toxic. |
| | | 5. Paris Green (Copper aceto-arsenite containing 50% plus of arsenious oxide.) | 1-lb. Paris green per acre. For hand or power dusting dilute to 5-10% with inert dusts such as road dust, fine sand, talc, hydrated lime, condemned flour. As an airplane dust dilute to 25%. Apply every 7-10 days. For control of *Anopheles* mos‑ | Very toxic if eaten. Non-toxic in water at recommended dosages. |

| | | | | |
|---|---|---|---|---|
| Mosquito larvae (cont'd) | | 6. DDT dusting powder (10% DDT). | Dilute 10% powder with several parts of any dry dust diluent and apply at rate of 0.2 lb. of DDT per acre with rotary duster or other suitable equipment. This material may be used safely on vegetation where oil preparations may cause damage. | None. |
| | | 7. Insecticide, DDT, Water-dispersable Powder. | Make 2½% suspension and apply as a spray at the rate of 0.2 lb. of DDT per acre. Keep well-agitated. | Non-toxic when used as recommended. |
| | | 8. Dieldrin. | 1% dieldrin-water emulsion may be used effectively as a spray to control species that are resistant to DDT. Apply in similar manner as for DDT oil solution above. | Studies indicate non-toxicity when used properly at recommended doses. |
| | | 9. Lindane. | Same as for dieldrin. | Same as above. |
| Fly larvae. | 1. Latrines. | 1. Petroleum Oils (kerosene, fuel oil, waste motor oil, etc.). | Thorough wetting the entire surface of the breeding media 3 or 4 times weekly, by means of a coarse spray will control most fly larvae. | Essentially non-toxic. |
| | | 2. Dieldrin or Lindane. | 1% water emulsion or wettable powder of either of these chemicals sprayed twice week as wet spray over the entire surface of the breeding media will give good control. | Same as for Dieldrin in mosquito control above. |
| | 2. Garbage dumps, rubbish heaps, and other breeding places. | 1. Dieldrin or Lindane. | Same as above for control in latrines. Note: Continued use of these materials may result in insecticide resistant strains. | Same as above. |
| Lice (cootie, grey-back). *Pediculus humanus* var. *humanus* and *capitis*; pubic louse (crab), *Phthirus pubis*. | 1. On body and clothing. | 1. DDT Powder (10% DDT in pyrophyllite or other inert dusts). | Mass Treatment. Thoroughly dust between inside garment and skin itself by applying dust gun at all openings of clothing. Use 1.5 ounces per individual. Body lice are most frequently found in the seams of clothing. Individual Treatment. Apply powder from sifter top can over the entire inner surface of underwear and treat seams on the inside of shirt and trousers, use one (1) ounce of powder. | Essentially non-toxic. |
| | | 2. Lindane dust (1% in inert dust). | Should be applied as described for DDT above. Three applications are recommended. Note: Not more than 60 grm. per application per person and applications not closer than 7 days apart. Particularly recommended where DDT resistent lice are encountered. | Studies indicate non-toxicity when used properly at recommended dosages. |
| | 2. Body. | 1. Insecticide Spray, Delousing (DDT, benzyl benzoate, benzocaine, and emulsifier). | Dilute concentrate 1 part with 5 parts of water and spray hairy parts of body with about 20 to 30 ml. of the liquid. | Essentially non-toxic. Protect eyes during application. |
| | 3. Clothing impregnation. | 1. DDT-Water Emulsion Concentrate. | Dilute to 2% DDT. Use ordinary laundry facilities. 1 pt. per suit of underwear. | Studies indicate non-toxicity when used properly at recommended dosages. |
| | 4. Mass clothing treatment. | 1. Methyl Bromide (danger). | 8 lbs. per 1000 cu. ft. for half hour. Use in specially constructed fumigators. To be used by experts only. Individual clothing and equipment fumigation may be done in special rubberized bags by breaking an ampule of methyl bromide in bag. | Very toxic. No warning odor. Safe dosage, 30 parts per million for operators. |

* Originally prepared by Captain W. N. Sullivan, Sn.C. Most of the research in the United States on the biological effects of DDT against insects affecting man and animals has been done by the Orlando Laboratory, Bureau of Entomology and Plant Quarantine, United States Department of Agriculture.

† United States Department of Agriculture Public Service Patent by Goodhue and Sullivan.

‡ DDT is an abbreviation for dichloro-diphenyl-trichloroethane.

Table 69 *The Chemical Control of Arthropods of Medical Importance** (Continued)

| ARTHROPOD | PLACE OF TREATMENT | CHEMICAL | AMOUNT AND METHOD USED | TOXICITY TO HUMANS |
|---|---|---|---|---|
| Fleas *Xenopsylla* spp., *Ceratophyllus* spp., *Pulex irritans*, etc. | 1. Rooms. | 1. DDT Oil Solution (5% DDT in kerosene). | 1 gal. 5% DDT in oil per 1000 sq. ft. will give good results. 2 lbs. DDT in 5 gallons oil. | Non-toxic at recommended dosages. |
| | | 2. Lindane Dust (1% in any inert diluent dust). | Dust lightly over floor and furniture with hand or rotary type duster. | Same as above. |
| | | 3. Insecticide Dust, Pyrethrins and/or Synthetics. | Same as No. 2 above. | Same as above. |
| | | 4. DDT Dust (10% in pyrophyllite). | Same as for lindane dust, No. 2 above. | Non-toxic if used as recommended. |
| | | 5. Napthalene (moth flakes). | 3 lbs. per 1000 cu. ft. Thorough dusting on floor, especially cracks. Overnight fumigation. | Non-toxic unless eaten. |
| | | 6. Paradichlorobenzene. | Same as No. 5 above. | Same as above. |
| | 2. Animals. | 1. DDT Dust (10% in pyrophyllite). | Light application over animal. Rub lightly into hair. | Slightly toxic to cats and other animals that lick themselves. |
| | | 2. Rotenone Dusts (Derris powders). | Thorough application over animal. Rub lightly into hair. | None. |
| | 3. Rat runways, rodent burrows, rubbish heaps, and other rodent- and flea-infested areas. | 1. DDT Dust (10% in pyrophyllite). | Dust lightly over entire area to kill fleas leaving rodents. Dust heavily in burrows and rat runways to kill fleas on rodents going through the dusted area. | None if used as recommended. |
| Bedbugs (Chinches) *Cimex* spp. | 1. Inclosed spaces. | 1. DDT Kerosene Solution (5% DDT in kerosene). | 1 qt. sprays 5 beds and mattresses. Thoroughly spray mattresses, beds, and into cracks and crevices in wall, with particular attention to springs and the corners of beds. Residual effect of a year or more. | Studies indicate non-toxicity when used properly at recommended dosages. |
| | | 2. Hydrogen Cyanide (Danger). | To be used by experts only. | Extremely toxic. |
| | | 3. Pyrethrum Extracts (1 lb. per gallon of kerosene). | Thorough wetting of cracks and crevices containing bedbugs. For minor infestations. Repeat. | None. |
| Roaches | 1. Inclosed spaces. | 1. Chlordane (2%) and DDT (5%) in kerosene. | Apply as wet spray directly to crack, crevices and behind objects, particularly in kitchens, food storerooms, and near water supplies. Also very effective against ants. | Toxic. Should be used according to recommendations. Protect foods and utensils. |
| | | 2. Chlordane (5% to 10% dust). | Thorough application to cracks, crevices, and all infested areas. Also very effective against ants. | Toxic. Protect food and utensils. |
| | | 3. Sodium Fluoride Dust (should be colored). | Thorough application to cracks, crevices and all infested areas. Keep dry. | Very toxic if eaten. |
| Mites (Chiggers, redbugs, harvest mites), *Trombicula* spp. (larvae). | 1. Body. | 1. Dimethyl Phthalate. | Barrier Treatment. Apply thin layer ½ in. wide along all openings of uniform and socks. Good until uniform is washed. Most rapid acting. | Non-toxic. |

| | | | |
|---|---|---|---|
| Mites (cont'd) | 2. Clothing impregnation. | 1. Dimethyl Phthalate Emulsion (90% DMP and 10% emulsifier) toxic to mites. | Clothing impregnation with 5% DMP emulsion in water gives excellent protection until clothes are washed. Mix 1 gal. of 90% emulsion conc. with 17 gal. water. Will treat 35 to 50 fatigue suits and socks. Wring out thoroughly and dry before wearing. | Non-toxic. |
| | | 2. Benzyl Benzoate-Dibutyl Phthalate, Emulsion (45% benzylbenzoate, 45% dibutylphthalate, 10% emulsifier), toxic to mites. | 1 gal. of emulsion conc. mixed with 17 gals. of water will treat 35 to 50 uniforms including socks. Will protect against chiggers after 2 washings in cold water. Impregnated uniforms protect the wearer by killing chiggers that crawl on treated cloth. Also effective against species that transmit scrub typhus. | Essentially non-toxic when used as directed. Not to be used on skin as mosquito repellents. |
| Scabies, mange. (*Sarcoptes scabiei*) | 1. Body. | 1. Insecticide Spray, Delousing (DDT, benzyl benzoate, benzocaine, and emulsifier). | Dilute 1 part concentrate and 5 parts water. Apply as spray or by hand over body except head. Plain benzyl benzoate at 25% dilution in alcohol is also effective; used same as above. | Non-toxic when used as recommended. |
| | | 2. Eurax Cream or Kwell ointment. | Thorough application to affected parts. | Non-irritating. |
| Ticks (most species). | 1. Animals. | 1. Toxaphene (0.5% emulsion in water). | Apply thoroughly as a spray to all parts of animal's body. Do not dip animals in this preparation. | Safe if used as recommended. |
| | | 2. Lindane-DDT (0.025% lindane and 0.5% DDT emulsion in water. | Same as for toxaphene above. | Same as for toxaphene. |
| | 2. Ground-dusting of infested areas. | 1. DDT Dust. | Use 4 lbs. of DDT, diluted with several parts of inert diluent, per acre, dusted thoroughly over all infested areas. Will give fair control for 1 season. | Non-toxic. |
| | | 2. Dieldrin Dust. | Use 0.5 to 1.0 lbs. of dieldrin, diluted with several parts of inert diluent, per acre, dusted thoroughly over all infested areas. Will give good control for one season. | Non-toxic when used as directed at recommended doses. |
| | 3. Clothing impregnation. | 1. N-Butylacetanilide (may also use preparation containing 3 parts of 2-butyl-2-ethyl-1,3-propanediol, N-butylacetanilide, and benzyl benzoate, and 1 part of an emulsifier (M-1960)). | Uniform and socks should be dipped in an emulsion of N-butyl-acetanilide so as to evenly distribute about 2 oz. of the chemical on the garments. Will give excellent protection to the wearer against ticks and chiggers for about 2 weeks, or until clothing is laundered. | Studies indicate non-toxicity when used properly at recommended dosages. Not recommended for direct application to skin. |
| Insect repellents (flies, mosquitoes, gnats, mites, sandflies, fleas, and possibly others.) | 1. Exposed surfaces of body and clothes. | 1. 6-2-2 (6 parts Dimethyl phthalate + 2 parts Indalone + 2 parts of 612, mixed mechanically). | Application on Skin. 1/2 teaspoonful into palm of hand, rub hands together and then apply in thin layer to face, neck, ears, hands and wrists. Lasts 1-2 hours. Care not to get in eyes and mouth. | Non-toxic. Very irritating to the eyes. |
| | | | On Clothes. Spray or apply by hands on clothes. Effective for a number of days. Best all around repellent. Combines good qualities of three ingredients. | |
| | | 2. Dimethyl Phthalate. | Particularly effective against *Anopheles* and larval mites (chiggers). Use same as (1) above. | Same as above. |
| | | 3. Indalone. | Same as (1) above. Best use against biting flies. | Same as above. |
| | | 4. 2-Ethyl Hexanediol-1-3 (repellent 612). | Same as (1) above. Particularly effective against *Aedes*. | Same as above. |

species are therefore classed as "wild." In temperate regions wild culicines may be further divided into "spring breeding" and "summer breeding" forms. In North America, *A. stimulans, A. canadensis* and *A. cinereus* are examples of the first group; *A. sollicitans, A. taeniorhynchus* and *A. cantator,* of the second.

The most important culicine is *Aedes aegypti,* which is known to be one of the principal vectors of dengue and yellow fever. It also serves as a vector of filariasis, certain of the encephalitides and may mechanically transmit tularemia.

*Aedes aegypti* is a day flier until it obtains its first blood meal, after which it is said to feed and fly principally at night. Consequently certain additional precautions are necessary if adequate control is to be achieved.

In areas where *A. aegypti* is prevalent, all buildings, especially hospital wards, should be sprayed two or three times daily. Fox holes and outdoor resting areas for troops should be treated at least once a day as conditions permit. Persons in mosquito-infested areas should remain fully clothed with sleeves rolled down and should make use of mosquito repellents continuously. At night all persons should sleep under mosquito bars. If mosquito bars are not available, or if one is required to be out of doors at night, repellents should be used (p. 751).

Control of *A. aegypti* centers around measures that are applicable to urban communities, as this mosquito is a household breeder. Its larvae are found in cisterns, barrels, clogged or defective roof gutters, tin cans, buckets or in any depression in which water remains for several days. Furthermore, this species may oviposit inside houses in water pitchers, slop jars, flower bowls and the like. Ornamental garden pools, unless adequately stocked with fish, are potentially dangerous. Flower vases in cemeteries are often the source of mosquitoes.

In all such instances the larvae may be controlled by the judicious application of larvicidal oils or dust (p. 742), or by the emptying and removal of small water containers. In many tropical cities it is part of the public health program (yellow fever campaign) to maintain crews of especially trained inspectors to enter all dwellings at frequent intervals in order to detect and destroy larvae of *A. aegypti.*

**Control of Other Culicines**   As previously pointed out, there are other culicine species which serve as vectors of disease: certain species of *Culex* are good vectors of Japanese B or endemic encephalitis and of filariasis bancrofti. In the United States culicines transmit the virus of western equine encephalomyelitis. In the *Mansonia* group (including the subgenus *Mansonioides*) are vectors of the filarial worm, *Wuchereria malayi.* In addition to these, many species of *Culex* and *Aedes* are exceedingly important as human pests. Some coastal regions are virtually uninhabitable by reason of the tremendous number of salt marsh-breeding forms.

Control measures against other culicines are similar to those already described for *Aedes* and *Anopheles*. Oils are useful, especially since culicine larvae, by reason of their resting position, tend to feed below the surface film.

The genus *Mansonia* presents a special problem in that the larvae and pupae of these mosquitoes secure their oxygen from the subsurface stems of aquatic plants such as water lettuce (*Pistia*) and are therefore not readily affected by surface treatment. Development is slow, requiring nearly a year. In areas where both plants and mosquitoes are abundant, control may best be achieved by destruction of the plant.

Measures summarizing the methods for controlling various arthropods of medical importance appear in Table 69, p. 748.

### Family Blepharoceridae (Net-Winged Midges)

This family is mentioned only because of a peculiar dimorphism found in the females of certain species, one type being blood sucking, while the other feeds upon the nectar of flowers.

## Suborder Brachycera

Although entomologists recognize at least seventeen families in this suborder we are here concerned with only two, the TABANIDAE (horsefly family) and RHAGIONIDAE (snipe flies). Their separation is relatively easy (Table 70):

*Table 70   Key for the Separation of Horseflies and Snipe Flies*

1   (2)   Third antennal segment made up of several subsegments. Squamae (transparent scales beneath base of wing) large . . . . . . . . . . . . . . . . . . . . . . . . . . . . . . . . . . . . . . . . . . . *Tabanidae*

2   (1)   Third antennal segment usually simple, rarely annulate, but if so bearing a terminal arista (bristle-like process). Squamae small to vestigial . . . . . . . . . . . . . *Rhagionidae*

### Family Tabanidae

This large family (2500 species), known variously as horseflies, deer flies, three-cornered flies, greenheaded flies, gadflies, mangrove flies, seroots, clegs, thunder flies, and breezes, is widely distributed throughout the world. All species are blood suckers. However, only the females bite, the males feeding on plant juices, or in rare instances, the juices of soft-bodied insects. The family includes more than sixty genera, but the great majority of species fall either in the genus *Tabanus* (horsefly group) or the genus *Chrysops* (deer flies). These two important genera represent separate subfamilies which may be distinguished by the following characters:

The Genus, *Tabanus* alone includes over 1000 species and is represented in almost every part of the world. They are large flies, with a wingspread ranging up to two and a half inches, and are always stoutly built. All members of the genus have the third antennal segment furnished with a conspicuous angular projection. The wings are usually uniform in color (Fig. 296).

The Genus *Chrysops* also has a world-wide distribution. Over seventy species are found in North America alone. These are smaller flies, rarely exceeding a half inch in length. The wings are marked with a dark band across the middle and frequently display a second spot at the tip (Fig. 297).

The Genus *Silvius*, rare in North America, is abundantly represented in the Australian life zone. *Haematopota*, scantily represented throughout the world, is especially abundant in Africa and in the Orient. *Diachlorus* is best represented in South America.

*Table 71    Key for the Separation of Horseflies and Deer Flies*

1  (2)  Hind tibiae with at least small spurs at the tips; ocelli usually present—Subfamily PANGONIINAE (includes *Chrysops, Goniops Pangonia, Silvius*).

2  (1)  Hind tibiae without spurs at their tips; ocelli absent or at most rudimentary—subfamily TABANINAE (includes *Tabanus, Haematopota, Diachlorus*).

**Medical Importance**    BITES. The TABANIDAE attack silently and inflict a painful bite. The bite is not poisonous, but due to the size of the puncture the site may continue to bleed for some time after the fly has taken its blood meal. As in the mosquitoes, the proboscis includes a labrum-epipharynx and a sheath-like labium. Unlike mosquitoes, however, the labium has labella provided with pseudotracheae which are rasping in function. The mandibles are hard, sharply pointed cutting blades, which serve to pierce and lacerate the skin. The maxillae are more complicated and are provided with small, recurved teeth. The hypopharynx fits against the labrum-epipharynx to form a blood canal and is itself provided with a channel, the salivary duct. The saliva probably functions as an anticoagulant, but differs from that secreted by mosquitoes (and other NEMATOCERA) in being non-irritating to man.

As VECTORS OF DISEASE. Two species of Mango flies, *Chrysops silacea* Austen and *C. dimidiata* v.d. Wulp, are proved vectors of *Loa loa* worms in various West African countries.

Tabanid flies function also as mechanical vectors of certain important diseases. This type of vectorship relates to the habit of feeding on a succession of animal hosts in securing a single blood meal. If disturbed while biting they usually proceed at once to a second host, carrying on the wet proboscis any micro-organisms present in the blood of the first. Both anthrax and tularemia may thus be transferred by direct inoculation. *Chrysops discalis* is the species most concerned with the transmission of tularemia in the western United

States, while in Russia certain species of *Tabanus* are more commonly involved. It has been shown that *Chrysops* may remain infective for at least eight days and in some instances, fourteen.

**Habits and Life History**  Most species of TABANIDAE deposit their eggs in the vicinity of water, in many cases gluing them to foliage overhanging a swamp or stream. However, marginal or emergent rocks are sometimes used, while a few species actually prefer dry

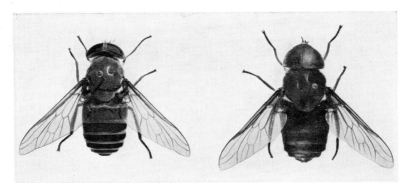

Fig. 296. The American horsefly, *Tabanus americanus* Ford. Female (left) and male (right). 2 ×. (Courtesy of Dr. C. Philip, Rocky Mountain Laboratory, U.S.P.H.S.)

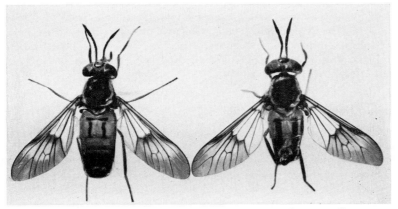

Fig. 297. Deer fly vectors of loiasis in West Africa: *Chrysops silacea* Austen (left) and *C. dimidiata* Wulp (right). (Courtesy of Dr. C. Philip, Rocky Mountain Laboratory, U.S.P.H.S.)

situations for oviposition. From 100 to 700 eggs are deposited in a single cluster, the whole being covered by a waterproof secretion. Hatching occurs in five to seven days. The larvae drop to the ground (or into the water) and develop either in mud, moist earth, leaf mold or rotting logs, the particular ecology depending on the species concerned. Tabanid larvae are soft, cylindrical, with 11 or 12 body segments and a very small head which bears a pair of pointed mandibles. Some species (especially *Chrysops*) feed on organic matter of vegetable origin, but others (most species of *Tabanus*) feed on insect larvae, earthworms, snails, crustacea and the like. A few are cannibalistic. There are four to nine larval molts and development requires several months. The pupal stage lasts from five days to three weeks, larger species tending to require the longer period. Emergence from the pupal skin is through a T-shaped slit along the dorsum of the thorax, as in other typical orthorrhaphous flies. The life-span of adult tabanids is relatively long, usually extending from four to eight weeks (Fig. 297).

**Control**   Repellents based on fish oils have been devised for the protection of domestic animals, but these are too malodorous for general use and are none too desirable in any case. Drainage of swamps has real value in reducing the numbers of TABANIDAE as shown by the very gratifying results obtained in northern Minnesota. Another practical procedure is the oiling of pools with kerosene. The adult flies are prone to visit quiet pools to drink, at which time they lower their bodies into the surface film. Large numbers are thus poisoned and will be found floating dead on the water a short time later. Incidental poisoning of great numbers of TABANIDAE has been reported more than once in connection with oiling operations aimed primarily at the control of mosquito larvae.

Natural control exists to a certain extent by reason of the activities of parasitic insects such as the hymenopterous species *Phanurus emersoni* Girault, which attacks the egg masses of *Tabanus punctifer* Sackin, an annoying species in the rice fields of California. Artificial dissemination of this parasite has been undertaken in Texas, with fairly satisfactory results.

### Family Rhagionidae (Leptidae)

This family is made up of small to medium sized flies with small heads, large eyes, long legs and a tapering abdomen. Blood-sucking forms are found in several genera. Only the females bite. They attack much as do common species of *Chrysops* (TABANIDAE), with a silent approach. The bite is sudden and painful but not poisonous. As yet no rhagionid has been incriminated as a transmitter of disease.

The larval habits vary, some species being aquatic, others terrestrial. Probably all are predaceous.

Species which have a reputation of being especially annoying to man are listed below:

| | |
|---|---|
| *Atherix longipes* Bell | Mexico |
| *Atherix variegata* Walker | Europe and N.A. |
| *Rhagio scolopacea* Linn. | Europe and N.A. |
| *Rhagio strigosa* Meigen | Europe |

*Spaniopsis longicornis* Ferguson . . . . . . . . .Australia
*Symphoromyia atripes* Bigot . . . . . . . . . . . .Western N.A.
*Symphoromyia hirta* Johnson . . . . . . . . . . .Rocky Mountain States
*Symphoromyia kincaidi* Aldrich . . . . . . . . .Pacific Coast, U.S.
*Symphoromyia pachyceras* Williston . . . . .Western N.A.

## Family Stratiomyiidae

*Parasitism by Larvae of Stratiomyiidae*   In addition to the two brachycerous families discussed above, the STRATIOMYIIDAE, or "soldier flies," are sometimes listed as of medical interest (though for very different reasons). The adults are of no medical importance. Their *larvae*, however, which develop normally in decaying fruit, vegetables or animal matter are sometimes taken by accident into the alimentary tract of man, usually with contaminated food. The patient suffers more or less disturbance of the stomach and intestines and may require treatment to get rid of the maggots. *Hermetia illucens* (Linn.) is the species most frequently concerned.

# Suborder Athericera (Cyclorrhapha)

These are the better known flies, and constitute a very large group. Even conservative taxonomists recognize no fewer than forty-three families, of which at least thirteen are of medical importance. So far as medically important forms are concerned, these may be separated by the following adult characters (Figs. 298, 299).

## Family Phoridae

This family is of interest because the larvae of at least one species, *Megaselia* (*Aphiochaeta*) *scalaris*, have been positively recorded as causing intestinal myiasis in man. There seems to be good evidence that these forms not only achieved maturity but actually reproduced within the human bowel.

## Family Syrphidae (Hover-flies)

The "rattail maggots" of the genera *Tubifera* (*Eristalis*) and *Helophilus* are capable of adapting themselves to the human intestinal tract. Nasal myiasis due to larvae of this group has also been recorded. The drinking of water from foul ditches or puddles is probably responsible for all cases of human infection. In nature the maggots hang head downward in the water, the posterior extremity of the elongate "tail-like" portion piercing the surface film. They thus derive oxygen from the atmosphere, but are otherwise completely submerged. The adult flies often show a remarkable resemblance to bees (see Fig. 304).

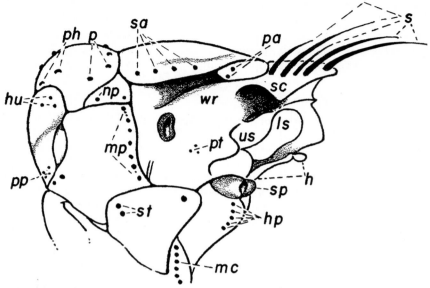

Fig. 298. Thorax of a typical higher fly (*Calliphora*); lateral view. *h*, halter; *hp*, hypopleural bristles; *hu*, humeral bristles; *ls*, lower squama (calypter, tegula, alula); *mc*, middle coxa; *mp*, mesopleural bristles; *np*, notopleural bristles; *p*, presutural bristles; *pa*, postalar bristles; *ph*, posthumeral bristles; *pp*, propleural bristles; *pt*, pteropleural bristles; *s*, scutellar bristles; *sa*, supra-alar bristles; *sc*, scutellum; *sp*, spiracle; *st*, sternopleural bristles; *us*, upper squama (calypter, tegula, alula); *wr*, root of wing.

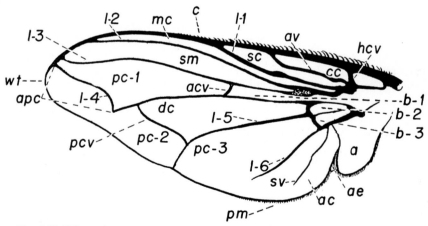

Fig. 299. Wing of a typical higher fly (*Calliphora*). *a*, alula (axillary lobe); *ac*, axillary cell; *acv*, anterior cross vein; *ae*, axillary excision; *apc*, apical cross vein; *av*, auxillary vein; *b-1, b-2, b-3*, basal cells by number; *c*, costa; *cc*, costal cell; *dc*, discal cell; *hcv*, humeral cross vein; *l-1, l-2, l-3, l-4, l-5*, longitudinal veins by number; *l-6*, sixth longitudinal (anal) vein; *mc*, marginal cell; *pc-1*, first posterior (apical) cell; *pc-2, pc-3*, posterior cells by number; *pcv*, posterior cross vein; *pm*, posterior margin of wing; *sc*, subcostal cell; *sm*, submarginal cell; *sv*, spurious vein; *wt*, tip of wing.

*Table 72  Key to Medically Important Families of Higher Flies*

1   (24)   Abdominal segments distinct; the two legs of each thoracic segment not widely separated . . . . . . . . . . 2

2   (3)   Wings with two distinct veins near the costal margin; other, lighter veins extending more or less in a posterior direction . . . . . . . . . . . . . . . . . . . . . . PHORIDAE†

3   (2)   Wings variously veined, but never as above . . . . . . . 4

4   (5)   Ocellar triangle very large, often extending to anterior margin of front; second basal cell not separated from discal cell by a cross vein; very small flies . . . . . . . . . . . . . . . . . CHLOROPIDAE (OSCINIDAE)\*

5   (4)   Ocellar triangle in normal proportion to surrounding structures; second basal cell separated from discal cell by a cross vein; small to very large flies . . . . . . 6

6   (7)   With a spurious vein usually present between third and fourth longitudinal veins . . . . . . . . . SYRPHIDAE†

7   (6)   Without such spurious vein. Antennae with a dorsal arista . . . . . . . . . . . . . . . . . . . . . . . . . . . . . . . . . . 8

8   (15)   Squamae (alulae; translucent scales, one beneath base of either wing) small or rudimentary; thorax without a complete transverse suture; subcostal vein sometimes vestigial or indistinct . . . . . . . . . . . . . . . 9

9   (10)   Legs long and stiltlike; proboscis short; first posterior (apical) cell constricted at wing margin
TYLIDAE (MICROPEZIDAE)†

10   (9)   Legs not especially long . . . . . . . . . . . . . . . . . . . . . . . .11

11   (12)   Subcostal vein complete to costa without break or scar in the latter at point of contact; palpi vestigial
SEPSIDAE†

12   (11)   Subcostal vein absent or vestigial or running very close to first longitudinal vein; first anal cell present, though quite small . . . . . . . . . . . . . . . . . . . . . . . . . .13

13   (14)   Arista plumose or pectinate; costa with two fractures
DROSOPHILIDAE†

14   (13)   Arista bare; subcosta, though very close to first longitudinal vein, distinct to tip . . . . . . . . . . PIOPHILIDAE†

15   (8)   Squamae (alulae) with at least the lower lobe conspicuously developed; thorax with a complete, transverse suture; subcostal vein distinct for its whole course . . . . . . . . . . . . . . . . . . . . . . . . . . . . . . . . . . . .16

16   (19)   Proboscis vestigial or much reduced; mouth opening small . . . . . . . . . . . . . . . . . . . . . . . . . . . . . . . . . . . . .17

17   (18)   Costa extending to tip of fourth longitudinal vein, the latter with a bend so that first posterior (apical) cell is narrowed in the margin (or petiolate)
OESTRIDAE†

*Table 72    Key to Medically Important Families of Higher Flies*
(Continued)

18    (17)    Costa ending slightly beyond tip of third longitudinal
vein, fourth longitudinal vein extending more or
less in a straight line to the margin
GASTEROPHILIDAE†

19    (16)    Proboscis well developed and functional; mouth opening normal . . . . . . . . . . . . . . . . . . . . . . . . . . . . . . . . . . .20

20    (21)    Hypopleural bristles absent, being represented by
nothing coarser than fine hairs.
MUSCIDAE (incl. of ANTHOMYIIDAE)†

21    (20)    Hypopleural bristles present; metanotum with not
more than a single convexity . . . . . . . . . . . . . . . . . .22

22    (23)    Body color in most cases showing metallic green, blue,
or yellow. Hindmost post-humeral bristle almost al-
ways on a lower level than the pre-sutural bristle
(side view) . . . . . . . . . . . . . . . . . . . .CALLIPHORIDAE†*

23    (22)    Body coloring predominantly gray, or silvery, sometimes golden pollinose; checker-board appearance
common. Hindmost post-humeral bristle on a level
with or a little higher than the presutural bristle
SARCOPHAGIDAE†*

24    (1)    Abdominal segments indistinct, the integument leathery; the two legs of each thoracic segment widely
separated; head sunk in an emargination of the
thorax . . . . . . . . . . . . . . . . . . . . . . . . . . . .HIPPOBOSCIDAE*

Note: Families indicated * contain species of medical importance in the *adult
state*. Those families designated † contain species in which the *larvae* are of medical
interest. It will be noted that in certain groups (CALLIPHORIDAE for example) both
larval and adult stages are concerned.

### Family Tylidae (Micropezidae)

The larvae of some members of the genus *Calobata* have been recorded as inhabiting the human intestinal tract. The family is best
represented in South America.

### Family Sepsidae

These small, slender flies live largely as scavengers, being found
about excrement, carrion, and decaying vegetation, in which their
larvae also live and grow. It is not strange that they have been reported as causative agents of intestinal myiasis in man.

### Family Piophilidae

A group very closely related to the Sepsidae with which they have
been combined by certain authors. Many of their larvae live in

cheese and preserved meats. The larva of *Piophila casei*, the well known "cheese skipper," has been repeatedly recorded as causing intestinal myiasis in man. The maggot, which attains a length of more than 5 mm., is rather conical, being pointed anteriorly and truncate posteriorly. The body is shining and smooth but the ventral travelling folds are roughened and the posterior segment bears small fleshy protuberances, four in number. The larva "jumps" by grasping the edge of the posterior segment with its mouth hooks and suddenly releasing it. Occasionally the larvae will pupate and develop into adults in the intestine of man. The patient usually suffers a severe colic, with headache, vertigo and nausea. The feces may contain blood.

### Family Chloropidae (Oscinidae of authors)

Medical interest attaches to the behavior of the adults, several species of which habitually feed on sores, open wounds and especially the secretions of the human eye. Outstanding in this respect is *Hippelates pusio* Loew, the "eye gnat" of the Coachella Valley, California, where it serves as the mechanical vector of epidemic conjunctivitis usually of a severe, follicular type. The species, however, is not confined to the western states, having been known for more than fifty years as a transmitter of conjunctivitis in Florida and elsewhere.

*Recognition Characters* *Hippelates pusio* is a small (2 mm.) blackish fly with yellowish legs. The head is relatively broad, the compound eyes conspicuous. Two beadlike antennal segments are visible, the second bearing a simple, hairlike arista. The thorax is somewhat narrower than either head or abdomen, and bears dorsally a number of very fine hairs. The wings lie scissor-like over the abdomen when at rest. There is a relatively long black spur on the distal extremity of each hind tibia.

*Habits and Life History* The adult flies are exceedingly fond of pus, blood, sebaceous material and lachrymal secretions. Though brushed away, they return again and again until thoroughly satiated. While they are not able to pierce the integument, they do possess tiny spines on the labellum, by means of which they are able to make minute, multiple incisions in mucous membranes. It is during this process of scarification that infective organisms may be introduced. Although breeding goes on more or less throughout the year, the adult flies are relatively inactive during the mid-summer, at which season they rest in the date gardens, hedge rows and shade of houses during the heat of the day, stirring abroad only during the morning and evening hours. From March to May, however, and again from August to October, they are exceedingly abundant and annoying (Fig. 300).

The white, curved, fluted eggs are deposited by preference in loose, cultivated soil with a high organic content. The plowing under of a cover crop or of a large amount of animal manure seems to provide ideal conditions. *Hippelates* will, however, breed in decaying vegetation and other organic media. Each female lays twenty to forty eggs and many individuals probably develop a second batch. Incubation requires not more than three days.

The larvae are short, cylindrical, whitish maggots, with rather conspicuous mouth hooks, by means of which they both feed and propel themselves. The larvae feed for five to ten days, the rate of development depending on the temperature. They then become sluggish and pass into the prepupal stage, rather shorter and flatter

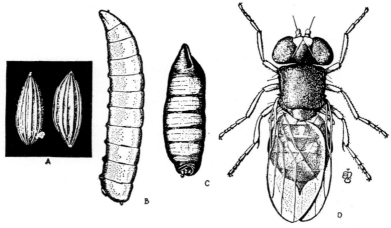

Fig. 300. The eye gnat, *Hippelates pusio. A*, Eggs; *B*, larva; *C*, pupa; *D*, adult. (Courtesy of Dr. D. G. Hall, Am. J. Hyg.)

than the active form and characterized by a somewhat yellowish color.

The pupal state follows in about twenty-four hours. The pupa is brown in color, flattened at the sides of one end, and is covered tightly by the last larval skin. Transformation usually requires about six days, though it should be noted that either the larva or the pupa may hibernate.

Besides serving as vectors of conjunctivitis, eye gnats may be of medical importance in other ways: *H. pallipes* is believed to be a mechanical vector of yaws in Jamaica, while *H. flavipes* probably functions in a similar capacity in Haiti. There is no cyclical development of the parasites, the spirochetes being digested in the stomach of the fly. *Siphunculina funicola* de Meyere is the common eye fly of India where it spreads both conjunctivitis and Naga sore. Trachoma may likewise be transmitted by chloropid flies.

At least one beneficial member of the family is known. *Pseudogaurax signata* Loew is predaceous in the larval state on the eggs of *Latrodectus mactans*, the black widow spider.

**Prophylaxis and Control**   Control is difficult, due to the fact that those agricultural practices best suited to the production of crops seem particularly encouraging to the development of the flies. Four approaches have been used:

1. Trapping and use of baits.
2. Sanitation and general clean up.
3. Modification of agricultural methods.
4. Use of chemicals (as baits, poisons, repellents).

Of these, the use of traps is most effective. Four features are essential: (*a*) a darkened bait chamber or entrance chamber, (*b*) a good bait (liver has proved to be the most efficient), (*c*) a glass jar or other light chamber near top of bait chamber, (*d*) all joints and cracks made "fly tight." Traps should be placed within a few feet of a windbreak or building, on the leeward side. The light chamber should face the strongest light. In the California experiments more flies were taken when the entrance chamber faced south or west.

## Family Drosophilidae

Known variously as "fruit flies," "pomace flies," or "banana flies," most members of this family breed in spoiled fruit, grape pomace and similar organic matter. The accidental ingestion of their larvae may result in infection of the alimentary tract (accidental myiasis). Both adults and larvae are very small (3 to 4 mm. in length).

## Family Muscidae (including Anthomyiidae of authors)

This family includes the house fly, *Musca domestica*, together with a very considerable number of related forms. Almost every conceivable medical relationship exists within the group. Some, like *Stomoxys*, are confirmed blood suckers, i. e., external parasites in the adult state. Others (*Glossina*) combine the same habit with the cyclical transmission of blood parasites (trypanosomes).

Filth breeding (and filth feeding) species act as mechanical vectors of bacteria, protozoal cysts and helminth eggs, while larvae of the same or other species not infrequently develop within the body of man, causing various types of myiasis, the nature of the parasitism depending on the adaptability of the species concerned. Whereas the genus *Musca* is world-wide in its distribution, other groups, like *Glossina*, are sharply limited to particular continents or parts thereof. The four most important genera (*Musca, Stomoxys, Glossina, Fannia*) are discussed here.

## Genus Musca

The best known species in this large genus is the much publicized "housefly" or "typhoid fly," *Musca domestica* Linn, referred to above. Of all flies taken in kitchens and pantries over a large portion of the United States, 98.8 per cent have proved to be of this species. In certain parts of the world, notably in Egypt, a variety, *Musca domestica vicina*, largely replaces the typical form. The same subspecies is common in India, as is *Musca nebulo*. *Musca sorbens* is a house visitor in Indonesia. This species, which occurs both in Ethiopian and Oriental life zones, shows great proclivity for feeding about the eyes, particularly if the latter are infected. For this reason it is believed responsible for the transmission of much trachoma and conjunctivitis.

The adults are approximately one-fourth of an inch in length, and are of a gray-brown color, save that the abdomen tends to be yellowish on the sides and still lighter below. Four longitudinal black stripes extend the length of the thorax (exclusive of scutellum) on the dorsal side. The eyes are reddish brown. The antennae are typically muscoid, extending vertically downward, within the facial depression. The third segment bears a typical dorsal *arista*, plumose practically to the tip. The wings diverge at an angle of nearly 60° when in the resting position. Vein 4 is bent forward near the extremity so as to contact the margin in advance of the apex and fairly close to longitudinal vein three.

**Medical Importance**   Because of their habits flies distribute an immense number of micro-organisms. There is positive laboratory proof for the transmission of thirty different diseases. Cholera, typhoid, amebic and bacillary dysentery, various diarrheas, tetanus, anthrax, trachoma, yaws, leprosy, tuberculosis and certain helminth infections (by eggs) are among the diseases listed.

In all this the vectorship of the fly is mechanical rather than cyclical in nature. There are at least four ways, however, in which the organisms may be conveyed:

1. By the general body surface and especially the hairs of the feet and legs. Particularly important are the sticky hairs of the *pulvilli* (pad-like structures situated close to the tarsal claws).

2. By feces, the organisms having passed through the alimentary canal of the fly. (This is sometimes accompanied by multiplication of the bacteria in the gut.)

3. By the vomitus, it being habitual with flies to regurgitate a portion of the contents of their crop, prior to the ingestion of food.

4. By metamorphosis, organisms taken up by the larval form being not infrequently present in the body of the adult fly, after emergence from the pupal case. The eggs of *Ascaris*, likewise the spores of anthrax and tetanus, are believed to be transmitted in this way.

**Habits and Life History**   The curved, whitish eggs are deposited in manure, garbage and other organic materials. Horse manure seems to be preferred, but cow, pig and chicken manure, as well as human excrement, are often used. A single female usually deposits about 120 eggs in a batch and individuals have been known to lay several batches with the total approaching 2400. Incubation requires eight to twenty-four hours, depending on the temperature.

The larvae, which measure only about 2 mm. at the time of hatching, grow rapidly, molt three times, and under favorable conditions reach maturity in six or seven days. As in many other muscoid species, house fly larvae are blind, footless maggots, with a pair of very small chitinized mouth hooks protruding downward from the tapering anterior end. The mouth hooks are really part of a somewhat elaborate pharyngeal skeleton largely concealed within the first two or three segments of the body. The larva is made up of twelve visible (thirteen actual) segments, the last bearing an obliquely tilted stigmal plate on which a pair of conspicuous, dark-colored spiracles may be easily observed. Maggots will not develop if the temperature is too hot, as at the center of a manure pile, neither can they survive if the medium becomes too dry, as in manure spread thinly upon an open field. (These facts have a bearing on practical methods of control.)

The pupal stage is passed inside the last larval skin, which becomes tightly contracted and takes on a reddish brown color. A pupal case formed in this manner is termed a *puparium*. Three to six days are required for transformation, after which the fly emerges by pushing off a circular cap (operculum) at the anterior end. This is accomplished by the pressure of a specialized bladder-like structure, the ptilinum, which, however, is withdrawn into the head a few hours after emergence.

After emergence from the puparium the adult flies require from two to twenty-four days before they are able to deposit eggs. The latter is unusual. In general, the warmer the temperature the shorter the preoviposition period. Many generations may occur in one year; therefore control measures, to be effective, must be applied relatively early in the season. Otherwise the problem becomes exceedingly difficult to handle so that even partially successful measures involve enormous labor and expense.

**Behavior of the Adult Fly**    Flies normally migrate but little from their place of origin, but studies on marked individuals indicate that they may travel as far as ten to fourteen miles either with, across or against the wind.

A fly population will be contaminated in inverse proportion to the degree of sanitation practiced in the homes and in the streets. In regions where the human feces are deposited directly upon the ground, the fly population becomes heavily laden, both externally and internally, with whatever infective organisms the human population may be harboring.

The size of the organisms capable of being taken into the fly's alimentary tract is of importance in that it constitutes a limiting factor in vectorship (Fig. 301).

The fly's proboscis has three well marked regions, a basal portion, the rostrum, which bears two small palpi, an intermediate portion, the haustellum, and a terminal sucking mechanism composed of two lobes or labella between which is a cleft (prestomum) leading directly to the food canal. Under ordinary circumstances, however, food material does not enter this aperture but is drawn in through the "interbifid grooves" of the pseudotrachea which run transversely across the free surface of the labella. These tiny orifices will not admit an object greater than 0.006 mm. in diameter; hence a majority of individuals only rarely take up items as large as pollen grains.

The act of feeding involves first a flattening of the oval lobes against the surface to be explored. Next, the fly regurgitates a portion

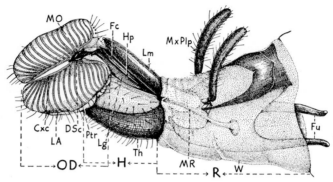

Fig. 301. Mouthparts of a non-biting fly, the housefly (*Musca*). *R*, Rostrum; *H*, haustellum; *OD*, oral disc; *MO*, mouth opening; *Cxc*, a main collecting channel of the pseudotracheae; *DSc*, discal sclerite; *Fc*, food channel between the hypopharynx (*Hp*) and the labrum (*Lm*); *Fu*, fulcrum seen in outline beneath the chitinous membrane (*W*); *Hp*, hypopharynx; *LA*, labella; *Lg*, labial gutter; *Lm*, labrum; *MR*, maxillary rods (stipes); *MxPlp*, maxillary palpi; *Ptr*, pseudotracheae; *Th*, theca; *W*, membrane of proboscis. (Matheson, R.: Medical Entomology. 2nd ed. Ithaca, N. Y., Comstock Publishing Co., 1950.)

of the contents of its crop, the vomitus serving to dissolve or at least emulsify the substance on which the fly is about to feed. This habit provides for generous contamination of the food substance by whatever organisms the fly may have swallowed during the past several days. Human food and drink may thus become inoculated by dangerous organisms, especially if the insect has fed recently on human excrement. When the food particles have passed into solution (or suspension) the fly sucks up the mixture of vomitus and nourishment, but the clean-up is incomplete and many contaminative organisms of course remain.

While feeding, the fly may also defecate at least once and this provides additional opportunity for infective organisms to leave its body. In general, however, vomit specks are probably much more important than fecal specks in the dissemination of disease, since by actual count they have been found to be from ten to one hundred times as numerous as the latter.

It has been shown that dysentery bacilli remain alive in the intestine of the fly at least four days and that cysts of *Endamoeba histolytica* may survive for forty-nine hours.

The foregoing account pertains particularly to the more or less cosmopolitan species *Musca domestica* Linn, including the common subspecies *M. domestica vicina* Macq. It is also essentially applicable to the closely related *Musca autumnalis* DeGeer (*M. corvina* Port. nec Fabr.) with which it is frequently confused. *Musca sorbens* Wied. (= *W. vetustissima* Walk.), common in houses in the East Indies, has somewhat different habits, already mentioned.

*Musca (Philaematomyia) crassirostris* Stein, which ranges from the Mediterranean into Oriental and Ethiopian regions, is a blood sucker. Its larvae, which normally develop only in fresh cow dung, have been known to cause myiasis in man, as have the larvae of *M. domestica.*

It should be pointed out that flies of other genera (*Fannia, Muscina*) and also of other families (CALLIPHORIDAE, SARCOPHAGIDAE) frequently breed and feed in filthy material, but that such species do not as a rule tend to enter houses or visit human food as frequently as does the housefly. They are therefore less likely to be a menace to human health. To be an important transmitter of infection a species must: (1) feed on human excrement; (2) visit houses, contaminate food and drink. Unless a species does both, it need give us no great concern.

**Fly Control**   Two principles are important to keep in mind: 1. If possible begin early in the season, before the fly population gets out of hand. 2. Concentrate primarily on prevention of breeding rather than on destruction of the adult fly.

The elimination of fly breeding areas involves at least three separate problems.

THE DISPOSAL OF ANIMAL MANURE. In military life this will be important if there are cavalry or artillery animals on the post, or if pack animals are maintained, as in the case of mountain troops. The most difficult problem arises in connection with animals kept by native populations living nearby. The following procedures are recommended:

1. Daily spreading of the manure on agricultural land. Where possible this is the best method of all since it allows no breeding opportunity to exist and utilizes the fertilizer at the most favorable time for benefiting the soil.

2. Storage of the manure in fly-tight boxes, or pits, preferably of concrete with wooden doors above, which of course are kept closed except when material is being put into the pit. A fly trap should be placed at the top to catch the flies produced by the small infestation which is always inevitable.

3. The piling of the manure in cubes or "ricks" with vertical sides. The heat of decomposition drives the maggots to the surface where they may be treated in various ways.

4. Treatment by use of chemicals:

*a.* HELLEBORE (must be fresh) one-half pound in ten gallons of water. The preparation should be allowed to stand for twenty-four hours and may then be sprinkled over the manure with a watering pot. This amount is sufficient for the treatment of eight bushels.

*b.* BORAX, eleven ounces in from two to ten gallons of water depending on the amount of moisture already present in the material to be treated. This amount also is sufficient to treat eight bushels and may be applied by sprinkling. There is a drawback to this method in that the borax may prove toxic to crops. Manure spread on fields, less than fifteen tons of treated manure per acre, is considered to be safe.

*c.* CALCIUM CYANAMIDE one-half pound, in combination with a like amount of *Superphosphate* (acid phosphate). This treats one bushel of manure and accomplishes complete control. It has the further advantage of adding both nitrogen and phosphorus to the soil.

*d.* CRANK-CASE OIL (or crude petroleum) may be used to destroy maggots, especially if the manure is not to be used for agricultural purposes.

*e.* COMMERCIAL SODIUM ARSENITE. Two pounds treat one ton of manure, which should be completely wetted by a 0.1 per cent solution of the salt; apparently it is not harmful to crops.

*f.* PARATHION. Use wettable powder and apply over surface of manure in concentration of 0.1 per cent.

5. "Maggot trap" method of storage. A slatted platform is arranged over a concrete pit which contains a certain amount of water. Heavy wetting of the manure will drive the maggots out, whereupon they fall into the water and are drowned. Third stage maggots, seeking a place in which to pupate, will likewise be captured. Frequent cleaning or flushing of the pit should be provided for. This is especially necessary in malarious areas, where a neglected pit provides an ideal situation for the development of certain species of mosquitoes.

It is needless to say that stables should be properly constructed and should receive thorough, daily care.

DISPOSAL OF HUMAN EXCREMENT. This involves:

1. The installation of a sanitary sewage disposal system (if possible).

2. The screening of all privies and latrines, with special attention to cracks, ventilation devices, and other apertures likely to be overlooked.

3. Sprinkling of *borax* over exposed feces at least every three or four days. Use enough to make the surface appear white.

4. Covering of feces with earth, as under field conditions where straddle trenches are in use. It is well to add oil, if possible, as flies will emerge through a considerable depth of loose soil.

DISPOSAL OF GARBAGE. 1. For temporary storage of garbage, watertight metal cans, with accurately fitting covers should be used.

2. For ultimate disposal nothing is superior to incineration, if equipment is available.

3. Conservation uses (require special care and supervision). These fall into four general categories:

*a.* Reduction in special plants, with salvage of useful chemical substances. This is practical only in very large municipalities where volume warrants the capital outlay. A market for the commercial products is also necessary.

*b.* Grinding of bones, for fertilizer.

*c.* Feeding of edible portions to swine. Hog farms are always a menace in the matter of fly production, and should be located beyond flight range of the community or camp.

*d.* Composting, with a view to future agricultural use. This is very desirable in certain Asiatic countries from an economic standpoint. Skillful supervision is necessary, however, to prevent fly breeding.

4. Burial of all garbage is usually very satisfactory if there is thorough compaction of both the garbage and the soil covering. The latter should be not less than one foot in depth, preferably two.

5. Removal of the garbage to sufficient distance so that it can be abandoned is the most economical procedure and, where there is but scant population in the area, it need not be too severely criticized.

MEASURES AGAINST THE ADULT FLIES. In spite of conscientious efforts to prevent the development of the larvae, at least a few flies will succeed in attaining maturity. Again (especially in the military service), the medical officer may find himself confronted with a problem of fly-borne disease in a region where he has had no opportunity to face the situation early in the season, and consequently finds a larger number of flies already on hand. The following procedures are of proved value:

SCREENS. In humid climates copper, bronze, alloy or plastic must be used, to avoid corrosion. In a very dry climate, however, galvanized screening is usually adequate. Painting of the screens also provides protection against weathering. A mesh of 14 wires to the inch will exclude houseflies, but it is better to use at least 18 mesh because of the desirability of controlling smaller insects at the same time. Accurate fitting of both screen doors and window screens is important. Doors should open outward. Foods likely to attract flies, such as hung meats, should, of course, be screened as well.

FLY TRAPS. A tremendous reduction in the fly population may be effected by the judicious placing of fly traps of suitable construction. A conical type, made of screen and baited with molasses, milk, or waste fruit, works very well. The flies enter from below and as a result of their tendency to fly upward, toward the light, pass through the narrow aperture at the apex of the cone into an upper chamber from which they are unable to escape. Frequent emptying of traps is desirable. Captured living flies should be killed before removal either with hot water or by means of a spray. Fly traps function best when set in the sun, in a place protected from the wind.

ELECTRICITY. When electric power is available it is sometimes practical to charge screen doors in such a manner that flies coming into contact with the metal are killed and fall to the floor. Such devices have proved of great value in controlling flies about stables and dairy barns.

SPRAYS. The application of sprays, either by hand spray-guns or power sprayers, is a useful procedure when flies are abundant. Such sprays are of two types, which may be combined, if desired.

1. Space Sprays. These act as contact poisons, and are especially useful indoors. Pyrethrum, if fortified by proper synergists, such as piperonyl butoxide, is an effective killing agent. Greaseless kerosene or other light, mineral oils are commonly used as carriers. Best effects are achieved if rooms can be tightly closed for at least a half hour after spraying.

2. Residual Sprays. In these sprays the toxic agent is applied to walls of buildings, both inside and out, to screens, and in the vicinity of garbage cans, privies, manure piles, and other places where flies are prone to congregate. Surfaces so treated remain toxic for long periods of time, sometimes for several months. Except when applied in great excess these substances are not repellent. The flies therefore alight in usual numbers, and are killed by contact. DDT was the first of this type of insecticide to be discovered, but benzene hexachloride, chlordane, toxaphene, methoxychlor, dieldrin and others are becoming as well known. Oil solutions, emulsions, and wettable powders have been used.

The great enthusiasm which greeted the discovery of residual insecticides has been largely dampened, at least so far as flies are concerned, with the development of highly resistant strains of flies in various parts of the world. Two or three successful seasons of control with any one preparation are all that may be hoped for in a given locality, after which many of the flies become highly resistant to it. Attempts to rotate the use of two or more insecticides have not been particularly successful, since flies resistant to one residual insecticide often prove quite refractory to others. The outlook for complete control of flies by residual insecticides, once thought possible, has become very poor. A renewed emphasis on the importance of basic sanitary practices, which were somewhat neglected during the early years of DDT, is still imperative.

3. Aerosols. Bombs containing pyrethrum, freon, and a synergist, with or without DDT, may be employed to produce a floating vapor, consisting of exceedingly fine particles, very useful in killing insects in a small, enclosed space. The interior of airplanes may be effectively treated in this way. The residual element, if present, collects eventually on walls and other surfaces, which thereby become toxic for a considerable period of time.

POISONS. Formalin, sodium salicylate, and various arsenic compounds have been used to poison flies, but only the first two are generally recommended since the use of arsenic about kitchens and homes is a dangerous procedure. Two teaspoonfuls of Formalin to one pint of milk or water, with a little brown sugar added, makes a good poison bait. It may be set out in an inverted tumbler resting in a saucer lined with blotting paper. The lip of the tumbler should be elevated at one point by a toothpick or a match stick, to provide for automatic renewal of whatever liquid may be lost through evaporation.

Sodium arsenate or arsenite, sprinkled on barn floors in a dilute solution of molasses makes an excellent bait. Only twenty-five per cent of the concrete surface need be covered, preferably in strips. In using arsenic compounds state and Federal recommendations should be followed.

STICKY FLY PAPERS of the tanglefoot variety are useful, even if somewhat unsightly. The spiral ribbon type, suspended from the ceiling, is most desirable for mess halls and barracks.

FLY SWATTERS, while of little influence when many flies are about, can be of real use early in the season when the killing of a single individual may forestall the development of thousands.

In conclusion, it should be pointed out that individual efforts to control the fly population may be of small avail unless the entire community is prepared to cooperate in the enterprise. A single, neglected breeding spot may completely nullify the effects of an otherwise excellent program. There exists the same necessity for co-operation between a military establishment and adjacent civilian communities, ranches, and farms.

### Genus Stomoxys

The best known species is the biting stable fly, or dog fly, *Stomoxys calcitrans* (Linn.). This form enjoys practically a world-wide distribution. Three other species, *S. nigra* Macquart, *S. omega* Newstead and *S. inornata* Grünberg are limited to the Ethiopian life zone. Since the habits of all are very similar, an account of the biology of *S. calcitrans* will suffice for an understanding of the group.

This species somewhat resembles the housefly, *Musca domestica*, but may be distinguished by the fact that the proboscis, instead of being expanded distally into a conspicuous pair of oral lobes, is slender at the tip, being adapted as an organ for piercing and sucking. The stable fly is also more robust than the housefly, and has a broader abdomen. Of the four thoracic stripes, the outside ones are broken at the middle. The abdomen has somewhat of a greenish yellow sheen and shows more or less of a checker-board pattern, after the manner of the SARCOPHAGIDAE. The arista is plumose on the upper side only, whereas in the housefly it is hairy both above and below. Also the third and fourth longitudinal veins are much more widely separated at their tips than in *M. domestica*.

**Medical Importance**    Although once thought to be concerned with the spread of poliomyelitis, these flies probably function but rarely in the transmission of human disease. They may occasionally act as mechanical vectors of anthrax, tetanus, yellow fever and possibly oriental sore. Such transmission is favored if the fly is interrupted during its blood meal and immediately thereafter attacks a second host, the proboscis being still wet with blood. On an experimental basis they have also been found capable of the mechanical transmis-

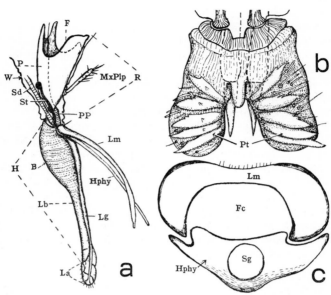

Fig. 302. Mouthparts of the biting stable fly (*Stomoxys*). *a*, Side view of the proboscis. *b*, The labella of the proboscis with the prestomal teeth exposed. *c*, Cross section of the labrum and hypopharynx near the middle of the proboscis. *B*, swollen base of the labium; *F*, fulcrum; *Fc*, food channel; *H*, haustellum; *Hphy*, hypopharynx; *La*, labellum; *Lb*, labium; *Lg*, labial gutter; *Lm*, labrum; *MxPlp*, maxillary palpus; *P*, pharynx; *PP*, prepharynx; *Pt*, prestomal teeth; *R*, rostrum; *Sd*, salivary duct; *Sg*, salivary duct in hypopharynx; *St*, stipes; *W*, chitinous membrane. (Matheson, R.: Medical Entomology, 2nd ed. Ithaca, N. Y., Comstock Publishing Co., 1950.)

sion of certain trypanosomes. So far as is known, *T. evansi*, the causative agent of surra, is transmitted in nature by the activity of biting flies.

*Stomoxys* flies are best known, however, by reason of their painful bites, and when present in great numbers, have been known to render recreational areas quite uninhabitable and even to cause demoralization among troops (Fig. 302).

The manner of feeding is as follows: The *labella* are small oval lobes which normally lie close together and conceal the biting structures. When about to feed, the fly expands its labella, exposing two rows of five teeth and in their midst a number of leaflike cutting blades. The teeth (and blades) effect a quick and rather rough puncturing of the skin, after which the labella are also forced into the wound. The blood is drawn up through a channel formed by the apposition of the *labrum-epipharynx* (above) and *hypopharynx* (below). Both males and females are vicious biters. Fortunately the bites are not poisonous and there are no unpleasant after effects.

**Habits and Life History**    The adult female requires a number of blood meals (three?) before she is able to develop her eggs. These are deposited in small batches up to a total of 120 or so before the female seeks another meal. A single fly may engage in at least three egg-laying episodes during the season, with a total production of well over 600 eggs. Their favorite breeding places are wet, rotting piles of hay, straw, lawn clippings or sea weed. Animal manure and vegetable rubbish are also used, but apparently this species has never been known to develop in human excrement.

The eggs require from two to five days for hatching, and, assuming a summer temperature of 75° to 80° F., the larvae mature in fourteen to twenty-one days. The third stage larva seeks a somewhat drier location for pupation, transformation requiring from six to twenty days more, depending on the temperature. The life cycle may thus be completed in as short a time as two weeks, though unfavorable conditions may prolong it to seven or eight. In North America either the larval or the pupal stage may undergo hibernation.

The adult flies tend usually to congregate in sunny places, such as on walls or fences, especially in the vicinity of stables and barnyards, where a food supply is usually available. They appear to feed indiscriminately on cattle, horses, small animals and man. In warm weather they are said to require two meals a day. On dark days (as also at night) they seek shelter in houses, barns and sheds. Before and during storms they are prone to bite fiercely, thereby creating the impression that meteorological conditions have caused the housefly to become a biter. This concept is entirely in error, as the housefly has no means of perforating the skin.

**Control**    The best control is obviously destruction of the breeding sites. If possible, straw intended for use in the bedding of animals should be baled and stored indoors. Straw stacks should be built with vertical sides and the top shaped so as to shed water. Old stacks should never be allowed to stand, as they become sodden and furnish ideal conditions for larval development. Lawn clippings and spoiled vegetables should be spread to dry rather than left in piles.

A special problem exists in the control of *Stomoxys* flies which develop in the drifts of sea weed ("bay grass") cast up by storms and tides. Spraying these masses or windrows with a mixture of creosote and oil (or creosote and sea water) seems to have been quite effective in controlling this species along the Florida coast. Barges equipped with pumps are maneuvered along shore, the sea water required for the mixture being drawn up from below. Both larvae and pupae are killed by the spray, and flies are probably discouraged from further oviposition. Bay grass treated with creosote and sea water remains free from larvae for at least a month.

A certain amount of protection against the bites may be achieved by the application of repellents, of which Indalone, pure or in mixture with 612 and dimethyl phthalate (6–2–2), is probably the best available.

There is record of the larva of *Stomoxys* being found in a lesion on the foot of a stable boy in South Africa. Ordinarily, however, the genus is not considered a myiasis-producing group.

### Genus Glossina

These are the tsetse flies, best known because of their role in the transmission of trypanosomes. The genus includes some twenty species, but not more than three or four are important vectors of human disease. *Glossina palpalis* (Rob.-Desv.) is the principal vector of *Trypanosoma gambiense*, with *G. tachinoides* Westwood in all probability a natural vector also. *Trypanosoma rhodesiense*, however, is transmitted by *G. morsitans* Westwood and *G. swynnertoni* Austen. *Glossina morsitans*, the "original" tsetse fly, is the principal vector of nagana, an important and usually fatal trypanosome disease of domestic animals.

The group is confined to tropical Africa, save that *G. tachinoides* has been recorded from Southern Arabia, an example of discontinuous distribution.

Tsetse flies are for the most part slender, wasplike insects of brownish coloration. The better known forms are very slightly larger than houseflies. Some of the rarer species are larger. The arista is distinctive, the ornamental bristles being secondarily branched. (As in *Stomoxys*, the arista is naked on the under side.) The proboscis is elongate and extends forward from the head like a bayonet when not in use. It is bulbous at the base and is normally enclosed by the palpi, each of which is grooved internally so that the two palpi, taken together, form a protective sheath. When engaged in feeding, the fly lowers the proboscis until the tip makes contact with the skin. The palpi, however, continue to extend horizontally. The wings of tsetse flies are folded, scissor-like, above the abdomen when not being used for flight, and in most species extend a considerable distance beyond the caudal extremity of the fly. The fourth longitudinal vein is curiously bent rather near its base, where it is tied to vein three by a very short cross-vein. This causes the *discal cell* to assume a peculiar shape, resembling somewhat the outline of a butcher's cleaver. The presence of this cleaver-shaped cell is diagnostic for the group. The several species, however, are difficult to identify and the physician would do well to utilize the services of a specialist when exact knowledge of the species is desired. (No key to species will be attempted here.)

**Habits and Life History**    Tsetse flies bite in the daytime and both males and females are voracious feeders. The labella are reduced in size and, after the inner "rasps" or "teeth" have perforated the integument, penetrate the wound, as in *Stomoxys*.

Tsetse flies by no means confine their attacks to man, all species being parasites primarily of game or reptiles. *Glossina tachinoides*, however, maintains itself very well in regions where man is the only available host.

A female *Glossina* does not deposit eggs, but retains the larvae within her uterus until ready for pupation. Only one larva is developed at a time, the fly "giving birth" every ten or twelve days throughout her adult life. The individual larva lies with its posterior spiracles in contact with the external os while the mouth remains in proximity to the so-called "milk glands" which are situated near the internal extremity of the uterine sac. All three larval stages are passed in this position, nourishment being derived from the "milk glands," oxygen from the outside. When first extruded, the larvae are a creamy white in color except for the posterior extremity, which portion is shining black, and consists largely of a pair of conspicuous, protruding knobs on each of which a spiracle is borne. The adult fly shows considerable discrimination in selecting an appropriate site for larviposition. Loose, pebbly soil, preferably in the shade and not too far from water, seems to be definitely preferred by *G. palpalis*, but the larvae of *G. morsitans* can survive in hard soil, wood ashes from forest fires, and in other situations. The flies appear consistently to avoid contact with manure and putrefactive material. The larvae, lacking strong mouth hooks, are unable to crawl, but do manage to burrow a few centimeters beneath the surface. Pupation usually takes place within an hour, the puparium gradually becoming dark brown in color. It may be easily recognized by the conspicuous caudal knobs, reminiscent of the larval state. Three to four weeks are usually sufficient for transformation, though at cool temperatures an even longer period may be required.

As in other muscoid genera the fly is provided with a *ptilinum* by which it effects the rupture of the pupal case.

The several species show marked differences in their choice of environment. *Glossina palpalis* breeds by preference on the shores of rivers and lakes, usually in dense undergrowth. It is found over an enormous range, but is most abundant in West Africa and in the Congo. Although it has been stated in literature that *G. palpalis* is primarily a reptile feeder, its preferred food seems to be the blood of man. It also feeds on many other warm-bloods, such as mongoose, waterbuck, bushbuck, hippopotamus, monkey, pig and goat. *Glossina morsitans* requires more open country, such as glades or plains where four-footed game animals may be found. Logs, rocks or trees must be in the vicinity, however, to provide breeding and resting places for the flies. This species also has an extensive distribution, but is of greatest importance in Rhodesia, Belgian Congo and the Sudan. *Glossina swynnertoni* tolerates still dryer situations than *G. morsitans*. It feeds by preference on wild game.

The transmission of trypanosomes by tsetse flies may be either mechanical or cyclical, though it is doubtful if the first is ever involved in the infection of the human host. Experimental work has shown that the flies are capable of transmitting the trypanosomes mechanically for not more than two days after feeding on an infected animal. They then become non-infective and there intervenes a period of some twenty days or more during which the parasites undergo cyclical development within the fly's alimentary tract. At the expiration of this time the flies become once more infective and so far as known continue to be so for the remainder of their lives. It has been demonstrated that trypanosomes are usually injected in large numbers as soon as the fly's proboscis penetrates the skin. Thus a *Glossina* which merely "probes," without remaining to feed, may nevertheless transmit infection. Adult tsetse flies live from ninety to 250 days or longer. Not all flies become infective even though they may feed freely on infected hosts. The trypanosomes are sometimes digested, sometimes swept out with the feces of the fly. Only those which succeed in reaching the salivary glands pass through the crithidial stage and so finally become infective, metacyclic forms.

**Prophylaxis and Control**    The control of tsetse flies presents a complex and difficult problem. Procedures applicable to the adult fly are limited, largely because of the insect's long flight range and its migration from one type of terrain to another in the change from the wet to the dry season. Since there is no free larval stage, it is impossible to apply measures calculated to interfere with larval development. Existing control practices fall under three heads:

1. Direct measures against the flies.

2. Indirect control by destruction or management of game animals (based largely on the suspected identity of the human trypanosomes with *Trypanosoma brucei*).

3. Prophylactic measures pertaining to the individual.

DIRECT MEASURES. Since most species tend to be restricted to definite "fly-belts," a certain measure of success has been achieved (especially against *G. palpalis* and *G. tachinoides*) by clearing the jungle for some distance back from water courses and around the native villages; 50 to 100 yards on each side of the breeding areas is recommended. Such strips are thus rendered unsuitable either for pupation or for the resting of the adult flies. Maintenance of such clearance, however, is difficult and expensive, and in some instances it has been found preferable to move entire human populations to a new location. Burning of grass lands has sometimes proved effective in reducing the numbers of *G. morsitans*, although in some localities the practice seems to have had an opposite effect. Trapping of the flies has been very successful in certain areas, the insects being best attracted by traps made to resemble game animals in size and shape. Trap breeding areas are also a possibility, the flies being encouraged to deposit their larvae in situations where the pupae may be readily collected and destroyed. The use of residual insecticides, now being promoted on an experimental basis, shows promise as a means of controlling tsetse flies. As yet this group has not manifested the resistance to these chemicals that has made the housefly so difficult to control.

INDIRECT MEASURES. The destruction of wild game has been advocated by some on the grounds that the natural reservoir for the trypanosomes might thereby be largely eliminated, causing infected flies to become a rarity. However, domestic animals may certainly function at least as a temporary reservoir and the risk to man would still exist. Again, in regions where domestic animals are few or absent, destruction of game tends actually to force the flies to seek man with greater frequency than before.

An alternative procedure would be to segregate the game into restricted areas, where the flies, seeking the blood of such hosts, might be trapped in large numbers and destroyed.

PROPHYLACTIC MEASURES. The risk of being bitten by an infected tsetse may be greatly reduced by any or all of the following practices:

1. The avoidance of fly belts.
2. The wearing of white clothing, it being well established that the flies much prefer to alight on darker surfaces.
3. Wearing of head nets, gloves, other protective clothing.
4. Proper screening of houses and verandas.

As yet no satisfactory repellent has been devised.

### Genus Fannia

The group to which this genus belongs is usually considered as constituting a separate family, the ANTHOMYIIDAE, distinguishable from the MUSCIDAE by the fact that the third and fourth longitudinal veins are more widely separated in the margin. However, since this is the only genus of sufficient medical importance to be considered in this work, we may conveniently regard the group as falling in the family MUSCIDAE, in the larger sense, along with *Musca, Glossina* and *Stomoxys*.

Two species are of importance to human health, *Fannia canicularis* (Linn.), the so-called "lesser housefly" and *F. scalaris* (Fabr.), the "latrine fly." Both are widely distributed through all but the colder regions of the world.

*Fannia canicularis* is a small, grayish fly distinguishable from the housefly not only by the wing character described above, but also by the fact that the antennal arista is naked while the dorsal thoracic stripes are but three in number. The legs are black and the halteres distinctly yellow. At times as many as 25 per cent of all flies found in houses may be of this species. They do not, however, tend to congregate on human food as eagerly as do houseflies.

The eggs of this species are laid on either decaying vegetable matter or animal manure, including human excrement. Piles of grass, especially lawn clippings, furnish an ideal breeding site. The eggs hatch in twenty-four hours and the larvae require at least seven days for development. They may be very readily identified by the large spinelike processes borne both dorsally and laterally by practically every segment of the body. The lateral processes are double or multiple. Unlike typical muscoid maggots these larvae are greatest in diameter at the middle, both anterior and posterior extremities being bluntly tapered. The entire larva is noticeably flattened dorsoventrally.

The pupal stage lasts approximately one week.

*Fannia scalaris*, the latrine fly, is very similar to the above species, but is usually a bit larger. The abdomen bears a dark median stripe, more or less interrupted by transverse bands. The effect is that of a series of dorsal, triangular spots. In males the tibia of the middle leg bears a fairly conspicuous tubercle.

The life history is similar to that of *F. canicularis*, but the fly seems to prefer excrement to vegetable matter as a site for oviposition. The egg usually hatches within twenty-four hours, after which the larva requires at least six days for development and the pupa usually nine. The larva differs from that of *F. canicularis* in that the lateral processes are single and conspicuously "feathered." The dorsal processes are very much reduced.

The larvae of both species have been repeatedly recorded as causing both intestinal and urinary myiasis in man (see Table 73, page 794). The parasites apparently gain access to the human host in two ways:

1. By way of the mouth, along with decaying fruit or on food soiled with human or other excrement. Either the eggs or the developing larvae are apparently infective.

2. By exposure of the anus or genitals in such a manner as to give the flies an opportunity to deposit ova in or near these apertures. This might occur either while the person is using an open privy or while resting or sleeping in a more or less unclothed condition. Any odor or lack of cleanliness would tend to attract the flies, infection being especially liable to occur when infants are left for sometime on the stool by careless or busy mothers. Urinary myiasis, as caused by these species, probably always originates by the external route rather than by migration through the tissues from the alimentary canal. Infection of the genito-urinary tract is more common in females than in males.

**Symptoms of Infection by Fannia Larvae**   GASTRIC MYIASIS   The presence of any considerable number of larvae in the stomach usually causes nausea, sharp pain, vertigo and sometimes violent vomiting. This often results in the expulsion of some of the larvae, on which diagnosis may be based.

INTESTINAL MYIASIS. Pain, diarrhea and hemorrhage from the

anus are possible indications of the presence of larvae in the intestinal tract. A certain number of larvae may eventually be expelled in the feces spontaneously. Headache, chronic constipation, furry tongue, sallow complexion and general nervousness have been reported in cases of repeated infection.

GENITO-URINARY MYIASIS. Victims of infection in these organs have been known to manifest albuminuria, dysuria, hematuria, pyuria and strangury. Spontaneous passage of the larvae, with complete termination of symptoms, is not uncommon.

**Treatment and Prophylaxis**   This depends on the location and abundance of the larvae. The use of emetics in the case of gastric myiasis and of purges and enemas in the case of intestinal infection is often helpful in eliminating the parasites. Vermifuges, as employed for helminth infections, are sometimes very effective also. The treatment of genito-urinary myiasis is difficult. Skillful use of the cystoscope has made possible removal of the parasites in some cases. It is usually best to treat the patient symptomatically until the infection terminates naturally.

Care should be taken to avoid reinfection, and the patient's personal habits should be carefully studied to ascertain if there is some factor predisposing to the acquisition of the parasites. Cleanliness, and the screening of houses and privies, are the best general prophylactic measures. When resting or sleeping one should either cover the body apertures or remain in quarters that are properly screened.

### Genus Muscina

Besides the four genera discussed above, it may be mentioned that the genus *Muscina* (non-biting stable fly) is sometimes of medical importance. Larvae of this genus have been found infesting open wounds (probably as secondary invaders) and have also been taken from the human intestinal tract.

### Family Gasterophilidae (Botflies, in part)

These are the botflies of horses, asses and related hosts. The larvae live normally within the alimentary tract of these animals, being attached by their mouth hooks to the gastric or intestinal mucosa. The exact location varies in accordance with the species concerned.

These flies deposit their eggs on the skin (hair) or lips of the animals, whence the larvae either burrow in or are swallowed, eventually arriving at their definitive location.

The distribution is world-wide. Human infection, though apparently accidental, is nevertheless fairly common, especially in warmer regions. In man, however, the larvae usually remain subcutaneous in position where they cause a "creeping eruption" somewhat similar to that brought about by the larvae of the dog hookworm *Ancylostoma braziliense*. There is at least one record of *Gasterophilus* larvae (*G. haemorrhoidalis* [Linn.]) being found in the human intestinal tract, but this condition appears to be exceedingly rare.

The adult flies of this group range from 9 to 18 mm. in length and are characterized by stout bodies rather densely clothed with fine hair. They somewhat resemble honeybees. True bristles are absent. The antennae lie well within the facial depression; the aristae are bare. The proboscis is short, the mouth parts being poorly developed. The palpi, though abbreviated, are considerably expanded in diameter. The wings are large and may be either hyalin or possessed of dusky spots, depending on the species. The apical cross vein is absent. The squamae are relatively small. In the genus *Gasterophilus* the fourth longitudinal vein extends in a straight line toward the margin. The abdomen (oval in the male sex) tapers conspicuously in females.

**Habits and Life History**    These flies are quite unable to bite; in fact they take very little food of any kind. They are nevertheless exceedingly annoying to horses, which seem to have an instinctive fear of them and sometimes become unmanageable in their presence. They glue their triangular (stalked) eggs to the hairs of the host animal, hatching being stimulated (at least in certain species) by friction against the teeth or tongue, as the horse bites or licks its legs. The egg of each species has a distinctive shape. Even the newly hatched larvae possess rather conspicuous, backwardly directed spines on most of the body segments. Later instars are larger, with a greater relative diameter, and bear heavier spines. After completing their development the larvae are passed in the animal's feces, and fall to the ground. Pupation takes place in dry horse dung or loose soil. The flies copulate soon after emergence and in a temperate climate oviposition normally takes place in early summer. The life cycle requires about a year.

**Symptoms of Parasitism in Man**    When eggs are laid on the human host the first stage larvae burrow into the skin as far as the stratum germinativum, after which they wander aimlessly about producing a form of cutaneous myiasis. They may survive for months. A tortuous inflammatory line marks the path of migration, the larvae being found just in advance of the progressive inflammation. Such an infestation is commonly termed "larva migrans." *Gasterophilus intestinalis* (De Geer) is the species most commonly involved, though *G. haemorrhoidalis* (Linn.) and *G. nasalis* (Linn.) also infect human hosts occasionally. Intense itching usually accompanies the infection and secondary sepsis from scratching is not uncommon.

**Diagnosis and Treatment**    The larva is usually found just in advance of the inflammatory line. It may be rendered visible by the application of a small amount of mineral oil, which causes the skin of the patient to become transparent. By use of a lens the backwardly directed spines, segmentally arranged, may be readily demonstrated, thereby establishing the dipterous nature of the parasite. (Hookworm larvae have no such structures.) Surgical extraction is relatively easy. Aseptic precautions should be observed.

### Family Oestridae (Botflies, concluded)

For practical purposes, the botflies other than the GASTEROPHILIDAE may be grouped in a single family, the OESTRIDAE.* In these forms the fourth longitudinal vein bends sharply forward, either joining vein three before the margin (*Oestrus*) or terminating in close proximity to it (*Dermatobia*). The mouthparts are vestigial. As in the GASTEROPHILIDAE, it is only the larval stage which is of medical importance. Most species normally parasitize animal hosts, the human subject being attacked but rarely. The following genera will be discussed: *Dermatobia, Cuterebra, Oestrus, Rhinoestrus, Hypoderma.*

### Genus Dermatobia

The only recognized species is the so-called "human botfly," *D. hominis* (Linn.). This species is native to Central and South America and Mexico, where its larvae are found parasitic in the skin of various mammals and birds as well as man. Domestic cattle are very frequently parasitized. The young larva is sometimes called *ver macaque*, later instars being known under the designation *torcel*, or *berne*. Another common name is *ver moyocuil*. The adult fly measures approximately 15 mm. in length, and is in general of a brownish gray color. The abdomen, however, is of a distinctly bluish cast, especially when viewed in reflected light. The legs and face are orange-yellow.

**Habits and Life History**    The adult fly does not seek its host directly, always utilizing some other species of insect for the transmission of its eggs. Mosquitoes of the genus *Psorophora* (*Janthinosoma*), particularly *P. lutzii* Theobald and *P. ferox* Humboldt, seem to be favorite carrier hosts in Central America and Northern South America, but in Brazil biting flies, such as *Stomoxys* and *Siphona* (*Haematobia*) are made use of and even *Musca* and *Anthomyia*, as well as certain species of ticks, are sometimes found with *Dermatobia* eggs glued fast to their bodies. The *Dermatobia* female usually captures the mosquito (or other species) in flight, and, while hovering, manages to fasten some fifteen to twenty-five whitish eggs to the abdomen of the carrier host without causing any injury to the latter. During oviposition the victim is held with the head forward and the dorsal surface close against the botfly's thorax. Upon release the burdened carrier then goes its own way, in the case of blood-sucking forms to seek a blood meal from an appropriate warm-blooded host,

---

* It is recognized that *Dermatobia, Cuterebra, Pseudogametes* and *Rogenhofera* are considered by certain authors as constituting a separate family, the CUTEREBRIDAE, with *Hypoderma* serving as the type of another natural group, the HYPODERMATIDAE. In the interest of simplification, however, the CUTEREBRIDAE and HYPODERMATIDAE are here included with the OESTRIDAE, in the broader sense.

in the case of non–blood-sucking species perhaps to rest on vertebrate skin.

The eggs which contain fully developed embryos are stimulated to hatch by the warmth of the host's body, the eggs being so placed that the end through which the larva emerges is directed away from the body of the carrier host. In penetrating the skin of the vertebrate host, the young larvae frequently make use of the feeding puncture of the carrier species, but are perfectly capable, if need be, of perforating the unbroken surface with their own mouth parts. This process, however, may require some time (up to ninety minutes under experimental conditions). It has been shown that larvae which do not have an opportunity to establish themselves on a suitable host may survive up to a maximum of twenty days.

The larvae, once established, do not migrate but remain in situ where they give rise to a boil-like swelling, open at the top. The larva (whose anterior segments become robust) is much attenuated posteriorly, particularly for the duration of the second instar. The caudal extremity bears a pair of large, functional spiracles which remain in contact with the exterior, thus insuring an adequate supply of air.

The parasites become larger, fatter and considerably more grub-like as time goes on. Conspicuous, backwardly directed spines adorn most of the forward segments. A few small spines, directed forward, occur on the two posterior segments, where they are believed to function in keeping open the aperture in the integument of the host. Development requires from fifty to one hundred days, after which the parasites extricate themselves from the host tissue, drop to the ground and pupate. The pupal state lasts from twenty-two to twenty-four days.

**Symptoms of Infection**    There is usually no sensation during the actual penetration of the skin by the first stage larvae. Experimental observers, however, report a sharp pricking sensation some thirty minutes later. During the first week there may be pruritis, particularly at night, and by the second week a serous exudate is frequently observed. After this the lesion begins to resemble a small furuncle which increases in size and becomes exceedingly painful by the beginning of the fourth week, continuing so until larval development is completed. Muscular soreness and stiffness may be continuously present, while attempts on the part of the parasite to rotate on its own axis frequently result in excruciating pain at the point of infection.

There is considerable destruction of local tissue and the appearance of the lesion may even resemble a local streptococcus infection, with associated lymphangitis. Inguinal lymphadenitis may likewise be evident, particularly if the lesion be located on or near the ankle.

Prior to the emergence of the larva, the swelling may attain the size of a pigeon's egg, but emergence itself seems to involve almost no pain or sensation of any sort.

Competent observers who have permitted the larvae to develop on themselves report mild toxic symptoms, especially drowsiness. With the termination of the infection, naturally or otherwise, such symptoms disappear. During most of the time there is sufficient annoyance from serum and exuding wastes to warrant continuous bandaging of the part involved.

Palpebral infections, though rare, have been recorded.

**Treatment and Removal of the Larva**    Several methods for removal of the parasites have been employed. Natives squeeze out the larva after opening the boil and applying tobacco juice. A good, modern technique involves the following steps:

1. Injection of a 2 per cent aqueous solution of procaine with a hypodermic needle both in and around the lesion as a preliminary procedure. Larva and host are thus both anesthetized. 2. The larva is then exposed by a linear incision, 4 or 5 cm. long if necessary. The parasite may be removed by forceps. Irrigation with sterile saline, followed by packing with a one-to-one mixture of sulfanilamide and sulfathiazole, is recommended. 3. If little or no secondary infection is present the wound may be closed with interrupted dermal sutures; otherwise it is best to apply a tight, dry dressing without suturing.

The patient usually experiences immediate relief.

**Prophylaxis and Control**    The use of repellents, screens and bed nets to prevent contact with the carrier hosts is undoubtedly the most practical means of avoiding parasitism by *Dermatobia*. Any small pimples which do not heal within a normal time should be carefully watched for evidence of parasites. Since cattle probably constitute the most important reservoir hosts, attention from a veterinary standpoint is particularly desirable, not only for the benefit of the animals themselves but also as a means of reducing the source of human infection. Investigations have shown that the feeding of powdered garlic, either as a drench or mixed with bran, will cause up to 99 per cent of the parasites to drop from the animals at once, regardless of the stage of larval development. Drenches have been found more effective than bran mixtures in all cases.

### Genus Cuterebra

This genus comprises a group of botflies whose larvae are normally parasitic beneath the skin of rodents and lagomorphs. There is at least one record of a *Cuterebra* larva infecting the maxillary sinuses of man. The adults of certain species resemble bumblebees.

### Genus Oestrus

This genus is of special interest because of the common head bot of sheep, *Oestrus ovis* (Linn.), whose larvae develop normally in the sinuses and nasal passages of the above-mentioned host. On occasion, however, the adult flies deposit first stage larvae in the human eye where they give rise to a painful and dangerous ophthalmomyiasis. They are also known to invade the nasal passages and sometimes the pharynx. The species is world-wide in distribution, occurring wherever sheep and goats are raised.

The adult fly is of a grayish brown color, intermediate in size between a housefly and a honeybee. The abdomen is darker than the thorax. The head is white or yellowish, and bulging. The antennae are exceedingly small, the mouth parts lacking. The transparent wings extend an appreciable distance beyond the caudal extremity of the body. The calypters (squamae) are conspicuous, being large and white in color. The entire body is clothed with very fine hair.

**Habits and Life History**     The fly normally deposits living maggots in the nostrils of sheep and goats. The young larvae work their way into the nasal and frontal sinuses where they may accumulate in such numbers as to cause their hosts considerable pain and discomfort, sometimes producing death. The symptoms may resemble "gid." (True gid of sheep is caused by a larval tape worm of the genus *Multiceps*). Larviposition takes place any time during the summer or early fall, the larvae remaining within the host until the following spring, when they will have attained a length of 25 to 30 mm. Two generations a year are possible in certain latitudes. They then wriggle out of the nostrils of the host and fall to the ground, where they undergo pupation. Transformation requires from three to seven weeks.

**Symptoms of Ophthalmic Infection in Man**     Almost immediately after larviposition the patient is conscious of severe pain, as the tiny larva proceeds to attach to the conjunctival membrane by means of its curving mouth hooks. The first stage maggot (see Fig. 304) has exceedingly large mouth hooks in proportion to its size, and the injury to the host tissue may be severe. If the larva is not removed at once a progressive conjunctivitis develops, leading in some cases to loss of sight. Infection by *Oestrus ovis* is to some extent an occupational condition, shepherds being very commonly attacked, especially in Palestine.

**Treatment**     Anesthesia may be effected by dropping cocaine into the eye, after which the larvae may be removed either by irrigation or by use of forceps.

**Prophylaxis and Control**     Reduction of the number of flies in sheep raising areas appears to be the best insurance against infection in man. Daily irrigation of the sheep's nostrils with benzine is the recommended procedure for expulsion of the "grubs." Salt holes (bored in logs), the edges of which are smeared with pine tar, are quite effective in keeping the animal's muzzles unattractive to the flies. "Hothouse" lambs are practically free from head grubs, since the flies never enter buildings for larviposition.

### Genus Rhinoestrus

This genus is best known from *R. purpureus* Brauer, the common head botfly of horses and asses in Europe, Africa and parts of Asia. The habits of the species are similar to those of the sheep botfly (*Oestrus ovis* [Linn.] ophthalmomyiasis in man being not infrequently the result of infection by this form. Removal of the parasites may be accomplished as indicated for *O. ovis* larvae.

### Genus Hypoderma

These are the cattle botflies or ox-warbles. Two species are especially well known, *H. lineata* (Villers) and *H. bovis* (Linn.). Both occur widely in Europe, Asia and North America, the second being restricted to somewhat more northerly latitudes. The "grubs" are found normally in tumorous swellings on the backs of cattle, but may occur as parasites of horses and sometimes occur in man.

**Habits and Life History** The hairy, beelike fly deposits up to 800 eggs, usually on the hairs of the cattle. The hatched larvae bore through the skin of the host, migrate through the tissues and eventually localize beneath the skin of the back. Later they escape through the skin and drop to the ground to pupate. The life cycle requires one full year.

**Symptoms of Infection in Man** The act of oviposition usually goes unnoticed. Several days later soreness and swelling may be apparent, the center of irritation shifting in accordance with the migrations of the larvae. There seems to be a tendency for the larvae to migrate upward "against the pull of gravity," a tropism which should bring them to their definitive location in the normal host, but which leads merely to aimless wandering in the case of man, whose upright posture seems to disorient the parasites. Migrations from knee to chin and from groin to scalp have been recorded.

Once the larvae approach the surface of the skin they usually move but little. Perforation may thus take place long before the larva is mature, which gives opportunity for recognition and removal of the parasite. Considerable muscular stiffness, with hernia-like swellings, has been reported in specific cases. Surgical removal with the usual aseptic precautions is the recommended procedure. If the larvae are full grown it is possible to distinguish the species, *H. bovis* having the last two segments entirely devoid of spines, while in *H. lineata* only the last segment shows this condition.

Since *Hypoderma* is but rarely a parasite of man, it will not be necessary to discuss control measures in this place. It should be remembered, however, that infestation with *Hypoderma* can be far more serious than the more commonly encountered parasitism by *Gasterophilus*.

### Family Calliphoridae* ("Blowflies" and Others)

This widely distributed family is made up of medium to large, robust, rather bristly flies, characterized for the most part by metallic green, blue or yellowish coloration, at least on the abdominal segments. As viewed from the side (Fig. 298) the hindmost post-humeral bristle (thorax) is almost always on a lower level than the pre-sutural bristle. None of these species is a blood sucker in the adult stage; all, however, may function as mechanical vectors of various disease organisms by means of their feces, vomitus or body hairs. Of particular interest is the fact that many of their larvae produce myiasis in man, some as specific parasites, others in a semi-specific or accidental capacity. The following genera will be discussed in turn: *Auchmeromyia, Cordylobia, Callitroga* (= *Cochliomyia*), *Chrysomya, Lucilia, Phormia, Calliphora.*

### Genus Auchmeromyia

The genus is well known from the "Congo floor maggot," *Auchmeromyia luteola* (Fabr.), a common species in tropical Africa. The large, brownish yellow flies deposit batches of eggs on the floor of native huts, on sleeping mats or on dry sand previously contaminated with human excreta. The larvae are extremely resistant to dryness and can survive long periods (30 days) without food. They remain hidden during the day, but become active at night, when they proceed to wander about in search of a blood meal. With their mouth hooks and body spines they perforate the skin of persons sleeping on the ground. With the anterior segments more or less embedded in the tissues, they engorge until their color becomes a reddish black. This process requires from fifteen to twenty minutes. They then detach and once more go into hiding in the soil or dust. If hosts are available for nightly feeding, larval development may be accomplished in as brief a period as two weeks; otherwise, as long a time as three months may be required. Pupation takes place on or in the ground and requires about twelve days. Parasitism is obligatory with this species. Such a type of myiasis differs from all others in that the larva remains external in its parasitic relationship and spends long periods of time apart from its host.

**Prophylaxis**  Avoid sleeping on the ground, especially the floors of native huts. Sleeping mats, as carried from village to village by native travelers, undoubtedly distribute eggs and larvae. The use of repellents applied, both to the skin and to the mats has been suggested.

---

* This family is with difficulty separated from the family SARCOPHAGIDAE (flesh flies); in fact the two are sometimes combined under the family name METOPIIDAE. The latter name, however, is rare in medical literature, and it is felt that separate treatment of the groups will better serve the purpose of this work.

#### Genus **Cordylobia**

*Cordylobia anthropophaga* (Grünberg) is a large, brownish yellow fly, distinguishable from *A. luteola* by the possession of a narrower front and more rounded abdomen. Another distinguishing feature is found in the fact that in *C. anthropophaga* all visible abdominal segments are of approximately the same length, whereas in *A. luteola* the second visible segment is noticeably longer than any of the others. This species is confined entirely to the African continent, where it is known under the name of "Tumbu fly." The female deposits her eggs in polluted soil or on clothing which bears an odor of perspiration. The larvae hatch in twenty-four to forty-eight hours and proceed to seek an appropriate mammalian host. After penetrating the unbroken skin (usually the feet in the case of man), they develop very much like *Dermatobia hominis*, the location of each parasite being marked by the presence of a furuncular swelling. Sloughing and even gangrene may be observed, particularly where a number of parasites localize in a restricted area. Fortunately, only eight to ten days are required for larval development, the parasites having by that time attained a length of 12 to 15 mm. Pupation takes place in the ground. The adults emerge from 22 to 24 days later.

**Treatment and Prophylaxis**   The application of mineral oil will usually cause the larvae to loosen their hold and leave the host, regardless of the stage of development.

Since rats constitute the principal reservoir for these parasites, rodent control is of importance in holding the species in check.

It may be noted that animals which have supported an infection appear to be relatively immune to subsequent attacks.

#### Genus **Callitroga** ( = **Cochliomyia**)

These are the screw worm flies of the western hemisphere. The adults are metallic green in color, resembling somewhat ordinary green bottle flies (*Lucilia*), but may be recognized by the dark stripes on the dorsal surface of the thorax. The sternopleural bristles are arranged two in front and one behind. Two species are of medical interest, *C. americana* C. and P. and *C. macellaria* (Fabr.), of which the first, though less common than the second, is of far greater importance from a medical standpoint. The two species sometimes may be distinguished in the female sex by the fact that in *C. americana* the small scale at the base of the costal vein is black, whereas in *C. macellaria* it is white or yellowish. Males may be distinguished by the copulatory organ (aedeagus) which in *C. americana* is robust and curved, in *C. macellaria*, slender and nearly straight.

*Callitroga americana* C. and P. is the "primary screw worm" of animals and man, found in the southern United States and throughout the American tropics. The flies are attracted by any open wound or discharging aperture, depositing their eggs in batches on the skin close by. A single fly may deposit as many as 300 eggs in five minutes' time. The larvae may either enter the wound or, in thin-skinned animals, such as rabbits and guinea pigs, penetrate the unbroken skin. It is not believed that they can perforate the unbroken skin of man. This species does not confine its activity to necrotic areas, preferring to burrow deeply into healthy tissue, sometimes penetrating cartilage and even bone. Deep, festering wounds of an extremely malodorous nature are characteristic of the infec-

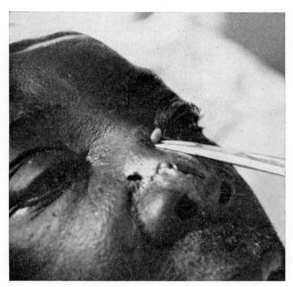

Fig. 303. Infection with *Callitroga americana*. Over 230 screw worm larvae were removed from this patient's nasal passages. (Courtesy Dr. W. E. Dove and associates, Bureau of Entomology and Plant Quarantine, U. S. Dept. of Agriculture.)

tion. One or two larvae alone rarely succeed in surviving as they cannot destroy sufficient tissue, especially when young, to offset the healing process. However, the fly's habit of laying eggs in batches usually insures the presence of a sufficiently large colony not only to keep the wound open, but continually to extend the area affected. Nasal and aural infections due to this species are truly dangerous, penetration of the brain, especially by way of the middle ear, being a not uncommon occurrence. The fatality rate of nasal and aural myiasis is given as approximately 8 per cent. Death occurs both from destruction of tissue and from absorption of poisons.

The larvae require up to three weeks (usually four to ten days) for development depending on the conditions encountered. When full-grown they are of a pinkish color and are about two-thirds of an inch in length. Advanced larvae will mature even after the death of the animal. Pupation takes place in the soil. Transformation requires from one week (in summer) to nearly two months (in colder weather).

**Symptoms of Infection in Man**   Nasal infection is the most common, but frequently goes undiagnosed for some time. There may be much local swelling and the patient usually complains of intense pain, together with a sensation of "crawling." Delirium is not uncommon. Rarely, some of the larvae may be sneezed out or emerge spontaneously. With proper illumination the physician may usually see the larvae in situ. Their mouthparts are normally embedded deep in the tissues, the posterior extremity (with its spiracles) being left free to insure a supply of air (Fig. 303).

**Treatment of Nasal Myiasis**   Three steps are involved:

1. Anesthetize the larvae (and the mucous membrane) by applying benzol, ether or chloroform, either on a cotton pledget or by use of an atomizer. Block nostrils with dry cotton for 2 or 3 minutes.

Irrigation with 20 per cent chloroform in sweet milk or 15 per cent chloroform in light mineral or vegetable oil is also an effective method of accomplishing anesthesia.

2. Remove the larvae by use of forceps and by having the patient blow his nose. Special care should be taken to avoid rupturing exposed blood vessels.

3. Give aftercare appropriate to any similar wound.

Two or three applications of the anesthetic may be necessary in the case of extensive infection.

At least one case of nasal infection in man was successfully treated by irrigation with a mixture of pine tar oil and sulfonated castor oil (turkey red oil) according to the following formula:

Destructively distilled pine oil (distilled largely from 199° to
216° C. at atmospheric pressure) ....................... 75%
Sulfonated castor oil, neutralized with ammonium hydroxide ... 25%

The maggots emerged spontaneously, by way of the nostrils and the throat. Such an effect is much more desirable than having the larvae die *in situ* where, if overlooked, their subsequent putrefaction may cause serious complications. The spines and mouth hooks can be especially irritating since their chitinous nature prevents them from being absorbed.

Pine tar oil is likewise of value in combating the offensive odor which is always present in an infection by this species.

**Prophylaxis and Control**   CONTROL OF ANIMAL INFECTION. Since human infection occurs largely in persons having frequent contact with domestic animals, the control of infection in animal hosts has much to do with lessening the hazard to man. The following methods are of value:

1. Confine branding, castrating and dehorning activities to fly-free seasons, or keep animals confined until wounds are healed.

2. Treatment of wounded animals: To prevent oviposition U.S. Dept. of Agr. Formula "E.Q. 335" is recommended. (Lindane 3%; pine oil 35%; white mineral oil 42%; commercial emulsifier 10%; silica gel 10%.) This treatment also eradicates infections already established.

3. Burning of the carcasses of dead animals not only prevents the maturing of any screw worm larvae present at death, but also eliminates the breeding of vast numbers of blowflies, of various types, which would otherwise oviposit on the carcass.

4. A certain amount of natural control is apparently effected by the activities of ants, attracted to carcasses. It has been recorded that only 4.1 per cent of *C. americana* larvae completed their development when ants were present, as compared with 93.1 per cent when ants were excluded.

PROTECTION OF THE INDIVIDUAL. 1. All persons who wish to sleep during the day in screw worm territory should be protected by screens or bed nets. This is especially important in the case of those who are wounded or who have active nasal catarrh, or discharges from the eyes.

2. Any bandages or clothing stained with blood should be promptly removed and destroyed.

3. Adequate screening of hospitals is essential.

*Callitroga macellaria* (Fabr.) was for many years confused with *C. americana*, since the larvae of both species are found frequently associated in the same wound. In such cases, however, *Callitroga macellaria* is always a secondary invader, being attracted apparently by the malodorous lesions created by the activities of *C. americana* larvae. *Callitroga macellaria* normally deposits its eggs in carcasses or in the diseased tissues of animals about to die. An infection with this species alone is not particularly serious (apart from the possibilities of secondary infection), since the larvae tend to confine their activities to necrotic tissue and thus "clean up" the wound rather than extend it.

### Genus Chrysomya

This genus is similar to *Callitroga* in that all species are medium-sized flies of bright metallic coloration. They may be distinguished, however, by the fact that the sternopleural bristles are arranged one in front and one behind. The *vibrissae* (large bristles of the face) are well above the oral margin. The genus is confined to Africa, Australia, parts of Asia, and various islands including the Philippines. *Chrysomya bezziana* (Villeneuve), known generally as the "old world screw worm fly," is similar in its habits to *Callitroga americana*, being not only an important pest of sheep, but also the causative agent of serious and disfiguring myiasis in man, especially in Asia. The maggots may occur in any portion of the body, but infections of the ophthalmic type are particularly serious. Erosion of bone is not uncommon. The larvae develop very rapidly, being ready for pupation on the sixth or seventh day. The adult fly is characterized by the presence of transverse abdominal bands.

Certain other species of the genus *Chrysomya* are believed to develop in animal excrement, but at least two or three have been reported from human tissue.

### Genus Lucilia (Green Bottle Flies)

These are medium-sized, metallic green or bluish flies distinguished from related genera by the fact that the sternopleural bristles are arranged two in front and one behind; also by the relatively robust dorsocentral and acrostical bristles. Thoracic markings are absent and the spiracles of the mesothorax are always black.

The genus is very widespread.

The females normally deposit their eggs on meat or dead animals. Not infrequently, however, they utilize open wounds or malodorous body apertures. *Lucilia sericata* Meigen, sometimes referred to the genus *Phaenicia*, is an important sheep maggot in the British Isles and elsewhere, damaging healthy tissue and endangering the life of animals. In man this species invades healthy tissue only in certain localities (China, N. Africa). In other regions the larvae restrict their activities to wholly diseased tissues. Such races were formerly used in the treatment of osteomyelitis. The same species, because of its abundance and filth-feeding habits, is frequently important in the mechanical transmission of intestinal diseases. *Lucilia caesar* (Linn.) is a well known species in the Old World, while *L. illustris* occupies a similar position in North America. *Lucilia cuprina* is the common sheep maggot of Australia. Larvae of this genus have been known to cause various types of myiasis in man, including cutaneous, intestinal and genito-urinary infections.

### Genus Phormia (Black Bottle Flies)

Flies of this group may be either shiny black, blue or green in color. They are distinguishable from species of *Lucilia* by the fact that the prothoracic spiracle is orange rather than black, and by various structural characters. A well known species is the "black blowfly," *Phormia regina* (Meig.), normally a breeder in decaying meat, but capable of causing traumatic myiasis in man. This species has also been used in the treatment of osteomyelitis.

### Genus Calliphora (Blue Bottle Flies)

Rather large flies of various metallic coloration, the common pattern consisting of a grayish thorax with the abdomen some shade of blue. The prothoracic spiracles are brownish red. The sternopleural bristles are arranged two in front and one behind. The distribution is world-wide.

As in related genera, blue bottles breed usually in the bodies of dead animals and doubtless have some sanitary value in thus hastening the destruction of putrefactive material. The larvae of some forms, however, develop as parasites on nestling birds. *Calliphora vicina* Robineau-Desvoidy (*C. erythrocephala* Meig.) and *C. vomitoria* (Linn.) are the best known members of the genus. *Calliphora livida* Hall is less common. All three are undoubtedly of some importance in the distribution of filth-borne infections. As with *Lucilia*, larvae of this genus may cause nasal, cutaneous, gastro-intestinal or genito-urinary myiasis in man.

### Family Sarcophagidae* (So-called "Flesh Flies")

This family includes a considerable number of small to large flies most of which present a remarkable uniformity of appearance. The prevailing color is gray (though a golden pollinose sheen is not infrequently observed on the abdominal segments). Dark longitudinal lines characterize the dorsal surface of the thorax. In almost all species the dorsal surface of the abdomen presents a striking "checker-board" appearance. For the most part, sarcophagids are "neatly tailored" flies, the males, especially, having the abdomen symmetrically tapered, so as to suggest a stream-line appearance. They may be distinguished structurally from the Calliphoridae by having the hindmost post-humeral bristle on a level with or a little higher than the presutural one. The arista is plumose for about two-thirds of its length or a little more. Two genera, *Sarcophaga* and *Wohlfahrtia* are of medical importance.

### Genus Sarcophaga

This is a very large genus, the adults of which are either filth feeders or flower feeders, while the larvae are found in a variety of situations, many feeding on the bodies of dead insects, carrion or animal excrement. Not a few, however, live as parasites in arthropod hosts. With such diversity of habit, it is not strange that they should sometimes develop on or in the bodies of vertebrate animals, including man. *Sarcophaga haemorrhoidalis* Fallen is a proved agent of intestinal myiasis, the eggs or larvae being ingested presumably along with food (fruit, meat) to which flies have been able to gain access. Other species are undoubtedly capable of similar adaptation. *Sarcophaga carnaria* seems to prefer the vaginal orifice for oviposition.

As in the following genus, larvae have been taken from wounds, cutaneous ulcers, nasal passages and sinuses, the adult flies being doubtless attracted in all cases by a malodorous discharge. *Sarcophaga dux* may cause tissue myiasis and *S. ruficornis* has been re-

* See note on family Calliphoridae, p. 786.

covered from wounds. *Sarcophaga fuscicauda* (*peregrina*) has been known to cause extensive traumatic myiasis of the face.

Mechanical vectorship by the adult flies is illustrated by the demonstration of plague bacilli in the dejecta of *S. carnaria* (Linn.).

### Genus Wohlfahrtia

This genus is very similar to the genus *Sarcophaga* except that the checkerboard pattern of the abdomen gives way to more or less of a black spotting in most of the species. *Wohlfahrtia vigil* (Walk.) and *W. opaca* Coquillet in North America, also *W. magnifica* (Schin.) in Europe and the Near East are frequent causative agents of myiasis of the integument and sense organs. All three are larviparous, and first stage maggots of *W. vigil* and *W. opaca* (= *W. meigenii* of authors), at least, are capable of penetrating the unbroken skin.

**Treatment and Removal of Sarcophagid Larvae**    Proceed as outlined for similar infections by larvae of MUSCIDAE, OESTRIDAE, GASTEROPHILIDAE and CALLIPHORIDAE.

### Family Hippoboscidae

A group of degenerate flies, best known from the so-called "sheeptick" or "ked," *Melophagus ovinus* (Linn.), a wingless species which feeds normally on the blood of sheep, but which may transfer itself to sheep handlers and cause some concern by crawling about on the human body. However, it practically never attempts to feed on human blood, hence may be regarded as of little or no medical importance. The group is interesting in that the females retain the larvae within their body until ready for pupation, somewhat after the fashion of *Glossina* flies. *Melophagus* is a proved vector of both rickettsial and trypanosomal infections in sheep.

# 73  Myiasis

As already mentioned (p. 650), myiasis (myasis) may be either specific, semi-specific or accidental in type. The various examples of infection, however, may also be classified according to the *portion of the body affected*, an approach which is frequently of greater value to the physician whose interest in the phenomenon is clinical rather than biological in nature. The outline on p. 797 will serve to clarify and integrate various statements of fact which occur scattered throughout the preceding discussion of the several families and genera concerned.

*Table 73  Types of Myiasis in Man*

SPECIFIC MYIASIS

| COMMON NAME OF SPECIES | SCIENTIFIC NAME (OR GROUP) | GEOGRAPHICAL DISTRIBUTION | RELATION TO HOST | CLINICAL PICTURE | RECOMMENDED PROCEDURE | REMARKS |
|---|---|---|---|---|---|---|
| Congo floor maggot | Auchmeromyia luteola | Tropical Africa | Sucks blood at night only | Perforation of skin | Avoid contaminated ground and native huts | Larvae hide in ground during daytime |
| Tumbu fly | Cordylobia anthropophaga | Tropical Africa | Young larvae invade unbroken skin (often of feet) | Furuncular swelling, with sloughing | Avoid contact with soil; mineral oil hastens emergence of larvae from tissue | Larvae leave normally after 8–9 days |
| Human botfly | Dermatobia hominis | Tropical South America, Central America, Mexico | Larvae invade exposed areas of skin | Throbbing pain, pruritus, oozing of blood | Adhesive tape; petroleum jelly on cotton; surgical removal | Fly glues eggs to mosquito or other "carrier" |
| Horse botfly | Gasterophilus spp. | World-wide | Larvae wander beneath skin; galleries small, superficial | Shifting, swollen skin lesions (creeping eruption); not serious | Remove larvae, using aseptic precautions | Three species are normal parasites in gut of horse |
| Cattle botflies (ox warbles) | Hypoderma spp. | World-wide | Larvae beneath skin; galleries large, deep; rarely cause ophthalmomyiasis interna | Larvae less motile than above; lesions sometimes furuncular; may be serious | Remove larvae, using aseptic precautions | Are normal parasites in backs of cattle |
| Sheep botflies | Oestrus ovis | World-wide | Pharynx, nose, conjunctival sac | Great irritation; may cause optic atrophy | Remove from eye by instruments; from nares by irrigation | Are normal parasites in head passages of sheep |
| Head botfly of horses | Rhinoestrus purpureus | Southern and eastern Europe; N. Africa; Asia Minor | Conjunctival sac, etc. | Inflammation of conjunctiva or lachrymal duct | Remove with aseptic precautions | "Russian gadfly;" normal in head passages of horse |
| Rodent botfly | Cuterebra sp. | Widespread (specific record from Virginia, U.S.A.) | Maxillary sinuses | Pain, congestion | Remove with aseptic precautions | Human infection very rare |
| Primary screw worm fly | Callitroga americana | Western hemisphere (tropical, subtropical and warm temperate) | Larvae invade nose, ears, sinuses, wounds (rarely unbroken skin) | Produce festering, deep, disfiguring wounds | Remove by aid of irrigations (chloroform in milk or oil) | Mortality 8% |
| Old World screw worm fly | Chrysomya bezziana | Oriental and Ethiopian life zones | Gums, nares, ears, conjunctiva, sinuses, vagina or lesion anywhere on body | Erode bone; produce foul-smelling lesions | Remove with aseptic precautions | Usually leave wound in 7–14 days |

| Flesh flies | *Wohlfahrtia magnifica* | Mediterranean, Near East, Russia Nearctic | Invades nose, ears, wounds of all types; Invades unbroken skin | Produces disfiguring wounds; Furuncular lesions | Remove by aid of irrigations; Remove, with aseptic precautions | May cause death; Parasitizes babies especially in neck region |
|---|---|---|---|---|---|---|
| | *W. vigil* | | Invades unbroken skin | Furuncular lesions | Remove, with aseptic precautions | Parasitizes babies especially in neck region }  All are larviparous |
| | *W. meigenii* (New World form) | Western U. S. | Invades unbroken skin | Furuncular lesions | Remove, with aseptic precautions | Parasitizes babies especially in neck region |

## SEMI-SPECIFIC MYIASIS

| Common screw worm fly | *Callitroga macellaria* | Western hemisphere widespread | Invades lesions, wounds (especially if malodorous) | Often complicates lesions of primary screw worm fly | Remove by irrigation, or mechanically | Normal in decaying flesh; really "saprozoic" |
|---|---|---|---|---|---|---|
| Green bottle flies | *Lucilia sericata* *Lucilia* spp. | World-wide | Invade wounds, cutaneous ulcers, malodorous apertures | Complicate existing lesions; induce purulent conditions | Removal, with aseptic precautions | Usually attack only diseased tissue; formerly used in surgery, treatment of osteomyelitis |
| Blue bottle flies | *Calliphora* spp. *Cynomyia* spp. | World-wide | Invade wounds, cutaneous ulcers, malodorous apertures | Complicate existing lesions; induce purulent conditions | Removal, with aseptic precautions | Usually attack only diseased tissue |
| Black bottle flies | *Phormia regina* *Phormia* spp. | World-wide | Invade wounds, cutaneous ulcers, malodorous apertures | Complicate existing lesions; induce purulent conditions | Removal, with aseptic precautions | Usually attack only diseased tissue; formerly used in treatment of osteomyelitis |
| Flesh flies | *Sarcophaga* spp. | World-wide | Invade wounds, cutaneous ulcers, malodorous apertures; may penetrate unbroken skin | May produce serious disfigurement | Removal, with aseptic precautions | Many species are larviparous |
| Stable fly | *Stomoxys calcitrans* | World-wide; (specific record from S. Africa) | Probably invades open wound | Aggravates existing lesion | Removal, with aseptic precautions | Very rare in man |
| Non-biting stable fly | *Muscina* spp. | World-wide | Probably invades open wound | Aggravates existing lesion | Removal, with aseptic precautions | Presumably a secondary invader |
| Houseflies | *Musca* spp. | World-wide | Probably invades open wound | Aggravates existing lesion | Removal, with aseptic precautions | Presumably a secondary invader |

Table 73 Continued

## ACCIDENTAL MYIASIS—INTESTINAL

| COMMON NAME OF SPECIES | SCIENTIFIC NAME (OR GROUP) | GEOGRAPHICAL DISTRIBUTION | RELATION TO HOST | CLINICAL PICTURE | RECOMMENDED PROCEDURE | REMARKS |
|---|---|---|---|---|---|---|
| Houseflies<br>Houseflies<br>Green bottle flies<br>Blue bottle flies<br>Flesh flies<br>*Latrine flies<br>*Lesser housefly<br>Non-biting stable fly<br>Cheese skippers<br>Rat tail maggot<br>Other syrphid flies | Musca crassirostris<br>M. domestica<br>Lucilia spp.<br>Calliphora spp.<br>Fam. Sarcophagidae<br>Fannia scalaris<br>F. canicularis<br>Muscina stabulans<br>Piophila casei<br>Tubifera (Eristalis) spp.<br>Helophilus sp. | India<br>{ More or less generally distributed throughout the world | Inhabit various portions of gastro-intestinal tract | Symptoms variable; distress, pain, anorexia, nausea, vomiting, cramps, diarrhea, melena | Vermifuges and purges sometimes effective; (spontaneous passage of larvae rather common) | Infection acquired by eating or drinking or by flies depositing eggs or larvae on anus during defecation |
| Soldier fly<br>Flies of the screw worm group<br>Wood gnats<br>Fruit flies | Hermetia illucens (Fam. Stratiomyidae)<br>Callitroga putoria<br>C. chloropyga<br>Rhyphus fenestralis (Fam. Anisopodidae)<br>Drosophila sp.<br>Calobata sp. (Fam. Micropezidae) | Records few and scattering | Inhabit various portions of gastro-intestinal tract | Symptoms variable; distress, pain, anorexia, nausea, vomiting, cramps, diarrhea, melena; rarely, ulcerative colitis | Vermifuges and purges sometimes effective; (spontaneous passage of larvae rather common) | Infection acquired by eating or drinking or by flies depositing eggs or larvae on anus during defecation |
| Hump back fly | Megaselia (Aphiochaeta) scalaris (Fam. Phoridae)<br>M. rufipes | West Indies, N.A., Belgian Congo; India, Burma; widespread (except Australian region) | Gastro-intestinal tract; larvae, pupae and flies passed in feces | Intestinal distress | Vermifuges and purges helpful | Also recorded from wounds. M. scalaris more common in man than M. rufipes |

## ACCIDENTAL MYIASIS—GENITO-URINARY

| COMMON NAME OF SPECIES | SCIENTIFIC NAME (OR GROUP) | GEOGRAPHICAL DISTRIBUTION | RELATION TO HOST | CLINICAL PICTURE | RECOMMENDED PROCEDURE | REMARKS |
|---|---|---|---|---|---|---|
| Houseflies<br>Cheese skippers<br>Moth flies<br>Rat tail maggots<br>Other syrphid flies<br>Latrine flies<br>Green bottle flies<br>Non-biting stable flies<br>Flesh flies<br>Blue bottle flies | Musca domestica<br>Piophila casei<br>Psychoda sp.<br>Tubifera (Eristalis) sp.<br>Syrphus sp. (Fam. Sepsidae)<br>Sepsis sp. (Fam. Sepsidae)<br>Fannia spp.<br>Lucilia sp.<br>Muscina sp.<br>Sarcophaga carnaria<br>Sarcophaga sp.<br>Calliphora sp. | Records few and scattering | Urinary tract, including bladder; genital passages of females | Obstruction, dysuria, hematuria, pyuria, strangury | Careful removal by use of cystoscope sometimes successful; (spontaneous passage of larvae is common) | Infection acquired by migration of larvae from intestinal tract or by flies depositing eggs or larvae on genital aperture, especially of females |

* Most commonly reported causative agents of intestinal myiasis in man.

1. **Specific Cutaneous Myiasis**
   *a.* Superficial—Example: *Auchmeromyia luteola*
   *b.* Typical
      (1) Non-migratory—Examples: *Cordylobia anthropophaga,*
          *Dermatobia hominis*
      (2) Migratory—Examples: *Gasterophilus, Hypoderma*
2. **Nasal, Stomatic, Ocular and Aural Myiasis** (flies attracted by malodorous breath or discharges)
   *a.* Usually ophthalmic—Examples: *Oestrus ovis, Rhinoestrus purpureus (nasalis)*
   *b.* Miscellaneous—Examples: *Callitroga americana, Chrysomya bezziana.* Various genera capable of facultative parasitism (see below)
3. **Traumatic Myiasis** (flies attracted to wounds, ulcers and malodorous skin, regardless of location) Examples: *Wohlfahrtia, Chrysomya bezziana, Callitroga macellaria, Phormia, Lucilia, Calliphora, Stomoxys* (rare)
4. **Gastro-intestinal Myiasis** Examples: *Fannia, Piophila casei, Tubifera (Eristalis), Megaselia (Aphiochaeta), Musca, Muscina, Sarcophaga*
5. **Genito-urinary Myiasis**
   *a.* By migration from alimentary tract—Example: *Psychoda*
   *b.* By oviposition in sexual apertures—Examples: *Fannia, Sarcophaga carnaria*

A recapitulation from the biological standpoint is provided in Table 73.

## Key for the Identification of Certain Dipterous Larvae Capable of Causing Myiasis in Man (Third Stage Only)

The following key, based partly on the study of available specimens, partly on data compiled from a variety of published sources, is at best somewhat inaccurate and incomplete. No attempt has been made to provide a key to first and second stage larvae, as the characters used for their separation are difficult of interpretation and do not lend themselves to presentation in simple form. Larvae which emerge from the host spontaneously are in most cases fully developed (third stage) and should in most cases be determinable according to the following characters. If a number of living specimens are recovered from any one case it is highly desirable to permit a few to pupate, with the purpose of rearing a small series of the adult flies. It will then be possible not only to determine with absolute certainty the species involved, but also to associate larval and adult characters more definitely than has usually been possible from the relatively incomplete records of the past. Only when a much larger amount of material has become available to students of these groups, will knowledge thereof reach the point where a complete and reliable classification may be assured (Fig. 304).

*Table 74   Key to Myiasis-Producing Larvae in Man*

| | | |
|---|---|---|
| 1 | (6) | Body with large spinose or fleshy processes extending laterally ................................... 2 |
| 2 | (3) | Posterior spiracles set in a depressed area (stigmal field) ..............*Chrysomya* (certain species) |
| 3 | (2) | Posterior spiracles set on small elevations ....*Fannia* 4 |
| 4 | (5) | Lateral processes not noticeably "feathered"; dorsal processes conspicuous ...............*F. canicularis* |
| 5 | (4) | Lateral processes conspicuously feathered; dorsal processes very small ......................*F. scalaris* |
| 6 | (1) | Body smooth or with short spines but never with long, fleshy lateral processes ........................ 7 |
| 7 | (8) | Small (4 mm.) dirty white larvae with small, pointed processes on the dorsum; processes sometimes hairy *Megaselia (Aphiochaeta)* |
| 8 | (7) | Not such larvae ............................... 9 |
| 9 | (10) | Small larvae with posterior spiracles at the end of peglike tubercles ......*Drosophilia, Sepsis, Piophila casei* |
| 10 | (9) | Larger larvae; spiracles variously borne but never at the end of peglike tubercles ....................11 |
| 11 | (12) | Body with a long, slender tail or caudal process capable of a certain amount of extension and retraction *Tubifera (Eristalis)*; also *Helophilus* |
| 12 | (11) | Body sometimes narrowed posteriorly, but never with a long, flexible caudal process .................13 |
| 13 | (26) | Larvae more or less grublike; in most species slightly flattened dorsoventrally ......................14 |
| 14 | (21) | Posterior spiracles each with three slits, all distinct ..15 |
| 15 | (18) | Slits of posterior spiracles straight, or very slightly curved ........................................16 |
| 16 | (17) | Spiracular slits short, thick (4 × 1) almost touching one another laterally. (Larvae external blood suckers.) .....................*Auchmeromyia luteola* |
| 17 | (16) | Spiracular slits more elongate (8 × 1); at most points separated from one another by at least the width of a single slit (larvae embedded in tissue) *Dermatobia hominis* |
| 18 | (15) | Slits of posterior spiracles conspicuously and sinuously curved ........................................19 |
| 19 | (20) | Each slit with a distinct bend at the middle, the ends being relatively straight .............*Gasterophilus* |
| 20 | (19) | Each slit with two or more bends, suggestive of a corkscrew ..................*Cordylobia anthropophaga* |

*Table 74*   Continued

21 (14)  Posterior spiracles each with a considerable number of small openings .............................22

22 (23)  Each posterior spiracle divided into a number of plates; each spiracular opening a small, curved, cross-barred slit ......................*Cuterebra*

23 (22)  Each posterior spiracle a single, solid plate at most but vaguely subdivided; individual apertures more or less circular without conspicuous cross-bars .......24

24 (25)  Button area part of the plate, usually central in position (See Fig. 304) ......... *Oestrus, Rhinoestrus*

25 (24)  Button area lying in an indentation of the plate.
*Hypoderma*

26 (13)  Larvae maggot-like, of typical "muscoid" shape, tapering anteriorly, broadly truncate at the posterior end; cross section more or less circular at all points ....27

27 (36)  Posterior spiracles with the button area well chitinized and the ring complete; spiracles never in a distinct pit or depression ...........................28

28 (31)  Button area a part of the ring .................29

29 (30)  Principal transverse subdivisions of spiracular slits well marked, usually not more than six in number; both ring and button heavily chitinized; accessory oral sclerite present ....................*Calliphora*

30 (29)  Transverse subdivisions of spiracular slits less distinctly marked, from six to twenty in number; ring and button less heavily chitinized; accessory oral sclerite absent ..........................*Lucilia*

31 (28)  Button area within the ring ..................32

32 (33)  Slits but slightly curved ..................*Muscina*

33 (32)  Slits sinuous, with at least a double curve ..........34

34 (35)  All three slits in the same open area .........*Musca*

35 (34)  Each slit separated from the other two by heavy chitinous bridges extending between the button and the ring .............................*Stomoxys*

36 (27)  Posterior spiracles with the button very slightly chitinized or absent, the ring being incomplete in the button area .................................37

37 (40)  Posterior spiracles in more or less of a distinct pit or depression .................................38

38 (39)  Integument spinulose at the incisures (lines of demarcation between segments); button usually absent ..............................*Wohlfahrtia*

*Table 74*   Continued

39  (38)  Integument rather smooth; vestigial button usually present ........................*Sarcophaga*

40  (37)  Posterior spiracles flush with surface or borne on slight elevations .................................41

41  (42)  Each spiracular slit ornamented with a chitinous, lateral loop ...................*Chrysomya bezziana*

42  (41)  Spiracular slits not ornamented with lateral loops ...43

43  (46)  Vestigial button usually present (though sometimes small and pale); walls of respiratory slits bearing semitransparent, lateral swellings, sometimes as long as the slit itself; surface of spiracular plate between ring and slits more granular than striated
*Callitroga* 44

44  (45)  Chitinous ring broad .................*C. macellaria*

45  (44)  Chitinous ring narrower ............ *C. americana*

46  (43)  Vestigial button usually absent; walls of spiracular slits without noticeable lateral swellings; surface of spiracular plate between ring and slits more striated than granular, the striations frequently arranged in fanlike patterns ......................*Phormia*

## Concluding Remarks on the Order Diptera

As indicated on foregoing pages, the medical relationships of the various species of flies are exceedingly complicated and diverse. Particularly is this true for the Suborder ATHERICERA (CYCLORRHAPHA) where, even in a single genus, a wide variety of disease relationships may be encountered. These facts tend to present a rather confusing picture unless one bears in mind a few simple principles, an understanding of which should enable the physician to comprehend and deal with whatever situations arise, in spite of the number of species and diversity of conditions involved:

1. In two of the three suborders (NEMATOCERA and BRACHYCERA) the blood-sucking habit is confined to the *female sex*. In blood-sucking ATHERICERA, however, *both sexes* bite. Thus all specimens of *Glossina palpalis* are potential vectors of trypanosomiasis, while *only females* of *Anopheles gambiae* transmit malaria.

2. The mechanical transmission of parasites of blood and other tissues by blood-sucking flies requires *prompt* feeding on a second host.

3. Cyclical and propagative transmission of blood and tissue parasites by blood-sucking flies requires typically a *lapse of time* during which interval the vector is usually *not infective*.

4. With certain rare exceptions (e.g., *Stomoxys*) *no* species which is a *blood sucker* in the adult state has *parasitic larvae*.

5. Conversely, species capable of causing myiasis do *not*, generally

speaking, possess *piercing* and *sucking* mouth parts as adult flies.

6. The mechanical transmission of bacteria, protozoa, helminth eggs, etc., by *non–blood-sucking* flies depends upon two factors:

*a.* contact with contaminative sources (feces, sputum, garbage);

*b.* contact with human food.

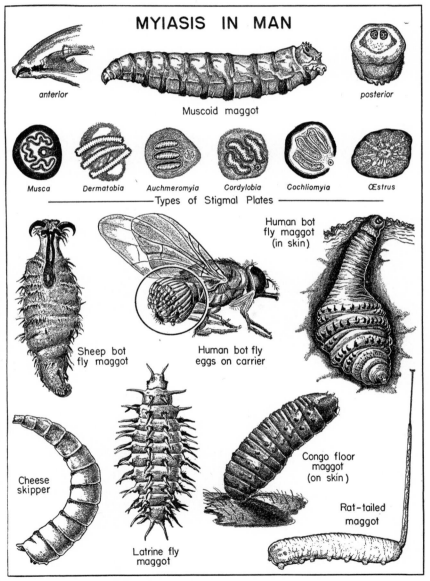

Fig. 304. Dipterous larvae causing myiasis in man.

**SOME LABORATORY DIAGNOSTIC METHODS**

# 74 Methods and Procedures

**803**

# General Procedures

### Introduction

This section gives concise instructions for performing some of the laboratory tests used in the diagnosis of important tropical diseases. Some examples have been chosen for their excellence in producing the desired results while others have been selected for their applicability to small laboratories with limited equipment. In fact, many of the tests may be performed in the field. For the details of elaborate laboratory procedures the reader is referred to standard texts on the subject.

### 1. Preserving and Packing Pathologic Tissues for Shipment

**a. Formalin Fixation**　　Blocks of tissue of about 0.5 cm. or less in thickness are dropped into 25 to 50 times their volume of 10 per cent Formalin solution in distilled water (formaldehyde 37 per cent by weight is 100 per cent Formalin). Fix for one or two days and transfer to 5 per cent Formalin.

**b. Zenker Fixation**　　Zenker's is one of the best fixatives for pathologic tissues in general.

　1. Fixing Solutions.

Solution A
| | |
|---|---:|
| Potassium dichromate ............................ | 25 gm. |
| Mercuric chloride ............................... | 50 gm. |
| Sodium sulfate (sometimes omitted) ................ | 10 gm. |
| Distilled water ................................. | 1000 ml. |

Solution B
　　Glacial acetic acid

Before use mix by volume—
| | |
|---|---:|
| Solution A ........................ | 95 parts |
| Solution B ........................ | 5 parts |

This mixture deteriorates upon standing.

2. Procedure. Blocks of tissue of 0.5 cm. thickness are left in fixative for 24 hours, then washed in running water for 24 hours. If piped water is not available the tissues may be washed in a brook in cheesecloth sacks; or, beakers containing tissues may be decanted frequently and refilled with water. After being washed, tissues are transferred to 50 per cent alcohol for 3 hours, then to 70 per cent for preserving and shipment. A pencilled note inside container should accompany tissue indicating its nature, fixing agent, and the fact that it is preserved in 70 per cent alcohol but has not been treated with iodized alcohol.

**c. Shipping** Fixed tissue blocks are wrapped in cheesecloth and either packed in cotton saturated with the preservative (usually 70 per cent ethyl alcohol) or placed directly in jars of the preservative which are completely filled with fluid and carefully stoppered.

## 2. Preserving and Packing Protozoa, Helminths and Helminth Eggs from Feces

**a. Protozoan Cysts and Worm Eggs in Feces** Dilute feces with tap water to a watery consistency, then pour simultaneously with an equal volume of hot (80° C.) 10 per cent Formalin into a separate vessel. Let stand a few hours, decant, and replace with 5 per cent Formalin. Bottle, pack, and ship. Formalinized protozoan cysts often do not float well in zinc sulfate solution (even when a solution with a specific gravity of 1.2 is used), but do stain well with iodine. Cysts and eggs remain well preserved for at least a year.

**b. Fecal Smears** Coverglasses with fecal smears fixed in Schaudinn's fluid (see p. 826) are packed for shipping in 70 per cent alcohol between lens paper in wide mouth bottles completely filled with the alcohol. Include data giving source of material, method of fixation, and whether it has been treated with iodine.

**c. Helminths** Dead helminths of all types obtained at autopsy or roundworms from stools need only be washed in lukewarm physiologic salt solution and dropped into hot (80° C.) 5 per cent Formalin for preservation.

Live worms such as large tapeworms or ascarids may be allowed to die in cold water before fixation in hot 5 per cent Formalin. If allowed to stand too long after death degenerative changes (such as blistering or fraying of cuticle) will occur. Tapeworms may also be washed in physiologic salt solution, wrapped around a spool or a glass plate while still alive, and immersed in 3 per cent Formalin. Small live nematodes and flukes will frequently become extremely distorted if dropped directly into fixatives, so a preliminary fatiguing process, consisting of prolonged shaking of the worms in physiologic salt solution, is sometimes necessary. When relaxed they are dropped into 70 or 80 per cent alcohol made up with 3 to 5 per cent Glycerin and heated to 60° C. The label should indicate the nature of the fixative so that the recipient of the shipment can mount the worms in glycerin merely by slow evaporation of the alcohol.

Pack for shipment as indicated on p. 805 for pathologic tissues.

### 3. Preserving and Packing Arthropods for Shipment

Insects and other arthropods of medical importance should be collected whenever possible for study and identification. Full data for each collection, such as date, locality, elevation, host, habitat and collector, should be included.

**a. Aquatic Larvae, Especially Mosquito Larvae**    (1). Kill in any manner to prevent distortion, such as immersion in hot water for ten to twenty seconds, or in a mixture of borax formaldehyde, and then transfer to 50 per cent and subsequently to 70 per cent alcohol.

(2). Pack carefully by placing larvae in small vial or in short lengths of ordinary glass tubing. Fill with alcohol and stopper with cotton, at both ends in the latter case, being careful to exclude *all* air bubbles. A number of such tubes may be packed in cotton in a larger alcohol-filled container which *should* contain an air bubble to allow for changes in pressure.

**b. Adult Diptera, Especially Mosquitoes**    (1). Collect at least 10 of each sex and kill with chloroform or cyanide collecting tube. Reared specimens should be kept alive for 5 or 6 hours to allow them to harden.

(2). Adults are delicate and must be packed as soon as possible after killing by placing in pill boxes or the like between layers of cellu-cotton, lens paper, cleansing or soft toilet tissue. Pack to prevent movement. *Do not use ordinary absorbent cotton.*

(3). The above applies also to gnats, sandflies and other mosquito-like insects.

**c. Other Arthropods**    1. Large forms such as house flies may be preserved in 70 per cent alcohol. Also use alcohol for all wingless forms such as hard ticks, mites, fleas, spiders and maggots. Soft ticks may be shipped alive in well stoppered vials.

**d. Shipping**    Pack carefully in such a manner as to avoid breakage and forward for identification.

### 4. Use of the Microscope

1. The first essential is proper illumination. Artificial light is better than daylight, because the intensity remains constant. For most purposes, each light should be filtered through Corning daylight glass, or cobalt glass. Use *flat* side of *mirror* (concave side is for use when the condenser is lacking). Center it so that source of light fills mirror.

2. See that lenses are *clean* especially upper lens of ocular and

lower lens of objective. To clean the lenses, use lens paper. A good technique is to breathe on the lens, then wipe off film of moisture with a fresh piece of lens paper.

3. See that condenser is used at *maximum elevation*. For high powers it is scarcely ever desirable to use the condenser in any other position. To cut down light, use the *iris diaphragm*. The sharpest definition is secured when the aperture is smallest.

4. *Manipulate the mirror* until *maximum intensity* of *illumination* is secured. Quality of image is reduced if mirror is used in any other position.

5. *Always* use *lowest power practicable,* as image is sharper and size of field is greater.

6. Always *remove immersion oil* from *oil immersion objective* before putting away microscope. If this is not done it will probably be overlooked next time, and *old immersion oil* will cause a *hazy image* until removed.

7. Not all instruments are parfocal. Use care in shifting from one objective to another.

8. Immersion oil is of two kinds: mineral oil and oil of cedarwood. The former will not gum or become sticky, but the latter gives slightly better optical results. Xylol (xylene) is a solvent for either kind of oil.

### 5. Care of Slides

*a. Uncovered* blood smears are cleaned by immersing for a few minutes in a jar of xylol and are then stood on end to dry. (They are left uncovered largely because they fade less rapidly.) Or, they may be flooded with xylol from a dropper bottle, and then cleaned by drawing a small strip of lens paper across the surface. *Never apply even a small amount of pressure to such smears, or use any other kind of paper on them.* Even though they do not appear to suffer damage from such treatment, microscopic examination will show many resulting scratches.

*b. Slides with covers* are never to be immersed in xylol. Oil should be wiped off with lens paper using only gentle pressure on cover so as not to injure smear or section underneath.

### 6. Making Blood Films

*a.* Cleanse ear lobe or fingertip with gauze saturated with 70 per cent alcohol. In an emergency rum or other strong spirits may be substituted. Dry with sterile gauze or allow to air dry.

*b.* Prick skin with Hagedorn needle or No. 11 Bard-Parker detachable blade deeply enough to cause free flow of blood. Discard first drop.

*c.* Collect three or four small drops in small area near one end of clean glass side. Stir them together with corner of another clean glass slide. Area covered by film should be the size of dime, thickness such that newsprint can barely be read through it.

*d.* Make thin smear on remaining slide surface.

*e.* Place in slide box and allow to dry thoroughly in horizontal position. Thick drop may require two hours or more to dry (especially in the tropics). Protect from dust, flies, cockroaches.

### 7. Use of Anticoagulants

If large numbers of smears are desired from the same patient or if clotting is to be prevented, one of several anticoagulants may be used as follows:

#### a. Heller and Paul Anticoagulant Mixture:

```
Potassium oxalate ..................... 0.8 gm.
Ammonium oxalate .................... 1.2 gm.
Water ...........................to 100 ml.
```

(1). Take 1 ml. of above in test tube and evaporate water in oven, leaving crystalline residue. (2). Add 10 ml. of blood to tube. This mixture has the advantage of preventing cell distortion.

**b. Heparin**    The exact quantity to be used is very small, not more than 2 mg. per cc. of blood. It may be dissolved in physiologic salt solution or alcohol, the liquid portion being subsequently evaporated as above. Tubes thus prepared are then ready for use.

**c. Citrate**    Two per cent sodium citrate in 0.85 per cent salt solution is an efficient anticoagulant. It is used in quantities up to 2 ml. per 8 ml. of blood (giving a 20 per cent solution of citrate). Blood thus rendered liquid may be used for parasite counts or other quantitative work only if the necessary mathematical adjustment due to its dilution is made. Other anticoagulants listed above do not alter the original blood volume significantly.

CAUTION: Large quantities of anticoagulant should not be used if blood is to be injected into experimental animals.

## Methods of Examining Smears, Blood and Other Tissues

### 1. Gram's Stain (From TM 8–227)

#### a. Materials

```
Ammonium oxalate–crystal violet solution:
   Crystal violet (85% dye content, certified) ..  4 gm.
   Ethyl alcohol (95%) ...................... 20 ml.
```

Dissolve the crystal violet in the alcohol.

```
Ammonium oxalate ........................... 0.8 gm.
Water ...................................... 80.0 ml.
```

Dissolve the ammonium oxalate in the water. Dilute the crystal violet solution 1:10 with distilled water. Mix 1 part of the diluted crystal violet solution with 4 parts of ammonium oxalate solution.

Iodine solution:
Iodine ........................................ 1 gm.
Potassium iodide .............................. 2 gm.

Dissolve in 5 ml. of distilled water, then make up to 240 ml. with water and add 60 ml. of 5 per cent aqueous sodium bicarbonate. Prepare fresh solution if color loss is noted on standing.

Counterstain:
Safranin (2.5% solution in 95% alcohol) ........... 10 ml.
Water ....................................... 100 ml.

**b. Procedure**   (1). Stain 1 minute with the crystal violet solution.
(2). Wash in water.
(3). Apply iodine solution for 1 minute.
(4). Wash in water.
(5). Decolorize in 95 per cent alcohol for 30 seconds with gentle agitation, or until violet dye fails to appear in the alcohol. Wash in water. Acetone or equal parts acetone and alcohol may be employed as decolorizing agents, but care should be taken to wash with water as soon as the violet dye stops running, usually within a few seconds after applying the decolorizer.
(6). Apply counterstain for 10 seconds.
(7). Wash in water; dry without blotting.

## 2. Giemsa's Stain for Blood Protozoa

### a. Stock Solution

Powdered stain ...................... 1.0 gm.
Glycerin (C.P.) ..................... 66.0 ml.
Methyl alcohol, absolute, acetone-free ... 66.0 ml.

Grind powdered stain and glycerin together. When well mixed, dissolve stain in glycerin in a water bath at 55° to 60° C. When cool add the methyl alcohol, allow to stand for 2 to 3 weeks, filter and store in small brown bottles.

**b. Preparation of Buffered Water**   For this purpose two buffer solutions have been adopted—$M/15$ $Na_2HPO_4$ (disodium phosphate, anhydrous) and $M/15$ $NaH_2PO_4.H_2O$ (sodium acid phosphate).

These are made up according to Table 75 and may be kept indefinitely in separate pyrex glass stoppered bottles.

### Table 75   Stock Buffer Solutions

$M/15$ $Na_2HPO_4$ (disodium phosphate, anhydrous).. 9.5 gm. per liter
$M/15$ $NaH_2PO_4.H_2O$ (sodium acid phosphate)..... 9.2 gm. per liter

From these stock solutions make (according to Table 76), the buffered water used in preparing stain and in rinsing stained specimens. Filter buffers before use. Buffered water is kept in well-stoppered glass bottles and made up fresh each week. The *p*H of these solutions should be checked occasionally.

### *Table 76   Buffered Water*

(formula for one liter)

| *p*H | M/15 Na$_2$HPO$_4$ | M/15 NaH$_2$PO$_4$.H$_2$O | Distilled water |
|------|--------------------|----------------------------|-----------------|
| 6.8  | 49.6 ml.           | 50.4 ml.                   | 900 ml.         |
| 7.0  | 61.1 ml.           | 38.9 ml.                   | 900 ml.         |
| 7.2  | 72.0 ml.           | 28.0 ml.                   | 900 ml.         |
| 7.4  | 80.3 ml.           | 19.7 ml.                   | 900 ml.         |

#### c. Staining Procedure*

(1). THIN SMEARS

(*a*). Fix smear by immersing in absolute methyl alcohol for a few minutes.

(*b*). Then place smear in diluted stock Giemsa, 1 ml. to 50 ml. buffered water *p*H 7.0, for 45 minutes. Older smears require a lower *p*H.

(*c*). Wash quickly in buffered distilled (or tap) water and stand on end to dry.

(*d*). If smear appears too red use a more alkaline buffer; if too dark use a more acid buffer.

(2). THICK SMEARS. Do not fix with methyl alcohol, but otherwise follow the procedure for staining thin smears. Wash gently for 2 minutes. Thick films are automatically laked while staining in an aqueous dilution of stain.

(3). THICK AND THIN SMEARS. These may be stained together on the same slide, using caution not to fix the *thick* smear; stain as outlined above.

#### 3. Leishman's Stain for Blood Protozoa

Leishman's stain is extensively used by the British. It is quite satisfactory for uses in which Giemsa's or Wright's stains might be employed; its chief disadvantage is that blood films stained with it fade rapidly.

**a. Stock Solutions**   The stain is prepared as follows:

```
Solution A
    Pure medicinal methylene blue ...................  1 gm.
    Sodium carbonate ............................... 0.5 gm.
    Distilled water ................................ 100 ml.
    Dissolve methylene blue in water and add sodium carbonate.
        Store at 65° C. for about 12 hours and then in the dark at
        room temperature for several days.
```

---

* The dilution of the stain and time required for fixing and staining may be varied considerably without changing the quality of the result very much. The *p*H of the buffer, age of smear, and brand of stain used are important factors which determine the quality of the result.

Solution B

Eosin ........................................... 0.1 gm.
Distilled water ................................. 100 ml.
Mix solution *A* and solution *B*. Allow to stand for about 12 hours until a precipitate forms and then filter. Dry the precipitate and dissolve in methyl alcohol as outlined below.

**b. Staining Procedure**   Prepared stain in powder or tablet form is usually employed due to its accessibility and ease of use. In the case of powder, 0.15 gm. is dissolved in 100 ml. methyl alcohol. This is allowed to ripen and then used in the manner of Wright's stain, i.e., the thick films are first laked in distilled water, while the thin films are *not* fixed in advance.

(1). 15 to 20 drops of the stain are placed on the slide.

(2). ½ minute later distilled water is added and allowed to stand for 5 or 10 minutes, being mixed by tilting the slide.

(3). It is then washed with water until pink.

In the tropics methyl alcohol should be procured in 10 ml. sealed ampules. Tablets of stain, 0.15 gm. each, are simply dissolved in this quantity of alcohol. Aging the stain at ice box temperatures for six to eight months improves the quality considerably.

### 4. Wright's Stain for Blood

#### a. Stock Solution

Stain (powdered) ............................... 0.3 gm.
Glycerin (C.P.) ................................ 3.0 ml.
Methyl alcohol, absolute, acetone free ............. 97.0 ml.

Grind powdered stain and glycerin together. When well mixed add the methyl alcohol and stir well. Place mixture in a tightly stoppered brown glass bottle for 2 to 3 weeks, then filter and the stain is ready for use. This stain improves considerably with age.

**b. Staining Procedure**   (1). THIN SMEARS (*a*). Rule off area covered by the blood film with a wax pencil.

(*b*). Cover dried film with stock stain for 1½ minutes (this fixes the blood film).

(*c*). Add an equal amount of freshly distilled or buffered water (*p*H 6.8). Stain for 3 minutes.

(*d*). Wash by flooding with distilled or buffered water. Stand on end to dry.

(2). THICK SMEARS. In staining thick smears, it is first necessary to lake the red blood cells. This is done by simply immersing thick film in $H_2O$ until the hemoglobin stops running out and smear appears gray. Allow to dry, then stain as for thin films.

### 5. Field's Rapid Method for Staining Malarial Parasites in Thick Blood Films

In this method thick blood films are stained in such a manner that the stained parasites and leukocytes are contrasted against a homogeneous background. After staining, differentiation of color is more clearly shown in lower edge of the film toward which the hemoglobin has drained.

Reduced hemoglobin content of the blood increases the staining time necessary to as much as ten seconds in cases of severe anemia.

***a. Preparation of the Blood Films***   Blood films should be about the size of a dime and not too thick. Films are ready to stain as soon as they are no longer obviously moist. Fixation is not necessary. Freshly prepared blood films stain better than when a day or two old.

***b. Preparation of the Stains***

Solution A

| | | |
|---|---|---|
| Methylene blue | 0.8 | gm. |
| Azur B (American stains) | 0.5 | gm. |
| Disodium phosphate (anhydrous) | 5.0 | gm. |
| Potassium phosphate, monobasic (anhydrous) | 6.25 | gm. |
| Distilled water | 500 | ml. |

Solution B

| | | |
|---|---|---|
| Eosin | 1.0 | gm. |
| Disodium phosphate (anhydrous) | 5.0 | gm. |
| Potassium phosphate, monobasic (anhydrous) | 6.25 | gm. |
| Distilled water | 500 | ml. |

The phosphate salts are first dissolved; then the stain is added. Solution of the granular Azur B is aided by grinding in a mortar with a small quantity of the phosphate solution. Solutions of stain should be set aside for twenty-four hours, when, after filtration, they are ready for use. The same solutions may be used for many weeks without deterioration, but the eosin solution should be renewed when it becomes greenish from a slight carry-over of methylene blue.

***c. Staining Procedure***   (1). Dip film for one second into solution *A*.

(2). Remove from solution *A* and immediately rinse by waving *gently* in clean water for a few seconds until the stain ceases to flow from the film and the glass of the slide is free from stain.

(3). Dip for one second into solution *B*.

(4). Rinse by waving *gently* for two or three seconds in clean water.

(5). Place vertically against a rack to drain and dry.

The concentration of the stain is adjusted for staining times of one second with an immediate wash of five seconds, but relative times may need slight adjustment to suit different batches of stain.

## 6. Hematoxylin Staining of Thick Films for Microfilariae

Hematoxylin stains the sheaths of microfilariae better than does Giemsa's stain.

***a. Preparation of Delafield's Hematoxylin***

| | | |
|---|---|---|
| Hematoxylin crystals | 4.0 | gm. |
| 95% ethyl alcohol | 25.0 | ml. |

Dissolve the crystals in the alcohol and mix the solution with 400 ml. of a saturated aqueous solution of ammonium alum.

Place in loosely capped container and keep in a light airy location for two weeks. Then add mixture of—

> Methyl alcohol (acetone-free) ...................... 100 ml.
> Glycerin ......................................... 100 ml.

Bottle and expose to direct sunlight for at least a month. Filter before use.

**b. Staining Procedure**    (1). Make a thick blood film as previously described or place centrifugalized sediment (see p. 808) on glass slide.

(2). When thoroughly dry, lake smear in tap water.

(3). Allow to air dry.

(4). Fix in equal parts of ether and 95 per cent alcohol for 10 minutes.

(5). Allow to air dry.

(6). Stain with Delafield's hematoxylin for 10 to 12 minutes.

(7). Destain in water made slightly acid with HCl.

(8). Wash in running water until blue color appears in film.

(9). Air dry. Mount in Clarite or any *neutral* mounting medium.

When microfilariae are observed in Giemsa's stained preparations they should be destained in acid alcohol, washed thoroughly, and then stained according to the above directions.

## 7. Modified Gram's Stain for Spirochetes

This stain was used originally for the spirochete of Vincent's infection, but can be used also for relapsing fever organisms.

**a. Procedure**    (1). Fix smear (as swab smears from Vincent's infection or laked thick blood smears) by passing once or twice through flame.

(2). Flood with gentian violet (1 per cent aqueous solution), add 5 drops of sodium bicarbonate (5 per cent solution, fresh or made previously with 1:20,000 merthiolate), allow to stand for 30 seconds.

(3). Wash quickly in water.

(4). Flood smear with iodine solution (iodine, 1 gm.; potassium iodide, 2 gm.; distilled water, 200 ml.) for 1 minute.

(5). Rinse slide in water, stand on end to air dry.

(6). Examine with oil immersion lens. Spirochetes and fusiform bacilli stain dark purple.

## 8. India Ink Method for Spirochetes and *Cryptococcus*

**a. Staining Procedure**    (1). Mix a bacteriologic loop of fluid containing spirochetes or fungi with a small drop of India ink.

(2). Smear and allow film to air dry.

(3). Examination reveals the general shape of the organism as a clear figure in a dark background. This is not a staining method in the true sense.

### 9. Macchiavello Stain for Rickettsiae

*a. Fixing and Staining Procedures* (1). Smear material to be stained on a clean glass slide.

(2). Fix the smear by heat.

(3). Flood with basic fuchsin 0.25 per cent for 5 minutes; drain.

(4). Flood with citric acid 0.5 per cent and wash immediately with tap water.

(5). Counterstain with methylene blue medicinal 1.0 per cent for 20 to 40 seconds. Rickettsiae appear bright red against a blue background. This stain is not useful in demonstrating rickettsiae of scrub typhus.

### 10. Examination of Fresh Blood

*a. Procedure* (1). Collect a small drop of blood from ear lobe or fingertip on slide.

(2). Superimpose cover glass immediately; press gently to distribute blood evenly and thinly. Examine with the microscope.

(3). Trypanosomes, microfilariae and spirochetes betray their presence by jostling the red cells. Malaria is recognized by pigment granules within the erythrocytes which, particularly in *Plasmodium vivax*, may be carried about by cytoplasmic streaming of the parasite.

### 11. Examination of Tissue Aspirates

*a. Procedure* (1). Fluid aspirated from lymph nodes may also be examined in the fresh state for trypanosomes or microfilariae.

(2). Aspirates from splenic punctures (kala azar) or from the indurated margin of ulcers (dermal leishmaniasis) should be smeared and stained as blood smears. Examine for leishmanial bodies.

### 12. Dark Field Illumination for Spirochetes and Leptospiras (from TM 8–227)

*a. General* Observation of living spirochetes in transmitted light is very difficult. Organisms should be brought into view by a special dark field condenser which gives concentrated oblique illumination, or by a "funnel stop" inside the oil immersion objective which reduces the amount of direct light. A special light source is needed as daylight is not sufficiently intense.

*b. Adjustment of Apparatus* (1). Remove the ordinary condenser and insert the dark-field condenser with its two lateral adjustment screws forward.

(2). Adjust the source of light until a bright ring or spot appears on the upper surface of the condenser; the plane mirror is used.

(3). With the low power objective, locate the top of the condenser and the ring etched on the surface of the condenser.

(4). Manipulate the lateral adjustment screws until the ring is brought into the center of the field.

(5). Remove the lower half of the oil immersion objective, insert the funnel stop with its small end towards the lens, and reassemble the objective.

**c. Procedure**    (1). Secure clean slides 1.45 to 1.55 mm. in thickness, and clean cover glasses.

(2). Rim the cover glass with a small amount of petroleum jelly.

(3). Place a small drop of the fluid to be examined on the center of the slide, apply the cover slip and press down to obtain a thin film, *avoiding bubbles*.

(4). Lower the substage slightly and place a drop of immersion oil, free of bubbles, on the upper surface of the condenser.

(5). Put the slide preparation on the mechanical stage and center the specimen.

(6). Raise the substage until the oil is spread by contact with the slide.

(7). Place a drop of immersion oil, free of bubbles, on the cover slip.

(8). Lower the oil immersion objective, focus on the micro-organisms which should appear as bright objects against a black background. Adjust the light for brilliant illumination, reducing, if necessary, with the condenser diaphragm.

### 13. Centrifugation Methods for Trypanosomes

**a. In Blood**    (1). Mix 9 ml. of blood and 1 ml. of 6 per cent sodium citrate.

(2). Centrifuge at 1500 r.p.m. for 10 minutes.

(3). Remove small amount of thin creamy layer between red cells and supernatant with a capillary pipette and examine; or

(4). Transfer leukocytic cream and supernatant to another tube and spin at 1800–2000 r.p.m. for 15 minutes.

(5). Examine sediment directly under microscope; or

(6). Make smears, lake, fix and stain with Giemsa's.

**b. In Cerebrospinal Fluid**    (1). Spin 5 ml. of spinal fluid at 1800 r.p.m. for 15 minutes.

(2). Examine sediment directly; or

(3). Make smears, lake, fix and stain.

### 14. Centrifugation Methods for Nematode Larvae in Blood and Spinal Fluid

**a. In Laked Blood**  KNOTT's MODIFIED SURVEY METHOD.    (1). Collect exactly 1 ml. of venous blood.

(2). Mix with 10 ml. of 2 per cent Formalin in a 15 ml. centrifuge tube. Blood lakes at once.

(3). Centrifuge, or allow to sediment for 15 to 18 hours.

(4). Decant supernatant fluid from sediment by quick tipping of tube so as to pour off surface bubbles.

(5). Holding tube inverted, aspirate sediment with a capillary pipette.

(6). Spread sediment into square area size of 22 mm. cover glass; air dry.

(7). Fix in equal parts of ether and 95 per cent alcohol for 10 minutes; air dry.

(8). Stain with Delafield's hematoxylin for 40 to 60 minutes.

(9). Rinse quickly in 0.05 per cent HCl.

(10). Wash in running water until blue color appears in film; air dry.

(11). Add immersion oil with or without cover glass and search for parasites under low power; confirm under oil.

**b. In Citrated Blood** (1). Mix 5 ml. of freshly drawn blood and 1 ml. of 2.0 per cent sodium citrate made up in 0.85 per cent sodium chloride solution.

(2). Centrifuge at 1000 r.p.m. for 10 minutes.

(3). Pass a fine pipette through the red cell sediment to remove material on bottom of tube.

(4). Spread this sediment on a glass slide and examine for active microfilariae with low power of the microscope; also examine the buffy coat for microfilariae.

**c. In Cerebrospinal Fluid** (1). Five to 15 ml. of fluid is centrifuged at 1000 r.p.m. for five or ten minutes.

(2). Examine sediment under low power of the microscope for living *Trichinella* larvae.

## 15. Examining for Superficial Fungi

**a. Procedure** Hair should be epilated from lesion by forceps; skin should be scraped from periphery of lesions or obtained from roof of vesicles with curved manicure scissors; nails should be scraped where friable or discolored and detritis beneath nail collected.

These materials may be placed between two sterile glass slides, wrapped in paper and allowed to desiccate from 5 to 7 days before culturing, or may be cultured directly after microscopic examination has revealed the presence of fungi.

**b. Microscopic Examination** (1) Clear collected material in 10 to 40 per cent potassium hydroxide by placing a small fragment of hair, skin or nail on slide in a drop of potassium hydroxide; add cover glass.

(2). Heat gently over a low flame of Bunsen burner or alcohol lamp to hasten clearing process.

(3). Examine under low or high dry power of a compound microscope; oil immersion is rarely needed.

From material found to contain fungi other specimens should be cultured on Sabouraud's glucose agar slants by placing two or three small fragments on each slant (see p. 838 for further details).

### 16. Examining for Systemic Fungi

Sputum, pus and spinal fluid should be examined in the fresh state without the addition of a clearing agent to avoid artifact formation. A loopful of sputum or pus should be placed on a slide and gently pressed to a thin film under a cover glass. Spinal fluid itself may be examined directly or the centrifuged sediment may be examined. These materials should be mixed with a drop of India ink to demonstrate capsule formation if *Cryptococcus neoformans* is suspected (see p. 814). Examine all preparations with reduced light from the microscope condenser.

All material should be cultured on Sabouraud's glucose agar at room temperature and beef infusion blood agar at 37° C. Hold all cultures for at least three weeks. If *Actinomyces bovis* is suspected, beef infusion glucose agar shake cultures should be inoculated to obtain a culture of this microaerophylic fungus (see p. 838 concerning cultures).

### 17. Lactophenol Cotton Blue for Staining Fungi

Lactophenol cotton blue is prepared as follows:

| | |
|---|---|
| Phenol crystals | 20 gm. |
| Lactic acid | 20 ml. |
| Glycerin | 40 ml. |
| Water | 20 ml. |

Heat gently under a hot water tap to dissolve. Add 0.05 gm. cotton blue ($C_4$ Poirrer).

Use as directed (see p. 838) for staining fungi.

## Examination of Feces for Protozoa and Helminths

### 1. Direct Smears

**a. Procedure**   (1). Emulsify a fecal sample composed of bits of the stool selected from scattered points in 0.85 per cent sodium chloride solution on a slide; add cover glass. Feces should be sufficiently comminuted to provide an even spreading of the smear. Newsprint should be just legible through the smear after applying cover glass.

(2). Examine under microscope.

(3). Prepare and examine at least three smears before rendering a negative report.

## 2. Iodine Stained Smears for Protozoan Cysts

Iodine staining will kill trophozoites of protozoa and is not recommended for identifying worm eggs, but is invaluable in studying amebic and flagellate cysts as nuclei and glycogen masses otherwise almost invisible are thereby stained. Such a procedure does not improve observation of diagnostic chromatoid bars so often visible in unstained cysts of *E. histolytica* and *E. coli*.

**a. Iodine Stains**　　(1). Prepare an iodine stain by mixing the following:

| | |
|---|---:|
| Potassium iodide | 1.0 gm. |
| Iodine crystals or powder | 0.5 gm. |
| Distilled water | 100.0 ml. |
| Glacial acetic acid | 1.0 ml. |

(2). D'Antoni's iodine solution is preferred by some.

(3). Lugol's iodine solution may be substituted for (1) or (2), and may be diluted with distilled water in a ratio of 1:10.

**b. Procedure for Immediate Examination**　　(1). Emulsify as when making a direct smear (*vide supra*) using a few drops of iodine solution in place of saline.

(2). Examine under microscope.

(3). Prepare several smears before making a negative report. In practice a saline smear may be made on one end of the slide and the iodine smear at the opposite.

**c. Procedure for Delayed Examination**　　(1). Use Lugol's or D'Antoni's iodine solution.

(2). Place a small quantity of the patient's stool in two or three times the quantity of iodine solution.

(3). Comminute thoroughly.

(4). Store and examine at convenience. The nuclei and glycogen will be stained by the iodine.

## 3. "MIF" Stain and Fixative for Intestinal Protozoa and Helminth Eggs (after Sapero and Lawless)

Both cysts and trophozoites are stained in a solution which also acts as an effective preservative.

**a. For Staining the Cysts and Trophozoites of Fecal Specimens Brought to the Laboratory**　　(1). PREPARATION. (*a*). Place in a Kahn tube 1 ml. of stain-fixative solution (sufficient for 25 fecal examinations) made up as follows: 0.125 ml. formaldehyde solution (USP); 0.775 ml. tincture of merthiolate (No. 99 Lilly 1:1000); and .10 ml., freshly prepared Lugol's solution 5 per cent (Merck Index). (Note: If Lugol's solution is over 1 week old, increase 0.10 ml. to 0.125 ml.;

if over 2 weeks old, increase to 0.15 ml. Reduce merthiolate in same amount that Lugol's solution is increased. Do not use Lugol's over 3 weeks old.)

(*b*). Place Kahn tube with 1 ml. of stain, and a second Kahn tube containing distilled water in a rack. Put medicine dropper in each tube.

(2). PROCEDURE. (*a*). Place a small drop of distilled water at one end of a glass slide; add equal size drop of stain solution. To this drop add feces and make a wet smear as described for the direct saline smear.

**b. For Collection and Preservation of Specimens in Survey Studies, Hospital Wards, Homes, and for Mailing to a Laboratory** (1). PREPARATION. Freshly prepare a 5 per cent Lugol's solution, and a stable stock "MF" solution containing 250 ml. distilled water; 200 ml. tincture merthiolate (No. 99 Lilly 1:1000); 25 ml. solution formaldehyde, USP; 5 ml. glycerin, to make 480 ml. stock "MF" solution (store in brown bottle).

(2). PROCEDURE. (*a*). Measure 2.35 ml. "MF" stock solution into a standard Kahn tube and stopper with cork.

(*b*). Measure 0.15 ml. Lugol's solution (5 per cent) into a second Kahn tube and stopper with a rubber cork. The two tubes represent a collection unit.

(*c*). Immediately upon collecting a stool, pour the "MF" solution into the Kahn tube containing the Lugol's solution. *The two solutions must not be combined until just prior to the addition of the fecal specimen.* Using an applicator stick, add and thoroughly stir into the solution a portion of feces about twice the volume of a medium-sized pea (about 0.25 gm.). Do not overload with feces. Stopper the tube and record pertinent data on label.

(*d*). To examine: With a medicine dropper, draw off a drop of fluid and feces from surface layer of sedimented feces. Observations indicate that most species of protozoa and helminth eggs tend to concentrate on the upper layer of the sedimented feces. Place drop on a glass slide. Mix the fecal particles in the drop thoroughly by means of an applicator stick, crushing any large particles. Cover and examine.

**c. Preservation of Larger Samples of Feces for Teaching Purposes, or for Helminth Eggs or Protozoal Concentration Procedures** (1). Use screw type cap vials to prevent evaporation. Feces, "MF" stock solution, and Lugol's solution, may be placed in vials in proportions as follows:

|  | AMOUNT OF FECES | "MF" SOLUTION | LUGOL'S SOLUTION |
|---|---|---|---|
| (small) | 0.25 gm. | 2.35 ml. | 0.15 ml. |
| (medium) | 0.50 gm. | 4.70 ml. | 0.30 ml. |
| (large) | 1.00 gm. | 9.40 ml. | 0.60 ml. |

Lugol's solution should not be over 3 weeks old and should never be added to "MF" stock solution until just before the feces is to be added.

Prior addition of iodine to "MF" stock solution will cause a dense precipitate to form upon standing.

(2). PROCEDURE. (*a*). Remove a drop of intermixed fluid and feces from sedimented surface layer, make coverslip preparation and examine. Preparation may be ringed with sealing materials.

(*b*). For flotation concentration of helminth eggs, replace supernatant fluid in vial specimen with saturated brine solution and proceed as usual for recovery of ova.

**d. *Important Principles in Usage of Technique; Staining Characteristics*** (1). By placing feces in solution *within 5 minutes of passage*, the major disadvantage of loss of organisms and morphology deterioration which occur in most all stools which are allowed to stand, may be prevented. As an example, *D. fragilis* and flagellates, frequently largely lost in iron-hematoxylin stained mounts, are recovered in undiminished density by immediate fixation in MIF solutions.

(2). STAINING. (*a*). Staining reaction comprises an initial iodine phase, as seen in ordinary iodine preparations with the exception that both cysts and trophozoites are stained, and a subsequent eosin stage which gradually replaces the iodine. A reversal to the iodine phase, if desired, may be accomplished by addition of fresh Lugol's to specimen, i.e., by adding a drop of fresh MIF solution. In trophozoites from cases of amebic dysentery, red blood cells are even more readily defined than in fresh saline preparations.

(*b*). Trophozoite forms stain immediately; cysts take stain more slowly. An increase in the strength of Lugol's, or use of a more freshly prepared Lugol's solution, will speed the staining time of cysts.

## 4. Concentration of Cysts and Eggs by Flotation

Salt, sugar, and zinc sulfate are the principal solutes used in preparing media for levitating protozoan cysts and worm eggs (except operculate and schistosome eggs). Saturated salt solution, while good for nematode eggs, plasmolyzes most protozoan cysts, so it is not generally useful. Various other methods for concentration of cysts and eggs from feces follow.

**a. *Zinc Sulfate Flotation*** (1) PROCEDURE. (*a*). Comminute a fecal sample the size of a pea in glass sputum cup or other suitable container.

(*b*). Nearly fill to top with $ZnSO_4$ solution; stir thoroughly.

(*c*). Fill brimful with $ZnSO_4$ solution; allow to stand for 20 minutes.

(*d*). Contact surface film with cover glass or slide.

(*e*). Place cover slip on microscope slide with adhering droplet down; or if slide was utilized, cover drop on slide with a cover glass.

(*f*). Examine under low or high dry powers of microscope for eggs or protozoan cysts.

If searching for protozoan cysts, add a small drop of iodine to the concentrate before examining under the microscope.

A $ZnSO_4$ solution with a specific gravity of 1.2 is recommended for use with Formalinized material.

### 5. Concentration of Cysts and Eggs by Zinc Sulfate Centrifugation-Flotation

This method is excellent for cysts of amebae and flagellates, and for eggs. It is stated that living *Strongyloides* larvae likewise are brought to the surface.

**a. Procedure** (1). Thoroughly comminute a stool sample the size of a pea in 2 or 3 ml. lukewarm tap water in a 13 by 100 mm. Wassermann tube. Occasionally it may be necessary to strain feces through gauze.

(2). Add water to one-half inch of the brim, stir thoroughly with applicator, centrifuge for 45 seconds at 1200 to 1800 r.p.m.

(3). Decant supernatant; fill with water and stir as before; centrifuge.

(4). Repeat (3); may omit if supernatant is clear.

(5). Decant water; replace with ¼ tube of zinc sulfate solution (Granular $ZnSO_4.7H_2O$ U.S.P.; dissolve 331 gm. in 1 liter of water, giving the solution a specific gravity of 1.180) stir thoroughly, fill to ¼ inch of brim of tube and spin at 2500 r.p.m. for 45 to 60 seconds. Allow centrifuge to stop smoothly.

(6). Using a 3/16-inch bacteriologic loop, transfer the surface film onto a glass slide, and apply small cover glass.

(7). Examine for cysts and eggs.

If the examination is intended for protozoan cysts, loop surface film into a drop of iodine solution.

### 6. Concentration of Cysts, Eggs and Larvae by Centrifugation-Sedimentation

**a. The 406th MGL Method—Formalin-Ether Sedimentation** (after Ritchie)  This method is recommended for general use. It concentrates helminth larvae, eggs and protozoan cysts.

(1). PREPARATION. Keep ether refrigerated except when in use. Prepare a 10 per cent solution of Formalin.

(2). PROCEDURE. (*a*). Partial comminution of entire stool, with an appropriate amount of water, can be accomplished in the stool container. Add enough water to make it possible to recover 10–12 ml. of strained emulsion, which when centrifuged, will yield ½ to 1 ml. of fecal sediment.

(*b*). Strain through two layers of gauze and collect in a 15 ml. centrifuge tube.

(*c*). Wash the emulsion with water by centrifugation (1½–2 minutes at 1700–2100 r.p.m.); decant.

(*d*). The remaining fecal sediment is thoroughly mixed with 10 ml. of 10 per cent Formalin. Allow 10–30 minutes for fixation, which reduces distortion of protozoan cysts.

(*e*). Add about 3 ml. of refrigerated ether to the Formalinized specimen; stopper and shake vigorously. Then centrifuge specimen at a relatively low speed for about 2 minutes. Free the superficial debris from the centrifuge tube with an applicator and decant until only sediment at the bottom of the tube remains. Swab tube down to the sediment with a cotton swab.

(*f*). Thoroughly mix the sediment remaining in the tube with the fluid that drains back from the tube wall and pour onto a glass slide. An applicator may be used to drag the few drops to the lip of the tube and is especially useful in controlling the amount of sediment that escapes onto the slide. An excess should be avoided. A small drop of 2 per cent iodine solution is placed near the drop of sediment and mixed with it by using the edge of the coverslip. Finally the edge of the coverslip is pushed into the drop, allowing the fluid to run under the coverslip, and, at the same time, pushing the coarse debris aside. This step is critical in obtaining a suitable microscopic preparation. Examine under the compound microscope.

**b. The AMS III Method—Acid–Sodium Sulfate–Triton NE\*–Ether Concentration** (after Hunter et al.)   This method is highly recommended for the detection of helminth larvae and eggs. It is the method of choice for the detection of schistosome eggs.

(1). PREPARATION. (*a*). Prepare by adding approximately equal amounts of hydrochloric acid of a specific gravity of 1.089 (45 ml. of concentrated HCl (37 per cent) and 55 ml. of water) and sodium sulfate solution of a specific gravity of 1.080 (9.6 gm. of anhydrous sodium sulfate to 100 ml. of water), the final mixture having a specific gravity of 1.080.

(*b*). In each solution, adjust to the proper specific gravity, if needed, before preparing the final mixture, which keeps four weeks or more.

(*c*). To insure the best possible results, it is advisable to dehydrate the sodium sulfate before using. Dry in a hot air oven for 2 hours at 130° C. and cool in a desiccator.

(2). PROCEDURE. (*a*). Partial comminution of the entire stool with an appropriate amount of water can be accomplished in the stool container. Add enough water so that it will be possible to recover 10–12 ml. of strained emulsion, which, when centrifuged, will yield 1–1.5 ml. of fecal sediment.

(*b*). Strain through 2 layers of gauze moistened with $HCl-Na_2SO_4$ mixture into a 15 ml. centrifuge tube.

(c). Wash 3 times by brief centrifugation ($1\frac{1}{2}$–2 minutes at 1700–2100 r.p.m.) with $HCl-Na_2SO_4$, decanting the supernatant each time and mixing the sediment with fresh $HCl-Na_2SO_4$.

---

\* Triton NE (Triton = X 30) is a wetting agent which may be secured from Rohm & Haas Co., Philadelphia, Penna., at a nominal cost.

(*d*). After decanting, add 5 ml. of HCl–Na$_2$SO$_4$ plus 3 drops of Triton NE plus 5 ml. of refrigerated ether. Shake for 30 seconds and centrifuge for one minute at 1700–2100 r.p.m.

(*e*). Remove tube, break ring at the interface with an applicator and decant. Swab the tube down to the sediment with a cotton swab.

(*f*). Add tap water to the 0.4 mark, mix sediment, and pour as much as can be read onto a slide; cover with a 24 or 40 mm. cover glass. An applicator may be used to draw the few drops of sediment to the lip of the tube, and is especially useful in controlling the amount of sediment that escapes onto the slide.

(*g*). Examine under the low power of compound microscope. There should be a minimum of debris and the eggs should stand out clearly. Some mature eggs will exhibit viable miracidia.

### 7. Concentration by Sedimentation (after Faust, Ingalls and See)

Sedimentation is not so efficient a procedure as flotation or centrifugation-flotation for concentrating cysts and eggs, but it concentrates somewhat and eliminates mucus and many bacteria which sometimes interfere with microscopic examination of fresh smears. The procedure is useful for concentrating operculate eggs, which are not adapted to flotation. If utilized to concentrate schistosome eggs an examination must be made within five hours to avoid hatching of eggs.

**a. Procedure** (1). Mix 10 to 100 gm. portion of stool to be examined in small amount of lukewarm tap water; dilute by stirring in cold water until sample has the consistency of a thin soup.

(2). Pour through a tea strainer (wire mesh) into a tall glass cylinder, or a large cone-shaped graduate; add 10 to 20 times volume of 0.5 per cent glycerinated tap water; allow to stand for one hour.

(3). Decant top three-fourths, refill with glycerinated water, stir well, and allow to stand for forty-five minutes.

(4). Repeat dilutions until supernatant is clear at thirty-minute intervals.

(5). Decant supernatant, transfer some of sediment to slide, cover and examine.

It is claimed that 10 per cent ethyl alcohol in water (sp. gr. 0.986) is superior to glycerinated tap water for the recovery of schistosome eggs.

### 8. Quantitative Diagnosis of Worm Infections by Egg Counts

Either Stoll's dilution method or Beaver's direct smear may be used for the estimation of worm burden. They are mostly used for the evaluation of hookworm, *Ascaris* and *Trichuris* infections but may be applied to any worm infection in which eggs or larvae are more or less continuously added to the bowel stream. The main advantages in the smear method are that it is rapid and that it requires no correction for stool consistency. The chief disadvantage in the smear is that a calibrated, specially adapted photoelectric light meter is required. However, since smears made by experienced technicians are fairly uniform and nearly always contain between 1 and 2 mg. feces, worm infections can be determined roughly as heavy, moderate and light without the use of a light meter. Counts should not be made by either method on stools that are not made up of more or less normal fecal elements.

  **a. Stoll Dilution Method**   (1). MATERIALS. (*a*). N/10 (0.4 per cent) sodium hydroxide solution.

  (*b*). Long-necked Erlenmeyer flask marked to indicate 56 ml. and 60 ml. levels.

  (*c*). Glass beads, slides and 22 x 30 mm. cover glasses.

  (*d*). Pipette calibrated to deliver 0.075 ml.

  (2). PROCEDURE. (*a*). Fill flask to 56 ml. mark with sodium hydroxide solution.

  (*b*). Add feces to bring contents up to 60 ml. mark.

  (*c*). Add glass beads or BB shot to nearly fill flask and stopper it.

  (*d*). Allow to stand 12–24 hours with occasional shaking.

  (*e*). Shake to thoroughly mix and withdraw exactly 0.075 ml.

  (*f*). Transfer to slide, cover and count eggs in entire preparation.

  (*g*). Eggs per preparation $\times$ 200 $\left(\text{i.e., } \dfrac{4}{60} \times \dfrac{75}{1000} = 200\right)$

gives eggs per ml. uncorrected.

  (*h*). Correct the count for stool consistency by multiplying uncorrected counts as follows: $\times$ 1, for hard-formed; $\times$ 1.5 for mushy-formed (can be cut with applicator but holds shape against stroke against container); $\times$ 2, for mushy (can be compressed by stroke against container; $\times$ 3, for mushy-diarrheic (takes shape of container but will not pour); $\times$ 4, diarrheic (can be poured).

  **b. Beaver Direct Smear Method**   The ideal fecal smear for most purposes contains about 1 mg. of feces in 1 drop of water or normal saline solution. Some workers prefer 2 mg. smears.

  (1). MATERIALS. (*a*). Any type of photo-electric light meter having the galvanometer dial and the cell window on the same face of the instrument, and calibrated.

  (*b*). An adapter (hand-made from wood or similar material having a thickness of about 18 mm.) to reduce the cell window to a circular opening 16 mm. in diameter.

  (*c*). Goose-neck or other type of vertically adjustable lamp.

  (2). CALIBRATION PROCEDURE. (*a*). Prepare 2N $Na_2SO_4$ and N/1 $BaCl_2$ solutions and mix each with ½ part pure glycerin.

  (*b*). Combine 1 part $BaCl_2$ mixture with 6 parts $Na_2SO_4$ mixture to give a white suspension of $BaSO_4$.

  (*c*) Place light meter apparatus directly under the lamp and adjust light to give an arbitrary whole number on the dial with a clean slide over the window.

(*d*). Deliver one drop (0.05 ml.) of the $BaSO_4$ suspension onto the slide above the window and spread just to cover the window.

(*e*). The amount of reduction in the dial reading produced by the spread suspension (as compared with the clean slide) is that which will be produced by 1 mg. of formed feces in one drop (0.05 ml.) of water or normal saline solution.

(*f*). Calibration of instrument for making 2 mg. fecal smears is as above except 3 parts glycerinated $Na_2SO_4$ mixture to 1 part of the $BaCl_2$ mixture are used to give a $BaSO_4$ suspension twice as heavy.

(3). Egg-count Procedure. (*a*). Adjust light over meter to give arbitrary pre-determined "zero point" with clean slide in place over window.

(*b*). Place one drop of water or normal saline solution on slide and spread to just cover the window.

(*c*). Add feces from applicator by stirring until dial is shifted to 1 mg. point (or 2 mg. as desired) determined by previous calibration.

(*d*). Cover with 22 x 22 mm. cover glass and count eggs in entire preparation.

(*e*). Counts can be recorded either as eggs/mg. or eggs/gm. (essentially the same as eggs/ml. corrected to the formed stool basis). Infections giving counts of less than 5 hookworm or whipworm eggs, or less than 20 *Ascaris* eggs per mg. feces generally are regarded as light; counts above 25 for hookworm or whipworm and 50 for *Ascaris* indicate heavy infections. Interpretations must vary somewhat with circumstances such as age and condition of the patient, average bulk of the stool and duration of the infection.

## 9. Rapid Iron-Hematoxylin Staining of Fecal Smears for Protozoa
(after Markey, Culbertson and Giordano)

This method is useful for rapid staining of protozoa when immediate results are desired.

### a. Staining Solutions

Schaudinn's Fluid
Saturated aqueous solution of mercuric chloride ...   60   ml.
95% alcohol .................................   30   ml.
Acetic acid, glacial ..........................   10   ml.

Mordanting Solution (Iron Alum)
Ferric ammonium sulfate ......................   5.0 gm.
Distilled water ..............................  100.0 ml.

Hematoxylin Solution
10 per cent solution of hematoxylin in 95% alcohol .   1.0 ml.
Acetic acid, glacial ..........................   2.0 ml.
Distilled water ..............................  100.0 ml.

### b. Procedure   (1). Fix smears of fresh feces in Schaudinn's fluid for 2 minutes or longer.

(2). Dip in 95 per cent ethyl alcohol 30 seconds.

(3). Wash in distilled water 3 times, rapidly but gently.

(4). Mordant in iron alum at 56° C. for 2 or 3 minutes.

(5). Wash in distilled water 3 times as in (3).

(6). Stain in hematoxylin solution for 1 or 2 minutes in a 56° C. water bath.

(7). Differentiate in tap water until smears are blue-black, changing water once or twice (for permanent mounts wash in running water 30 minutes).

(8). Dip in 95 per cent alcohol for 1 minute.

(9). Dip in absolute alcohol (or acetone) 1 minute.

(10). Clear in xylol 1 or 2 minutes.

(11). Mount in balsam, Clarite, or Permount.

NOTES: (1). Smears must not be permitted to dry before or after any step in the entire process.

(2). Overstaining may occur. In such cases dip slide into mordant diluted one-half with distilled water until proper intensity of stain is attained in parasite. Then proceed as in (7).

## 10. Iron-Hematoxylin Staining of Fecal Smears (Long Method)

This is the best method of staining protozoa in feces. Properly prepared slides last many years.

### a. Staining Solutions

Schaudinn's Fluid
Saturated $HgCl_2$ solution in distilled water ........ 64 ml.
Absolute (or 95%) alcohol .................... 32 ml.
Acetic acid, glacial .......................... 4 ml.

Hematoxylin Stain—Stock solution:*
Hematoxylin powder ......................... 10 gm.
Absolute ethyl alcohol ........................ 100 ml.

Mordanting Solution (Iron Alum)
Ferric ammonium sulfate ..................... 4 gm.
Distilled water ............................... 100 ml.

**b. Procedure** (1). Make a thin fecal smear with a toothpick or applicator on a clean side or cover glass.

(2). Before drying occurs, gently lower slide, smear downwards, onto surface of Schaudinn's fluid (in a flat dish and heated to 45° C.) and fix for 5 to 15 minutes.

(3). Pass through the alcohol series as follows:

| | |
|---|---|
| 35% | 3 to 5 minutes |
| 50% | 3 to 5 " |
| 70% plus iodine (wine color) | 5 " |
| 70% | 5 " |
| 85% | 3 to 5 " |
| 95% | 30 " |
| 85% | 3 " |
| 70% | 3 " |
| 35% | 3 " |

* Dissolve powder in alcohol. Keep several weeks to ripen before use. Make staining solution by mixing 10 ml. of stock solution with 90 ml. of distilled water.

(4). Mordant in iron alum ...................12 to 24 hours
(5). Wash in distilled water .................2 minutes
(6). Stain with hematoxylin ...............12 to 24 hours
(7). Wash in tap water ......................5 minutes

(8). Smears are now overstained. Destain in 2 per cent solution of iron alum, until the nuclear chromatin stands out under high-dry lens.

(9). Stop destaining by washing slide in gently running tap water overnight.

(10). Pass through ascending series of alcohols, clear in xylol and mount.

### 11. Polyvinyl Alcohol–Fixative Method for Trophozoites of Intestinal Protozoa (after Brooke and Goldman)

This method is specifically designed to preserve trophozoites of amebae for long periods of time in a condition suitable for permament staining. It can also be used to prevent the washing-off during the staining process of amebae occurring in liquid stools or in cultures. It is fairly satisfactory for the detection of protozoan cysts.

**a. Preparation**   Add 5 gm. of polyvinyl alcohol* to a mixture at room temperature of 1.5 ml. glycerol, 5 ml. glacial acetic acid, and 93.5 ml. of Schaudinn's solution (2 parts of saturated aqueous mercuric chloride to 1 part of 95 per cent ethyl alcohol). Heat gently while stirring to about 75° C. or until the solution clears. Solution keeps for several months at least.

**b. Procedure**   (1). FIXATION IN VIAL. (*a*). Thoroughly mix one part of specimen in a vial containing three parts or more of PVA-fixative.

(*b*). Films for staining may be prepared immediately or months later by spreading a drop or two of the mixture on a microscope slide and allowing the smear to dry thoroughly (preferably overnight at 37° C.). Films should be of moderate thickness.

(2). FIXATION ON MICROSCOPE SLIDES. (*a*). Mix thoroughly one drop of specimen with about three drops of PVA-fixative on a microscope slide.

(*b*). Spread the mixture over approximately one-third of the surface of the slide and allow to dry thoroughly.

(3). STAINING OF ORGANISMS IN PVA FILMS. (*a*). Place the dried smear in 70 per cent alcohol containing iodine for 10 minutes or longer in order to remove crystals resulting from mercuric chloride fixation.

(*b*). Stain with any standard hematoxylin procedure in the usual manner for fecal smears.

(*c*). Smears may be removed from staining solutions and allowed

---

* Polyvinyl alcohol may be obtained from E. I. du Pont de Nemours & Co., Wilmington 98, Del., under the trade name of Elvanol. Grade 90–25 (medium viscosity, complete hydrolysis) has given the best results.

to dry at any point in the procedure except during dehydration in graded alcohols after staining. Occasionally, films may wrinkle around the edge or in the middle during prolonged exposure to aqueous solutions. This tendency may be minimized by preparing relatively thin, rectangular smears. To prevent the loss of a wrinkling film, the slide may be laid flat in a 37° C. incubator and allowed to dry before continuing the staining process.

(*d*). Examine for trophozoites and cysts.

## 12. Diagnosis of Pinworm Infection

*a. Procedure*    The most satisfactory means of diagnosing pinworm infection is by the recovery of eggs or female worms from the perianal region, as only 5 to 10 per cent of infected persons pass eggs in their stools.

(1). SCOTCH TAPE METHOD (after Graham). (*a*) Hold a 2- to 2½-inch long strip of Scotch tape, sticky side out, with a pair of forceps or place over butt end of a test tube or tongue depressor.

(*b*). Swab Scotch tape gently but firmly around the perianal rugae of the patient, preferably in the morning before the patient has defecated.

(*c*). Place Scotch tape, sticky side down, in a drop of toluene on a clean glass slide and examine for pinworm eggs and adults.

(*d*). This preparation may be forwarded to a central laboratory for confirmation.

## 13. Fixing and Staining Trematodes

Many of the techniques recommended for one group of worms can be employed with equally satisfactory results for others. Some are outlined.

### a. Fixing Solutions

(1). Corrosive-Acetic Fixative
Saturated aqueous solution mercuric chloride ....... 95 ml.
Acetic acid ................................... 5 ml.
(2). Formalin ................................... 5–8%
(3). Bouin's-Solution A. Saturated aqueous solution—picric acid.

Solution B
Formalin .............................. 5 ml.
Acetic acid ............................ 1 ml.
Mix solutions A and B before use:
Solution A ............................. 75 ml.
Solution B ............................. 30 ml.

### b. Staining Solutions    Any of these will give consistently good results.

(1). Semichon's Acetic Carmine
Acetic acid ............................ 50 ml.
Distilled water ........................ 50 ml.

Place in small flask; add excess carmine powder. Stopper flask with pierced stopper with thermometer, place in water bath, heat to 100° C. for fifteen minutes. Cool, allow to settle, decant supernatant and filter.

(2). Delafield's hematoxylin (see p. 813)
(3). Alum cochineal
Potassium alum .............................. 30 gm.
Cochineal ................................... 30 gm.
Distilled water .............................. 400 ml.

Boil for one hour; cool and filter. Boil filter paper in 200 ml. distilled water for 30 minutes; filter; add to first filtrate; boil 30 minutes. Filter and make up to 400 ml. with distilled water.

**c. Procedure**   (1). Relax flukes by shaking vigorously in bottle half-filled with 1.0 per cent salt solution for 3 minutes.

(2). Pour off liquid, replace with equal parts of 1 per cent salt solution and 1 part fixative; shake vigorously for 3 minutes.

(3). Drop the fixed trematodes into undiluted fixative for 3 to 12 hours.

(4). Place in 70 per cent alcohol colored like port wine with iodine for 12 hours.

(5). Place in 70 per cent alcohol for several hours to remove iodine.

(6). Stain (diluted half and half with distilled water). The interval will vary with the stain used and the size of the specimen.

(7) Decolorize in 70 per cent alcohol made slightly acid with a few drops of hydrochloric acid (about 0.5 to 1 per cent) until the internal structures are visible in transmitted light. Neutralize by repeated washings in 70 per cent alcohol.

(8). Pass through 85 per cent, 95 per cent, and 100 per cent alcohols, allowing at least a half hour in each.

(9). Mount in balsam, clarite or other neutral mounting medium.

## 14. Fixing and Staining Cestodes

### a. Fixing Solution

Alcohol—Formol—Acetic
Alcohol, 95 per cent ........................... 24 ml.
Formalin ...................................... 15 "
Acetic acid, glacial .......................... 5 "
Glycerin ...................................... 10 "
Water ......................................... 46 "

**b. Procedure**   (1). Allow worms to lie in cold water until contractions have ceased, or wrap the worm about a spool (or glass plate) after washing in physiologic saline.

(2). Drop into fixative.

(3). Cut out selected proglottids with sharp scalpel, and place in water a few minutes before staining.

(4). Proceed as described above for flukes, beginning with (6) p. 830, using Delafield's hematoxylin or Semichon's acetic carmine.

## 15. Fixing and Examining Nematodes

### a. Fixing and Clearing Solutions

(1) Lacto-phenol
Phenol ...................................... 10 gm.
Glycerin ................................... 10.6 ml.
Lactic acid ................................ 8.2 ml.
Distilled water ............................ 10 ml.
(2) Formalin ................................ 5–8%
(3) Glycerin-Alcohol
Ethyl alcohol 70–80% ....................... 96 ml.
Glycerin ................................... 4 ml.

**b. Procedure for Small Nematodes** (1). Fix in warm solution of Formalin and preserve.

(2). Transfer to drop of lacto-phenol for examination; add cover glass.

**c. Procedure for Larger Nematodes** (1). If worms are alive, shake vigorously in a bottle half-filled with physiologic saline solution for 3 to 4 minutes.

(2). Drop worms into glycerin-alcohol fixative heated to 60° C. in a small evaporating dish.

(3). Set evaporating dish in a warm place to permit slow evaporation of the alcohol.

(4). When alcohol appears to have entirely evaporated mount nematodes on slides in glycerin jelly.

The intestinal structures will ordinarily stand out clearly. Staining nematode worms is ordinarily not too successful and is not necessary.

## Methods of Examining Urine

### 1. Examining Urine for Schistosome Eggs

**a. Procedure** (1). Collect urine sample for examination of eggs at end of micturition in sedimentation glass.

(2). Allow to settle; pipette off bottom sediment to slide.

(3) Examine microscopically.

In infections with *Diotophyme renale,* a kidney worm rarely infecting man, eggs may be found in urine sediment. Occasionally microfilariae of *W. bancrofti* have been recovered from urine in cases of filariasis with chyluria.

### 2. Examining Urine for Spirochetes

Spirochetes of relapsing fever, *Leptospira icterohaemorrhagiae* or *L. canicola* sometimes may be found in urine.

**a. Procedure** (1). Collect 30 to 50 ml. of urine in a sterile vessel.

(2). Centrifuge at 2000 r.p.m. for 30 minutes.

(3). Examine sediment under a dark field for spirochetes.

Refrigerate (but do not freeze) urine sample if urine must be transported great distances.

## Methods of Examining Sputum

### 1. Examining Sputum for Helminth Eggs and Larvae

*a.* Mix sputum and 3 per cent sodium hydroxide solution in equal amounts.

*b.* Centrifuge at high speed.

*c.* Decant supernatant.

*d.* Examine sediment for eggs and larvae.

### 2. Antiformin Concentration Method for Acid Fast Bacilli

#### a. Materials

```
(1). Liquor sodae chlorinatae
     Sodium carbonate ........................... 600 gm.
     Chlorinated lime ............................ 400 gm.
     Distilled water ............................. 4000 ml.
(2). Sodium hydroxide ....................... 15% solution
```

Mix equal parts of (1) and (2); this is antiformin. Place in dark bottle and keep in cool place.

**b. Procedure**   (1). Place equal parts of 24-hour sputum sample and 50 per cent antiformin solution in suitable container.

(2). Incubate at 37° C. for 30 minutes; stir occasionally to insure liquefaction.

(3). Dilute with 3 volumes sterile water.

(4). Centrifuge for 10 to 30 minutes; decant supernatant.

(5). Repeat until all fractions have been centrifuged; decant.

(6). Add distilled water, stir sediment; centrifuge; decant supernatant.

(7). Transfer sediment to slides.

(8). Make smears and stain as for acid-fast bacilli.

### 3. Ziehl-Neelsen Stain for Acid-Fast Bacilli (from Manual of Methods for Pure Culture Study of Bacteria)

This stain is used to differentiate acid-fast and non–acid-fast organisms and depends upon a primary stain, decolorizer and counterstain.

#### a. Materials

(1). ZIEHL'S CARBOL FUCHSIN

```
Solution A
  Basic fuchsin (90% dye content) ................ 0.3 gm.
  Ethyl alcohol (95%) ........................... 10.  ml.
Solution B
  Phenol ........................................ 5.0 gm.
  Distilled water ............................... 95.0 ml.
  Mix solutions A and B
```

(2). Loeffler's Alkaline Methylene Blue

> Solution A
> Methylene blue (90% dye content) .............. 0.3 gm.
> Ethyl alcohol (95%) ........................ 30.0 ml.
> Solution B
> Dilute KOH (0.01% by weight) .............. 100. ml.
> Mix solutions A and B

**b. Procedure** (1). Stain dried smears 3–5 minutes with Ziehl's carbol fuchsin, applying enough heat for gentle steaming.

(2). Rinse in tap water.

(3). Decolorize in 95 per cent ethyl alcohol containing 3 per cent by volume of concentrated HCl, until only a suggestion of pink remains.

(4). Wash in tap water.

(5). Counterstain with Loeffler's alkaline methylene blue.

(6). Wash in tap water.

(7). Dry and examine. Acid-fast organisms stain red, others blue.

## Culture Methods

### 1. Boeck-Drbohlav's Locke-Egg-Serum Medium

This medium may be employed for the cultivation of *Endamoeba histolytica*, *E. coli*, *Endolimax nana*, *Dientamoeba fragilis*, *Chilomastix mesnili* and *Trichomonas hominis*. Transfers are made every 48 hours, except in the case of *E. coli* which requires transfers every 72 hours. About 0.5 ml. of the fluid medium at the bottom of the tube is used for each transplant.

**a. Materials Required**

(1). Eggs.

(2). Sterile Ringer's Solution. This is prepared according to the following formula:

| | | |
|---|---|---|
| Sodium chloride | (NaCl) | 8.0 gm. |
| Potassium chloride | (KCl) | 0.2 gm. |
| Calcium chloride | (CaCl$_2$) | 0.2 gm. |
| Magnesium chloride | (MgCl$_2$) | 0.1 gm. |
| Monosodium phosphate | (NaH$_2$PO$_4$) | 0.1 gm. |
| Sodium bicarbonate | (NaHCO$_3$) | 0.4 gm. |
| Distilled water | (H$_2$O) | 1000 ml. |

It is then autoclaved at 15 pounds pressure for 20 minutes and allowed to cool.

(3). Modified Sterile Ringer's Solution. Prepared by adding 0.25 gm. of Loeffler's Dehydrated Blood Serum* to 1000 ml. of Ringer's solution which should be made up in addition to the

* Instead of the Loeffler's Dehydrated Blood Serum sterile human serum or sterile horse serum (inactivated and tri-cresol free) may be used, in which case the modified Ringer's solution should consist of 1 part serum to 8 parts of Ringer's solution. This solution is sterilized by passing through a Berkefeld filter and incubated at 37.5° C. to determine sterility before pouring onto egg slants.

Ringer's solution of (2). Boil serum and Ringer's solution for one hour to facilitate solution of serum, filter, and autoclave for 20 minutes at 15 pounds pressure.

(4). STERILE CHINESE RICE FLOUR. The rice flour is sterilized by placing about 5 gm. in a test tube and plugging it with cotton. It is distributed evenly and loosely over inner surface of tube by shaking, and then sterilized in horizontal position in dry heat at about 90° C. for 12 hours, using intermittent sterilization and allowing four hours for each period; flour remains white if not overheated.

**b. Procedure**   Wash four eggs thoroughly, rinse, and brush well with 70 per cent ethyl alcohol. Break into sterile Erlenmeyer flask containing glass beads and 50 ml. of Ringer's solution. Emulsify completely by shaking. Place about 4 ml. of this material in each test tube and sterilize as follows (using autoclave as inspissator): Place tubes in a preheated autoclave in such a position as to produce a slant of about 1 to 1.5 inches, close the door and vacuum exhaust valve, turn on the steam and open the outside exhaust valve. When steam appears from this valve, close it and allow the pressure to rise to 15 pounds; then shut off steam and allow pressure to decline to zero; remove media from autoclave. Repeat on three successive days, storing media at room temperature between sterilization.

To these sterile solid slants add enough modified Ringer's solution (about 5 or 6 ml.) to cover egg slant completely. Incubate at 37.5° C. for 24 hours to determine sterility before adding the sterile Chinese rice flour. Flour is added by taking up 0.25 ml. into a clean, sterile, dry, wide bore, 1 ml. pipette and discharging it into the liquid medium by tapping the pipette against the inside wall of the tube. The tubes are again incubated at 37.5° C. for 24 hours to test for sterility

## 2. Cleveland and Collier's Medium for Cultivation of Amebae

### a. Materials

> Bacto-Entameba Medium
> Horse Serum
> NaCl

**b. Procedure**   (1). Suspend 33 gm. of the Bacto-Entamoeba in 1000 ml. distilled $H_2O$ and heat to boiling to dissolve medium completely.

(2). Place in tubes and autoclave at 15 pounds pressure (120° C.) for 20 minutes.

(3). Slant tubes. Test for sterility. Overlay slants with sterile horse serum–saline solution (1:6 dilution). Add a 5 mm. loop of sterile rice flour.

## 3. Egg-Yolk Medium for the Cultivation of Amebae (after Balamuth)

### a. Materials

> Dehydrated or fresh egg yolk
> Liver extract (Lilly, No. 408)

Dibasic potassium phosphate (K$_2$HPO$_4$)
Potassium acid phosphate (KH$_2$PO$_4$)
Sodium chloride
Rice flour

**b. Procedure**    (1). Mix 36 gm. of dehydrated egg yolk or the crumbled yolks of 4 hard-boiled eggs with 36 ml. of distilled water.

(2). Add 125 ml. of 0.8 per cent NaCl and mix with a rotary beater or Waring Blendor.

(3). Heat the mixture over boiling water for 20 minutes after the temperature has reached 80° C. and add distilled water to offset the loss by evaporation.

(4). Filter. The mixture of the dehydrated yolks is difficult to separate through a Buchner funnel but may be passed through a double layer of muslin instead. If fresh eggs are used the mixture may be filtered by suction through a Buchner funnel using ordinary filter paper.

(5). Bring the filtrate to a volume of 125 ml. by adding 0.8 per cent NaCl.

(6). Autoclave at 15 pounds (120° C.) for 20 minutes.

(7). Cool to below 10° C. and filter through a Buchner funnel.

(8). Add to the filtrate an equal amount of M/15 potassium buffer adjusted to *p*H 7.5, prepared by diluting 1:15 a solution of M/1 dibasic potassium phosphate 4.3 parts and M/1 potassium acid phosphate 0.7 parts.

(9). Add a 5 per cent crude liver extract (Lilly, No. 408) to give a final concentration of 0.5 per cent in order to insure rapid growth.

(10). Autoclave and then refrigerate until dispensed in tubes containing 7 to 10 ml.

(11). Prior to inoculation add a 5 mm. loop of sterile rice flour.

## 4. Alcoholic Extract Medium for the Cultivation of Amebae (after Nelson)

### a. Materials

Finely divided tissue or egg yolk
95% Ethyl alcohol
Agar
Sodium chloride
Rice flour

This medium is recommended because of its simplicity and because it does not grow *Blastocystis hominis* or a heavy bacterial population.

**b. Procedure**    (1). Extract one part of finely divided tissue (such as liver) or egg yolk with 9 parts of 95 per cent ethyl alcohol for 48 hours.

(2). Evaporate the alcohol from the stock extract in a boiling water bath and add twice the volume of 2 per cent agar in buffered 0.5 per cent sodium chloride solution (*p*H 7.4).

(3). Tube, autoclave and slant.

(4). Cover the slants with buffered 0.5 per cent sodium chloride solution. The addition of 0.025 per cent of agar to the overlay is beneficial.

(5). Sterile rice flour is added at the time of inoculation.

## 5. NNN Medium for *Leishmania*

### a. Materials

| | |
|---|---|
| Bacto-Agar ..................................... | 14 gm. |
| Sodium chloride ................................ | 6 gm. |
| Distilled water ................................. | 900 ml. |
| Sodium hydroxide solution ...................... | N/1 |
| Rabbit (or guinea pig) defibrinated blood ........... | 10 ml. |

### b. Procedure

To a flask containing 900 ml. of distilled water add 14 gm. of Bacto-Agar and 6 gm. of sodium chloride. Bring to a boil and then neutralize with N/1 NaOH. Place 150 ml. of the medium in 6 Erlenmeyer flasks and sterilize in autoclave for one-half hour at 12 pounds pressure. Store in refrigerator. Stock medium will keep for several months if stored at ice box temperatures.

Place one of the flasks containing 150 ml. of stock medium in a boiling water bath and when agar has melted cool medium to 50° to 55° C. and, using sterile technique, add 10 ml. of defibrinated rabbit blood, mixing thoroughly. Pipette 5 ml. of this medium into test tubes and slant tubes so as to produce a long slant. When slants have hardened, paraffin the cotton plugs and place in refrigerator for 12 hours, subsequently incubating tubes at 37.5° C. for 24 hours to test for sterility.

## 6. Diphasic Blood-Agar Medium for Trypanosomes and Leishmanias (NIH Method)

### a. Materials

| | |
|---|---|
| Bacto-Beef (Difco) ............................ | 25.0 gm. |
| Neopeptone (Difco) ........................... | 10.0 gm. |
| Bacto-Agar (Difco) ........................... | 10.0 gm. |
| Sodium chloride .............................. | 2.5 gm. |
| Distilled water ............................... | 500 ml. |

### b. Procedure

(1). Infuse Bacto-Beef and distilled water in water bath for 1 hour; heat mixture for 5 minutes at 80° C. to coagulate a portion of the protein.

(2). Filter, using ordinary grade of filter paper.

(3). Add Neopeptone, Bacto-Agar and sodium chloride.

(4). Adjust the *p*H to 7.2–7.4 with NaOH.

(5). Autoclave at 15 pounds, 120° C. for 20 minutes.

(6). Cool until mixture may be held comfortably in the hand

and add 10 per cent defibrinated rabbit blood. (For *Trypanosoma lewisi* add 30 per cent defibrinated rabbit blood.)

(7). Dispense 5 ml. per test tube, slant and cool.

(8). Before inoculating overlay the slants with 2 ml. of sterile Locke's solution prepared by the following formula:

| | |
|---|---|
| Sodium chloride .............................. | 8.0 gm. |
| Potassium chloride ........................... | 0.2 gm. |
| Calcium chloride ............................. | 0.2 gm. |
| Potassium phosphate (monobasic) ............... | 0.3 gm. |
| Dextrose .................................... | 2.5 gm. |
| Distilled water .............................. | 1000 ml. |

## 7. C.P.L.M. (Cysteine-Peptone-Liver-Maltose) Medium for the Cultivation of *Trichomonas vaginalis* (after Johnson and Trussell)

### a. Materials

| | |
|---|---|
| Bacto-Peptone .............................. | 32.0 gm. |
| Bacto-Agar ................................. | 1.6 gm. |
| Cysteine HCl ................................ | 2.4 gm. |
| Maltose .................................... | 1.6 gm. |
| Liver infusion (Difco) ....................... | 320 ml. |
| Ringer's solution | |
| (NaCl 0.6%, NaHCO₃, KCl and CaCl₂ 0.01% each) . | 960 ml. |
| Sodium hydroxide N/1 ........................ | 11–13 ml. |

**b. Procedure** (1). Heat the mixture in a boiling water bath to melt the agar and filter through coarse filter paper.

(2). Add 0.7 ml. of 0.5 per cent aqueous methylene blue. Adjust the $p$H to 5.8 to 6.0 with N/1 HCl or N/1 NaOH.

(3). Tube in 8 ml. amounts and autoclave.

(4). Cool; add 2 ml. of sterile human serum.

(5). Incubate for sterility for at least 4 days at 37.5° C. and store at room temperature until used.

## 8. Barret and Yarbrough's Medium for *Balantidium coli*

### a. Materials

| | |
|---|---|
| Inactivated human serum ....................... | 1 part |
| Sodium chloride solution, 0.5% .................... | 16 parts |

Sterilize by filtration and distribute in 8 ml. portions in test tubes.

**b. Procedure** (1). Inoculate tubes by adding 0.1 ml. of feces containing organisms at bottom of tubes with a pipette.

(2). Incubate at 37° C. and examine in 24 hours.

(3). Make transfers every 24 or 48 hours, using media near bottom of tubes. Cysts also appear in culture. Substitution of Locke or Ringer's solution without dextrose gives better results than salt solution.

## 9. Media for Fungi

### a. Materials

Sabouraud's glucose medium:

| | |
|---|---|
| Glucose (maltose) | 40.0 gm. |
| Peptone | 10.0 gm. |
| Agar | 20.0 gm. |
| Water | 1000.0 ml. |

Keep in 10 ml. quantities in stab tubes. Melt and allow to cool to 45°C., add 10 units of penicillin and 30 units of streptomycin per ml. of agar. Allow to slant while hardening or pour into sterile petri dishes. Actidione, 0.1 mg./ml. also may be added. Final *p*H should be 5.6.

Sabouraud's conservation medium:

| | |
|---|---|
| Peptone | 40.0 gm. |
| Agar | 20.0 gm. |
| Water | 1000.0 ml. |

Beef infusion blood agar (*p*H 7.4 to 7.6):

| | |
|---|---|
| Beef infusion broth | 1000.0 ml. |
| Peptone | 20.0 gm. |
| Sodium chloride | 5.0 gm. |
| Agar | 20.0 gm. |

Keep in 100 ml. quantities in flasks. Melt and allow to cool to 45° C., add 5 ml. of sterile blood, mix and pour into tubes for slants or sterile Petri dishes for plates. Test for sterility by incubating at 37.5° C. for 24 hours.

Penicillin and streptomycin also may be added to this medium.

Littman's Oxgall Agar (Difco) is a useful medium for use in the tropics where saprophytic fungi tend to overgrow cultures.

Maintain cultures at room temperature for 2 or 3 weeks. Transfers of growth from any bit of inoculum are made to fresh tubes for pure cultures. Cultures which cannot be readily identified should be maintained on Sabouraud's conservation medium to prevent degenerative loss of diagnostic morphologic characters.

**b. Procedures**   Yeastlike cultures are best examined by placing a bit of the culture on a slide in drop of water and adding coverslip to the preparation. Filamentous cultures should be examined in a mounting medium. These cultures are examined by picking small fragments of the aerial growth from the agar surface by means of a straight inoculating wire bent slightly at the end. Place material on slide in a drop of lactophenol cotton blue (see p. 818), tease or spread out gently with dissecting needles and add cover glass. Gentle heating of such a preparation will drive out air bubbles and allow greater penetration of the stain.

## 10. Fletcher's Medium (after TM 8–227)

### a. Materials

| | | |
|---|---|---|
| 12% Sterile rabbit serum in sterile distilled water | 100. | ml. |
| 2% Nutrient agar | 7.5 | ml. |

**b. Procedure**   (1). Heat rabbit serum solution to 50° C.

(2). Add melted nutrient agar.

(3). Tube in 5 ml. quantities and sterilize by heating at 56° C. for 1 hour on 2 successive days.

(4). Incubate for sterility.

(5). Inoculate with 0.03 ml. of blood and incubate at 30° C.

(6). Examine for leptospira on a darkfield microscope on the seventh, fourteenth, twenty-first and twenty-eighth day. Then discard.

## Serologic and Immunologic Methods

### 1. Methods of Collecting Materials for Laboratory Diagnosis of Neurotropic Virus Diseases

*a. Blood for Complement Fixation and Neutralization Tests* (1). As soon as possible after the onset of illness, then again after approximately three and six weeks, collect 25 ml. blood samples using sterile precautions.

(2). Whole blood may be shipped, except in areas where sustained temperatures over 100° F. prevail.

(3). In the latter case separate blood and serum using aseptic technique.

(4). Blood is shipped in 30 ml. vacuum tubes if collected in them; blood or serum, in sterile Wassermann tubes with sterile rubber or cork stoppers sealed with adhesive.

CAUTION: The specimen should not be frozen.

*b. Specimens for Isolation of the Virus*  BLOOD. (1). Withdraw 12 ml. of blood in dry, sterile syringe and distribute equally in three sterile Pyrex Wassermann tubes. Stopper tubes with sterile corks and seal with adhesive tape or fire seal if equipment is available.

(2). Freeze contents by immersing tubes in a mixture of alcohol and dry ice. Rotate tubes while freezing; this distributes the contents over a greater surface area and prevents breakage from expansion of fluid. Wrap the tube or tubes in cotton and pack carefully in a vacuum bottle. Fill remainder of vacuum bottle with small pieces of dry ice. (Dry ice may be broken up by wrapping it in a piece of cloth and then crushing with a hammer.)

CAUTION: Do not touch dry ice with fingers. Use a forceps or spoon to fill bottle. Cut a small V-shaped slot longitudinally in vacuum bottle cork or place a large bore venipuncture needle through center of cork to allow escape of gaseous $CO_2$. A tiny hole should also be punched in the outer metal cap of bottle.

(3). Stopper bottle and pack carefully.

SPINAL FLUID. About 3 ml. of spinal fluid should be placed in each of 3 sterile Pyrex Wassermann tubes. Stopper, freeze, and label as directed for blood.

BRAIN. (1). As soon as possible after death remove brain, with sterile precautions, before thorax and abdomen are opened.

(2). Take several generous blocks from (I) temporal lobe including hippocampus, (II) motor cortex, (III) midbrain, (IV) thalamus, (V) pons and medulla, (VI) cerebellum, and (VII) cervical spinal cord.

(3). Blocks of tissue for virus studies may be shipped frozen in dry ice or unfrozen in sterile 50 per cent buffered glycerin solution (see below). Freezing is preferable. Individual blocks of tissue are placed in separate small wide-mouth sterile bottles without added fluid, stoppered with sterile corks and sealed with adhesive tape. Freeze and pack in vacuum bottle as described for blood.

If shipment cannot reach the laboratory within 24 to 36 hours the tissues should be shipped in buffered 50 per cent glycerin in a sterile stoppered container.

**c. Preparation of Sterile Buffered Glycerin**    (1). Citric acid 21 gm. in 1000 ml. double distilled water.

(2). Anhydrous $Na_2HPO_4$ 28.4 gm. to 1000 ml. double distilled water.

(3). Take 9.15 ml. of (1) and 90.85 ml. of (2) to make 100 ml. of buffered solution $pH$ 7.4.

(4). Mix equal parts of (3) and C. P. glycerin; fill specimen bottles half full, stopper with corks and sterilize at 15 lb. steam pressure for 30 minutes.


## 2. Methods of Collecting Material for Laboratory Diagnosis of Rickettsial Infections

Excised tissue blocks (such as brain or testis) and blood specimens are frozen and packed as described above for suspected virus infections.


## 3. The Weil-Felix Reaction

**Theoretical Considerations**    The Weil-Felix reaction is based on the agglutination of the "O" variant of certain strains of *Proteus X*. These strains appear in two growth phases designated as "H" (Ger. *Haut*) and "O" (Ger. *ohne Haut*). The H motile, flagellar form spreads rapidly over the surface of the medium while the O nonmotile form grows in discrete colonies. The flagellar antigen possesses a component in common with *Proteus vulgaris* and is, therefore, "non-specific," while the somatic O antigen is "specific" for the typhus-like diseases. The flagellar antigen is heat labile but gives rise to agglutinins which are heat stable. On the other hand the somatic "O" antigen is heat stabile and gives rise to agglutinins that are heat labile. Consequently, sera to be used in the Weil-Felix reaction should not be "inactivated" as in the Wassermann test, as some of the "specific" agglutinins are thereby destroyed.

The three type strains of *Proteus X* in general use are X2, X19 and XK.

The first two were isolated from the urine of patients ill with classic typhus: They originally appeared in the O phase. XK, the origin of which is not entirely clear, was received by Dr. Kingsbury in Malaya from the National Type Cultures in London (the "K" denoting the so-called Kingsbury strain). An additional strain, XL, isolated by Dr. Lima in an endemic center of "exanthematic typhus" at São Paulo, Brazil, is also frequently used. This strain is, according to Felix, of the X19 type but also produces agglutinins for XK, which is not true of the original X19 strain.

X19 is of the greatest diagnostic importance in louse- and flea-borne typhus.

XK is the only strain agglutinated in the scrub typhus group.

In the Weil-Felix reaction for the spotted fever group OX2 as well as OX19 should be used as some sera agglutinate only the X2 strain and not infrequently the agglutinin titer for OX2 is as high or higher than for OX19.

Strains of *Proteus X* have also been recovered from the brain, bone-marrow, spleen, liver, kidney, bile and heart blood. The organism is considered by Felix as the cultivable saprophytic stage of the specific infecting agent.

**Cultivation of Proteus X Strains** The strains should be carried on fresh meat infusion agar adjusted to $p$H 6.8. All strains are in some degree unstable, i. e., there is a tendency to an O–OH (non-motile to motile) reversion. This is most marked in the XK strain and least in the X2. Excess moisture hastens the reversion. Consequently, it is of greatest importance that all O variants be carried on a medium from which excess moisture has been removed, by drying in the incubator for several days. To assure H variants, on the other hand, it is just as important that the medium has its full moisture content. Although media made from dehydrated preparations support a fairly heavy growth, cultures carried on such media may show a decreased agglutinibility.

**The Test** In the usual macroscopic tube test 0.5 ml. of serial serum dilutions, 1:10, 1:20, etc., are placed in a series of agglutination tubes and 0.5 ml. of a 24-hour suspension of organisms killed by alcohol, phenol, Formalin or by heat and standardized to MacFarland nephelometer reading No. 3 or to a "500" silica standard are added to each tube, thereby doubling the dilutions. The rack is shaken gently, placed at 37° C. for 2 hours and stored in the ice box for 48 hours. Twenty-four hours at ice box temperature gives only a slightly lower reading. Usual controls should always be included.

The O agglutination results in a fine granular deposit often adhering to the walls of the tube. The H-agglutination appears in large flocculi and is massed at the bottom of the tube.

**Interpretation** Normal sera may show a low agglutinin titer for OXK or OX19, seldom for OX2. If 2 or more successive serum samples are available, a sharp rise in titer is of definite significance. As a rule, serum taken during the first week will not show a titer higher than 1:80 or 1:160. This titer will then serve as a basis for later tests. When possible, second and third samples should be tested, the second taken on or about the tenth day, and the third at the end of the second or during the third week of the disease, or during early convalescence.

It must be remembered that, as in any serologic test, the Weil-Felix reaction is only an aid to diagnosis. It is only a part of the picture and should be interpreted as such. An occasional serum may show a relatively high titer in the absence of any apparent rickettsial infection.

Sera of infected guinea pigs do not give a Weil-Felix reaction.

### 4. Hemagglutination-Inhibition Test for the Diagnosis of Virus Influenza (after the AMSGS)

#### a. Materials

> Physiologic saline made with freshly boiled distilled water.
> Standard 0.5% suspension of type "O" human red cells; fresh or preserved in dextrose (2.05%), sodium citrate (0.80%) and sodium chloride (0.42%).
> Standard lyophilized virus antigens for influenza A, A', B, and C.
> Standard chicken antisera against the viruses.
> Hemagglutination tubes (13 × 75 mm.)
> Wire test tube support which will permit observation of tests from below.

#### b. Preparation of Material for Influenza A, A', and B   (1). Rehydrate the antigens with sterile distilled water as directed on the label. Rehydrated antigens are stable for a period of months at —20° C. and for at least 3 weeks at 4° C.

(2). Titrate the antigens to determine the hemagglutinating unit of each. The unit is 0.5 ml. of the highest dilution of antigen which completely agglutinates 0.5 ml. of standard human erythrocyte suspension in $1\frac{1}{4}$ hours.

(3). Each antigen for use in the test is to contain 4 units in 0.25 ml. This is $\frac{1}{8}$ the highest dilution of antigen which showed complete agglutination in the antigen titration.

#### c. Procedure for Influenza A, A', and B   (1). 0.3 ml. amounts of each serum to be tested are inactivated at 56° C. for 30 minutes.

(2). Dilute each serum 1:8 by adding 2.1 ml. physiologic saline.

(3). Set up identical series of twofold serial dilutions of each serum for each antigen such that each tube contains 0.25 ml. and the serum dilutions range from 1:8 to 1:4096.

(4). Add 0.25 ml. of test antigen to each tube of a series.

(5). Shake well.

(6). Add 0.5 ml. of the standard erythrocyte suspension to each tube.

(7). Shake well and incubate at 22 to 25° C. for 60 minutes without disturbing the racks. The tests are read and recorded in terms of degree of inhibition of agglutination by each serum using each antigen. The titer of a given serum using a given antigen is defined as the highest dilution of serum which effects complete inhibition of agglutination.

(8). CONTROLS: (*a*). Antisera from roosters immunized against the viruses used in the test are used for control purposes. The tests with positive control sera serve (1) to confirm the identity of the antigen used; and (2) to further test the specificity and quantity of the reacting materials in the test antigens.

(*b*). The test antigens must be retitrated at the same time that the hemagglutination-inhibition tests are performed. The initial dilution is, however, the dilution of the test antigen. These retitrations are read after 65 to 75 minutes. Complete agglutination should occur in the first four tubes of each antigen tested and there should be less than complete agglutination in the fifth and remaining tubes.

**d. Procedure for Influenza C**  Since influenza C virus rapidly elutes from red blood cells at room temperature, all tests with the C agent are performed with chilled reagents and incubation is carried out in the refrigerator (4 to 6° C.) for 80 to 90 minutes. With these exceptions, the procedures as outlined in section **c** are followed.

**e. Interpretation**  Results are reported in terms of the titers of each of the paired sera obtained with each antigen. A four fold or greater increase in titer during convalescence is considered of diagnostic significance. Influenza vaccination histories should be ascertained. A rise in titer to both type A and type B virus should be suspected of being due to recent vaccination and a thorough check should be made. Concurrent infection in a single individual with both type A and type B influenza virus is a rare occurrence.

Individual diagnoses on a representative group of individuals are usually sufficient to detect the existence of an epidemic of influenza.

## 5. Methods of Collecting Material for Laboratory Diagnosis of Spirochetal Infections

**Blood**  *Spirillum minus* of rat-bite fever does not live long after blood has been drawn, so animal inoculations have to be made almost immediately. The relapsing fever spirochetes and *Leptospira icterohaemorrhagiae,* however, remain viable for a long time in sterile drawn blood, so that samples of whole blood for animal inoculation may be taken at the height of the febrile reaction and shipped in 30 ml. vacuum collecting tubes or in sterile Wassermann tubes as described above for blood for complement fixation and neutralization tests in neurotropic viruses. Refrigeration, but not freezing, of the blood samples is recommended. When the samples reach the laboratory, grind clot in a mortar under sterile conditions in physiologic salt solution and inoculate into mice or other experimental animals.

**Cerebrospinal Fluid**  In cases of relapsing fever and *Leptospira icterohaemorrhagiae* infection showing meningeal symptoms, the cerebrospinal fluid may contain spirochetes. Like blood, it is collected aseptically and shipped in sterile tubes to the laboratory where it is centrifuged for a half hour at 2000 r.p.m., and the sediment examined in the dark field for spirochetes.

### 6. The Complement Fixation Test for Leptospirosis (after the AMSGS)

*Introduction*   The complement fixation test for leptospirosis employs the standard Kolmer technique, utilizing sonic vibrated leptospiral antigens. Since these antigens have broad spectrums and antibodies are produced by the various species of leptospirae, they will cross in the test. It is recommended that sera be tested against a battery of three antigens, *L. icterohaemorrhagiae, L. hyos* and *L. grippotyphosa.* This combination of antigens has been found to detect antibodies against all species of leptospirae which have been tested.

*Preparation of Sera*   Inactivate cell-free serum (0.75 ml.) in water bath (56° C. for 30 minutes).

*Reagents*   (1). An 0.85 per cent sodium chloride solution containing 0.1 gm. magnesium sulfate per liter (Kolmer saline).

(2). A 2.0 per cent sheep cell suspension.

(3). Antigens. *L. icterohaemorrhagiae, L. hyos* and *L. grippotyphosa* antigens should be rehydrated according to the procedure recommended by the manufacturer.

(4). Stock dilution of 1:100 hemolysin.

(5). Complement. Rehydrate lyophilized complement by dissolving in the prescribed amount of buffered diluent supplied with it and store under refrigeration at all times.

*Titration of Hemolysin*   Hemolysin is titrated according to standard Kolmer technique. The unit is read as the highest dilution of hemolysin that gives complete hemolysis. Two units contained in 0.5 ml. are used in the complement titration and in the test.

*Titration of Complement*   Complement is titrated according to standard Kolmer technique. The smallest amount of complement giving complete hemolysis is the exact unit. The next larger amount (0.05 more) is the full unit. Use two *full units* contained in 1.0 ml. in the test.

*Complement Fixation Test for Leptospirosis*   (1). The tests are conducted in one-half volume by reducing the amounts of reagents and sera by half. The hemolysin and complement, however, are titrated at full volume as described for the regular test. The table on p. 845 should be followed in performing the test.

(2). Controls of positive and negative sera for each antigen should be included.

(3). After addition of hemolysin and corpuscles mix contents of each tube by thorough shaking of the rack and place in the water bath at 37° C. for 10 minutes longer than the time required for the antigen controls to clear.

| TUBE NO. | KOLMER SALINE SOLUTION | ANTIGEN | | | COMPLE-MENT (2 FULL UNITS) | | HEMOL-YSIN 2 UNITS | COR-PUSCLES 2% |
|---|---|---|---|---|---|---|---|---|
| | | *L. ictero.* | *L. grippo.* | *L. hyos* | | | | |
| *Patient's Serum* 1. 0.1 ml. | ml. None | ml. 0.25 | ml. None | ml. None | ml. 0.5 | | ml. 0.25 | ml. 0.25 |
| 2. 0.1 ml. | None | None | 0.25 | None | 0.5 | | 0.25 | 0.25 |
| 3. 0.1 ml. | None | None | None | 0.25 | 0.5 | | 0.25 | 0.25 |
| 4. 0.1 ml. | 0.25 | None | None | None | 0.5 | | 0.25 | 0.25 |
| *Controls* 5. *L. ictero.* antigen | 0.25 | 0.25 | None | None | 0.5 | | 0.25 | 0.25 |
| 6. *L. grippo.* antigen | 0.25 | None | 0.25 | None | 0.5 | | 0.25 | 0.25 |
| 7. *L. hyos* antigen | 0.25 | None | None | 0.25 | 0.5 | | 0.25 | 0.25 |
| 8. Hemolytic system | 0.5 | None | None | None | 0.5 | | 0.25 | 0.25 |
| 9. Corpuscle | 1.25 | None | None | None | None | | None | 0.25 |

*(center vertical note: Refrigerate at 6° to 8° C. for 15 to 18 hours; then place in 37° C. water bath for 10 minutes)*

(4). Read as negative, 1, 2, 3, or 4 plus according to standard methods of reading of complement fixation tests.

(5). The above procedure is a screening test and all sera showing 2 plus or greater fixation of complement must be titrated to determine the exact titer.

**Interpretation**    Leptospiral complement fixing antibodies are usually demonstrable by the eighth and may appear as early as the fourth day of the disease. The maximum titer (in the order of 1:128–1:512) is usually attained during the second week of illness. Complement fixing antibodies remain in detectable levels for periods varying from 3 to over 12 months. For this reason, demonstration of a rise in titer is essential to the confirmation of the clinical diagnosis of acute leptospirosis. Since it is impossible to determine the infecting strain by the examination of sera with antigens of this type, positive results should be reported as "Complement fixation test for leptospirosis: positive (indicate titer) or negative."

**7. Dye Test or Cytoplasm-Modifying Test for Toxoplasmosis** (after Sabin and Feldman)

**a. Reagents**    (1). TOXOPLASMA. The strain used should multiply extensively in the peritoneal cavity of mice in 3 to 4 days.

(2). ACCESSORY FACTOR. Human serum which in the fresh state

can be incubated with *Toxoplasma* at 37° C. for 1 hour without affecting the staining of the cytoplasm by methylene blue at *p*H 11; this may be stored for at least four years in dry ice.

(3). POSITIVE CONTROL SERUM. Any human or animal serum that has been found to have cytoplasm-modifying antibodies.

(4). METHYLENE BLUE AT *p*H 11. Prepared daily by mixing 3 ml. saturated alcoholic solution of methylene blue with 10 ml. of buffer at *p*H 11. (9.73 ml. of 0.53 per cent sodium carbonate plus 0.27 ml. of 1.91 per cent sodium borate [$Na_2B_4O_7 \cdot 10H_2O$]). Commercially available buffer tablets (*p*H 10.8) can be used to make the buffer solution.

(5). ANTICOAGULANT. A 1 per cent solution of heparin in 0.9 per cent solution of sodium chloride.

**b. Procedure**    (1). Each serum should be screened by testing the 1:16, 1:64 and 1:256 dilutions. Fourfold dilutions of the test serums in 0.1 ml. amounts, prepared in 0.9 per cent solution of sodium chloride, should be ready before the *Toxoplasma* suspension is prepared.

(2). The *Toxoplasma* suspension for use in the test is prepared by mixing 0.2 ml. of undiluted peritoneal exudate with 0.02 ml. of 1 per cent heparin and 0.8 ml. of the normal human serum containing the accessory factor. This mixture should be put in a refrigerator immediately after preparation, but the whole test should be set up within 1 hour after peritoneal exudate is removed from the animal.

(3). A preliminary examination of the condition of the *Toxoplasma* organisms is made by adding 0.1 ml. of this mixture to 0.1 ml. of 0.9 per cent solution of sodium chloride, incubating at 37° C. for 20 minutes and examining with the dye to make certain that the cytoplasm of at least 90 per cent of the extracellular *Toxoplasma* organisms are well stained.

(4). 0.1 ml. of the *Toxoplasma*-accessory factor mixture is added to 0.1 ml. of the various serum dilutions in small tubes.

(5). After incubation for 1 hour at 37° C. in a water bath, 0.02 ml. of the methylene blue is added to each tube.

(6). One drop from each tube is put on a slide, covered with a coverslip, and examined with the high power lens of a microscope.

(7). The number of extracellular *Toxoplasma* organisms with stained or unstained cytoplasm is determined. The highest dilution of serum in which 50 per cent or more of the organisms have unstained cytoplasm is the titer. Ordinarily the cytoplasm-modifying antibody develops within 10 to 20 days. Titers of 1:256 to 1:4000 or higher can persist for at least five years.

## 8. Napier's Aldehyde (Formol-Gel) Test for Kala Azar

This is a test for euglobulin, which is increased in kala azar as well as in some other diseases.

The test in kala azar is not ordinarily of diagnostic value until after the third to fifth month of the disease, and the reaction may remain positive for about four months after recovery.

*a. Procedure* To 1 ml. of clear serum of the patient add 1 or 2 drops full strength commercial Formalin.

If serum becomes solidified and opaque like boiled egg white within fifteen minutes it is read as a strong positive. If a similar result is obtained within twenty-four hours the reaction is still considered positive. If serum solidifies without becoming altogether opaque the interpretation is doubtful. When serum remains clear it is read as a negative even though solidification occurs.

## 9. Chopra's Antimony Test for Kala Azar

This test gives a positive result earlier in kala azar than does the aldehyde test, but false positives may occur in sera from patients with splenomegaly due to other causes.

*a. Procedure* (1). Half fill small test tube (made by sealing one end of a piece of 4 to 5 mm. glass tubing 2½ to 3 inches long) with patient's serum diluted 10 times with distilled water.

(2). Add, by means of capillary pipette, an equal amount of a 4 per cent solution of urea stibamine.

(3). Rotate tube between palms to mix the two solutions.

A heavy flocculent precipitate denotes a strong positive reaction, absence of precipitate a negative reaction.

## 10. Euglobulin Precipitation Test for Kala Azar and Schistosomiasis (after Sia)

An excess of serum euglobulin is produced in kala azar, chronic schistosomiasis and other diseases.

Mix 10 to 20 cu. mm. of patient's blood with 0.6 ml. of distilled water in small test tube by gentle agitation. If positive, a cloudy precipitate forms. Since this test is not specific, the clinical findings must supplement differentiation between kala azar and schistosomiasis.

## 11. Precipitin Test to Determine Source of Mosquito Blood Meals

(1). Collect engorged female mosquitoes early in morning. Transport to laboratory in vials kept iced in vacuum jug.

(2). Kill mosquito by chloroforming; place it on its back, head pointing away. With a small curved tissue forceps take hold of mosquito near anterior end of abdomen, and push lower abdomen against a small strip of filter paper of the harder sort (as Whatman No. 5), rupturing abdomen wall and stomach in such a manner that blood will be spread and absorbed by paper.

(3). Write pertinent data as to date and place of collecting on remainder of the strip of filter paper.

(4). Store strips in dry, cool insect-proof place until tests can be made.

(5). Cut off blood spot on filter paper into 2 to 3 ml. of physiologic salt solution, and allow to soak for 1 hour at room temperature, shaking from time to time. If blood spot is unusually small, a smaller amount of saline solution should be used. It is not necessary to filter this solution but it should stand a while before the supernatant fluid is drawn off for precipitin test.

(6). A few cubic millimeters of diluted, previously prepared anti-human serum is carefully pipetted into a small serum tube so as not to wet the sides above the serum level.

The dilution of the anti-human serum depends on its known titer. If the titer is from 3000 to 4000, a titer rarely attained in the rabbit, the serum should be diluted about 1:7. Sera of lower titer are diluted correspondingly.

(7). The supernatant fluid from (5) is carefully layered onto the anti-human serum.

(8). A cloudiness or opalescence at the interphase of the two fluids denotes a positive precipitin test, indicating that the mosquito had probably bitten man.

(9). If the reaction does not occur immediately, inspect at intervals of 10 minutes for one hour.

(10). Similar tests can be made with anti-horse, anti-pig, etc., sera.

## 12. Flocculation Test for Trichinosis (after Suessenguth and Kline)

### a. Materials

Antigen emulsion of cholesterol crystals coated with trichina larvae antigen extract.

### b. Procedure
(1). Pipette 0.05 ml. of inactivated test serum into a cell of a Boerner glass microslide.

(2). Allow a drop of antigen emulsion to drop into the serum from a 26 g. needle with syringe.

(3). Rotate the slide on a flat surface 4 minutes at 150 rotations per minute.

(4). Examine the mixture at once through a compound microscope at a magnification of 100 times.

The test is reported in terms of pluses according to the degree of clumping and the size of clumps.

## 13. Intradermal Test for Trichinosis

### a. Materials

Stock antigen prepared from lyophilized adult *Trichinella spiralis*.

### b. Procedure
(1). Dilute stock trichina antigen 1:10,000 with physiologic saline and keep refrigerated until use.

(2). Inject 0.1 ml. of antigen intracutaneously on one forearm and an equal amount of saline control on the other forearm. In positive reactions a white swelling surrounded by an unraised irregular erythematous area of about 5 cm. in diameter appears at the site of injection. The reaction reaches its maximum in 10 minutes and begins to fade in 15 to 20 minutes. In negative tests, there is no reaction to the antigen.

#### 14. Intradermal Test for Echinococcus Infection

##### a. Materials
Stock antigen of purified, powdered hydatid fluid.

**b. Procedure**   (1). Dilute the stock antigen 1:10,000 with physiologic saline.

(2). Inject 0.2 ml. of antigen intradermally on the upper arm and 0.2 ml. of saline control on the other arm. In positive cases a wheal develops at the site of injection of antigen within 30 minutes.

## Miscellaneous

### 1. Parasite Counts in Malaria (after Wilcox)

**a. Procedure**   There are both thick smear and thin smear methods of enumerating malaria parasites, but the former is recommended even for relatively inexperienced workers.

(1). Make a thick smear at the same time the blood is drawn for a white count.

(2). Fix and stain the thick film.

(3). Count one hundred white cells (or multiples of one hundred) on the thick film.

(4). Count the malaria parasites seen in the same microscopic fields with the white cells.

(5). Calculate the parasites per cubic millimeter of blood as follows:

$$\frac{x \text{ (No. of parasites per cu. mm.)}}{\text{White cell count per cubic mm.}} = \frac{\text{No. of parasites counted in the same fields with 100 white cells}}{\text{No. of white cells counted (100 in this case)}}$$

$x =$ No. of parasites/cu. mm. of blood

Example:
$$\frac{x}{4000} = \frac{1200}{100}$$
$$100x = 4,800,000$$
$$x = 48,000$$

#### 2. Examination of Female Anopheline Mosquitoes for Malarial Parasites

It is desirable to know under certain conditions whether or not mosquitoes contain oocysts on the stomach wall or whether the salivary glands contain sporozoites.

**a. Procedure**   (1). Kill female mosquitoes a few at a time with chloroform, carbon tetrachloride or tobacco smoke and identify species. It may be desirable to mount identical specimens for subsequent confirmation.

(2). Do not dissect recently engorged mosquitoes. Remove legs and wings, dip quickly into 35–50 per cent alcohol and place at edge of drop of physiologic saline with head pointing away.

(3). STOMACH DISSECTION. Nick both sides of body wall of next to last abdominal segment so as partially to sever chitinous wall.

(4). Transfix posterior thorax with needle, placing free needle on partially severed terminal abdominal segments and exert gentle intermittent traction to draw out stomach, attached malpighian tubules and ovaries.

(5). Carefully set aside thorax and head of mosquito in saline for subsequent examination.

(6). Sever gut posterior to stomach, discarding attached malpighian tubules, intestine, ovaries and débris; transfer to a clean drop and carefully lower cover glass onto stomach.

(7). Examine stomach wall for oocysts which may be recognized as follows:

(*a*). *Young oocysts* are clear, round, oval bodies, 6 to 12 microns in diameter, are more refractile than stomach cells, and contain minute pigment granules.

(*b*). *Intermediate oocysts* are denser than stomach cells, measure 12 to 40 microns in diameter, and contain clumps of pigment.

(*c*). *Mature oocysts* are 30 to 80 microns in diameter, show fine striations owing to enormous numbers of attenuated, spindle-shaped sporozoites 12 to 44 microns in length. Pigment granules are not readily visible.

CAUTION: Protruding unpigmented stomach cells may be confused with immature oocysts of *Plasmodium.*

(8). SALIVARY GLAND DISSECTION. Place head and thorax (or entire mosquito with wings and legs removed if it is being examined only for sporozoites) in a drop of physiologic saline tinted with methylene blue, with body pointing away.

(9). Exert gentle pressure on anterior thorax so that neck bulges slightly, place second needle behind head and draw away from thorax.

(10). Transfer head and attached tissue to a fresh drop of saline and search for blue-stained salivary glands under dissecting binocular or hand lens.

(11). Tease out one or both trilobed glands and transfer carefully to a fresh drop on same slide; gently lower cover glass.

(12). Examine all 3 lobes of each gland carefully under a high dry lens for the characteristic sporozoites. If necessary confirm with oil immersion objective.

(13). Crush glands by exerting pressure on cover with clean instrument; search again.

(14). If glands are positive remove cover glass and allow material on it and slide to dry. Fix both in methyl alcohol and stain with Giemsa's or Wright's stain. If desired, cover glass may be mounted smear side up on slide. Examine with high dry and oil immersion objective for sporozoites, which appear as slender blue-staining spindles with a central red chromatin dot.

### 3. Examination of Mosquitoes for Filarial Worms

In areas where filariasis is endemic it is sometimes desirable to dissect mosquitoes to determine the per cent infected.

*a. Procedure* (1). Proceed as in (1) and (2) above.

(2). Sever head and place in separate drop of saline. Carefully dissect thorax, teasing all tissues apart, add cover glass and examine for developing parasites.

(3). Carefully dissect proboscis and head for presence of infective larvae, which are usually 0.1 mm. or more in length.

### 4. Rearing Entomologic Specimens

*a. Mosquito Larvae* It is often desirable to rear mosquito larvae to maturity in order to identify the species concerned, or to obtain a disease free stock for experimental purposes.

(1). PROCEDURE. (*a*). To transport live larvae from the field to the laboratory they should be placed in a container provided with a small glass tube extending through the stopper to supply oxygen and prevent injury due to slopping.

(*b*). Larvae are placed in shallow open pans containing mud and water from same locality. These should be set in a partially shady humid environment.

(*c*). Feed on fragments of stale toast, a 50:50 mixture of brewer's and baker's yeast or pulverized Purina duck chow.

(*d*). Change water if it becomes turbid or covered with scum.

(*e*). Remove pupae once a day and place in beaker in screened mosquito cage, small screened cage that fits snugly over beaker, or in individual cotton-stoppered test tubes.

(*f*). Kill adults 5 to 6 hours after emerging by transferring to chloroform tube if raised for identification.

(*g*). Mount as described on p. 852.

*b. Fly Larvae* Fly maggots and other insect larvae recovered in stools, urine, vomitus, or from human or animal tissue may often be induced to pupate by placing them in a cage with a quantity of slightly moistened sand. Frequent inspection is desirable in order that the adult insects may be studied before they have had opportunity to damage their wings, legs and antennae by battering them against the sides of the container.

## 5. Mounting Entomologic Specimens for Study

**a. Whole Mounts**   Mosquito larvae, lice, fleas, mites, bedbugs and other small specimens not too heavily pigmented are usually cleared and mounted on glass slides for study by transmitted light. The following procedure, applicable specifically to mosquito larvae, may be modified, as necessary, for other forms:

(1). USE OF POTASSIUM HYDROXIDE. Opaque or heavily chitinized specimens may require preliminary soaking in a 10 per cent solution of potassium hydroxide. Such treatment takes from a few minutes to several hours, depending on the condition of the specimens.

(2). MOUNTING IN BALSAM. (*a*). Kill larvae by dropping into steaming hot water (150° to 160° F.).

(*b*). Dehydrate in alcohol as follows:

> 50% alcohol—15 minutes*
> 70% alcohol—15 minutes
> 85% alcohol—15 minutes
> 95% alcohol—15 minutes
> absolute alcohol—10 minutes

* These time intervals are minimum—longer periods in each alcohol may result in better preparations.

(*c*). Clear in xylene for approximately ten minutes.

(*d*). Mount in balsam under a cover glass. This technique produces good permanent mounts.

If Euparal or Diaphane is used, the procedure is the same except that specimens do not require clearing in xylene but may be mounted directly from absolute alcohol.

(3). MOUNTING IN BERLESE'S MEDIUM. (*a*) FORMULA:

> Gum arabic ....................................... 8 gm.
> Water (distilled) ................................. 8 ml.
> Glycerin ......................................... 5 ml.
> Chloral hydrate .................................. 70 gm.
> Glacial acetic acid ............................... 3 ml.

Dissolve gum arabic in water and add other ingredients in order. Strain through muslin before use.

(*b*). PROCEDURE. Specimens may be mounted in Berlese's medium directly from water, or if preserved in alcohol may be mounted after rinsing in water. This produces good mounts of a semi-permanent nature.

**b. Maggots**   Only the mouth hooks and posterior spiracles of most maggots are dissected off and mounted.

**c. Ticks**   Ticks may be punctured, cleared and mounted as above. Live mounts, the specimens being placed between a slide and a strip of adhesive tape, are often more satisfactory. Some specimens should be placed in a dorsal position, others in a ventral position, so that all structures may be seen.

**d. Pinned Specimens**   Adult specimens of mosquitoes, flies, bees, wasps, ants, beetles, bugs and other groups may be mounted on insect pins, in any of several ways. Such specimens require no special preservation and if kept in pest-proof boxes remain suitable for study for many years. The following techniques are recommended:

(1). For larger insects (except COLEOPTERA), direct impalement through center of thorax is the most desirable procedure. Specimen is pushed up to within a quarter of an inch of pinhead. This allows ample room below for small labels on which are written date and place of collection, collector's name and other pertinent data.

(2). For beetles procedure is same, save that pin passes through base of right elytron (wing cover).

(3). For smaller forms two techniques are employed:

(*a*). With small bugs, beetles and other species characterized by fairly rigid chitin and absence of body hair, use of small cardboard points is preferred. Thrust pin through broader end of point; add a small drop of shellac or similar material to fasten extremity of point to right side of insects' thorax.

(*b*). With more delicate forms possessing an abundance of hair on wings or body, very fine pins, termed "minuten nadeln," are recommended. Minuten, which are approximately half an inch in length, are thrust up through one end of a small bit of cork, balsa wood or especially prepared cardboard which in turn is impaled on a standard pin in usual manner. Point of minuten is usually thrust up through specimen from below, though some prefer insects be mounted in a lateral position.

**e. Alcoholic Specimens**  Most ticks, spiders, scorpions, centipedes and larger larvae of all types do not lend themselves either to pinning or to mounting on slides. These are best preserved in vials containing 70 per cent alcohol or 4 per cent formaldehyde. For study they may be transferred to a watch glass and examined with a hand lens or binocular microscope.

# Index

**855**